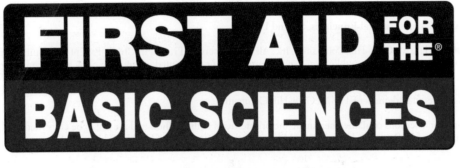

FIRST AID FOR THE® BASIC SCIENCES

General Principles

Second Edition

SENIOR EDITORS

TAO LE, MD, MHS
Associate Clinical Professor of Medicine and Pediatrics
Chief, Section of Allergy and Immunology
Department of Medicine
University of Louisville

KENDALL KRAUSE, MD
Resident, General Preventive Medicine/Public Health
Colorado School of Public Health

EDITOR

VINITA TAKIAR, MD, PhD
Resident, Radiation Oncology
University of Texas, MD Anderson Cancer Center

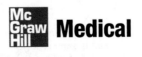

Medical

New York   Chicago   San Francisco   Lisbon   London   Madrid   Mexico City
Milan   New Delhi   San Juan   Seoul   Singapore   Sydney   Toronto

First Aid for the® Basic Sciences: General Principles, Second Edition

5 6 7 8 9 0   CTP/CTP   18 17 16 15

ISBN 978-0-07-174388-4
MHID 0-07-174388-X

NOTICE

Medicine is an ever-changing science. As new research and clinical experience broaden our knowledge, changes in treatment and drug therapy are required. The authors and the publisher of this work have checked with sources believed to be reliable in their efforts to provide information that is complete and generally in accord with the standards accepted at the time of publication. However, in view of the possibility of human error or changes in medical sciences, neither the authors nor the publisher nor any other party who has been involved in the preparation or publication of this work warrants that the information contained herein is in every respect accurate or complete, and they disclaim all responsibility for any errors or omissions or for the results obtained from use of the information contained in this work. Readers are encouraged to confirm the information contained herein with other sources. For example and in particular, readers are advised to check the product information sheet included in the package of each drug they plan to administer to be certain that the information contained in this work is accurate and that changes have not been made in the recommended dose or in the contraindications for administration. This recommendation is of particular importance in connection with new or infrequently used drugs.

This book was set in Electra LH by Rainbow Graphics.
The editors were Catherine A. Johnson and Peter J. Boyle.
The production supervisor was John Williams.
The illustration manager was Armen Ovsepyan.

The designer was Alan Barnett.
Project management was provided by Rainbow Graphics.
China Translation & Printing, Ltd., was printer and binder.

The following material was reproduced, with permission, from Le T, et al. *First Aid for the USMLE Step 1*, New York: McGraw-Hill, 2011:
Figures 1-3, 1-7, 1-18, 1-19, 1-21, 1-23, 1-24, 1-26, 1-27, 1-29, 1-30, 1-32, 3-5, 3-7, 3-8, 3-9, 3-14, 3-15, 3-16, 3-17, 3-26, 3-27, 3-34, 3-42, 3-45, 3-48, 3-49, 3-53, 3-59, 3-68, 3-69, 3-72, 3-105, 3-124, 3-125, 3-126, 3-127, 3-128, 4-3, 4-5, 4-6, 4-11, 4-25, 5-7, 5-8, 5-40, 5-41, 5-43, 6-5, 6-9, and 6-10; Tables 3-19, 3-28, 4-7, 5-52, 6-10, 6-14, and 6-16.

Library of Congress Cataloging-in-Publication Data

Le, Tao.
 First aid for the basic sciences. General principles / Tao T. Le, Kendall Krause. — 2nd ed.
    p. ; cm.
 General principles
 Includes bibliographical references and index.
 ISBN-13: 978-0-07-174388-4 (pbk. : alk. paper)
 ISBN-10: 0-07-174388-X (pbk. : alk. paper)
1. Medical sciences—Outlines, syllabi, etc. 2. Medical sciences—Examinations, questions, etc. 3. Physicians—Licenses—United States—Examinations—Study guides. I. Krause, Kendall. II. Title. III. Title: General principles.
 [DNLM: 1. Biological Science Disciplines—Outlines. 2. Medicine—Outlines. WB 18.2]
 R834.5.F57 2012
 616.02′52—dc23

                                    2011026446

DEDICATION

To the contributors to this and future editions, who took time to share their
knowledge, insight, and humor for the benefit of students.

and

To our families, friends, and loved ones, who supported us
in the task of assembling this guide.

Contents

CONTRIBUTING AUTHORS

Raj J. Chovatiya
Yale School of Medicine
Medical Scientist Training Program

Daniel J. Durand, MD
Instructor and Fellow
Radiology and Radiological Sciences
Johns Hopkins University School of Medicine

Aaron Feinstein
Yale School of Medicine
Class of 2012

Peter M. Gayed
Yale School of Medicine
Class of 2016
Yale Graduate School of Arts and Sciences
Class of 2015

John W. Gilbert
Yale School of Medicine
Class of 2012

Jose Luis Gonzalez
Yale School of Medicine
Class of 2012

Hadiza S. Kazaure
Yale School of Medicine
Class of 2012

Lauren Michal de Leon, MD
Intern, Department of Internal Medicine
Alpert Medical School of Brown University

Seenu Susarla, MD, DMD, MPH
Resident, Departments of Surgery/Oral-Maxillofacial Surgery
Massachusetts General Hospital
Harvard Medical School

Rany Woo
Yale School of Medicine
Class of 2012

James S. Yeh, MD
Resident, Clinical Fellow in Medicine
Cambridge Health Alliance
Harvard Medical School

FACULTY REVIEWERS

Steven I. Aronin, MD, FACP
Chief, Section of Infectious Disease
Hospital Epidemiologist
Waterbury Hospital
Associate Clinical Professor of Medicine
Yale School of Medicine

Susan Baserga, MD, PhD
Professor of Molecular Biophysics and Biochemistry, Genetics,
  and Therapeutic Radiology
Yale School of Medicine

Choukri Ben Mamoun, PhD
Associate Professor of Medicine and Microbial Pathogenesis
Yale School of Medicine

Sheldon Campbell MD, PhD
Associate Professor of Laboratory Medicine
Yale School of Medicine

Oscar R. Colegio, MD, PhD
Associate Professor of Dermatology
Yale School of Medicine

Frantz Hastrup, MD
Chief of Critical Care Medicine
Instructor in Medicine
Cambridge Hospital
Harvard Medical School

Shanta Kapadia, MBBS, M Surg
Lecturer, Section of Anatomy
Department of Surgery
Yale School of Medicine

Michael Kashgarian, MD
Professor Emeritus of Pathology
Senior Research Scientist
Department of Pathology
Yale School of Medicine

Richard J. Pels, MD
Associate Chief of Medicine
Internal Medicine Residency Program Director
Director of Graduate Medical Education, Cambridge
  Health Alliance
Assistant Professor of Medicine
Harvard Medical School

Steve Sazinsky, PhD
Postdoctoral Fellow
Boston University

Howard Steinman, PhD
Assistant Dean for Biomedical Science Education
Professor of Biochemistry
Albert Einstein College of Medicine

Richard Sutton, MD, PhD
Associate Professor of Internal Medicine
Yale School of Medicine

Preface

With this second edition of *First Aid for the Basic Sciences: General Principles*, we continue our commitment to providing students with the most useful and up-to-date preparation guides for the USMLE Step 1. For the past year, a team of authors and editors have worked to update and further improve this second edition. This edition represents a major revision in many ways, including:

- Every page has been carefully reviewed and updated
- New high-yield figures, images, tables, and mnemonics have been added
- Hundreds of user comments and suggestions have been incorporated
- Increased emphasis on integration and linkage of concepts

These books would not have been possible without the help of the hundreds of students and faculty members who contributed their feedback and suggestions. We invite students and faculty to please share their thoughts and ideas to help us improve *First Aid for the Basic Sciences: General Principles*. (See How to Contribute, p. xiii.)

Tao Le
Louisville

Kendall Krause
Denver

Acknowledgments

This has been a collaborative project from the start. We gratefully acknowledge the thoughtful comments and advice of the residents, international medical graduates, and faculty who have supported the editors and authors in the development of *First Aid for the Basic Sciences: General Principles.*

We wish to extend sincere and heartfelt thanks to our managing editor, Isabel Nogueira, who, once again, was truly the backbone of this project. Without her enthusiasm and commitment, the extensive update of this project would not have been possible. For support and encouragement throughout the process, we are grateful to Thao Pham and Louise Petersen.

Furthermore, we wish to give credit to our amazing editors and authors, who worked tirelessly on the manuscript. We never cease to be astounded by their dedication, thoughtfulness, and creativity.

Thanks to Catherine Johnson and our publisher, McGraw-Hill, for their assistance and guidance. For outstanding editorial work, we thank Linda Davoli. A special thanks to Rainbow Graphics for remarkable production work.

We also thank the faculty at Uniformed Services University of the Health Sciences (USUHS) for use of their images.

Tao Le
Louisville

Kendall Krause
Denver

How to Use This Book

Both this text and its companion, *First Aid for the Basic Sciences: Organ Systems*, are designed to fill the need for a high-quality, in-depth, conceptually-driven study guide for the USMLE Step 1. They can be used either alone, or in conjunction with the original *First Aid for the USMLE Step 1*, *First Aid Cases for the USMLE Step 1*, or *First Aid Q&A for the USMLE Step 1*. In this way, students can tailor their own studying experience, calling on either series, according to their mastery of each subject.

Medical students who have used the previous edition of this guide have given us feedback on how best to make use of the book.

- **It is recommended that you begin using this book as early as possible** when learning the basic medical sciences.
- As you study each discipline, **use the corresponding section in *First Aid for the Basic Sciences: General Principles*** to consolidate the material, deepen your understanding, or clarify concepts.
- As you approach the test, use *First Aid for the Basic Sciences: General Principles* and *First Aid for the Basic Sciences: Organ Systems* to review challenging concepts.
- Use the margin elements (ie, Flash Forward, Flash Back, Key Fact, Clinical Correlation, Mnemonic) to test yourself throughout your studies.

To **broaden** your learning strategy, you can **integrate** your *First Aid for the Basic Sciences: General Principles* study with *First Aid for the USMLE Step 1*, *First Aid Cases for the USMLE Step 1*, and *First Aid Q&A for the USMLE Step 1* on a chapter-by-chapter basis.

How to Contribute

To continue to produce a high-yield review source for the USMLE Step 1, you are invited to submit any suggestions or corrections. We also offer paid internships in medical education and publishing ranging from three months to one year (see below for details). Please send us your suggestions for:

- New facts, mnemonics, diagrams, and illustrations
- High-yield topics that may reappear on future Step 1 examinations
- Corrections and other suggestions

For each entry incorporated into the next edition, you will receive a $10 gift certificate, as well as personal acknowledgment in the next edition. Diagrams, tables, partial entries, updates, corrections, and study hints are also appreciated, and significant contributions will be compensated at the discretion of the authors. Also let us know about material in this edition that you feel is low yield and should be deleted.

The preferred way to submit entries, suggestions, or corrections is via our blog:

www.firstaidteam.com.

Otherwise, please send entries, neatly written or typed, or on disk (Microsoft Word), to:

First Aid Team
914 N. Dixie Avenue, Suite 100
Elizabethtown, KY 42701
Attention: First Aid General Principles

NOTE TO CONTRIBUTORS

All entries become property of the authors and are subject to editing and reviewing. Please verify all data and spellings carefully. In the event that similar or duplicate entries are received, only the first entry received will be used. Include a reference to a standard textbook to facilitate verification of the fact. Please follow the style, punctuation, and format of this edition, if possible.

AUTHOR OPPORTUNITIES

The author team is pleased to offer opportunities in medical education and publishing to motivated medical students and physicians. Projects may range from three months (eg, a summer) up to a full year. Participants will have an opportunity to author, edit, and earn academic credit on a wide variety of projects, including the popular First Aid series. English writing/editing experience, familiarity with Microsoft Word, and Internet access are required. Go to our blog **www.firstaidteam.com** to apply for an internship. A sample of your work or a proposal of a specific project is helpful.

Anatomy and Histology

Cellular Anatomy and Histology

THE CELL

A cell is considered the most basic structural and functional unit of life. Living organisms, with the exclusion of viruses, are composed of cells, which may exist as independent units or form more complex organisms. Each cell is a collection of diverse components; each component contributes to the integral biochemical processes that sustain the life of the organism. The most important eukaryotic cellular components will be covered in the following sections.

Plasma Membrane

Every eukaryotic cell is enveloped by an asymmetrical lipid bilayer membrane. This membrane consists primarily of two sheets of **phospholipids**, each one molecule thick. Phospholipids are **amphiphilic** (also referred to as amphipathic) molecules, containing both hydrophilic and hydrophobic regions (Figure 1-1).

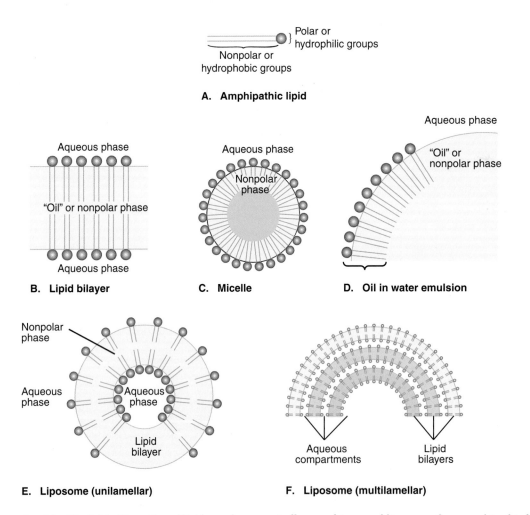

FIGURE 1-1. **Amphipathic lipids.** Formation of lipid membranes, micelles, emulsions, and liposomes from amphipathic lipids (eg, phospholipids). (Modified with permission from Murray RK, Granner DK, Rodwell VW. *Harper's Illustrated Biochemistry*, 27th ed. New York: McGraw-Hill, 2006: 130.)

- The **hydrophilic** portions (ie, phosphate groups) of the outer layer face the extracellular environment, and those of the inner layer face the cytoplasm.
- The **hydrophobic** portions of each layer (ie, fatty acid chains) intermingle within the center of the membrane.

This bilayer membrane also contains **steroid** molecules (derived from cholesterol), glycolipids (fatty acids with sugar moieties), sphingolipids, proteins, and glycoproteins (proteins with sugar moieties). The cholesterol and glycolipid molecules alter the physical properties of the membrane (eg, increase the melting point), in relative proportion to their presence. The proteins serve important and specific roles in the transport and trafficking of nutrients across the membrane, signal transduction, and interactions between the cell and its environment.

The cell membrane performs the following functions:

- Enhancing cellular structural stability.
- Protecting internal organelles from the external environment.
- Regulating the internal environment (chemical and electrical potential).
- Enabling interactions with the external environment (eg, signal transduction and cellular adhesion).

Nucleus and Nucleolus

The nucleus is the control center of the cell. The nucleus contains genetically encoded information in the form of DNA, which directs the life processes of the cell. It is surrounded by two lipid bilayers: The inner membrane defines the boundaries of the nucleus, and the outer membrane is continuous with the **rough endoplasmic reticulum (RER)** (Figure 1-2). In addition to DNA, the nucleus houses a number of important proteins that enable the maintenance (protection, repair, and replication), expression (transcription), and transportation of genetic material (DNA, RNA).

Most of the cell's **ribosomal RNA (rRNA)** is produced within the nucleus by the **nucleolus.** The rRNA then passes through the **nuclear pores** (transmembrane protein complexes that regulate trafficking across the nuclear membrane), to the cytosol, where it associates with the RER.

Rough Endoplasmic Reticulum and Ribosomes

As previously described, the RER is home to the majority of the cell's ribosomes. (The *rough* in rough endoplasmic reticulum comes from the many ribosomes that stud the membrane of the RER.) These rRNA doublets associate with **transfer RNA (tRNA)** to translate **messenger RNA (mRNA)** into amino acid sequences, and, eventually, into proteins (Figure 1-3). The RER functions primarily as the location for membrane and secretory protein production as well as protein modification (Figure 1-2). The RER is most well developed in cell types that produce proteins for secretion (pancreatic acinar cells or plasma cells).

Smooth Endoplasmic Reticulum (SER)

The SER is the site of fatty acid and phospholipid production as seen in the cells of the adrenal cortex and steroid secreting cells of the ovaries and testes. Most eukaryotic cells have a relatively small SER, with some exceptions. For example, hepatocytes, constantly engaged in detoxifying hydrophobic compounds through conjugation and excretion, have well-developed SER.

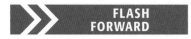

KEY FACT

Proteins comprise transmembrane transporters, ligand-receptor complexes, and ion channels; protein dysfunction underlies many diseases.

FLASH FORWARD

Genetic mutations may cause dysfunction of regulatory proteins, especially repair mechanisms, often leading to debilitating diseases, such as xeroderma pigmentosum.

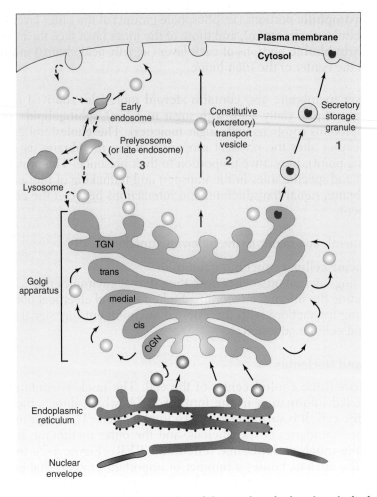

FIGURE 1-2. **Diagrammatic representation of the rough endoplasmic reticular branch of protein sorting.** Newly synthesized proteins are inserted into the endoplasmic reticulum membrane or enter the lumen from membrane-bound polyribosomes, depicted as small black circles studding the endoplasmic reticulum. Those proteins are then transported out of the endoplasmic reticulum (solid black arrows). The proteins then pass through, and are modified in, the various subcompartments of the Golgi apparatus. Proteins are segregated and sorted in the trans-Golgi network (TGN). Secretory proteins accumulate in secretory storage granules, from which they may be expelled (1). Proteins destined for the plasma membrane or those that are secreted in a constitutive manner are carried out to the cell surface in transport vesicles (2). Some proteins enter prelysosomes (late endosomes) and fuse with endosomes to form lysosomes (3). Retrieval from the Golgi apparatus to the endoplasmic reticulum is not considered in this scheme. CGN = cis-Golgi network. (Modified with permission from Murray RK, Granner DK, Rodwell VW. *Harper's Illustrated Biochemistry*, 27th ed. New York: McGraw-Hill, 2006: 508.)

Golgi Apparatus

Shortly after being synthesized, proteins from the RER are packaged into transport vesicles and secreted from the RER. These vesicles travel to and fuse with the **Golgi vesicles.** Within the lumen of this organelle, secretory and membrane-bound proteins undergo modification. Depending on their final destination, these proteins may be modified in one of the three major regions or Golgi networks: **cis (CGN), medial (MGN),** or **trans (TGN).** These proteins are then packaged in a second set of transport vesicles, which bud from the trans side and are delivered to their target locations (eg, organelle membranes, plasma membrane, and lysosomes; Figures 1-2 and 1-4).

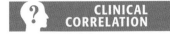

CLINICAL CORRELATION

I-cell disease, also known as mucolipidosis type II, results from the failed modification of lysosomal proteins. Rather than being targeted for the lysosome through the addition of mannose-6-phosphate, enzymes are secreted from the cell, thus hindering the disposal of intracellular waste. Coarse facial features and restricted joint movements result.

FUNCTIONS OF THE GOLGI APPARATUS

- Distributing proteins and lipids from the endoplasmic reticulum to the plasma membrane, lysosomes, and secretory vesicles.
- Modifying N-oligosaccharides on asparagines.
- Adding O-oligosaccharides to serine and threonine residues.
- Assembling proteoglycans from core proteins.
- Sulfating sugars in proteoglycans and tyrosine residues on proteins.
- Adding mannose-6-phosphate to specific proteins (targets the proteins to the lysosome).

Lysosomes

The lysosome is the **trash collector** of the cell. Bound by a single lipid bilayer, the lysosome is responsible for hydrolytic degradation of obsolete cellular components. Extracellular materials, ingested via endocytosis or phagocytosis, are enveloped in an endosome (temporary vesicle), which fuses with the lysosome, leading to enzymatic degradation of endosomal contents. Lysosomal enzymes (nucleases, proteases, and phosphatases) are activated at a pH below 4.8. To maintain this pH, the membrane of the lysosome contains a hydrogen ion pump, which hydrolyzes ATP to move protons against the concentration gradient.

Mitochondria

This is the primary site of **ATP** production in aerobic respiration. The proteins of the **outer membrane** enable the transport of large molecules (molecular weight ~10,000) for oxidative respiration. The **inner membrane**, separated from the outer by the **intermembranous** space, is selectively permeable (Figure 1-5). Although the inner membrane's surface area is greatly increased by numerous folds, known as **cristae**, its selectivity is maintained by transmembrane proteins. These transmembrane proteins, which constitute the electron transport chain, maintain a proton gradient between the intermembranous

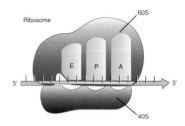

FIGURE 1-3. Schematic representation of ribosomal RNA (rRNA). Here, the 40S and 60S subunits of rRNA are shown, translating a portion of mRNA in the 5′ to 3′ direction. Many of these ribosomes are located within the membrane of the rough endoplasmic reticulum (RER) so that their initial protein product ends up within the lumen of the RER, where it undergoes further modification. **E** site = holds Empty tRNA as it Exits; **P** site = accommodates growing **P**eptide; **A** site = incoming **A**minoacyl tRNA.

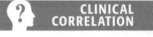

CLINICAL CORRELATION

A number of lysosomal storage diseases, such as Tay-Sachs disease, result from lysosomal dysfunction.

CLINICAL CORRELATION

Chédiak-Higashi disease, resulting from abnormal microtubular assembly, leads to decreased polymorphonucleocyte (PMN or neutrophil) phagocytosis and frequent infections.

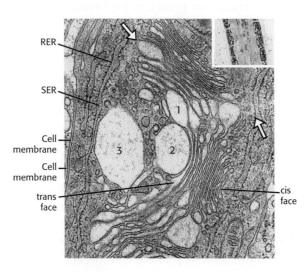

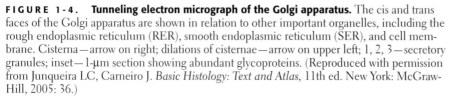

FIGURE 1-4. Tunneling electron micrograph of the Golgi apparatus. The cis and trans faces of the Golgi apparatus are shown in relation to other important organelles, including the rough endoplasmic reticulum (RER), smooth endoplasmic reticulum (SER), and cell membrane. Cisterna—arrow on right; dilations of cisternae—arrow on upper left; 1, 2, 3—secretory granules; inset—1-μm section showing abundant glycoproteins. (Reproduced with permission from Junqueira LC, Carneiro J. *Basic Histology: Text and Atlas*, 11th ed. New York: McGraw-Hill, 2005: 36.)

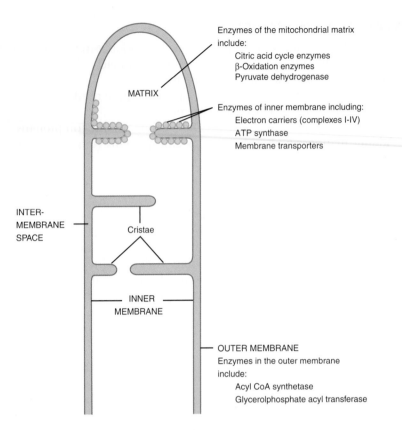

FIGURE 1-5. **Structure of the mitochondrial membranes.** The inner membrane contains many folds, or cristae, and the enzymes for the electron transport chain used in aerobic cellular respiration are located here. (Modified with permission from Murray RK, Granner DK, Rodwell VW. *Harper's Illustrated Biochemistry*, 27th ed. New York: McGraw-Hill, 2006: 101.)

space and the lumen of the inner membrane. The role of the electron transport chain is to generate energy for storage in the bonds of ATP.

Microtubules and Cilia

Microtubules are aggregate intracellular protein structures important for cellular **support, rigidity,** and **locomotion.** They consist of α- and β-tubulin dimers, each bound to two guanosine triphosphate molecules, giving them a positive and negative polarity. They combine to form cylindrical polymers of 24-nm diameter and variable lengths (Figure 1-6A). Polymerization occurs slowly from the positive end of the microtubule, but depolymerization occurs rapidly unless a GTP cap is in place.

Microtubules are incorporated into both flagella and **cilia.** Within cilia, the microtubules occur in pairs, known as **doublets.** A single cilium contains nine doublets around its circumference, each linked by an ATPase, **dynein** (Figure 1-6B). Dynein, anchored to one doublet, moves along the length of a neighboring doublet in a coordinated fashion, resulting in ciliary motion.

Epithelial Cell Junctions

Transmembrane proteins mediate intercellular interaction by providing cellular adhesion and cell signaling. Cellular adhesion and communication is vitally important to both the integrity and the function of an organ.

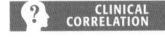

KEY FACT

Drugs that act on microtubules:

Drug	Disease
Mebendazole/ thiabendazole	Parasitic infections
Taxol	Breast cancer
Griseofulvin	Fungal infections
Vincristine/ vinblastine	Cancers
Colchicine	Gout

CLINICAL CORRELATION

A number of diseases arise from ineffective or insufficient ciliary motion.

Kartagener syndrome: A dynein arm defect that causes recurrent lung infections due to decreased mucus clearing, hearing loss, and infertility.

Dextrocardia: Proper directional flow does not occur during embryogenesis; therefore, internal organs, including the heart, are organized in the mirror image of normal.

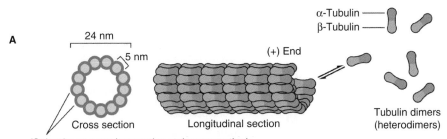

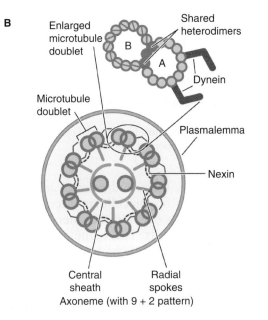

FIGURE 1-6. **Microtubules.** (A) Structure. The cylindrical structure of a microtubule is depicted as a circumferential array of 13 dimers of α- and β-tubulin. The tubulin dimers are being added to the positive end of the microtubule. (B) Ciliary structure. Nine microtubule doublets, circumferentially arranged, create motion via coordinated dynein ATP cleavage. (Modified with permission from Mescher AL. *Junqueira's Basic Histology: Text and Atlas,* 12th ed. New York: McGraw-Hill, 2010: Figure 2-31.)

Organs and tissues exposed to the external environment are the most resilient. These tissues are referred to as **epithelial,** primarily due to their embryologic origin. The epithelial cells of these external tissues contain an array of **cell junctions** that mediate cellular adhesion and communication processes. There are five principal types of cell junctions: **zona occludens (tight junctions), zona adherens (intermediate junctions), adherens junctions (desmosomes), hemidesmosomes,** and **gap junctions (communicating junctions)** (Figure 1-7).

ZONA OCCLUDENS

Tight junctions, also referred to as occluding junctions, have the following two primary functions:

- Determine epithelial cell polarity, separating the apical pole from the basolateral pole.
- Regulate passage of substances across the epithelial barrier (**paracellular transport**).

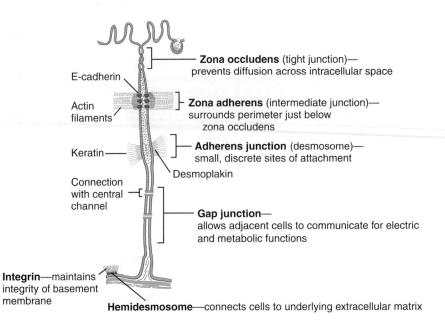

FIGURE 1-7. **Epithelial cell junctions.** Five types of epithelial cell junctions are depicted along with their supporting and component proteins.

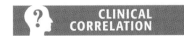
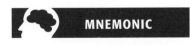
MNEMONIC

CADHErins are **C**alcium-dependent **ADHE**sion proteins.

In a typical epithelial tissue, the membranes of adjacent cells meet at regular intervals to seal the inter- or paracellular space, thus surrounding the cell like a belt. These connections occur at the interaction of the junctional protein complex of neighboring cells. This complex is composed of the proteins **occludin,** a four-span transmembrane protein, and **claudin.**

ZONA ADHERENS

Intermediate junctions are located just below tight junctions, near the apical surface of an epithelial layer. Like the zona occludens, the zona adherens occurs periodically along the circumference of the cell, in a beltlike distribution. Inside the cell, these transmembrane protein complexes are associated with actin microfilaments. Outside the cell, **cadherins** (see mnemonic) from adjacent cells use a calcium-dependent mechanism to span wider intercellular spaces than can the zona occludens.

ADHERENS JUNCTIONS

As opposed to the beltlike distribution of the zona occludens and adherens, desmosomes resemble spot welds—single rivets erratically spaced below the apical surface of the epithelium. Intracellularly, they are associated with keratin intermediate filaments, providing strength and rigidity to the epithelial surface. Like the zona adherens, adherens junctions are also mediated by calcium-dependent cadherin interactions.

HEMIDESMOSOMES

These asymmetrical anchors provide epithelial adhesion to the underlying connective tissue layer, the **basal lamina,** or **basement membrane.** The hemidesmosomes contain **laminin 5** (instead of cadherins), an anchoring protein filament that binds the cell to the basal lamina. Although the intracellular portion structurally resembles that of the desmosome, none of the protein components are conserved, except for the cytoplasmic association with intermediate filaments.

GAP JUNCTIONS

These intercellular junctions allow for rapid transmission of electrical or chemical information from one cell to the next. A connexon is formed from a complex of six **connexin** proteins. Each single **connexon** exists as a hollow cylindrical structure spanning the plasma membrane. When a connexon of one cell is bound to a connexon of an adjacent cell, a gap junction is formed, creating an open channel for fluid and electrolyte transport across cell membranes.

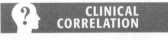

>> **FLASH FORWARD**

Gap junctions allow for "coupling" of cardiac myocytes, enabling the rapid transmission of electrical depolarization and coordinating contraction during the cardiac cycle.

HEMATOPOIESIS

Hematopoietic cells are primarily individual cells engaged in processes of cellular interaction, physiologic transport, and immune surveillance.

Blood

Blood is a connective tissue composed of cells suspended in a liquid phase. This liquid phase, which consists of water, proteins, and electrolytes is known as **plasma**. The O_2-carrying red blood cells, known as **erythrocytes,** make up about 45% of blood by volume (this percentage is known as the **hematocrit**). Erythrocytes can be separated from white blood cells, or **leukocytes,** and **platelets** by centrifugation. The erythrocytes form the lowest layer, and the leukocytes form the next layer, also known as the **buffy coat.** Plasma from which the platelets and clotting factors have been extracted is called blood **serum.**

The Pluripotent Stem Cell

The hematopoietic stem cell is the grandfather of all major blood cells. These cells reside within the bone marrow, where **hematopoiesis** (blood cell production) occurs. They are capable of asymmetrical reproduction: simultaneous self-renewal and differentiation.

- **Self-renewal,** integral to the maintenance of future hematopoietic potential, preserves the pool of stem cells.
- **Differentiation** leads to the production of specialized mature cells, necessary for carrying out the major functions of blood.

Two differentiated cell lines derive from the pluripotent stem cell: **myeloid** and **lymphoid** (Figure 1-8). These cells are considered **committed;** they have begun the process of differentiation and no longer have the potential to become any blood cell. The myeloid lineage produces six colony-forming units (CFUs), each ending in a distinct mature cell: erythroid (producing erythrocytes), megakaryocyte (producing platelets), basophil, eosinophil, neutrophil, and monocyte (differentiates into macrophage). The lymphoid lineage produces two cell lines: T cells and B cells.

? **CLINICAL CORRELATION**

Red cell cytoskeletal abnormalities (eg, hereditary spherocytosis, elliptocytosis) and hemoglobinopathies (eg, thalassemias, sickle cell anemia) cause significant morbidity and mortality.

Erythrocytes

Erythrocytes are nonnucleated, biconcave disks designed for gas exchange. These cells measure 7.8 μm in diameter, and their biconcave shape increases their surface area for gas exchange. These cells lack organelles, which are jettisoned shortly after they enter the bloodstream. Instead, they contain only a plasma membrane, a cytoskeleton, hemoglobin, and glycolytic enzymes that help them survive via **anaerobic respiration** (90%) and the hexose monophosphate shunt (10%). This limits the red blood cell life span to approxi-

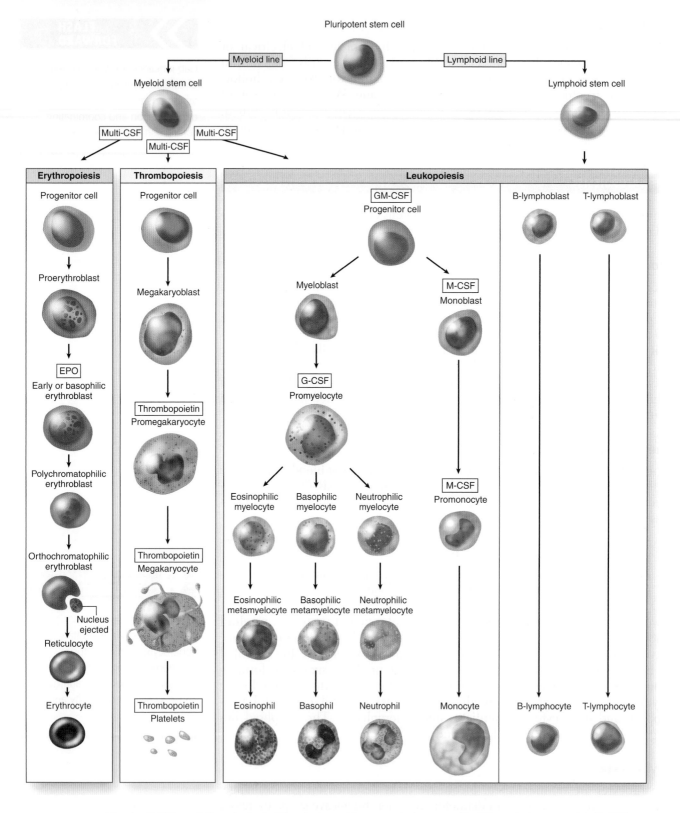

FIGURE 1-8. Blood cell differentiation. A chart of the pluripotent hematopoietic stem cell's differentiation potential. G-CSF, granulocyte colony-stimulating factor; GM-CSF, granulocyte–macrophage colony-stimulating factor; M-CSF, macrophage colony-stimulating factor; EPO, erythropoietin. (Reproduced with permission from Mescher AL. *Junqueira's Basic Histology: Text and Atlas*, 12th ed. New York: McGraw-Hill, 2010: Figure 13-1.)

mately 120 days, after which they are mainly removed via macrophages in the spleen and to a lesser extent via the liver. Mature erythrocytes are replaced by immature **reticulocytes** produced in the bone marrow. Reticulocytes are distinguished from mature erythrocytes by their retained nucleus and slightly larger diameter. Within 1–2 days after entering the circulation, they expel their nucleus and mature.

Erythrocyte metabolism begins with the transport of glucose across the red cell membrane via the **glucose transporter (GLUT1) protein.** At this point, glycolytic enzymes produce ATP and lactic acid via anaerobic metabolism. Important aspects of erythrocyte metabolism are listed in Table 1-1.

Leukocytes

Leukopoiesis is the process of white blood cell production from hematopoietic stem cells. **Neutrophils, basophils, mast cells,** and **eosinophils** develop through a common promyelocyte lineage. **Monocytes** develop from a monoblast. Lymphocytes, although separate from myeloid cells, are also considered leukocytes, and arise from the lymphoid stem cell.

> **CLINICAL CORRELATION**
>
> Reticulocyte counts increase when the bone marrow increases production to replenish red cell levels in the blood in response to bleeding or a hemolytic process.

TABLE 1-1. Important Aspects of Red Blood Cell (RBC) Metabolism

The RBC is highly dependent on glucose as its energy source; its membrane contains high-affinity glucose transporters.
Because RBCs have no mitochondria, there is no production of ATP via oxidative phosphorylation.
The RBC has a variety of transporters that maintain ionic and water balance.
Production of 2,3-bisphosphoglycerate by reactions closely associated with glycolysis, is important in regulating the ability of hemoglobin (Hb) to transport O_2.
The pentose phosphate pathway is operative in the RBC (it metabolizes about 5%–10% of the total flux of glucose) and produces the reduced form of nicotinamide adenine dinucleotide phosphate (NADPH); hemolytic anemia due to a deficiency of the activity of glucose-6-phosphate dehydrogenase is common.
Reduced glutathione is important in the metabolism of the RBC, in part to counteract the action of potentially toxic peroxides; the RBC can synthesize glutathione and requires NADPH to return oxidized glutathione (G-S-S-G) to the reduced state.
The iron of Hb must be maintained in the ferrous state; ferric iron is reduced to the ferrous state by the action of an NADH-dependent methemoglobin reductase system involving cytochrome b_5 and cytochrome b_5 reductase.
Synthesis of glycogen, fatty acids, protein, and nucleic acids does not occur in the RBC; however, some lipids (eg, cholesterol) in the RBC membrane can exchange with corresponding plasma lipids.
The RBC contains certain enzymes of nucleotide metabolism (eg, adenosine deaminase, pyrimidine nucleotidase, adenylyl kinase); deficiencies of these enzymes are involved in some cases of hemolytic anemia.
When RBCs reach the end of their life span, the globin is degraded to amino acids (which are reused in the body), the iron is released from heme and also reused, and the tetrapyrrole component of heme is converted to bilirubin, which is mainly excreted into the bowel via the bile.

(Reprinted with permission from Murray RK, Granner DK, Rodwell VW. *Harper's Illustrated Biochemistry*, 27th ed. New York: McGraw-Hill, 2006: 619.)

KEY FACT

Leukos = Greek for white.
Cytos = Greek for cell.

All leukocytes are involved in some aspect of the immune response:

- **Neutrophils** affect **nonspecific innate immunity** in the acute inflammatory response.
- **Basophils and mast cells** mediate **allergic responses**.
- **Eosinophils** help fight **parasitic infections**.
- **Lymphocytes** are integral to both **cellular** and **humoral immunity**.

NEUTROPHILS

These products of the myeloid lineage act as acute-phase granulocytes. They begin in the bone marrow as myeloid stem cells (Figure 1-8) and mature over a period of 10–14 days, producing both primary and secondary granules (promyelocyte stage; Figures 1-9 and 1-10). Once mature, these leukocytes are vital to the success of the innate immune system and are especially prominent in the acute inflammatory response.

Histologically, these cells are distinguished by their large spherical size, multilobed nuclei, and **azurophilic** primary granules **(lysosomes)**. These cells have earned the alternative name **polymorphonucleocytes (PMNs)** due to their multilobed nucleus. The key to their immune function, however, lies not in the nucleus, but in the ability of PMNs to phagocytose microbes and destroy them via **reactive oxygen species** (superoxide, hydrogen peroxide, peroxyl radicals, and hydroxyl radicals). Neutrophils contain several enzymes, most notably **NADPH oxidase,** which produces O_2^- radicals, directing the oxidative burst, as well as the **myeloperoxidase system (MPO),** which uses hydrogen peroxide and chloride to generate hypochlorous acid (HOCl), a potent bactericidal oxidant.

EOSINOPHILS

Eosinophils follow the same pattern of maturation as neutrophils, beginning in the bone marrow as eosinophilic CFUs. Eosinophils also contain azurophilic granules with myeloperoxidase. However, they differ in that they are larger than neutrophils with cationic proteins, such as **major basic protein (antibacterial)** and **eosinophilic cationic protein** (antiparasitic) within aci-

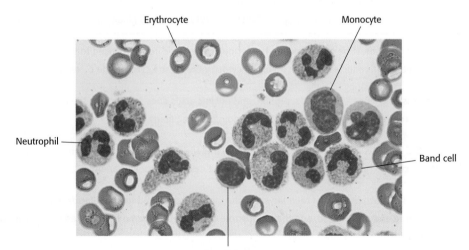

FIGURE 1-9. Peripheral blood smear with neutrophilia. This peripheral blood smear displays an extreme leukemoid reaction (neutrophilia). Most cells are band and segmented neutrophils. Two monocytes and a lymphocyte are also in the field. (Reproduced with permission from Lichtman MA, Beutler E, Kipps TJ, et al. *Williams Hematology*, 7th ed. New York: McGraw-Hill, 2006: Plate VIII-1.)

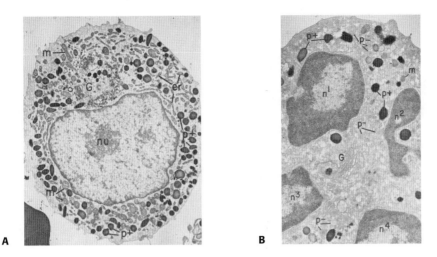

A   B

FIGURE 1-10. **Electron microscopy of neutrophils.** (A) Electron micrograph of mature neutrophil reacted for peroxidase. (B) Electron micrograph of a mature neutrophil from normal human marrow reacted for peroxidase. er = endoplasmic reticulum; G = Golgi apparatus; m = mitochondria; nu = nucleus; p = peroxisome. (Part A reproduced with permission from Lichtman MA, Beutler E, Kipps T, et al. *Williams Hematology*, 7th ed. New York: McGraw-Hill, 2006: 833. Part B reproduced with permission from Lichtman MA, Beutler E, Kipps T, et al. *Williams Hematology*, 7th ed. New York: McGraw-Hill, 2006: 833, 835.)

dophilic granules. Once fully mature, eosinophils possess a large, bilobed nucleus and sparse endoplasmic reticulum and Golgi vesicles (Figure 1-11).

BASOPHILS AND MAST CELLS

Distinguished by large, coarse, darkly staining granules, basophils produce peroxidase, **heparin,** and **histamine** (Figure 1-12). Basophils also release **kallikrein,** which acts as an eosinophil chemoattractant during hypersensitivity reactions, such as contact allergies and skin allograft rejection. Because they share a great deal of structural similarities, basophils can be considered the blood-borne counterpart of the **mast cell,** which resides within tissues, near

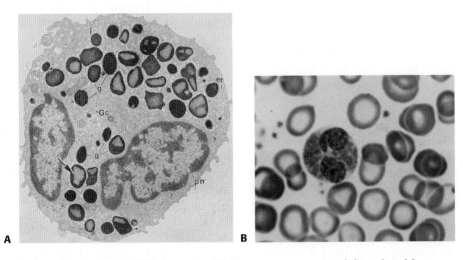

A   B

FIGURE 1-11. **Eosinophil microscopy.** (A) Human mature eosinophil incubated for peroxidase. (B) Light micrograph of a mature eosinophil with characteristic bilobed nucleus (stained purple). g = granules (arrows); er = rough endoplasmic reticulum; pn = perinuclear cisterna = Gc, Golgi cisternae. (Part A reproduced with permission from Lichtman MA, Beutler E, Kipps T, et al. *Williams Hematology*, 7th ed. New York: McGraw-Hill, 2006: 839. Part B adapted with permission from Lichtman MA, Shafer JA, Felgar RE, Wang N. *Lichtman's Atlas of Hematology.* New York: McGraw-Hill, 2007: Figure 11.D.2.)

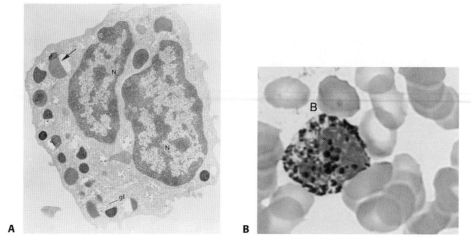

FIGURE 1-12. **Basophil microscopy.** (A) Electron micrograph of a mature basophil from human blood reacted for peroxidase. gl = glycoprotein; N = nucleus; arrow = speckled basophil. (B) Light micrograph of a mature basophil with tetra lobed anatomy. (Reproduced with permission from Lichtman MA, Beutler E, Kipps T, et al. *Williams Hematology,* 7th ed. New York: McGraw-Hill, 2006: 840 [A] and Plate VII-4 [B].)

blood vessels. Mast cells, although similar to basophils, are typically larger and contain **serotonin** (ie, **5-HT**), which basophils lack. Mast cells degranulate during the acute phase of inflammation, acting, via their released granule contents, on the nearby vasculature. This leads to vasodilation, fluid transudation, and swelling of interstitial tissues.

Monocyte Lineage

MONOCYTES

Monocytes are the myeloid precursor to the mononuclear phagocyte, the tissue macrophage. Morphologically, they appear as spherical cells with scattered small granules, akin to lysosomes. The blood monocyte is a large (10–18 μm), motile cell that marginates along the vessel wall in response to the expression of specific cell adhesion proteins. During an inflammatory response, these cell adhesion proteins (namely, platelet endothelial cell adhesion molecule, or **PECAM-1**) facilitate monocyte **diapedesis** (transmigration) across vessel walls into surrounding tissues. Once in close proximity to the inflammatory foci, the monocyte differentiates into a macrophage with increased phagocytic and lysosomal activity (Figures 1-9 and 1-13).

MACROPHAGES

During differentiation, monocyte cell volume and lysosome numbers increase. These lysosomes, which fuse with phagosomes, degrade ingested cellular and noncellular material. Macrophages (20–80 μm) also contain a large number of cell surface receptors. These differ, depending on the tissue in which the macrophage matures, contributing to the diversity of macrophage functions (Table 1-2).

As described in Table 1-2, several organs are involved in macrophage distribution. Similarly, connective tissues, such as the skin and bones, contain monocyte-derived cells, termed *tissue resident macrophages,* which are structurally related to macrophages. These cells are typically derived from monocytes that have taken up residence in the tissue in question. Alternatively, monocytes can migrate into tissues during an acute inflammatory response and, there, transform into reactive macrophages to aid the innate immune system. Once

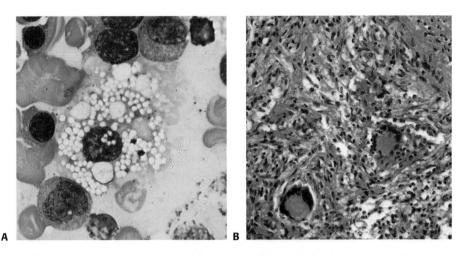

FIGURE 1-13. **Macrophage microscopy.** (A) Active macrophage and (B) multinucleated giant cell. (Part A reproduced with permission from Lichtman MA, Beutler E, Kipps T, et al. *Williams Hematology*, 7th ed. New York: McGraw-Hill, 2006: Plate-IX-1. Part B reproduced with permission from USMLERx.com.)

out of the circulation, monocytes have a half-life of up to 70 hours. Their numbers within inflamed tissues begin to overcome those of neutrophils after approximately 12 hours.

MULTINUCLEATED GIANT CELLS

At sites of chronic inflammation, such as tuberculous lung tissue, macrophages sometimes fuse to produce multinucleated phagocytes (Figure 1-13). These microbicidal cells can be produced in vitro via interferon-γ (IFN- γ) or interleukin-3 (IL-3) stimulation.

DENDRITIC CELLS

Antigen-presenting cells (**APCs**) are essential to the adaptive immune system. These monocyte-derived phagocytic cells take up antigens (primarily protein particles), process them, display them bound to the **major histocompatibility complex (MHC) II** cell surface marker, and travel to lymph nodes, where they recruit other cells of the immune system into action. Dendritic cells are especially important in the initial exposure to a new antigen. Successful dif-

TABLE 1-2. **Distribution of Mononuclear Phagocytes**

Marrow	Monoblasts, promonocytes, monocytes, macrophages
Blood	Monocytes
Body cavities	Pleural macrophages, peritoneal macrophages
Inflammatory tissues	Epithelioid cells, exude macrophages, multinucleated giant cells
Tissues	Liver (Kupffer cells), lung (alveolar macrophages), connective tissue (histiocytes), spleen (red pulp macrophages), lymph nodes, thymus, bone (osteoclasts), synovium (type A cells), mucosa-associated lymphoid tissue, gastrointestinal tract, genitourinary tract, endocrine organs, central nervous system (microglia), skin (dendritic cells)

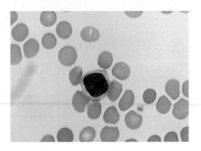

FIGURE 1-14. Light microscopy of a lymphocyte from a blood smear. Medium-sized agranular lymphocyte (stained purple) with a high nuclear to cytoplasmic ratio and an ill-defined chromatin pattern. (Adapted with permission from Lichtman MA, Shafer JA, Felgar RE, Wang N. *Lichtman's Atlas of Hematology.* New York: McGraw-Hill, 2007: Figure II.G.3.)

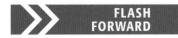

FLASH FORWARD

Dendritic cells are the most important antigen-presenting cells in the body and they are responsible for initiation of adaptive immunity.

ferentiation from monocytes depends on an endothelial cell signal that is secondary to foreign antigen exposure. In the absence of this second signal, these sensitized monocytes transform into macrophages.

Lymphocytes

Lymphocytes are easily distinguished from other leukocytes by their shared morphology (Figures 1-9, 1-14, and 1-15). After differentiating from lymphoblasts within the marrow, they migrate to the blood as spherical cells, 6–15 μm in diameter. Typically, the nucleus contains tightly packed chromatin, which stains a deep blue or purple and occupies approximately 90% of the cell cytoplasm.

As the primary actors in the adaptive immune response, lymphocytes undergo biochemical transformation into active immune cells via coordinated stimulatory signals. These activated lymphocytes then enter the cell cycle, producing a number of identical daughter cells. They eventually settle into G_0 as a memory cell while they await the next stimulation event. Alternatively, following replication, daughter cells can become terminally differentiated lymphocytes, primed for effector and secretory roles in immunologic defense of the host organism.

B CELLS AND PLASMA CELLS

B cells are the "long-range artillery" in the adaptive immune response. After the lymphoblast stage, the lymphocyte lineage diverges into B cells and T cells, each performing separate roles in the adaptive, or **humoral, immune response.** Once committed, **B** cells develop in the **B**one marrow and then migrate to other lymphoid organs. As they develop, B cells express immunoglobulins (IgM and IgD) on their surface, in association with costimulatory proteins. These **B-cell antigen receptor complexes** allow for the recognition of foreign antigens and subsequent activation of the B cell. Downstream cell signaling leads to the expression of necessary genes for terminal differentia-

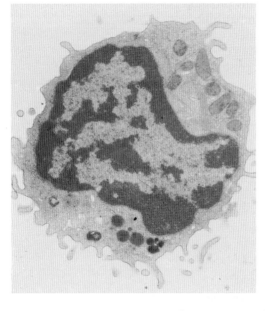

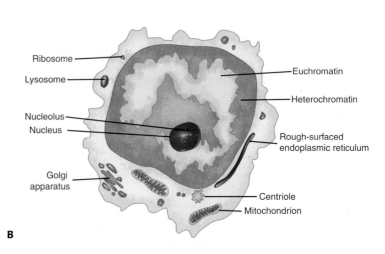

Ribosome

Lysosome

Nucleolus

Nucleus

Golgi apparatus

Euchromatin

Heterochromatin

Rough-surfaced endoplasmic reticulum

Centriole

Mitochondrion

A **B**

FIGURE 1-15. Lymphocytes. (A) Electron micrograph of a normal human lymphocyte (× 12,000). (B) Diagrammatic representation of a normal lymphocyte with organelles labeled. (Modified with permission from Lichtman MA, Beutler E, Kipps T, et al. *Williams Hematology,* 7th ed. New York: McGraw-Hill, 2006: 1024.)

tion to **plasma cells** that produce and secrete antibodies to aid the specific immune response. B cells that recognize self-antigens are triggered to undergo programmed cell death, or **apoptosis,** to reduce the chance of autoimmunity.

T CELLS

T cells are the "infantry" of the adaptive immune response. During maturation in the **Thymus,** early T cells begin expressing several surface receptors simultaneously, including the T cell receptor (**TCR**), **CD4,** and **CD8.** If one of these CD receptors recognizes **receptors** of thymic APCs, either major histocompatability complex (**MHC**) **II** or **I,** respectively, then this T cell is **positively selected,** proliferates, and matures. If a T cell recognizes self-antigen, then it is **negatively selected,** and undergoes apoptosis.

HELPER T CELLS

Two subtypes of T helper cells are derived from the CD4+ progenitor: T_H1 and T_H2. T_H1 responses occur in the presence of intracellular pathogens. Helminthic or **parasitic infections,** on the other hand, drive T_H2-mediated immune responses.

Helper T cells spring into action when they recognize foreign antigens bound to MHC II. Once activated, they secrete **cytokines,** chemical messengers that recruit and activate other immune effector cells. These cytokines, also called **interleukins,** specifically attract B cells, which, in turn, divide and differentiate into plasma cells. After the immune response is complete, some helper T cells become **memory cells**—quiescent immune cells that retain their specificity in case of a rechallenge with the same antigen in the future. The presence of memory cells increases the speed and efficiency of future immune responses.

CYTOTOXIC T CELLS

CD8+ T cells also proliferate in response to cytokines; however, they only recognize antigens in association with class I MHC. These cells are actively involved in immune surveillance of intracellular pathogens.

Every human cell contains MHC I, but only APCs contain MHC II.

- A cell infected by an intracellular pathogen (ie, a virus) processes viral proteins and presents them on the surface via MHC I.
- A roving CD8+ cell recognizes this signal and attaches to the infected cell via cell adhesion molecules.
- The activated cytotoxic T cell releases **perforins,** which are proteins that form holes in the plasma membrane of targeted cells.

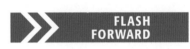

KEY FACT

Helper T cells "help" by mediating the specificity of the adaptive immune response. They act as a messenger between APCs and B cells, triggering humoral immunity.

FLASH FORWARD

Cytotoxic T cells also destroy target cells via the **Fas-Fas ligand** interaction. The interaction of Fas ligand of CD8+ T cells with the Fas receptor of the infected cell leads to apoptosis.

KEY FACT

T_H1 cells are associated with **innate** immunity and **cytolytic** responses. T_H2 cells are associated with **humoral** immunity and **asthma.**

Gross Anatomy and Histology

ABDOMINAL WALL ANATOMY

Layers of the Abdominal Wall

The layers of the anterior abdominal wall, penetrated during surgical incision or sharp trauma, differ, depending on their location with respect to the midline and the umbilicus. They are listed in Table 1-3 and depicted in Figure 1-16.

TABLE 1-3.   Layers of the Abdominal Wall

MIDLINE RELATION	UMBILICAL RELATION	LAYERS
Midline	Above or below	■ Skin ■ Camper's fascia—superficial layer of subcutaneous tissue ■ Scarpa's fascia—deep layer of subcutaneous tissue ■ Linea alba ■ Transversalis fascia ■ Parietal peritoneum
Anterolateral	Above or below	■ Skin ■ Camper's fascia—superficial layer of subcutaneous tissue ■ Scarpa's fascia—deep layer of subcutaneous tissue ■ Rectus sheath, composed of muscular aponeuroses ■ Transversalis fascia ■ Parietal peritoneum
Flank	Above or below	■ Skin ■ Camper's fascia—superficial layer of subcutaneous tissue ■ Scarpa's fascia—deep layer of subcutaneous tissue ■ External oblique muscle ■ Internal oblique muscle ■ Transverse abdominal muscle ■ Transversalis fascia ■ Parietal peritoneum

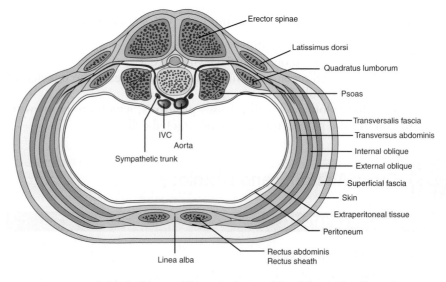

FIGURE 1-16.   Abdominal layers. The major layers of the abdominal wall are shown, as well as the relation of several retroperitoneal structures. IVC = inferior vena cava.

In addition to the differences displayed in Table 1-3, the abdominal muscle aponeuroses composing the rectus sheath differ above and below the umbilicus. Above the umbilicus, the external oblique and anterior internal oblique aponeuroses are found anterior to the abdominis rectus muscle. The posterior rectus sheath is made of the posterior internal oblique and transverse abdominis aponeuroses. Below the umbilicus, the anterior rectus sheath is composed of all three abdominal muscle aponeuroses (external oblique, internal oblique, and transverse abdominis). Deep to the muscle layer is the preperitoneal fat and fascia. The parietal peritoneum is deep to that fascia.

Inguinal Canal

The canal is an oblique, inferomedially directed channel, allowing the testes and its vessels and nerves contained in the abdominal cavity during development to traverse the abdominal wall to reach the scrotum (Figure 1-17). As the testes descend it carries a sheath of peritoneal sac (tunica vaginalis) into which it invaginates acquiring a partial covering. The canal lying superior and parallel to the **inguinal ligament,** allows the passage of the **round ligament** of the uterus in females and the **spermatic cord** (ductus deferens and testicular vessels) in males. The canal has two openings: the **internal** (or **deep**) and **external** (or **superficial**) **inguinal rings.** The transversalis fascia evaginates through the abdominal wall and continues as a covering of structures passing through the abdominal wall. The superficial ring is actually an opening through the external oblique aponeurosis. An indirect inguinal hernia occurs when there is a patent peritoneal sac between the deep and superficial rings that allow a loop of gut to enter the scrotal sac traversing the inguinal canal. A direct inguinal hernia occurs where there is a weakness in the muscle layers of the abdominal wall causing a hernia through the superficial inguinal ring but with no peritoneal sac involved. If the protrusion occurs at the site of the deep inguinal ring, the hernia is indirect. If the weakness occurs medial to the inferior epigastric vessels, the hernia is direct (Figure 1-17).

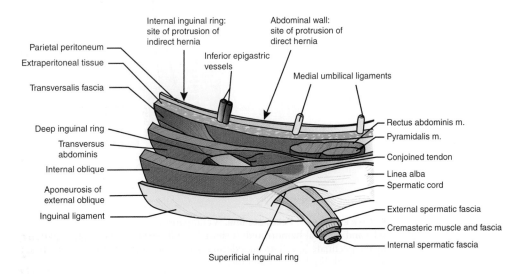

FIGURE 1-17.   Inguinal canal. The location and contents of the male inguinal canal, as well as the abdominal wall layers it traverses, are shown. Other important anatomic relations are also highlighted, including umbilical ligaments and inferior epigastric vessels. The locations of direct and indirect hernias are also labeled.

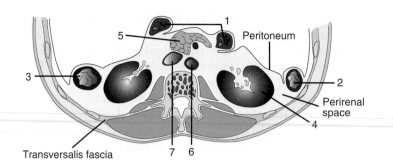

FIGURE 1-18. Retroperitoneal structures. The anatomic relations of important retroperitoneal structures are shown, including the duodenum (1; second, third, and fourth sections), descending colon (2), ascending colon (3), kidney and ureters (4), pancreas (5; head and neck), aorta (6), and inferior vena cava (7). The adrenal gland and rectum are not shown.

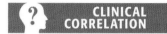
Retroperitoneum

The posterior abdominal cavity contains several important structures situated between the parietal peritoneum and the posterior abdominal wall. This region, the retroperitoneum, contains portions of the gastrointestinal, genitourinary, endocrine, and vascular systems (Figure 1-18).

The Pectinate Line

The pectinate line is the mucocutaneous junction where the endoderm meets the ectoderm in the anal canal. In the developing embryo, the endodermally derived hindgut fuses with the ectodermally derived external anal sphincter (Figure 1-19). Tissues on each side of this boundary are fed by separate neurovascular sources (Table 1-4).

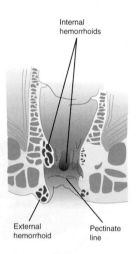

FIGURE 1-19. Pectinate line. A comparison of internal hemorrhoids (internal rectal vessels) and external hemorrhoids (external rectal vessels) is shown, highlighting their separation by the pectinate line. The endodermal and ectodermal origins of these structures underlie the anatomic distinction between them.

TABLE 1-4. Pectinate Line

CHARACTERISTICS	ABOVE	BELOW
Cell types	Glandular epithelium	Squamous cells
Cancer type	Adenocarcinoma	Squamous cell carcinoma
Innervation	Visceral	Somatic
Hemorrhoids	Internal (painless)	External (painful)
Arterial supply	Superior rectal artery (branch of inferior mesenteric artery)	Inferior rectal artery (branch of internal pudendal artery)
Venous drainage	Superior rectal vein → inferior mesenteric vein → portal system	Inferior rectal vein → internal pudendal vein → internal iliac vein

SPLENIC ANATOMY

The largest secondary lymphatic organ, the spleen, is located in the upper left quadrant of the peritoneal cavity. It is completely surrounded by peritoneum, except at its hilum, where the vasculature enters and exits. It is normally opposed to the underside of the diaphragm, where it rests against the posterior portions of ribs 9–11. Anterior to the spleen lies the stomach. Inferiorly lies the left colic flexure, and medially is the left kidney. It is attached to the stomach by the **gastrosplenic ligament** and to the posterior abdominal wall by the **splenorenal ligament.** The splenic artery and vein are located within the splenorenal ligament. The spleen is made up of two parenchymal tissues: **red pulp** and **white pulp.** The red pulp aids the hematopoietic system by removing senescent and damaged erythrocytes from the circulation. The white pulp provides a location for the hematogenous activation of the humoral immune system.

Red Pulp

The **splenic sinusoids** make up an interconnected network of vascular channels. These are lined by elongated endothelial cells and a discontinuous basement membrane made of reticular fibers (Figure 1-20). The walls separating the sinusoids are called **splenic cords** (cords of Billroth). The splenic cords contain plasma cells, macrophages, and blood cells supported by a connective tissue matrix. Macrophages adjacent to the sinusoids recognize opsonized bacteria, adherent antibodies, foreign antigens, and senescent red cells as they filter through the spleen.

White Pulp

The white pulp is made up of immunologic reinforcements. Arranged around a **central arteriole,** the white pulp contains immune cells in a specific orientation that facilitates immune activation via hematogenously delivered antigens. As an antigen enters the central arteriole, the vasculature branches into radial arterioles (emanating from the central arteriole like spokes of a wheel), and the antigen passes through a surrounding sheath of T cells. This region, known as the periarterial lymphatic sheath, allows for sampling of the arteriolar contents.

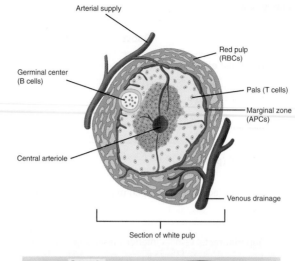

A

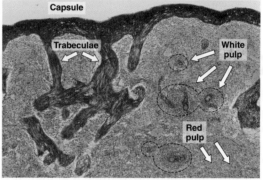

B

FIGURE 1-20. **Diagram and histologic section depicting splenic sinusoids.** (A) Schematic diagram of splenic sinusoids. Here, the important regions of the splenic sinusoid are delineated. A central arteriole is surrounded by the T-cell periarterial lymphatic sheath, which is itself surrounded by B cells. A third concentric ring of tissue, the red pulp, contains antigen-presenting cells (APCs) and macrophages to aid in innate and humoral immunity. RBCs = red blood cells. (B) Section of spleen. The capsule is illustrated, sending trabeculae to the interior of the organ. The red pulp occupies most of the microscopic field. Note the white pulp with its arterioles. (Reproduced with permission from Mescher AL. *Junqueira's Basic Histology: Text and Atlas*, 12th ed. New York: McGraw-Hill, 2010: Figure 14-23.)

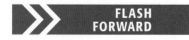

CLINICAL CORRELATION

Disordered red cell removal occurs in sickle cell anemia, leading to autosplenectomy and immunodeficiency (against encapsulated bacteria).

FLASH FORWARD

Acute lymphadenitis occurs when brisk germinal center expansion in response to a local bacterial infection (eg, teeth or tonsils) leads to painfully swollen lymph nodes.

If an APC is present, it may activate a number of T cells, which then travel to the adjacent **lymphatic nodule** for B-cell activation. This process produces active germinal centers where B cells mature. Mature B cells, or plasma cells, defend the host via soluble immunoglobulins secreted into the circulation.

The radial arterioles, which branch from the central arteriole, empty their contents into the **marginal zone.** This region of sinusoids between the red pulp and white pulp contains a high concentration of phagocytic APCs (Figure 1-20).

THE LYMPHATIC SYSTEM

The Lymph Node

Like **little spleens** dispersed along the lymphatic system, these small secondary lymphatic organs aid regional adaptive immune responses by housing APCs, T cells, and B cells (Table 1-5). Each node possesses multiple afferent lymphatic channels, which enter the node through its capsule near the cortex. The efferent lymphatics exit at the hilum, along with an artery and vein

TABLE 1-5.   Lymph Node Organization

REGION	DIVISIONS	CONTENTS AND FUNCTION
Cortex	Follicle (outer cortex)	▪ Primary follicles contain dormant B cells. ▪ Secondary follicles contain active germinal centers.
	Paracortex	▪ Helper T cells reside between follicles and the splenic medulla. ▪ High endothelial venules allow lymphocytes to enter circulation.
Medulla	Sinus	▪ Reticular cells and macrophages communicate with efferent lymphatics.
	Cords	▪ Closely packed lymphocytes and plasma cells.

(Figure 1-21). From the afferent lymphatics, antigens and APCs in the lymph enter the **medullary sinus.** There, free antigens meet macrophages for phagocytosis and presentation in association with MHC II for T-cell activation. Activated APCs bypass the adjacent **medullary cords** to reach the **paracortex,** where T cells await stimulation. Activated T cells move to the adjacent **cortical follicle,** where B cells await costimulatory signals. Once activated, mature B cells travel back to the medullary cords, where they develop into plasma cells and secrete immunoglobulins into the adjacent vascular supply.

Lymphatics

As part of the cardiovascular system, the lymphatic vessels **drain interstitial fluid from surrounding tissues** (Tables 1-6 and 1-7). They are also integral to the process of transporting fats and fat-soluble nutrients and facilitating the humoral immune response. Their role in immunity involves carrying foreign antigens and APCs to lymph nodes for T- and B-cell activation.

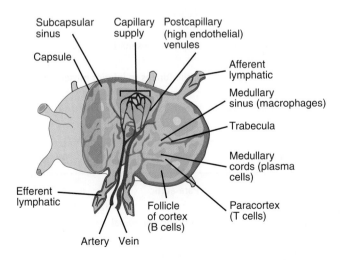

FIGURE 1-21.   Lymph node. Schematic representation of the lymph node structure shows the major divisions of the node. The medulla consists of cords of plasma cells and sinuses of macrophages. The cortex consists of dormant and activated B-cell follicles, as well as a T-cell paracortex.

TABLE 1-6.   Primary Lymph Drainage Routes

DRAINAGE ROUTE	ANATOMIC REGIONS DRAINED
Right lymphatic duct	Right arm, right half of head and right thorax
Thoracic duct	All other regions

The lymph vessels are analogous to veins in their structure and organization. However, rather than originating from capillary systems, they begin as blind sacs. The walls of the lymphatic capillary are made up of a layer of loosely bound endothelial cells, lacking tight junctions and bound to an incomplete basal lamina. This allows fluid to enter the lumen via hydrostatic pressure. As distal lymphatic capillaries merge, they produce larger vessels containing valves, just like veins, that maintain the direction of flow. In addition to interstitial hydrostatic pressure, muscular contractions aid the flow of lymph.

During its course back to the systemic circulation, lymphatic fluid is filtered through lymph nodes for immune surveillance. The remaining lymph reaches the bloodstream via one of two major routes: The larger **thoracic duct** or the smaller **right lymphatic duct**.

TABLE 1-7.   Drainage Routes for the Major Lymph Nodes

ANATOMIC REGION	MAJOR LYMPH NODES
Head and neck	Submental, submandibular, retroauricular, parotid, occipital, superficial and deep cervical
Lateral breast, upper limb	Axillary (pectoral, subscapular, humeral, apical, central)
Parasternal breast	Supra- and infraclavicular
Stomach	Celiac
Duodenum, jejunum, perineum	Superior mesenteric
Sigmoid colon	Colic (drains to inferior mesenteric)
Rectum (lower), anal canal above pectinate line	Internal iliac
Anal canal below pectinate line	Superficial inguinal
Testes	Para-aortic
Scrotum and thigh	Superficial inguinal
Lateral side of dorsum of foot	Popliteal

PERIPHERAL NERVOUS SYSTEM

Nerve Cells

During embryonic development, **neural crest cells** migrate into the peripheral tissues, where they differentiate into **neurons** of the following tissues:

- Sensory neurons of the dorsal root ganglia.
- Neurons of the cranial nerve ganglia.
- Neurons of the autonomic system.
- Neurons of the myenteric (Auerbach) and Meissner's plexus.

Neuronal cells contain three major parts: the cell body, or **soma, dendrites,** and **axons.**

- The soma houses the organelles (including the notable nucleus and the well-developed RER, referred to as the **Nissl body**).
- Dendrites are cytoplasmic processes arising from the soma that provide increased surface area for axonal synaptic connections, thus facilitating the reception and integration of information.
- Each neuron, in addition to multiple dendrites, has one axon, sprouting from the soma at the **axon hillock** and ending in a **synaptic terminal,** or **bouton.**

Because neurons are specialized for signal transduction, they can secrete several different **neurotransmitters.** These peptide molecules are produced in the RER, stored in secretory vesicles, transported through the axon along microtubules via molecular motors, and eventually released from the axon into the **synaptic cleft.** The synaptic cleft is the junction between the synaptic terminal and an adjacent cell. This vesicular secretion, which is triggered by a transmitted action potential, is the primary method of neural control.

Neuroglia

The **Schwann cell,** also a descendent of neural crest cells, envelops peripheral nervous system neurons by extending cytoplasmic processes that wrap themselves tightly around an axon. This encapsulation produces segments of **myelin sheathing** (Figure 1-22) that extend from the axon hillock to the axon terminal. Between each segment is a naked region of the axon called the **node of Ranvier;** each myelinated segment is referred to as an **internode.**

Peripheral Nerve

The peripheral nerve consists of a bundle of neuronal axons, Schwann cells, and protective connective tissues. It carries impulses from the central nervous system to the most distal parts of the body and everywhere in between. Although individual neurons are surrounded by Schwann cells, a nerve fiber is more complex (Figure 1-23). The most external layer of a nerve, known as the **epineurium,** is a dense connective tissue layer that covers the entire nerve, including its vascular supply. Beneath this layer lie the vessels and the **perineurium.** The perineurium acts as a permeability barrier, regulating nutrient transport from capillaries to the nerve fibers beneath. The perineurium invests a number of nerve **fascicles,** bundles of individual nerves surrounded by the **endoneurium.** This final connective tissue layer maintains the Schwann cells, which create the **myelin sheaths** and **nodes of Ranvier,** necessary for fast neuronal conduction.

CLINICAL CORRELATION

Myelin proteins can be highly antigenic, leading to autoimmune disorders, such as Guillain-Barré syndrome.

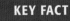 **KEY FACT**

Following trauma, the perineurium must be repaired via microsurgery to ensure proper nerve regeneration and functional restoration.

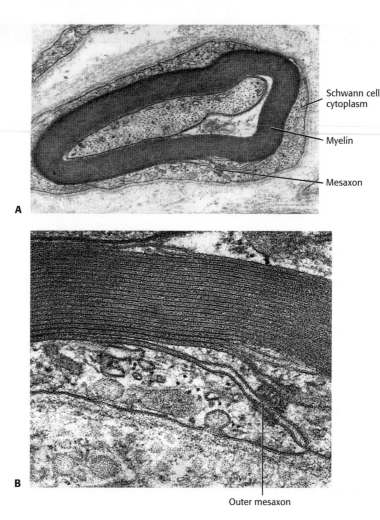

FIGURE 1-22. **Electron micrographs of a myelinated nerve fiber.** (A) ×20,000. (B) ×80,000. (Reproduced with permission from Junqueira JC, Carneiro J. *Basic Histology: Text and Atlas*, 11th ed. New York: McGraw-Hill, 2005: 173.)

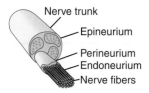

FIGURE 1-23. **Peripheral nerve layers.**

Brachial Plexus

The motor portions of spinal nerves are organized differently from the sensory neurons. Instead of clear divisions organized by spinal level that serve successively distal regions of the body, a great deal of mixing of neurons from each spinal level produces a single nerve supplying a specific muscle group. The upper extremity's **brachial plexus** is a prime example. As motor neurons exit the spinal column between C5 and T1, the ventral rami begin to exchange individual fibers. These rami are considered the **roots** of the brachial plexus (Figure 1-24). As the five roots reach the inferior portion of the neck, C5 and C6 unite to form the **superior trunk,** as C8 and T1 unite to form the **inferior trunk,** leaving C7 as the **middle trunk.** These three trunks pass beneath the clavicle, where they each split into **anterior** and **posterior divisions.** The anterior divisions of the superior and middle trunks merge to form the **lateral cord** of the brachial plexus, and the anterior division of the inferior trunk becomes the **medial cord.** Both of these cords eventually supply the muscles of the anterior compartments of the upper limb. All three posterior divisions merge to form the **posterior cord,** which supplies the posterior compartments of the upper limb. From cords, the plexus divides further into its terminal infraclavicular **branches.** The major infraclavicular and supraclavicular nerve

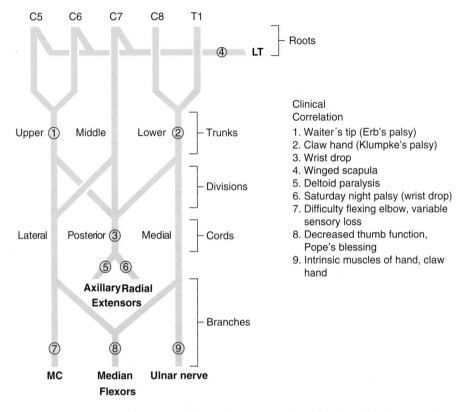

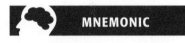

FIGURE 1-24.   Brachial plexus. Schematic representation of the brachial plexus on the left. To the right are clinical correlations to some common brachial plexus injuries and the location of nerve lesions that create them. MC = musculocutaneous nerve; LT = long thoracic nerve.

branches are listed in Table 1-8. Common injuries associated with the brachial plexus are listed in Table 1-9.

Dermatomes

Usually, successive spinal levels innervate successive caudal regions. Figure 1-25 displays the dermatomal organization of the body, as projected on the skin.

THE INTEGUMENTARY SYSTEM

Skin

The skin has several functions:

- Mechanical protection
- Moisture retention
- Body temperature regulation
- Nonspecific immune defense
- Salt excretion
- Vitamin D synthesis
- Tactile sensation

MNEMONIC

Organization of the brachial plexus—

Randy Travis Drinks Cold Beer:

Roots
Trunks
Divisions
Cords
Branches

TABLE 1-8. Principal Branches of the Brachial Plexus

BRANCH	ROOT	INNERVATION
Long thoracic	Ventral rami of C5–C7	Serratus anterior.
Suprascapular	Superior trunk, C4–C6	Supraspinatus, infraspinatus.
Musculocutaneous	Lateral cord, C5–C7	Coracobrachialis, biceps brachii, brachialis.
Median	Medial and lateral cords, C6–T1	All forearm flexors (except flexor carpi ulnaris) including lateral half of flexor digitorum profundus, abductor pollicis brevis, opponens pollicis, flexor pollicis brevis, first and second lumbricals.
Ulnar	Medial cord, C7–T1	Flexor carpi ulnaris, medial half of flexor digitorum profundus, other intrinsic hand muscles.
Axillary	Posterior cord, C5, C6	Teres minor, deltoid.
Radial	Posterior cord, C5–T1	Triceps brachii, brachioradialis, extensors.

TABLE 1-9. Common Brachial Plexus Injuries

LESION LOCATION	SYNDROME	DEFICITS
Superior trunk C5/C6	Erb-Duchenne palsy ("waiter's tip").	▪ Abduction (deltoid). ▪ Lateral rotation (infraspinatus, teres minor). ▪ Supination (biceps) and supinator muscle.
Inferior trunk C8/T1	Interphalangeal joint flexion and metacarpophalangeal joint extension paralysis (full "claw hand").	Intrinsic muscles of hand, forearm flexors of hand.
Posterior cord C5/C6/C7/C8	Axillary and radial nerve paralyses.	Same as for axillary and radial nerves.
Long thoracic nerve T1	Winged scapula.	Serratus anterior paralysis.
Axillary nerve	Deltoid paralysis.	Abduction.
Radial nerve	"Saturday night palsy."	Wrist drop (supinator, brachioradialis, triceps, extensors of wrist/fingers).
Musculocutaneous nerve	Biceps paralysis.	Elbow flexion, arm sensation.
Median nerve	"Pope's blessing" on making a fist.	Thumb abduction, thumb opposition, fourth/fifth digit extension.
Ulnar nerve	Fourth/fifth digit paralysis (partial "claw hand").	Grip strength, fourth/fifth digit flexion/extension, intrinsic muscles of hand.

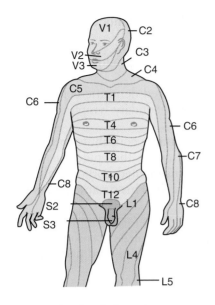

FIGURE 1-25.   **Landmark dermatomes.**

Important Dermatomes	
Forehead	V1
Nipples	T4
Umbilicus	T10
Anus	S5
Thumb	C6
Knee	L3/4
Great toe	L5

The skin is composed of three layers: The **epidermis** (ectodermally derived), the **deep dermis,** and the **hypodermis,** or subcutaneous tissues (the latter two of which are mesenchymally derived).

EPIDERMIS

The epidermis is predominantly made of **keratinocytes,** or epithelial cells named for the intermediate filament protein **keratin.** The epidermis is organized into five layers (Figure 1-26).

The **stratum basalis** is composed of columnar keratinocytes bound to a basement membrane via hemidesmosomes. Cellular proliferation occurring at this level maintains the population of epidermal stem cells, replenishes sloughed skin cells, and contributes to epidermal wound healing. These columnar keratinocytes undergo a process of differentiation, during which time they become progressively flattened and superficially located. At the level of the **stratum spinosum,** keratinocytes have a flattened polygonal shape and an ovoid nucleus. By the time they reach the **stratum corneum,** they are completely flattened and lack nuclei.

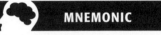

MNEMONIC

Layers of the epidermis—

Californians Like Girls in String Bikinis:

Stratum **C**orneum
Stratum **L**ucidum
Stratum **G**ranulosum
Stratum **S**pinosum
Stratum **B**asalis

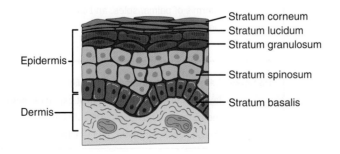

Stratum corneum
Stratum lucidum
Stratum granulosum
Stratum spinosum
Stratum basalis
Epidermis
Dermis

FIGURE 1-26.   **Epidermis layers.**

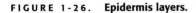

The epidermis also contains other cell types: **melanocytes, Langerhans cells,** and **Merkel cells.**

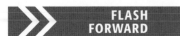

FLASH FORWARD

A deficiency in **tyrosinase** leads to **albinism,** a congenital lack of melanin.

- Melanocytes, derived from the neural crest, produce **melanin,** a tyrosine derivative responsible for skin pigmentation.
- Langerhans cells are bone marrow–derived dendritic cells residing in the skin. Once activated, they migrate to secondary lymph organs to present antigens to T cells.
- Merkel cells, found in the stratum basalis, contribute to the function of the numerous **mechanoreceptors** present in the epidermis. A myelinated sensory axon actually ends in an unmyelinated portion, called the **nerve plate,** which synapses on the Merkel cell. This synapse allows the Merkel cell to signal tactile sensation.

In addition to Merkel cells, two other specialized sensory structures exist within the body: **Meissner corpuscles** in the dermis and **pacinian corpuscles** in the deep tissues (Figure 1-27).

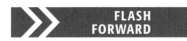

FLASH FORWARD

Autoantibodies against cellular adhesion molecules lead to debilitating blistering diseases such as bullous pemphigoid.

Dermis

The epidermis is anchored to its basement membrane by hemidesmosomes. Two indistinct layers, the **papillary layer** and the **reticular layer,** reside just below. The papillary layer (primarily loose connective tissue) consists of fibroblasts, collagen, and elastic fibers; the reticular layer contains mostly collagen and elastic fibers.

Skin Appendages

Skin appendages (**hair follicles, sweat glands,** and **sebaceous glands**) are present in the dermis, as is the blood supply to the skin (Figure 1-28). Hair shafts are made of hardened keratin, and the follicular bulb where the hair originates contains stem cells capable of repopulating the follicular shaft, or even the epidermis following injury. Sebaceous glands are oil-producing glands that actually empty their contents into the hair follicle, the tubular invagination that the hair shaft follows as it grows to the surface. Sweat glands occur in two forms: (1) The **eccrine** sweat gland is a ubiquitous coiled gland innervated by sympathetic cholinergic nerves and used in temperature regulation. (2) The **apocrine** glands, regulated by adrenergic stimuli, only become

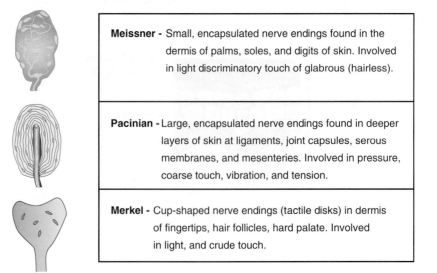

Meissner - Small, encapsulated nerve endings found in the dermis of palms, soles, and digits of skin. Involved in light discriminatory touch of glabrous (hairless).

Pacinian - Large, encapsulated nerve endings found in deeper layers of skin at ligaments, joint capsules, serous membranes, and mesenteries. Involved in pressure, coarse touch, vibration, and tension.

Merkel - Cup-shaped nerve endings (tactile disks) in dermis of fingertips, hair follicles, hard palate. Involved in light, and crude touch.

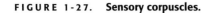

FIGURE 1-27.   Sensory corpuscles.

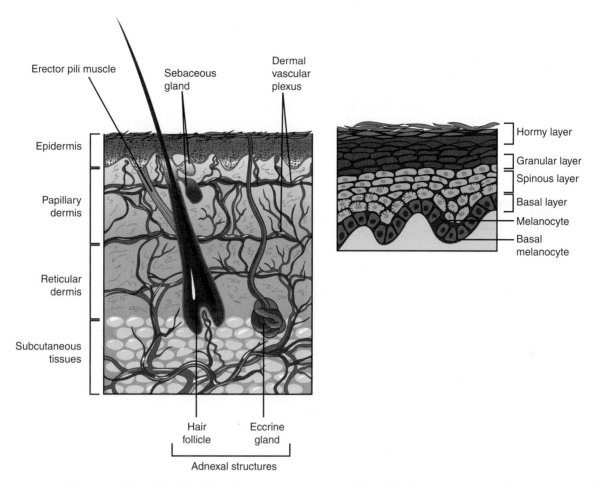

FIGURE 1-28. **Skin appendages.** The histologic schematic representation of skin (left) demonstrates a complex organization of cells, connective tissue, blood vessels, and adnexal structures. The drawing (upper right) depicts the orderly maturation of keratinocytes in the epidermis.

active following puberty. These coiled glands are found in the axilla, mons pubis, and circumanal regions.

THE RESPIRATORY SYSTEM

Respiratory Histology

Once air has traveled through the **air-conducting** channels (nasal cavities, nasopharynx, oropharynx, larynx, trachea, bronchi, and bronchioles), it enters the **respiratory tissues.** These include the respiratory bronchioles, alveolar ducts, alveolar sacs, and alveoli.

BRONCHI AND BRONCHIOLES

Except for their smallest divisions, these airways are involved in conducting inhaled air to the lung, rather than gas exchange. Primarily, the walls of the conducting airways contain a **pseudostratified columnar ciliated epithelium,** composed of three cell types:

- **Ciliated epithelial cells:** Coordinated ciliary motion helps to expel respiratory secretions that have collected pathogens and debris from inspired air.
- **Goblet cells:** Produce mucus and protect the airway and lung tissue from inspired particles.
- **Basal cells:** Provide structural support to the airway.

KEY FACT

Type II pneumocytes produce surfactant and have the ability to differentiate into Type I pneumocytes.

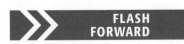

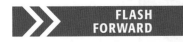

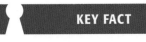

ALVEOLUS

Despite the many subdivisions of lung tissue, the basic functional unit is the alveolus. The lungs contain about 300 million alveoli, which increase the surface area for gas exchange to approximately 75 m². Each alveolar wall consists of two cell types, **type I** and **type II alveolar cells,** with each serving separate physiologic functions (Figure 1-29).

Continuous with the low cuboidal epithelium of the adjacent respiratory bronchiole, 90% of the alveolar surface is covered with type I alveolar cells. This anatomic arrangement allows deoxygenated blood to come into close proximity with O_2 inhaled from the environment. In fact, the primary function of the type I alveolar cell, a simple squamous epithelial cell, is to form the first layer of the **air-blood barrier.** Below the type I cells is a layer of dual basal lamina and endothelial cells of the alveolar capillaries, completing a semipermeable barrier that allows O_2 and CO_2 diffusion.

The type II alveolar cell's primary function is the production of pulmonary surfactant. Type II alveolar cell's also retain the ability to differentiate into type I alveolar cells if there is an injury to the lung. Clara cells, also known as C cells, also help produce surfactant in the lungs. C cells act as stem cells, which means they can differentiate and replace other damaged lung cells. Finally, C cells contain enzymes that can detoxify noxious substances in the lungs.

Lung Anatomy

The lungs are enveloped in serosal tissue, known as **pleura,** which has two layers. Apposed directly to the lung is the **visceral pleura.** The **parietal pleura** is adherent to the chest wall. Fluid within the potential space between the visceral and parietal pleura, the pleural space, allows respiratory tissues to slide effortlessly as the lung expands.

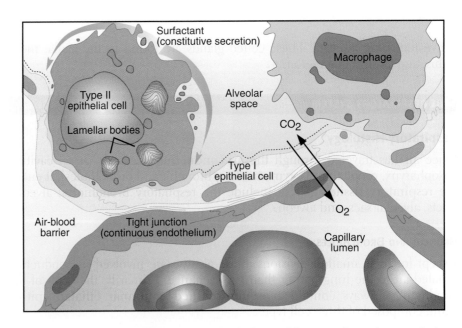

FIGURE 1-29.   **Gas exchange barrier.** The thickness of the gas exchange barrier is highlighted, as well as the anatomic relations of important cell types: type I and type II epithelial cells, endothelial cells, macrophages, and red blood cells.

Each lung is divided into **lobes,** which are further divided into **bronchopulmonary segments.** Each bronchopulmonary segment corresponds to a branch of the **bronchial tree** that delivers O_2 to the lung. The right lung is composed of three lobes, and the left lung, two. However, the superior lobe of the left lung contains a region, the **lingula,** which is analogous to the right lung's middle lobe. The **cardiac notch,** into which the apex of the heart protrudes, replaces the middle lobe. The bronchial tree begins at the trachea, which branches into right and left **main-stem bronchi.** The left is slightly longer, and the right makes a shallower angle (runs more vertically), with the trachea at its bifurcation.

The major vascular supply to each lung begins as a single branch of the **pulmonary artery** (carrying deoxygenated blood) and ends as two **pulmonary veins** (carrying oxygenated blood to the left atrium). Between these large vessels, the vasculature branch into intrasegmental pulmonary arteries, which travel with branching airways. The pulmonary veins are along the boundaries of the bronchopulmonary segment. Both end in a capillary network, within the alveolar septae, that facilitate gas exchange. In addition to the pulmonary vessels, the **bronchial circulation** aids in supporting the respiratory tissues. Originating from the aorta, blood from the bronchial circulation is dumped into the pulmonary venous circulation after passing through the lung. Although it is relatively deoxygenated, it mixes with recently oxygenated blood and is delivered to the left atrium.

ANATOMIC RELATIONS

The lungs reside within the rib cage, under the protection of the bony skeleton. The apices are at the level of the first rib, and the bases rest in the left and right costodiaphragmatic recesses. Along the midclavicular line, the lungs can be auscultated from just above the clavicle to the seventh or eighth rib anteriorly. Posteriorly, the lungs extend more distally, deep into the costodiaphragmatic recess, at the 11th or 12th rib. Within the chest, each of the three lung surfaces (**mediastinal, costal,** and **diaphragmatic**) are in close proximity to important structures.

- **Mediastinal surface:** Marks the lateral extent of the **mediastinum,** which houses the heart, great vessels, esophagus, trachea, thoracic duct, bronchial hilum, and hilar lymph nodes, as well as the vagus and phrenic nerves.
- **Costal surface:** Primarily contacts the inside of the chest wall. As mentioned previously, two layers of pleura exist between the functional lung tissue and chest wall.
- **Diaphragmatic surface:** The diaphragm resides just below each lung.

The diaphragm, a thin sheet of muscle separating the thorax and abdomen, and the main muscle for respiration, is innervated by the **phrenic nerves,** which originate from cervical roots C3, C4, and C5. A number of vital structures cross the diaphragm to pass from the thoracic to the abdominal cavity. In particular, the **aorta, esophagus,** and **inferior vena cava** (IVC) each pierce the diaphragm at different thoracic vertebral levels. The IVC, the most anterior of the three structures, crosses at the level of T8. The esophagus crosses at T10, and the aorta crosses at T12 (Figure 1-30).

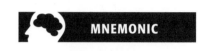

KEY FACT

Divisions of the bronchial tree:
Trachea
Right and left main bronchi
Lobar bronchi
Segmental bronchi
Bronchioles
Terminal bronchioles
Respiratory bronchioles
Alveolar ducts
Alveoli

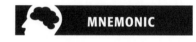

MNEMONIC

C3, 4, 5 keep the diaphragm alive!

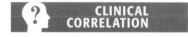

MNEMONIC

Structures that cross the diaphragm—

I 8 10 EGGs AT 12

I = **I**VC
8 = T**8**
10 = T**10**
EG = **E**sopha**G**us
G = va**G**us nerve
A = **A**orta and **A**zygos vein
T = **T**horacic duct
12 = T**12**

CLINICAL CORRELATION

Visceral diaphragmatic pain is conferred by nerves from C5. Because these nerves also supply the shoulder, pain can be referred to the shoulder.

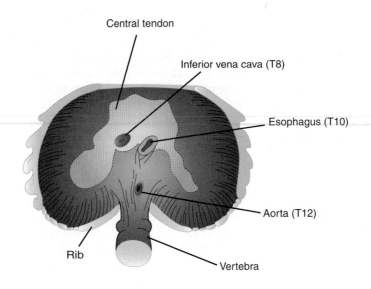

Central tendon

Inferior vena cava (T8)

Esophagus (T10)

Aorta (T12)

Rib

Vertebra

FIGURE 1-30. **Diaphragm structures.** Inferior view.

THE GASTROINTESTINAL SYSTEM

Small Intestinal Layers

The small intestine, the major organ of nutrient absorption from the gut, is composed of several layers, each contributing to the coordination of digestion and transport.

- **Mucosa:** Absorption.
- **Submucosa:** Vascular and lymphatic supply.
- **Muscularis externa:** Mechanical mixing, dissociation, and propulsion.
- **Serosa:** Protection.

MUCOSA

The intestinal mucosa, the absorption barrier of the alimentary canal, is composed of polarized epithelial cells specialized in transport and uses several molecular and structural adaptations that allow it to efficiently extract nutrients from food.

Structurally, the mucosa has four adaptations that increase the absorptive surface area:

- **Plicae circulares** (circular folds, or **valves of Kerckring**)
- **Intestinal villi**
- **Intestinal glands**
- **Microvilli** on the apical epithelium

A plicae circularis is a permanent folding of the mucosa and submucosa into the lumen of the intestine. Their distribution is not uniform throughout the intestine, but instead begins within the duodenum, peaks at the duodenojejunal junction, and ends at the mid ileum. Intestinal villi, on the other hand, are near-uniform finger-like projections of the mucosa into the lumen. These projections extend deep into the mucosa, to the **muscularis mucosa,** the boundary between the mucosa and the submucosa and ending in **intestinal glands** known as **crypts of Lieberkühn.** These glands are not actually secretory glands, but rather exist to enhance absorption.

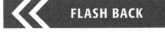

FLASH BACK

Molecularly, the intestinal epithelium employs cell adhesion molecules to determine polarity and maintain the physical barrier between the body and the intestinal lumen (external environment).

Finally, each **enterocyte,** or intestinal epithelial cell, contains microvilli on its apical border. This **brush border** increases the surface area approximately 30-fold. Microscopically, the microvillus contains a core of parallel cross-linked actin filaments bound to cytoskeletal proteins. The brush border is coated in a **glycocalyx,** a surface coat of glycoproteins excreted by columnar secretory **goblet cells.** In addition, the luminal membrane contains several intramembranous enzymes (eg, maltase, lactase, enterokinase) integral to digestion and small-molecule absorption. Intracytoplasmic enzymes break down absorbed di- and tripeptides.

SUBMUCOSA

The submucosa is the site of vascular and lymphatic supply to the intestine. This layer, composed of loose connective tissue, contains a vascular plexus that extends capillaries into the surrounding layers. The lymphatic drainage of the submucosa begins as blind-ended channels, known as **lacteals,** within the core of the intestinal villi. These lacteals empty into a submucosal lymphatic plexus that shuttles antigens to nearby lymphatic nodules and emulsified fat-soluble nutrients to the liver.

Within the **duodenum,** the submucosa contains **Brunner glands,** tubuloaci-nar mucus glands that produce an alkaline (pH ~ 9) secretion to neutralize acidified chyme from the stomach. Within the **ilium** reside the lymphatic nodules that provide immunologic surveillance to the intestines. These nodules, also known as **Peyer patches,** or **gut-associated lymphoid tissue (GALT),** contain a germinal center of B cells surrounded by specialized APCs: **M cells** and dendritic cells. Antigens enter the Peyer patch through antigen presentation via M cells and dendritic cells. The B cells of the GALT germinal center are specialized; they produce a specific immunoglobulin, **IgA,** which can be secreted into the intestinal lumen to neutralize pathogens before they invade the epithelium.

The submucosa also houses one of the two neural plexuses located within the small intestine. Considered part of the autonomic system, these neural networks receive a great deal of intrinsic input from the intestinal parenchyma. This allows the gut to operate nearly independently from the central nervous system, although its action can be modulated via extensive extrinsic neural input. Two networks control the activity of the small intestine: the submucosal **plexus of Meissner** and the **myenteric plexus of Auerbach** (Figure 1-31). They are extensively interconnected and probably equally modulate mucosal and muscular activity, coordinating action to maximize digestion.

MUSCULARIS EXTERNA

Intestinal motility is controlled by two layers of smooth muscle. One circular layer is surrounded by a second longitudinal layer (Auerbach's plexus resides between these two layers). Coordinated muscular contraction produces two types of mechanical results: **propulsion** and **segmentation.**

- **Propulsion** occurs when proximal contraction is coordinated with distal relaxation. This leads to increased upstream pressure, which slowly propels food through the digestive system. Contraction of proximal sphincters ensures that the food bolus only moves distally.
- **Segmentation** occurs when a bolus of food is mechanically compressed and split into two portions as the lumen constricts near the bolus center, not merely proximal to it. If this contraction is not coordinated with distal relaxation, the bolus cannot be propelled forward. Instead, its contents are mixed by the muscular contractions.

FLASH FORWARD

Defects in lactase activity lead to lactose intolerance. Loss of other intramembranous enzymes (eg, enterocyte toxicity following chemotherapy) leads to osmotic diarrhea.

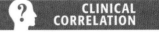

CLINICAL CORRELATION

Invasive adenocarcinomas that reach the submucosa are able to metastasize via the rich lymphatic and vascular plexus.

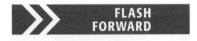

FLASH FORWARD

Dysfunction of the plexus, due to either congenital absence (Hirschsprung disease) or neurologic injury (diabetic neuropathy), leads to decreased intestinal motility.

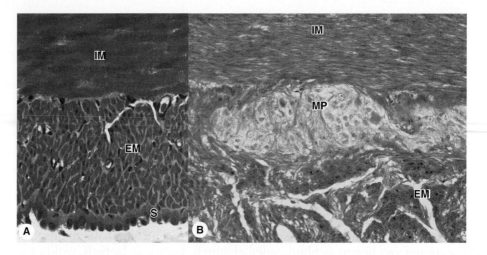

FIGURE 1-31. **Histologic section of intestinal layers.** (A) Transverse sections of the wall of the small intestine. The internal smooth muscle layer (IM) is predominantly circular, whereas the external smooth muscle layer (EM) is longitudinal. The serosa (S) is a thin connective tissue covering the small intestine, composed of squamous epithelium. (B) Pale-staining neurons and other cells in one myenteric plexus (MP) are seen between the two muscle layers. (Reproduced with permission from Mescher AL. *Junqueira's Basic Histology: Text and Atlas*, 12th ed. New York: McGraw-Hill, 2010: Figure 15-35.)

SEROSA

The serosa is composed of visceral peritoneum covering the small intestine. It is lined by a simple squamous epithelium (Figure 1-31A).

THE ADRENAL SYSTEM

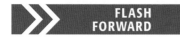

FLASH FORWARD

Deficiencies in enzymes of the adrenal gland lead to defects in physiology and sexual development.

MNEMONIC

The deeper you go, the sweeter it gets:
Zona glomerulosa: **Salt** hormones (aldosterone)
Zona fasciculata: **Sugar** hormones (glucocorticoids)
Zona reticularis: **Sex** hormones (androgens)
Or think of kidney **GFR** (**G**lomerular **F**iltration **R**ate), which adrenal gland sits above: **G**lomerulosa, **F**asciculata, **R**eticularis.

Adrenal Gland

Situated atop the kidney, the adrenal gland has an outer **cortex** surrounding an inner **medulla.** The mesodermally derived cortex produces **steroid hormones,** and the neuroectodermally derived medulla produces **catecholamines.**

CORTEX

The cortex is a three-story steroid hormone factory. Each of the three layers of the cortex (Figure 1-32) expresses specific enzymes for producing steroid hormones built from a cholesterol precursor.

- **Zona glomerulosa:** The outermost layer, which produces salt-regulating aldosterone.
- **Zona fasciculata:** The middle layer, which produces the stress hormone cortisol.
- **Zona reticularis:** The innermost layer, which produces sex hormones (androgens).

The zona glomerulosa is a region of concentrically arranged secretory epithelial cells, surrounded by a vascularized stroma. Residing just below the protective fibrous capsule of the gland, these cells are marked by a well-developed SER producing the mineralocorticoid aldosterone. **Angiotensin II,** produced in the lung, can trigger both release of aldosterone and hypertrophy of the zona glomerulosa.

The functional distinctions between the zona fasciculata and zona reticularis are less well developed, as are their morphologic boundaries. These regions

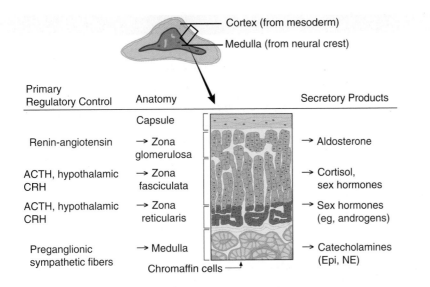

FIGURE 1-32. **Schematic depiction of the cortex of the adrenal gland.** ACTH = adrenocorticotropic hormone; CRH = corticotropin-releasing hormone; Epi = epinephrine; NE = norepinephrine.

are often treated as a functional unit. The columns of polygonal cells in the zona fasciculata occupy the majority of the cortex. Fenestrated capillaries intersperse these fascicles, delivering **adrenocorticotropic hormone (ACTH)** to regulate cortisol secretion back into the capillaries for systemic delivery. The zona reticularis, rather than forming columns or concentric circles, forms a network of cells, also surrounded by fenestrated capillaries for regulation by plasma ACTH.

MEDULLA

The adrenal medulla oversees the systemic stress response. **Epinephrine** and **norepinephrine** (NE), two tyrosine-derived chemical messengers of the systemic stress response, are produced here. Although NE is also released within the synaptic cleft of adrenergic neurons, these catecholamines are released in bulk into the venous sinusoids of the medulla. In fact, the adrenal medulla, like the autonomic nervous system, is derived from the neuroectoderm. They also receive innervation from sympathetic presynaptic neurons, thus acting as a modified sympathetic postganglionic neuron.

The medullary secretory cells, **chromaffin cells,** synthesize either epinephrine (80%) or norepinephrine (20%), but not both. These secretory products are produced from tyrosine, rather than cholesterol, as in the cortex.

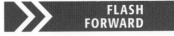

Catecholamine breakdown products, vanillylmandelic acid (VMA) and metanephrine, can be measured in the urine to determine systemic catecholamine levels.

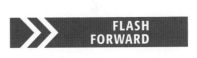

The most common tumors of the adrenal gland are adenomas from the cortex, neuroblastomas from medullary neural crest cells, and pheochromocytomas arising from the medullary chromaffin cells.

NOTES

Behavioral Science

Epidemiology

Increasingly, emphasis has been placed on the concept of evidence-based medicine. Every year, more questions about the techniques used to conduct research and interpret basic tests appear on Step 1. An understanding of the methodology and interpretation of research studies and the significance of diagnostic test results is very helpful.

Common types of questions include:

- Given a description of the population studied and the methods used, what type of study is this?
- Given a description of the study population and the goals of the research, what type of study is most appropriate?
- Perform common calculations and understand the mathematical definitions and significance of terms such as *false-positive* and *false-negative*.

> **KEY FACT**
>
> Epidemiologic questions are easy points, but only if students know the definitions and understand the basic calculations.

STUDY METHODS

Studies can be divided into two types: purely observational and experimental. **Observational studies** look at events that happen with little or no manipulation by the researcher. **Experimental studies** often require the researcher to assemble subjects, design a study protocol, and perform some type of intervention.

Observational Studies

CASE STUDY OR CASE SERIES

These studies are written descriptions of a patient or particular problem, generally used to document a unique manifestation of a disease, a previously unrecognized association or risk factor, the first incidence of a new disease, or some clinical presentation that might be of interest to other physicians. A case series is simply a collection of case studies, typically consecutive, that document a similar patient presentation or disease manifestation.

Example: Case studies documented rare opportunistic infections in apparently healthy young patients and were some of the earliest documentations of HIV/AIDS before the disease was recognized.

CROSS-SECTIONAL STUDY

A cross-sectional study collects data at a particular point in time from a group of people to assess the frequency of disease and related risk factors. It answers basic questions, such as, "In a given population, how many people have a disease?" or "How many people have risk factors in population X?"

Example: In the 1980s, some physicians noticed that hemophiliacs had a high incidence of AIDS. To determine what proportion of hemophiliacs had HIV/AIDS in 1988, a cross-sectional study, or survey, could be performed in this population.

CASE-CONTROL STUDY

A case-control study compares a group of people who already have a disease or condition with a group that does not to determine disease risk factors. Once a person with the condition is identified (a case), he or she is matched with one or more demographically similar person without the condition (control). The two groups are then compared for differences that may provide insight into possible causes or risk factors, as illustrated in Figure 2-1.

Example: To determine why some hemophiliacs contracted HIV/AIDS in the 1980s when many others did not, a case-control study was performed. In this study a group of HIV-positive hemophiliacs was matched by age-, sex-, race-, and location with a control group of hemophiliacs who did not have the disease. When the data were analyzed for differences between the two groups, it was found that the HIV-positive hemophiliacs were far more likely to have received more blood transfusions than the controls.

COHORT STUDY

A cohort study examines a large group and watches it evolve over time. It includes people with different exposures and follows all of these people to see which ones will develop the disease. At the outset, the participants do not usually have the condition or disease being studied. It is expected that some individuals in the study will develop the condition or complication being studied (Figure 2-2).

Example: To determine the risk of HIV transmission in IV drug users, identify a cohort of HIV-negative IV drug users and follow them for 10 years.

Experimental Studies

CLINICAL TRIAL

A clinical trial is a direct test of a drug, technique, or other intervention. Subjects are divided into at least two groups: one group acting as a control receives either a placebo or the current standard of care treatment; the other group is given the intervention being studied (Figure 2-3). Often, such trials are double-blind, meaning that neither the subjects nor the experimenters know who is receiving the actual treatment and who is receiving the placebo.

Example: To test a new HIV drug, similar HIV subjects are recruited and divided randomly into treatment and placebo groups. Experimenters do not know who is receiving the actual drug versus the placebo. At the end of the experiment, the group assignment is revealed to allow for comparison of the outcomes.

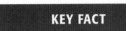

KEY FACT

In a case-control study, the cases already have a condition or illness, and controls generally are chosen **retrospectively.** In a cohort study, participants do not yet have a condition or illness; thus, they are generally observed **prospectively.**

KEY FACT

The Framingham Heart Study is a very well known cohort study that has followed the residents of Framingham, Massachusetts, for decades. More than 1000 papers on cardiac health have come out of this study.

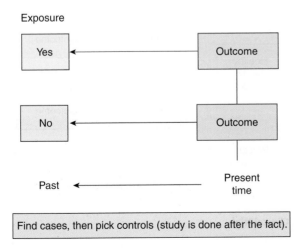

FIGURE 2-1. Case-control study.

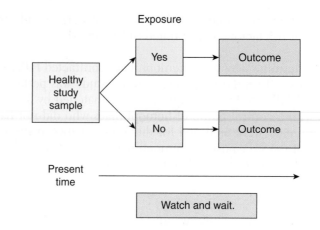

FIGURE 2-2. **Cohort study.**

CROSSOVER STUDY

Participants are randomized into one of two treatment groups, with the control group often given a placebo. After the experiment is performed once, however, participants are switched, or crossed over, into the opposite treatment group, and the experiment is run again. Thus, each participant receives both treatments at different times and can act as his or her own control. In essence, this is a variation of a case-control study; it is illustrated in Figure 2-4.

Example: A drug that may temporarily raise CD4 T-cell counts in HIV-positive individuals is being tested. Half of the subjects are assigned to a treatment group and the other half to a placebo group; then effects are measured. Because the effect is not permanent, one could repeat the experiment with switched groups. One can compare each subject's response to the drug and the placebo.

META-ANALYSIS

A meta-analysis combines the data from many preexisting studies on the same topic to produce what is essentially one big study. It is not necessary to understand the statistical techniques for the USMLE.

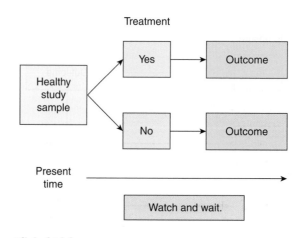
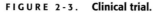

FIGURE 2-3. **Clinical trial.**

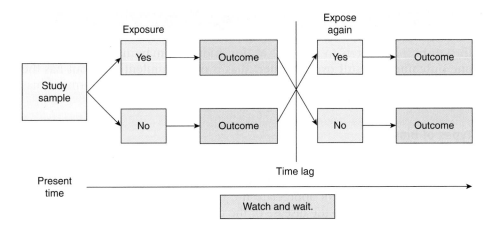

FIGURE 2-4. Crossover study.

Example: Many studies have assessed the effectiveness of treatments to prevent immunosuppression in HIV. However, no one study is large enough to state unequivocally that the treatment is truly effective. By combining the results of multiple studies, more definitive conclusions are possible.

Any time studies are combined, think meta-analysis. A meta-analysis is only as good as the studies it combines. Even when the studies are based on good data, it is hard to accurately combine studies because the methodology of each must be controlled.

All studies described earlier are compared in Table 2-1.

TABLE 2-1. Comparison of Study Types

Case Studies/Case Series	Cross-Sectional Studies
▪ Easy.	▪ Fairly easy.
▪ Purely descriptive.	▪ Purely descriptive.
▪ Do not address causality.	▪ Do not address causality.
▪ Do not provide prevalence statistics or other epidemiologic data.	▪ Do provide prevalence statistics or other epidemiologic data.
Case-Control Studies	**Cohort Studies**
▪ Retrospective.	▪ Prospective.
▪ Can be quick.	▪ Can take a long time.
▪ Do not provide prevalence statistics or other epidemiologic data.	▪ Do provide prevalence statistics or other epidemiologic data.
▪ Good for rare diseases.	▪ Not good for rare diseases.
Clinical Trials	**Crossover Studies**
▪ Good if effect is permanent.	▪ Good if the effect is temporary.
▪ Prone to bias.	▪ Prone to bias and unanticipated permanent effects.
▪ Gold standard if randomized and blinded.	

BIAS

In statistics, bias refers to any part of the study that **may inadvertently favor one outcome or result over another.** Bias is often unintentional, but has the potential to invalidate conclusions. It is possible to detect certain forms of bias by analyzing the study in question.

Types of Bias

CONFOUNDING BIAS

A confounding bias can occur when one variable is closely related to another. If the researcher does not appreciate the relationship, the incorrect variable may be thought to cause the disease or the condition being studied.

Example: A scientist notes that certain people stand outside every day during their breaks at work. He also notices that these same people often develop lung cancer. He collects data and finds that the more time one spends standing outside during work breaks, the more likely one is to develop lung cancer. He concludes that being outside causes lung cancer. In reality, of course, the people who stand outside a lot develop lung cancer because they smoke.

SAMPLING BIAS

Sampling bias occurs when the sample of people chosen for the study (or one group within the study) is not representative of the pool from which they were chosen.

Example: To test a new treatment for diabetes, 1000 men over the age of 65 are enrolled in a study. The drug appears to be effective in controlling symptoms. However, when marketed to the general population, the results are less favorable because the original study excluded younger patients or females, who respond poorly to the medication.

RECALL BIAS

When people are asked to recall information retrospectively, their responses are often influenced by knowledge gained after the fact, such as whether they received a placebo or a real drug.

Example: At the end of a study, a group of patients is told that they received the real drug and not a placebo. When asked if the drug worked, the patients are more likely to say "yes" if their personal bias going into the study was that the drug would work.

SELECTION BIAS

When the investigators or clinicians choose how to group participants for the purposes of the study, a selection bias results. In this situation, the distribution of subjects within the groups is often not random.

Example: Investigators or the patient's treating clinician are given the choice of whether subjects with cancer receive the standard chemotherapy treatment or an experimental treatment. The investigators or clinicians disproportionately choose the experimental treatment for subjects with advanced cancer because they know that the standard treatment is ineffective for late-stage cancer. Those receiving the experimental treatment might do worse on average, due not to the inherent ineffectiveness of the drug, but to the disproportionate number of very sick patients who received this treatment.

LATE-LOOK BIAS

The results in studies with a late-look bias are recorded at the wrong time, skewing the outcomes.

Example: Persons with a certain stage of colon cancer have, on average, 5 months to live. Half are given an experimental treatment, and they are found to have lived an average of 3 months. The investigators conclude that the treatment actually shortens life expectancy by 2 months. However, they overlooked the fact that treatment itself took 3 months. In this situation, the treated group actually lived 1 month longer!

Reducing Bias

Two common ways to reduce bias include **blinding** and **randomization.**

BLINDING

In blinded studies, participants or the investigators may not be told which intervention is being given. In a single-blind study, either the participants or the researchers performing the test are not told the intervention. In a double-blind study, neither party is aware who is receiving which intervention. Blinding **prevents recall bias.**

Example: A **placebo** is the classic way to blind participants in a study. A placebo is an inactive treatment that looks, tastes, and feels identical to the actual drug; thus, participants do not know which treatment they are receiving.

RANDOMIZATION

Participants are grouped randomly into study groups. Randomization **prevents selection bias** because neither subjects nor study conductors participate in the decision of whether subjects receive the experimental treatment.

Example: After a pool of subjects for a study is chosen, the subjects are placed in the intervention group or the placebo group, based on some random method such as a coin toss. Potential differences between subjects that may skew results are more likely to be randomly distributed into both groups.

Prevalence, Incidence, and Duration

Prevalence is how many people in a sample group have a condition **at a certain point in time.** Often written as a ratio, such as "1 in 4 persons over the age of 40 has high cholesterol."

Incidence is how many people will **newly acquire** a condition in a given period, such as "1 in 50 per year."

Duration is how long a given condition lasts, on average.

These three terms are related by the formula:

$$\text{Prevalence} = \text{Incidence} \times \text{Duration}$$

Example: In a given population, 1 in 100 persons acquires a new plantar wart each year (incidence). On average, the wart will last two years (duration). Survey this population in any given year, and roughly 2 in 100 persons will have a plantar wart (Incidence × Duration = Prevalence).

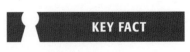

MNEMONIC

Don't be BIASeD:
Bad sample
Incorrect variable
After-the-fact recall bias
Selection bias
Delayed/late-look bias

KEY FACT

Randomized, double-blind clinical trials are the gold standard for robust studies.

KEY FACT

For diseases of very short duration, incidence = prevalence.

KEY FACT

Shorten the disease duration OR reduce the incidence to reduce the prevalence.

Sensitivity, Specificity, and Predictive Value

When a patient is given a test to determine the presence of a condition, the test most often yields one of two results: positive or negative. However, no test is 100% accurate. Thus, there are four possibilities:

- **True-positive (TP)** is a positive test result in a person who has the condition.
- **False-positive (FP)** is a positive test result in a person who does not have the condition.
- **True-negative (TN)** is a negative test result in a person who does not have the condition.
- **False-negative (FN)** is a negative test result in a person who does have the condition.

True-positives and **false-negatives** actually have the condition being tested for. **True-negatives** and **false-positives** do not have the condition (Figure 2-5). False-positive rate = 1 – Specificity.

These four outcomes for any test are used to calculate **sensitivity, specificity,** and **predictive values.**

Sensitivity and specificity describe the accuracy of a diagnostic test.

Sensitivity is a measure of how often a given test will detect the presence of disease *in those who have the disease.* In other words, it is a measure of how reliable the test is in identifying the disease. It is the percentage of positive test results (TP) among a population with the tested condition (TP + FN). It measures the percentage of those who have the condition that test positive in the test.

Specificity is a measure of how often a given test will detect the absence of a disease *in those who do not have the disease* (that is, true-negatives). It is a measure of how well the test identifies disease-free individuals. It is the percentage of negative test results (TN) among a population without the tested condition (TN + FP). It measures the percentage of those who do not have the condition that test negative in the test.

Predictive value describes the likelihood that a patient has (or does not have) the disease in question, based on the results of the diagnostic test.

Positive predictive value is the likelihood that a positive test result truly means that a patient has a given condition, that is, the number of correct positive tests (TP) out of the total number of positive tests (TP + FP).

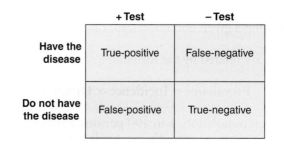

	+ Test	**– Test**
Have the disease	True-positive	False-negative
Do not have the disease	False-positive	True-negative

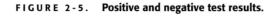

FIGURE 2-5.   **Positive and negative test results.**

Negative predictive value is the likelihood that a negative test result truly means that a patient does not have a given condition, that is, the number of correct negative tests (TN) out of the total number of negative tests (TN + FN).

The interrelationships between these values are depicted in Figure 2-6.

Steps to solve the common board questions related to sensitivity and specificity:

- Pick an easy number to use for the sample patient population (any number works).
- Use prevalence to calculate how many in the sample do and do not actually have the disease.
- For those who do have the disease, use the test's sensitivity to determine how many would test positive (true-positives) and how many would test negative (false-negatives).
- For those who do not have the disease, use specificity to calculate how many will test negative for the disease (true-negatives) and how many will test positive (false-positives).
- Calculate the positive predictive value by dividing the true-positives by all positive test results. Calculate the negative predictive value by dividing the true-negatives by all negative results.

KEY FACT

The lower the prevalence of a disease, the lower the positive predictive value, even if the test's sensitivity and specificity are high! Remember there can't be many true-positives if there aren't many patients.

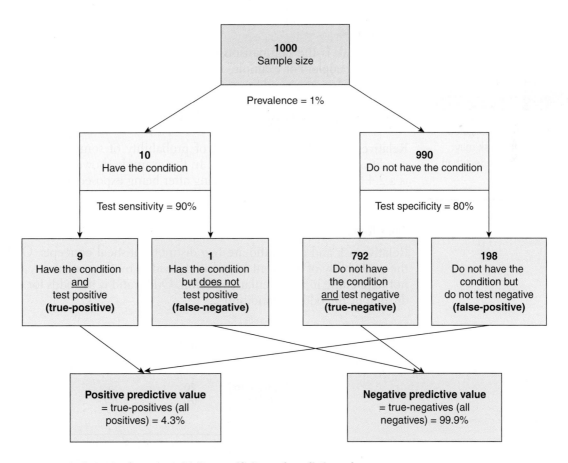

FIGURE 2-6.   **Integrating prevalence, sensitivity, specificity, and predictive values.**

Odds Ratio and Relative Risk

Odds ratios and **relative risk** express how much more likely something is to occur if a certain condition is met, such as a patient being exposed to an illness or receiving a particular treatment. These are calculated based on known outcomes, as in the example in Figure 2-7.

ABSOLUTE RISK

Relative risks and odds ratios are calculated from a chart similar to Figure 2-7 using **absolute risk,** which is the likelihood of an outcome over time without comparison to another group. That is, it is the probability of something occurring. The risk is not compared to any other risks.

$$\text{Absolute Risk (of dying if exposed)} = A / (A + B)$$
$$\text{Absolute Risk (of dying if not exposed)} = C / (C + D)$$

ATTRIBUTABLE RISK

Absolute risk (if not exposed) demonstrates that some subjects will have the outcome being studied, even when the condition is not met. To calculate how much risk is actually due to the condition being studied, use **attributable risk.**

$$\text{Attributable Risk} = \text{Absolute Risk (if exposed)} - \text{Absolute Risk (if not exposed)} = A / (A + B) - C / (C + D)$$

RELATIVE RISK

Relative risk is the comparison of risks between two different conditions or groups of people. For example, the relative risk of developing lung cancer for nonsmokers as compared to smokers is different.

$$\text{Relative Risk} = (A / (A + B)) / (C / (C + D))$$

Relative risk is the measurement of probability of something happening in condition 1 relative to condition 2. In the example shown in Figure 2-7, there is a 2.4 times greater chance of dying after being exposed to the pathogen versus not being exposed.

ODDS RATIO

Relative risk and odds ratio are two distinct statistical concepts. Odds ratio is the probability of an event happening divided by the probability of an event not happening in a particular condition. Odds ratio is the odds for condition 1 divided by the odds of condition 2.

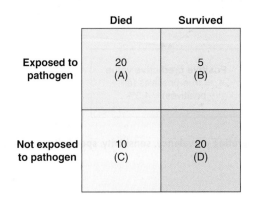

	Died	Survived
Exposed to pathogen	20 (A)	5 (B)
Not exposed to pathogen	10 (C)	20 (D)

FIGURE 2-7.   Outcomes matrix for a patient exposed to a pathogen.

In our example, if people are exposed to a particular pathogen, the odds of dying is 20/5 = 4. The odds of dying without exposure is 10/20 = 0.5.

Thus, the odds of dying if one is exposed to the pathogen compared to not having been exposed is 8 times higher (4/0.5 = 8).

$$\text{Odds Ratio} = (A / B) / (C / D)$$

Studies that **create a sample population based on outcome,** such as case-control studies, must **use odds ratios.**

Studies that create a **sample population based on exposure or treatment,** such as a controlled trial or cohort study, can **use relative risk.**

KEY FACT

If the outcome investigated is very rare, odds ratio ~ relative risk.

Precision, Accuracy, and Error

Precision, accuracy, and **error** describe the quality of measurements, such as those produced by a laboratory test.

- **Precision** is the reproducibility of a measurement.
- **Accuracy** is how close a measurement is to the true value.
- **Systematic errors** are errors that **occur the same way every time** a measurement is taken. As a result, the measurements are wrong in the same way each time and thus are not accurate, but are precise.
- **Random error** is unavoidable error that is **different each time a measurement is taken.** This reduces precision. It also reduces accuracy if the amount of error is large.

These differences are shown in Figure 2-8.

KEY FACT

Systematic errors decrease **accuracy.** Random errors decrease **precision.**

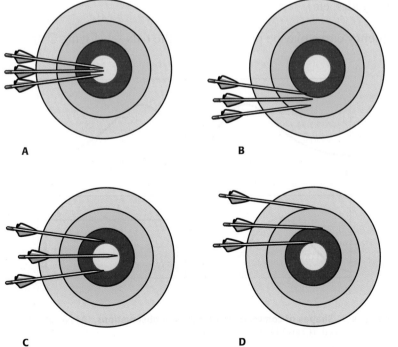

A   **B**   **C**   **D**

FIGURE 2-8.   Relationship of error to precision and accuracy. (A) High precision and high accuracy; low random error and low systematic error. (B) High precision, but low accuracy; low random error, but high systematic error. (C) Low precision, but high accuracy; high random error, but low systematic error. (D) Low precision and low accuracy; high random error and high systematic error.

Statistics

MEASURES OF CENTRAL TENDENCY AND STATISTICAL DISTRIBUTION

The term *distribution* describes the **frequency** of observations in a population or data set as plotted on a graph.

Distribution of a set of observations is defined by the measures of central tendency:

- **Mean (arithmetic mean** or **average)** is the most common measure of central tendency. It represents the ratio between the sum of all individual observations (ΣX) over the number of observations (n):

$$\text{Mean} = \Sigma X / n$$

  The mean, however, may not be an appropriate measure of central tendency for skewed distributions or in data sets that contain outliers.
- **Median (middle observation)** represents the **50th percentile of a distribution,** or the point at which half of the observations are smaller and half are larger. The median is often a more appropriate measure of central tendency for skewed distributions or in situations with large outliers.
- **Mode** represents the most frequent value in a distribution and is commonly used for a large number of observations to identify the value that occurs most frequently.

All three are used for continuous data (ie, data that can be expressed along a numerical continuum, such as weight); the median may also be used for categorical data (eg, grades of cancer, blood type groupings, ethnicity, asthma severity grades, etc).

A **frequency curve** may be produced from the data set (Figure 2-9).

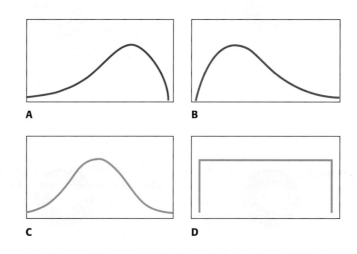

FIGURE 2-9. **Shapes of common distributions of observations.** (A) Negatively skewed. (B) Positively skewed. (C and D) Symmetrical.

> **KEY FACT**
>
> Continuous and categorical data are levels of measurements.
> **Continuous data:** Variables that can take on any range of values (eg, 0, 1, 2, 2.5, 2.6, 3, etc).
> **Categorical data:** Variables that are not quantitative and take a value of one of several possible categories (eg, a piece of rock can be categorized as metamorphic, igneous, or sedimentary).

Terms that describe the curves created include:

- **Gaussian:** Also known as a "normal," or "bell-shaped," curve. It indicates **symmetrical distribution** of the observations.
  - The mean, median, and mode are identical.
- **Bimodal:** The curve produces two "peaks" due to two separate areas of increased frequency of data in the population or data set. These curves may indicate **symmetrical** or **asymmetrical distribution** of observations.
- **Positive skew:** **Asymmetrical** curve with the tail on the **right** side of the graph. It indicates a large number of outlying values.
  - **Mean > median**
  - **Mean > mode**
- **Negative skew:** **Asymmetrical** curve with the tail on the **left** side of the graph. It indicates a small number of outlying values.
  - **Mean < median**
  - **Mean < mode**

STATISTICAL HYPOTHESIS

A statistical hypothesis is a formal statement regarding the expected outcome of an experiment. There are two major types of hypotheses, differentiated by how the statement is framed:

- **Null hypothesis (H_0):** A statement that suggests that there is **no difference**, or association **between two or more variables.** In medicine, this normally relates to disease and risk factors. H_0 is tested for possible rejection under the assumption that the hypothesis is true.
- **Alternative hypothesis (H_1):** A statement that suggests that **there is an association between two or more variables,** and contrary to the null hypothesis, the observations are the result of a real effect (Figure 2-10).

Type I Error (α)

Type I error results when one states or determines that there **is** an effect or difference when in reality one does not exist. Stated another way, the **alternative** hypothesis is accepted when in actuality the **null** hypothesis is correct. Type I error is also known as a **"false-positive."**

- This error is a **preset** level of significance, denoted as the Greek letter α, which is **defined as the probability of making a type I error.**
- The normal accepted α is usually < 0.5, which means that there is a less than 5% chance of making a type I error, or that the data will show something that **is not really true.**

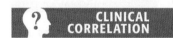
CLINICAL CORRELATION

An example of a null hypothesis is, "There is no association between sodium intake and hypertension."

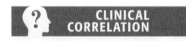
CLINICAL CORRELATION

An example of an alternative (H_1) hypothesis is, "Increased sodium intake leads to increased blood pressure."

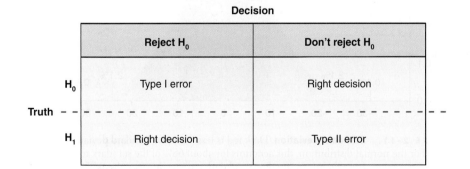

	Decision	
	Reject H_0	**Don't reject H_0**
H_0	Type I error	Right decision
Truth		
H_1	Right decision	Type II error

FIGURE 2-10. **Summary of possible results of any hypothesis test.**

Type II Error (β)

Type II error results when one states or determines that there **is not** an effect or difference when in reality one does exist. In other words, the **null** hypothesis is accepted when in actuality the **alternative** hypothesis is correct (Figure 2-10). Type II error is also known as **"false-negative."**

Power

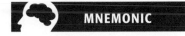

MNEMONIC

Power is **increased** by sample size; **there is power in numbers.**

Power is the probability of rejecting the null hypothesis when it is in fact false. The power can be manipulated by changing the sample size as well as by difference in compliance between sample groups. The power is calculated by subtracting the type II error (β) from 1.

$$\text{Power} = 1 - \beta$$

STANDARD DEVIATION VERSUS ERROR

Standard deviation is a statistical measurement used to describe the deviation, or the variability, from the central tendency within a statistical distribution (Figure 2-11). It is used to describe the spread of values within a particular distribution.

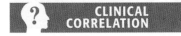

KEY FACT

SEM $< \sigma$ and **SEM decreases** as n increases.

All forms of measurement have some inherent error. For this reason, the **standard error of the mean** (SEM) is used to estimate the standard deviation of error in that particular method.

$$\text{SEM} = \sigma / \sqrt{n}$$
$$\sigma = \text{standard deviation}$$
$$n = \text{sample size}$$

Confidence Intervals

A confidence interval (CI) is a range, with upper and lower values, in which a specified probability of the means of the repeated samples would be expected to fall. It is used to indicate the reliability of the measurement.

CLINICAL CORRELATION

A *t*-test is useful when comparing the means of two groups (placebo vs. treatment) to see if a statistical significance exists between the mean clinical outcomes of the two groups.

The CI can be determined by using both the standard deviation and the SEM.

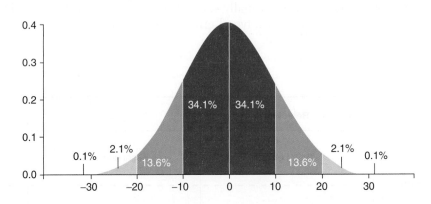

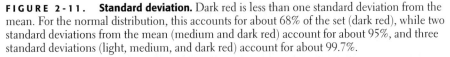

FIGURE 2-11. **Standard deviation.** Dark red is less than one standard deviation from the mean. For the normal distribution, this accounts for about 68% of the set (dark red), while two standard deviations from the mean (medium and dark red) account for about 95%, and three standard deviations (light, medium, and dark red) account for about 99.7%.

For a 95% confidence interval, that is the interval within which 95% of the sample means lie it can be calculated as:

$$CI = \text{mean} \pm 1.96\ (SEM), \text{ or } CI = \text{mean} \pm 1.96\sigma$$

- If the CI includes zero, the null hypothesis is **accepted** (ie, there is **no difference** between the variables).
- If the CI does not contain zero, the null hypothesis is **rejected** and the alternative hypothesis is accepted (ie, there **is a difference,** or association, between the variables).

Knowing the CI is important because it gives an estimate of how likely a value is to be true. Thus, if a number falls between the upper and lower limits of a 95% confidence interval, one can be confident that the data are correct 95% of the time.

Example: Imagine a study in which a group of people in a certain town have their blood pressure measured several times over the course of a year (independent samples taken repeatedly from the same population). The results of the blood pressure measurements would be reported by giving a range. It is best to express this range as a CI because it tells readers that a value falling within that range was similar to the blood pressure of 95% of the patient population.

t-TEST, ANOVA, AND CHI-SQUARE (χ^2)

t-Test

The *t*-test is used to determine the difference between the mean values of two groups of observations. This test is based on the *t* distribution, which involves **degrees of freedom (df).**

- For **groups with a large df** value, the *t* distribution is indistinguishable from the normal distribution.
- As the **df decreases,** the *t* distribution becomes increasingly spread out.
- The *t* distribution can be determined using a mathematical equation and correlated to a *P* value using the appropriate table.

ANOVA

ANOVA is used to determine the statistical difference between the means of three or more groups of observations.

Chi-Square (χ^2)

Chi-square is used to determine the statistical difference between two or more percentages or proportions of categorical outcomes (not mean values). It is a categorical test used to determine the probability that the observed distribution of data is due to chance (sampling error).

CORRELATION COEFFICIENT

The **correlation coefficient (*r*)** is a numerical value that always falls between 1 and –1. It indicates the strength and direction of a linear relationship (correlation) between two or more different and independent variables. Values approaching 1 indicate a strong correlation between the variables. A value of 0 indicates no correlation, and values approaching –1 indicate an inverse relationship.

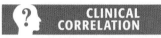

CLINICAL CORRELATION

Use paired *t*-tests when comparing two small sets of quantitative data when data in each sample set are related in a certain way. For example, the blood pressure difference before and after treatments using a new experimental drug is measured in subjects who received the drug. The paired *t*-test is used when comparing this difference between subject 1 versus subject 5.

CLINICAL CORRELATION

Use independent *t*-tests when comparing two small sets of quantitative data when samples are collected independently of one another. For example, differences in blood pressure due to a new experimental drug are compared between the group that received the drug and the control group.

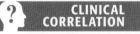

MNEMONIC

Mr. **T** is **mean.**

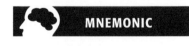

MNEMONIC

ANOVA = **AN**alysis **O**f **Va**riance of three or more variables.

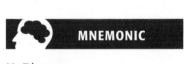

KEY FACT

χ^2 = compares percentages (%) or proportions.

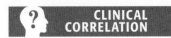

CLINICAL CORRELATION

An example of the chi-square test is a clinical trial comparing a 28-day survival rate of subjects in a treatment group versus those in a control group. The percentage of survivors versus controls can be compared using this test.

The **coefficient of determination** (R^2) is the proportion of **variability** (or **sum of squares**) in a data set that is accounted for by a statistical model, using regression analysis. It helps to determine whether a linear relationship exists between the response variable and the "regressors."

If $R^2 = 1 \rightarrow$ there **is a linear relationship** between the independent and dependent variables.

If $R^2 = 0 \rightarrow$ there **is no linear relationship** between the response variable and regressors.

Disease Prevention

FORMS OF DISEASE PREVENTION

Public health officials try to limit the spread of disease through primary, secondary, or tertiary prevention.

Primary Disease Prevention

Primary disease prevention stops the disease before it starts. For example, vaccination is used to build immunologic resistance and thus limit the infectivity and spread of a disease. Examples are human papillomavirus (HPV) vaccination for the prevention of cervical cancer. Other vaccines (eg, pneumococcal, tetanus, diphtheria, mumps-measles-rubella) also fall under the heading of primary disease prevention because these interventions occur before the host has become infected.

Secondary Disease Prevention

Secondary disease prevention seeks to detect disease early in its course before it becomes clinically apparent to reduce the associated morbidity and mortality. Examples of secondary disease prevention include cervical cancer screening through Papanicolaou (Pap) smears, which detect HPV viral DNA; colonoscopy for the detection of colon cancers; and mammogram screening for the detection of breast cancers. Early detection can reduce the morbidity and mortality of the disease and also prevent epidemics.

Disease screening tests usually are very **sensitive** in order to retain a high true-positive rate, but may result in many false-positives. **Sensitivity** is defined as

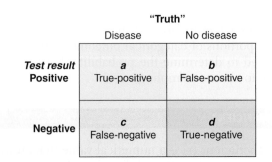

FIGURE 2-12. **Diagnostic testing and disease state.** (Modified with permission from Greenberg RS, Daniels SR, Flanders WD, et al. *Medical Epidemiology*, 4th ed. New York: McGraw-Hill, 2005: 94.)

the number or percentage of individuals with the disease who have a positive test result. Because screening methods err on the side of casting a very wide net to identify as many individuals with the disease as possible (remember, **sensitivity** rules people **in**), it may include more false-positives (individuals who do not have the disease, but have a falsely-positive test result). See Figure 2-12.

$$\text{Sensitivity} = \text{True-positives} / (\text{true-positives} + \text{false-negatives}) \times 100 = a / (a + c) \times 100$$

$$\text{Specificity} = \text{True-negatives} / (\text{true-negatives} + \text{false-positives}) \times 100 = d / (d + b) \times 100$$

Tertiary Disease Prevention

Tertiary disease prevention aims to reduce the disability or morbidity resulting from disease. Examples include exogenous insulin for diabetes and surgical treatment of cancers. Tertiary disease prevention aims to treat the disease through available medical or surgical management.

REPORTING AND MONITORING DISEASE

Reportable Diseases

By requiring clinicians to report certain infectious diseases, public health officials can monitor, track, and try to control the spread of contagious diseases. **Reportable infectious diseases** are shown in Table 2-2, and leading causes of death are reported in Table 2-3.

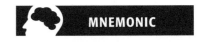
MNEMONIC

Be A S-S-S-M-MART CHICKEN or you're GONe:
Hep **B**
Hep **A**
Salmonella
Shigella
Syphilis
Measles
Mumps
AIDS
Rubella
Tuberculosis
CHICKENpox
GONorrhea

TABLE 2-2. Reportable Diseases

DISEASE	CAUSATIVE AGENT	COMMUNICABILITY
Acquired immune deficiency syndrome (AIDS)	HIV retrovirus	Spread by sexual contact, parenteral exposure, perinatal exposure where there is contact with blood or blood products.
Chickenpox	Varicella zoster virus (VZV)	Spread by inhalation of vesicles or close contact.
Gonorrhea	Gram-negative diplococcus *Neisseria gonorrhoeae*	Sexual contact.
Hepatitis A	Hepatitis A virus (HAV)	Fecal-oral route.
Hepatitis B	Hepatitis B virus (HBV)	Sexual contact, parental exposure.
Measles (rubeola)	Paramyxovirus	Inhalation of respiratory droplets.
Mumps	Paramyxovirus	Inhalation of respiratory droplets.
Rubella (German measles)	Togavirus	Inhalation of respiratory droplets.
Salmonella	Negative bacilli *Salmonella typhi*	Contaminated food or water.
Shigella	*Shigella dysenteriae*	Contaminated food.
Syphilis	Spirochete *Treponema pallidum*	Sexual contact, perinatal exposure.
Tuberculosis	*Mycobacterium tuberculosis*	Skin-to-skin contact and droplet transmission.

TABLE 2-3. Leading Causes of Death in the United States by Age

Age Group	Leading Cause of Death
Infants	▪ Congenital anomalies ▪ Short gestation/low birth weight ▪ Sudden infant death syndrome ▪ Maternal complications ▪ Respiratory distress syndrome
Age 1–14	▪ Injuries ▪ Cancer ▪ Congenital anomalies ▪ Homicide ▪ Heart disease
Age 15–24	▪ Injuries ▪ Homicide ▪ Suicide ▪ Cancer ▪ Heart disease
Age 25–64	▪ Cancer ▪ Heart disease ▪ Injuries ▪ Suicide ▪ Stroke
Age 65+	▪ Heart disease ▪ Cancer ▪ Stroke ▪ Chronic obstructive pulmonary disease (COPD) ▪ Pneumonia ▪ Influenza

Medical Surveillance

The effort to continuously monitor and detect the occurrence of health-related events is known as medical surveillance. Through **medical surveillance,** it is possible to determine the **incidence rate** of disease (the rate of new disease in a given period), the number of deaths resulting from the disease (**case fatality**), the **mortality rate** (combination of incidence rate and case fatality), **rate ratios** (a ratio of the incidence rates of two different groups, resulting in a comparison of the rate of disease occurrence), and **mortality patterns.** Figures 2-13, 2-14, and 2-15 show examples of incidence rates, mortality rates or patterns, and rate ratios, respectively.

GOVERNMENT FINANCING OF MEDICAL INSURANCE

Medical costs can be paid several ways: out-of-pocket payments, individual private insurance, employment-based private insurance, or government financing (Figure 2-16). The two major types of government financing are Medicare and Medicaid.

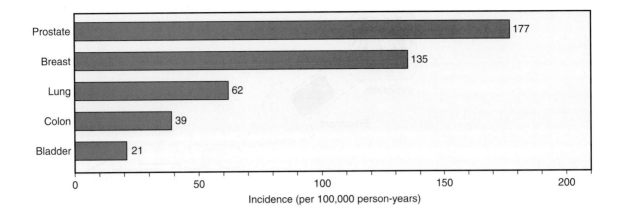

FIGURE 2-13. **Example of age-adjusted incidences rates.** Age-adjusted incidence rates of the leading cancers in men and women in the United States from 1996–2000. (Data from Ries LAG, Melbert D, Krapcho M, et al. *SEER Cancer Statistics Review, 1975–2000.* National Cancer Institute, 2003.) (Modified with permission from Greenberg RS, Daniels SR, Flanders WD, et al. *Medical Epidemiology,* 4th ed. New York: McGraw-Hill, 2005: 50.)

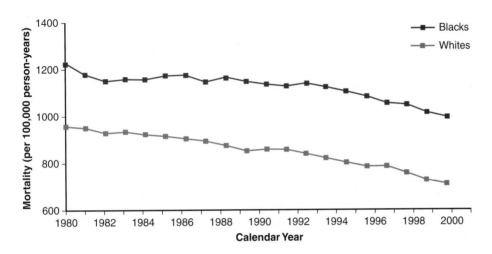

FIGURE 2-14. **Example of age-adjusted total mortality rates.** Age-adjusted total mortality rates by calendar year and race in the United States, 1980–2001. (Data from National Center for Health Statistics: National Vital Statistics Report, 2003.) (Modified with permission from Greenberg RS, Daniels SR, Flanders WD, et al. *Medical Epidemiology,* 4th ed. New York: McGraw-Hill, 2005: 58.)

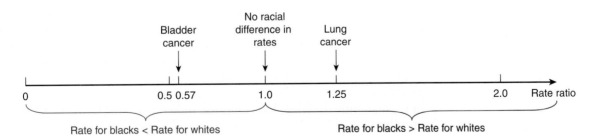

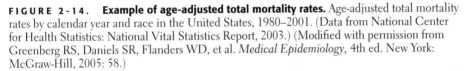

FIGURE 2-15. **Example of incidence rate ratio.** Schematic representation of black-to-white incidence rate ratio for cancers of the lung and bladder in the United States. (Data from Ries LAG, Melbert D, Krapcho M, et al. *SEER Cancer Statistics Review, 1975–2000.* National Cancer Institute, 2003.) (Modified with permission from Greenberg RS, Daniels SR, Flanders WD, et al. *Medical Epidemiology,* 4th ed, New York: McGraw-Hill, 2005: 52.)

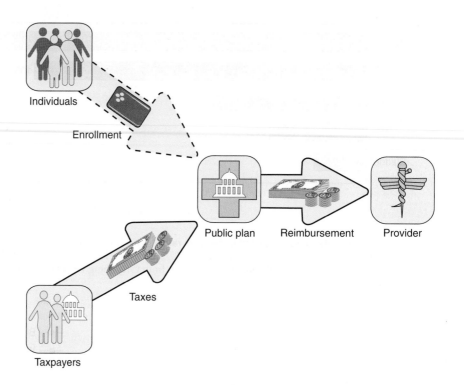

FIGURE 2-16. Government-financed insurance. Medicare and Medicaid are examples of government-financed insurance. (Modified with permission from Bodenheimer TX, Grumbach K. *Understanding Health Policy: A Clinical Approach,* 4th ed. New York: McGraw-Hill, 2005: 12.)

Medicare and Medicaid

Medicare is a government-sponsored program financed through Social Security, federal taxes, and monthly premiums that provides financial coverage for hospital and physician services for persons 65 years and older. It consists of **Medicare Part A** and **Medicare Part B.**

MEDICARE PART A

This portion covers **certain costs for hospitalization, skilled nursing facilities, home health care, and hospice care.** The amount that Medicare Part A will reimburse varies with the length of stay at the facility.

Example: For a hospitalization, Medicare Part A will pay for the first 60 days except a deductible per stay. After the first 60 days, Part A will cover all expenses except a daily deductible. Individuals older than 65 can enroll in Medicare Part A by paying a monthly premium. The program is also available to those who have chronic renal disease and are in need of dialysis or transplantation. It is also possible to enroll in Medicare Part A if a person is totally or permanently disabled. However, the individual must wait 24 months before enrollment.

MEDICARE PART B

Medicare Part B is available for patients who elect to pay a separate monthly premium. The rest of the program is financed through federal taxes. Medicare Part B covers **medical expenses for physician services; physical, occupational, and speech therapy; medical equipment; diagnostic tests; and preventive care** (eg, Pap smears, mammograms, vaccinations). Outpatient medications, along with eye, hearing, and dental services, are **not** covered.

MEDICARE PART D

Medicare Part D, which went into effect in 2006, is administered by private insurance companies to cover prescription drugs. It is only available to those who are eligible for Medicare Parts A or B. To receive the benefit the person must enroll in one of the many available prescription plans offered by the numerous private insurance companies and pay a separate monthly premium.

MEDICAID

Medicaid is a state-sponsored program, although the federal government contributes 50–80% of the funds (more money comes from the federal government in poorer states, as measured by per capita income). Medicaid provides **coverage for a number of services,** including **hospital fees, physician services, laboratory services, radiographs, prenatal care, preventive care, nursing home care, and home health services.** Requirements that need to be met to qualify for Medicaid vary from state to state. However, typically, low-income families with children, individuals (disabled, blind, or elderly) who receive cash assistance under the Supplemental Security Income (SSI) program, and pregnant women whose family income is less than or equal to 133% of the deferral poverty level are eligible.

KEY FACT

Medi**CARE** takes **CARE** of the elderly.

KEY FACT

Medi**AID** helps the state and federal government **AID** those in need.

Ethics

AUTONOMY

Patient autonomy is the right of patients to actively participate in and make final medical decisions that affect their health. Autonomy and justice are the most deeply seated principles in bioethics (and in the U.S. legal system) regarding medical decision making. Autonomy means that people have **the right to choose** (accept or refuse) treatment.

Example: A police officer does not have the right to search an individual's home without a warrant. Similarly, a doctor does not have the right to perform a lung biopsy without the patient's consent.

- **Patients** have **the right to accept or refuse treatments** that the physician may recommend because the patient "owns" his or her body and therefore has the right to make his or her own choices regarding health care.
- **Physicians** have an **obligation to respect patients' autonomy,** and they must honor patient preferences for care.

A patient's autonomy can be **breached** under the following circumstances:

- The patient is infected with a highly infectious and dangerous disease (eg, TB).
- The patient has greatly impaired decision-making capacity (eg, a delusion impairing understanding of the decision).
- The patient's autonomy is legally waived by the U.S. government (eg, epidemics).

Justice Cardozo established the legal medical autonomy standard in the 1914 case of ***Schloendoff vs. Society of New York Hospital*** (105 N.E. 92). The case involved a patient who consented to an examination of a fibroid tumor under ether, but explicitly denied consent for surgery. The surgeons performed the operation during the ether examination without her consent or knowledge.

Justice Cardozo stated, "Every human being of adult years and sound mind has a right to determine what shall be done with his own body; and a surgeon who performs an operation without his patient's consent, commits an assault, for which he is liable in damages."

This is true except in cases of emergency, when the patient is unconscious, and situations in which it is necessary to take action before consent can be obtained (life-threatening events).

INFORMED CONSENT

Informed consent implies that the patient must have been fully informed of all options (benefits and risks) by the physician. This principle is ethically rooted in the concept of respect for the patient's autonomy.

This legally requires the physician to:

- Discuss relevant information, including the risks and benefits of treatment, as well as the possible effect of no treatment.
- Obtain an agreement with the patient.
- Allow a patient's decision to be made free of coercion.
- Make sure the patient understands the risks, benefits, and alternatives, which include no intervention.

Informed consent requires the presence of three related factors:

- The patient must have voluntarily chosen to seek treatment and must have the capacity to reasonably make decisions.
- The patient must receive full objective disclosure of all of the necessary information; however, recommendations and an assurance of full patient understanding about each choice should be made by the physician. In general, physicians should give patients the amount of information an average, reasonable patient would want.
- The idea is for the patient and physician to engage in a conversation in which negotiation and conflict resolution of differences are welcomed to enhance patient autonomy.

For example, the patient should always feel free to obtain a second opinion.

A decision and authorization from the patient are necessary to carry out the procedure, **unless the patient is a minor,** and therefore may not have decision-making capacity. This differs depending on the kind of decision being made.

Key facts to remember about informed consent:

- An exception to consent is made in the case of an emergency, where consent is **implied.**
- Consent is necessary for **each** specific procedure.
- The health care worker performing the procedure **should** be the one to obtain consent.
- Beneficence (acting in what you believe to be the patient's best interest) does **not** obviate the need for consent.
- Consent received via the telephone **is** legitimate, but must be documented.

- Pregnant women **can** refuse therapy for their fetus (once the child is born, life-saving therapy cannot be refused).
- Decisions made by patients at a time when they were competent **continue** to be valid, even when they have lost the capacity to consent (ie, loss of consciousness).
- A health care proxy, living will, or medical durable power of attorney is the best method of obtaining consent (beforehand) from someone who has **lost** capacity.
- Informed consent must come from a parent, legal guardian, third-party court-appointed individual, or "substituted judgment" (an individual who ideally knows the patient well and can make decisions based on what he or she believes the patient would want). This prior preference may not be known for a **continuously** incompetent person (eg, patients with severe Down's syndrome). Then, the risk and benefits predominate.

INFORMED ASSENT

Informed assent consists of a **child's agreement** to medical procedures in the situation that he or she is not legally authorized or does not have the capacity to give consent competently (eg, participation in clinical trials, terminal illness).

In line with the WHO Research Ethics Review Committee (ERC), the following recommendations must be honored:

- Before seeking consent and assent to involve children in research, it must be demonstrated that comparable research cannot be done with adults to the same effect and scientific effect.
- Researchers must obtain consent from a parent or guardian on an Informed Consent Form (ICF) for all children.
- Research supported by the WHO follows the **Convention on the Rights of the Child,** where "child" means "every human being below the age of eighteen years" unless under the law applicable to the child, majority age is attained earlier.
- Children should be provided with detailed information and a description of the research to be conducted, geared to the child's age, and should have their questions and concerns addressed. They have the right to express their agreement or lack of agreement to participate.
- Researchers should consider asking for assent from children older than 7 years, while taking assent from all children older than 12 years.
- Children express their agreement to participate on an informed assent form (IAF) written in age-appropriate language. This form is **in addition to,** and **does not replace,** parental consent on an ICF.
- **Assent that is denied by a child should be taken very seriously.**

DECISION-MAKING CAPACITY

Question of decision-making **capacity** arises when there is a conflict of ethical principles between autonomy and beneficence. Beneficence is the concept of doing what is in the best interest for the patient. Health care professionals are often faced with the difficult task of determining if a patient has or does not have the capacity to make decisions.

The components of capacity include "**CRAM**":

- The patient **Communicates** a stable choice.
- The patient understands the **Relevant** information.
- The patient can **Appreciate** the situation and the consequences of the choice.
- The patient can **Manipulate** the information.

Example: A patient who is refusing psychiatric hospitalization often needs a psychiatric evaluation to determine if he or she has the capacity to make medical decisions. This may be the case even when a patient is involuntarily hospitalized because of a suicide attempt, for instance, or because of other circumstances in which he or she possess a danger to self or others.

LEGAL COMPETENCE

The components of legal competence generally include:

- The patient has the capacity to understand the material information and the ability to state a preference.
- He or she can reason through a logical decision and make a judgment about the information in light of his or her values.
- The patient intends a certain outcome.
- The patient is able to freely communicate his or her wish to caregivers or investigators.

> **KEY FACT**
>
> Competency is different from capacity. Competency is a legal determination.

Although some ethical principles consider that individuals can fall anywhere on a spectrum, **competence is an "all or nothing" concept.** The patient is either competent or not. Thus, the process for determining that a patient is indeed **incompetent** is often painstaking.

Case 1: Mrs. Jones is a 78-year-old woman with metastatic breast cancer who is intubated in the ICU. She can communicate through writing or pointing to a picture board. She is tired of heroic measures and wants to be at peace. She indicates her wish to withdraw respiratory support, but her husband knows that such an action will hasten her death.

Although the husband is reluctant to follow her wishes, the principle of autonomy suggests that a **competent patient** such as his wife should be able to make her own decisions.

Case 2: Mr. Smith is an 82-year-old man with Alzheimer's disease who was recently diagnosed with lung cancer. His short-term memory and cognition are severely affected by his dementia, but he firmly states that he does not want chemotherapy when the doctor asks him about treatment options.

- **This patient may or may not be legally competent** to make medical decisions.
- **If he is not competent,** the decision about his treatment plan will depend on an advance directive or the statement of a person he has designated as having medical power of attorney, if he did this before becoming incompetent.

ADVANCE DIRECTIVE

Advance directives are written while a person is competent and are used to direct future health care decisions. Thus, patients can maintain autonomy even when they lack legal competence.

Types of Advance Directives

There are two types of advance directives:

- A **living will** is a statement of exactly which procedures are acceptable or unacceptable, and under what circumstances. It describes the types of treatments the patient wishes to receive or not receive if he or she becomes incapacitated and cannot communicate about treatment decisions.
- **Medical durable power of attorney** grants a specific surrogate person the authority to perform certain actions on behalf of the person who signs the document. The surrogate acts as the health care proxy on behalf of the person. The health care proxy retains the power unless it is revoked by the patient. It is more flexible than a living will.

Case 2 continued: Mr. Smith never wrote an advance directive because he always thought he would "get around to it one day," but he never did. Fortunately, he **did appoint his son to have medical durable power of attorney** during the early, more lucid stages of his Alzheimer's dementia. The oncologists were able to call his son to ask for guidance in his father's care.

Oral Versus Written Advance Directives

Oral advance directives are taken from an incompetent patient's previous oral statements. These should be written in the patient's chart whenever possible.

Example: A patient who watched her mother die after a prolonged period on a ventilator may have said to her family members that she would never want to be on a ventilator.

Recollecting this desire could act as an **oral advance directive** if the patient is incapacitated and faced with a similar situation.

Unfortunately, people can often misinterpret an incapacitated person's previous statements. Thus, the following criteria add more validity to oral statements:

- The patient is informed.
- The directive is specific.
- The patient makes a choice.
- The decision is repeated over time.

Written advance directives are preferred because they provide stronger evidence of the patient's wishes.

One source lists these **problems with advance directives:**

- Relatively few persons have them.
- Designated decision makers may be unavailable or incompetent, or have a conflict of interest (eg, inheritance).
- Some people change their treatment preferences, but do not change the legal document.

- State laws often severely restrict the use of advance directives.
- They leave no legal basis for health care providers to overturn instructions that turn out not to be in the patient's best medical interest, although the patient could not have reasonably anticipated this circumstance while competent.

Case 2 continued: Mr. Smith's son had no written advance directive on which to base his decision regarding his father's chemotherapy. His mother suffered through chemotherapy for lung cancer, and he remembers that his father often remarked that he would rather die peacefully than endure chemotherapy.

Although the son cannot be sure that his father understood the oncologist's question about treatment, he can confidently make a decision based on an oral advance directive from his father's previous aversion to chemotherapy.

BENEFICENCE

Beneficence is **"the principle of doing good."** Physicians have a special ethical responsibility to act in the patient's best interest. This is known as a **fiduciary** relationship because the physician has a commitment to the patient.

Patient autonomy may conflict with beneficence. If the patient makes an informed decision, then ultimately the patient has the right to decide what is in his or her best interest.

The practice of doing whatever the physician feels is best for the patient without consideration of the patient's wishes is called **paternalism.** This old form of medical practice is no longer acceptable in most circumstances.

Case 3: An intern is riding the subway home after a long shift at the hospital. She witnesses one of her fellow passengers falling onto the floor because of a cardiac arrest.

Although the exhausted intern is now off duty, she is **morally obligated** to help the unfortunate passenger **within the limits of her expertise and the established guidelines of care.** This obligation to act is often referred to as the **"good Samaritan principle."**

NONMALFEASANCE

The principle **"first do no harm"** is derived from *primum non nocere* in the Hippocratic oath. Nonetheless, if the benefits of an intervention outweigh the risks, ethically, the physician must act, as when there is an emergency.

Key issues that can be addressed by this principle include:

- Killing versus letting die.
- Intending versus foreseeing harmful outcomes.
- Withholding versus withdrawing life-sustaining treatment.
- Extraordinary versus ordinary circumstances.

Many of these issues center on the terminally ill and the seriously ill and injured.

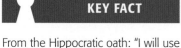

KEY FACT

Four general obligations for beneficence:

1. One ought not to inflict evil or harm (what is bad).
2. One ought to prevent evil or harm.
3. One ought to remove evil or harm.
4. One ought to promote or do good.

KEY FACT

From the Hippocratic oath: "I will use treatment to help the sick according to my ability and judgment, but I will never use it to injure or wrong them."

CONFIDENTIALITY

Confidentiality in the medical setting refers to keeping secret any personal information a patient discloses to his or her physician. Clinicians must respect the patient's privacy and autonomy, thus building a doctor-patient relationship based on trust. Patients may specify any information that they would like the physician to share with their family; anything that is not so specified should be kept confidential.

Certain **exceptions exist to the rule of confidentiality.** Such exceptions include:

- The patient indicates that he or she may harm himself or someone else.
- Child abuse and elder abuse require mandatory reporting. Mandatory reporting for spousal abuse varies depending on the state.
- Infectious diseases: The physician must report certain infectious diseases that pose significant public health risks. In addition, for some diseases, individuals at risk must be notified (ie, sexual partners of someone newly diagnosed with HIV), an action referred to as **"contact tracing."**
- Patients driving under the influence.
- Protection of individuals at risk for some harm that cannot be accomplished by some other means than by breaking confidentiality.
- Cases in which there is a reasonable chance that by breaking confidentiality the physician may be able to prevent some harm.

In the *Tarasoff* case, a jealous lover indicated to his therapist that he intended to shoot his flirtatious girlfriend. The therapist did not warn the girlfriend or her family out of respect for the patient's confidentiality. The man killed the girlfriend, and her family sued the University of California for her preventable death. The *Tarasoff* decision states that if a threat is revealed by a patient, a clinician must take some action, such as warning a threatened person of potential danger, regardless of the clinician's duty to confidentiality.

Case 4: A 47-year-old woman is diagnosed with metastatic breast cancer and is told she will probably not survive more than one year. She does not wish for her family to know about her disease or prognosis. The physician feels certain that the patient and her family will benefit by knowing the truth so that the family can support the patient and so they can make the most of their last months together.

What should the physician do?

The physician **may certainly urge** the patient to consider informing her family, but the **physician should not break her confidence.**

MALPRACTICE

Medical malpractice is a civil suit that is taken out by patients or their family members against a physician or other health professional due to some form of **negligence,** malfeasance, or nonfeasance (inaction that allows or results in harm to a person) by the physician or a direct subordinate that has caused some type of harm to the patient. Causes can be a direct act or an omission by the medical team that results in a deviation from the standard accepted practice and results in a negative consequence.

KEY FACT

The *Tarasoff* case: This classic case took place in California in 1976. This case highlighted the limits of confidentiality and established that therapists are allowed to breach confidentiality if someone else is in danger.

KEY FACT

The suicidal or homicidal patient may be held against his or her will.

Four conditions must be met for the plaintiff (patient or family member) to prove that malpractice has occurred, which together are known as **the four D's of malpractice.**

1. **Duty:** The physician accepts a duty to the well-being of the patient when taking on the medical care of that patient.
2. **Dereliction:** This duty to the patient is not fulfilled when the accepted standards of medical care are not followed (resulting in a dereliction of one's duties).
3. **Damage:** Because of a dereliction of one's duty to the patient, a direct harm, or damage, occurs.
4. **Direct:** The dereliction of one's duty directly results in the damage that the patient has received.

Without the fulfillment of these four criteria, malpractice cannot be proven in a court of law, and the physician is **not legally liable** for the damages that the patient has received.

It must be remembered that accidents that can cause harm frequently occur. Not all of these accidents result in malpractice suits; however, for a case to be made, all four conditions must have occurred.

Case 5: Samantha is an 8-year-old girl with a sore throat, fever, and painful submandibular lymph nodes. Her parents take her to the doctor's office, where Dr. Clark orders a rapid streptococcal throat swab, which is positive. **Samantha has never taken antibiotics before,** and Dr. Clark prescribes penicillin V 25 mg/kg PO BID for 10 days. The next morning, Samantha is taken to the emergency department by her parents and is in anaphylactic shock. Her parents sue Dr. Clark for malpractice.

- **Damage** was caused when Samantha took penicillin and had an allergic reaction.
- Dr. Clark is found **not guilty** because he was fulfilling his **duty** to the patient by treating her for streptococcal pharyngitis within the accepted medical guidelines.
- Therefore, there was no **dereliction** of duties that **directly** resulted in damage to the patient.

Life Cycle

DEVELOPMENT

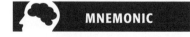

MNEMONIC

How My Recently Produced (Good) Baby Appears:

Heart rate (pulse)
Movement (activity)
Response to **P**rovocation (**G**rimace)
Breathing (respiration)
Appearance

Apgar Score

- The Apgar system is named after Dr. Virginia Apgar, a famous anesthesiologist. Each letter in the acronym Apgar stands for a sign assessed in newborns, as summarized in Table 2-4.
- The Apgar examination is fast, easy to perform, and helpful for determining whether medical intervention, including resuscitation, is needed. However, it is not particularly accurate as a prognostic indicator.

SCORING

The Apgar score is determined at 1 and 5 minutes after birth. Reassessment may be performed after 5 minutes, and thereafter, if the Apgar score is abnormal.

TABLE 2-4. **Apgar Signs and Scoring Criteria**

Sign	0 Points	1 Point	2 Points
Appearance (skin color)	Cyanotic appearance throughout (pale, bluish-gray appearance)	Normal color except for cyanotic extremities	Normal color
Pulse	Absent	< 100	≥ 100
Grimace (reflex irritability/response to stimulation)	No response	Grimace	Grimace and cough, pull away and/or sneeze
Activity (muscle tone)	None	Some	Active movement
Respiration	None	Weak, irregular	Strong, regular

- Each of the five signs is scored as 0, 1, or 2; the Apgar score is the sum of the five scores.
- 8–10: Normal; however, a perfect score of 10 is not typically given.
- 4–7: Some resuscitation may be needed.
- 0–3: Immediate resuscitation is necessary. In general, a low score is related to inadequate ventilation, as opposed to cardiac pathology.

LOW BIRTH WEIGHT

Low birth weight (LBW) is defined as birth weight below 2500 g and is caused by premature birth or intrauterine growth restriction (IUGR). LBW infants are at increased risk for the following complications:

- **Sepsis:** With possible sequelae of septic shock and disseminated intravascular coagulation (DIC).
- **Infant respiratory distress syndrome:** Also known as **hyaline membrane disease.** In this disorder, the infant's lungs produce inadequate surfactant, a protein normally secreted by type II pneumocytes in mature lungs. Surfactant (short for "surface active agent") facilitates inflation of alveoli and helps prevent alveolar collapse.
- **Necrotizing enterocolitis:** This is the most common neonatal gastrointestinal emergency; its cause remains uncertain, but is thought to be multifactorial. Possibilities include immaturity of the intestinal mucosa, compromise of the intestinal blood supply, and the presence of abnormal intestinal flora.
- **Intraventricular hemorrhage:** This may result in long-term complications including cerebral palsy and delayed development.
- **Persistent pulmonary hypertension:** Also called **persistent fetal circulation.** Increased pressure in the pulmonary vasculature causes shunting of deoxygenated blood into the systemic circulation, resulting in hypoxemia.

>> **FLASH FORWARD**

Infants born at 37–42 weeks' gestation are designated **term** infants; those born before 37 weeks' gestation are considered **premature.** An **LBW** infant need not be premature; he or she may have experienced IUGR or inappropriately low growth for gestational age.

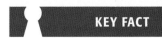

MNEMONIC

My Baby's Primary Reflexes:
Moro
Babinski's
Palmar
Rooting

KEY FACT

In general, motor development proceeds cephalocaudally head to toe, from medial to lateral and from proximal to distal. Ulnar precedes radial, grasp precedes release, and pronation precedes supination.

KEY FACT

In general, emotional differentiation proceeds as follows:
- Excitement → distress or delight at 2–3 weeks
- Distress → fear/anxiety and anger by 2–3 months
- Delight → joy and affection by 2–3 months

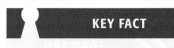

KEY FACT

Normal children progress at different rates, and variation may be considerable.

REFLEXES OF THE NEWBORN

Infants exhibit characteristic reflexes at birth that fade and then vanish at certain points in development.

- **Moro:** Infant spreads, then unspreads the arms when startled. Generally disappears around three months; persists in certain conditions, such as cerebral palsy.
- **Babinski:** Toes fan upward upon plantar stimulation. Generally disappears around 12–14 months; persists in certain neurologic conditions.
- **Palmar:** Infant grasps objects that come in contact with the palm. Generally disappears around 2–3 months.
- **Rooting:** Nipple seeking. Generally disappears around 3–4 months.

DEVELOPMENTAL MILESTONES

Developmental milestones are skill sets (described in Tables 2-5, 2-6, and 2-7) acquired by children at certain ages and are useful for determining whether a child is progressing at the expected rate. Variation among normal children can be considerable.

INFANT DEPRIVATION

History: In the 1950s, psychologist Harry F. Harlow demonstrated that rhesus monkeys deprived of affection and physical contact developed abnormally. Later studies have suggested the existence of a similar phenomenon in humans: Long-term infant deprivation results in multiple long-term sequelae.

Major effects of long-term infant deprivation:

- **Illness:** Increased vulnerability to physical ailments.
- **Floppy:** Decreased muscle tone.
- **Wordless:** Language deficiencies.
- **Mistrust:** Difficulty in forming emotional bonds, sense of abandonment.
- **Thin:** Weight loss, failure to thrive.
- **Withdrawn:** Deficient socialization skills.
- **Anaclitic depression:** Relating to one person's physical and emotional dependence on another person (eg, infant's dependence on mother).

TABLE 2-5. Infant Developmental Milestones

AGE (MONTHS)	MOTOR MILESTONE	SOCIAL/COGNITIVE MILESTONE	LANGUAGE MILESTONE
3	Holds head up, Moro's reflex disappears.	Social smile.	Begins babbling, turns head toward sound.
4–5	Rolls front to back, sits with support.	Recognizes people.	
7–9	Sits alone, transfers object from hand to hand.	Stranger anxiety, orients to voice.	Expresses joy and displeasure with voice.
12–14	Babinski's reflex disappears.	Imitates gestures, finds hidden objects.	Says "Dada"/"Mama," tries to imitate words.
15	Walks alone.	Separation anxiety.	Speaks a few words.

TABLE 2-6. Toddler and Preschool Developmental Milestones

Age	Motor Milestone	Social/Cognitive Milestone	Language Milestone
18 months	Stacks two blocks, runs while looking at ground.	Recognizes self in mirror or pictures, competes with other children for toys.	Speaks 8–10 words clearly, protests when frustrated.
2 years	Feeds self with spoon, stacks 3–4 blocks, walks backward.	Takes turns in play with other children, imitates parents.	Uses 2- to 3-word sentences, tries to hum or sing, listens to short rhymes.
3 years	Rides tricycle, copies line or circle, uses toilet with help.	Group play, knows first and last name.	Uses 3- to 5-word sentences, understands pronouns, asks short questions.
4 years	Simple drawings, hops on one foot, stacks 7–9 blocks, uses toilet alone.	Cooperative play, knows age, plays with imaginary objects.	Uses 5- to 6-word sentences, tells stories, uses past tense, enjoys rhyming.

The term *anaclitic depression* was used by Renee Spitz, a Hungarian-American psychoanalyst, to refer to the deteriorated psychological and physical health of infants who are separated from their caregivers and placed in cold, unstimulating institutional environments. Deprivation for > 6 months can lead to irreversible changes, such as withdrawn state, unresponsiveness, failure to thrive, and in severe cases, death.

MNEMONIC

Infant Fraught With Major Trouble When Deprived:

Illness
Floppy
Wordless
Mistrust
Thin
Withdrawn
Anaclitic **D**epression

CHILD ABUSE

Abuse of children by caregivers can be physical, emotional, or sexual; physical and sexual abuse are covered in Table 2-8. In addition, caregivers may commit neglect by failing to provide for a child's basic needs, such as food, clothing, and safety.

TABLE 2-7. School-Age and Adolescent Developmental Milestones

Age (Years)	Physical Development	Social/Cognitive Milestone
6–11	Improving muscle coordination, maturation of eye function.	Development of conscience (superego), same-sex friends, identification with same-sex parent.
11 (girls) / 13 (boys)	Development of secondary sex characteristics.	Abstract reasoning (formal operations), formation of personality, development of meta-cognition.

TABLE 2-8. **Characteristics of Child Abuse**

PHYSICAL ABUSE	SEXUAL ABUSE
Injuries intentionally caused by a caretaker that result in morbidity and mortality.	A child's involvement in an activity for purposes of adult sexual gratification.
Features include fractures visible on radiography, cigarette burns, iron burns, subdural hematomas, bruises on the back, retinal hemorrhage, and psychiatric symptoms (eg, anxiety, depression, withdrawal).	Features include genital/anal trauma, urinary tract infections (UTIs), sexually transmitted diseases (STDs), inappropriate social behavior for age (eg, flirtatiousness in a young child), and psychiatric symptoms (eg, anxiety, depression, withdrawal, discomfort around sexual impulses).
Abuser is usually female, young (< 30), and the primary caregiver.	Abuser is usually male and known to the victim.
~ 3000 deaths annually in the United States; approximately half the children brought for physical abuse–related medical attention are < 1 year.	Peak incidence at ages 9–12 years.

NORMAL CHANGES OF AGING

As adults move from early to late adulthood, certain patterns of physiologic and psychological change are notable.

- Sexual changes (male): Slower erection and ejaculation; longer refractory periods.
- Sexual changes (female): Vaginal shortening, thinning, and dryness.
- Sleep pattern changes: Decreased rapid eye movement (REM) and slow-wave sleep, and increased sleep latency. The sleep period, or time from sleep onset to morning awakening, does not decrease. However, true sleep time does decrease due to increased awakening during the night.
- Certain medical conditions become more common: heart disease, some cancers, arthritis, hypertension, cataracts.
- Psychiatric problems, such as depression, are more common.
- Higher suicide rate.
- Thinking becomes less theoretical and more practical.

NORMAL GRIEF

Elisabeth Kübler-Ross defined the stages of grief in her landmark book, *On Death and Dying*. (Victims of physical or psychological trauma [eg, rape] and various forms of personal loss may also experience these stages.) Although this order is typical, some individuals experience these stages in a different sequence. More than one stage may be present at a given time, and not all individuals experience all five stages.

- **Denial:** The reality of the loss is denied initially in an attempt to avoid emotional distress. One might understand the situation intellectually without experiencing the full emotional and psychological impact.
- **Anger:** Anger and resentfulness are experienced and possibly expressed toward the departed, family and friends, or caregivers. It is important for physicians to see the anger as normal and to not personalize it.
- **Bargaining:** The bereaved may try, in essence, to "make a deal," on the assumption that circumstances might improve if he or she alters his or her

behavior or attitudes. In this stage, patients and family members may try excessively to be "good."

■ **Despair** or **depression:** The loss is now acknowledged, with a passive, sad emotional response.

■ **Acceptance:** One integrates the experience into his or her world and copes successfully.

Psychology

INTELLIGENCE QUOTIENT (IQ)

Intelligence testing originated in the early 20th century for the purpose of identifying intellectually deficient children who would benefit from enrollment in special education programs.

IQ is:

■ Correlated with genetic factors.
■ More highly correlated with educational achievement and socioeconomic status.
■ Generally stable throughout life.

Commonly used IQ tests:

■ **Stanford-Binet:** Tests verbal, spatial, and memory functions.
■ **Wechsler Adult Intelligence Scale (WAIS):** Assesses verbal and nonverbal reasoning, as well as efficiency of processing of information.
■ **Wechsler Intelligence Scale for Children (WISC):** Similar to the WAIS, but created for children.
■ **Wechsler Preschool and Primary Scale of Intelligence (WPPSI):** Used for preschoolers.

In addition to IQ tests, assessment of one's actual living skills is sometimes performed and is required for the diagnosis of mental retardation. This refers to one's abilities in such areas as self-care, self-direction, social functioning, and communication. The Vineland Adaptive Behavioral Scale, which is based on information provided by a close observer, such as a parent or teacher, is one such test.

Interpretation of IQ tests:

■ All major IQ tests use deviation IQs, measuring the degree to which an examinee deviates from the normal performance for his or her age.
■ Mean = 100.
■ Standard deviation = 15.
■ Mental retardation is defined as an IQ less than 70 (> 2 SDs below the mean).
■ Mental retardation comes in four degrees of severity, as described in Table 2-9.
■ IQ tests are often administered with achievement testing to children who perform poorly in school. A specific learning disability is defined as past learning in reading, math, or writing that is significantly below that expected for the person's IQ and cannot be accounted for by other factors, such as ill health or lack of educational opportunity.

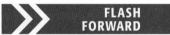

FLASH FORWARD

Mental degeneration can be assessed by administering an IQ test and comparing the result with that expected for the patient's educational level and occupational achievement. Pathology may be harder to detect in individuals with a high baseline IQ because their scores may appear normal despite a decline from their previous levels.

KEY FACT

The mean IQ is 100, the standard deviation is 15, and mental retardation is defined as an IQ > 2 SDs below the mean.

TABLE 2-9. Degrees of Mental Retardation and Corresponding IQ Ranges

DEGREE OF RETARDATION	IQ RANGE
Mild	55–69
Moderate	40–55
Severe	25–40
Profound	< 25

ERIK ERIKSON'S PSYCHOSOCIAL DEVELOPMENT THEORY

Erikson's theory outlines eight stages through which a normal individual proceeds, as shown in Table 2-10. Each stage consists of a **basic crisis** that must be successfully overcome to proceed to the next stage. Although the stages correspond approximately to certain chronologic phases of life, the rate of progression varies among individuals.

CONDITIONING

Conditioning is the alteration of behavior by consequences.

Classical Conditioning

Classical conditioning was first described by the Russian physiologist Ivan Pavlov. An **unconditioned stimulus (UCS)**, known to elicit a characteristic response (the **unconditioned response, or UCR**) is paired with a new, neutral stimulus (the **conditioned stimulus, or CS**) so that eventually the new stimulus alone elicits the same or a similar response. The response is known as the **conditioned response (CR)** when elicited by the CS alone. For the CS to effectively elicit a CR, it must precede the UCS during the conditioning phase.

TABLE 2-10. Erikson's Stages of Psychosocial Development

STAGE	BASIC CRISIS
Infancy	Trust versus mistrust.
Early childhood	Autonomy versus shame and self-doubt.
Play age	Initiative versus guilt.
School age	Industry versus inferiority.
Adolescence	Identity versus role confusion.
Young adulthood	Intimacy versus isolation.
Adulthood	Generativity versus stagnation.
Late adulthood	Integrity versus despair.

Example: A young child naturally cries (UCR) in response to sharp pain (UCS). If the child is brought to a physician's office for a vaccination, sees the syringe, and immediately experiences sharp pain from the needle, the child will associate the needle with the pain and cry (CR) in response to the mere sight of the needle (CS), even before the vaccination is given.

Operant Conditioning

Operant conditioning was first described by B. F. Skinner, who observed that the likelihood of voluntary behavior is increased by subsequent **reinforcement** or decreased by subsequent **punishment**. Both reinforcement and punishment can be **positive** or **negative**.

- **Positive reinforcement:** A pleasant experience occurs (eg, wages).
- **Negative reinforcement:** An unpleasant experience is removed (eg, relief from household chores).
- **Positive punishment:** An unpleasant experience occurs (eg, extra homework).
- **Negative punishment:** A pleasant experience is removed (eg, loss of days off).

Beware of confusion between punishment and negative reinforcement. Any reinforcement, both positive and negative, encourages the reinforced behavior.

Extinction is the process by which a previously reinforced behavior is no longer reinforced, leading to its elimination. For example, in classical conditioning, visits to the doctor who no longer gives shots will lead to decreased association of the needle with pain. In operant conditioning, a rat that no longer receives food when pressing a bar will stop associating this behavior with food and stop responding. In other words, conditioned behavior can be unlearned as well as learned.

Reinforcement Schedules

The two main categories of reinforcement schedules are **ratio** and **interval**. In the ratio schedule, reinforcement occurs based on behavioral events, regardless of time intervals. In the interval schedule, reinforcement occurs based on time intervals, regardless of the frequency of behavioral events. In either category, reinforcement can be **fixed** or **variable**.

> **KEY FACT**
>
> Reinforcement is most effective when presented in such a way that the individual can clearly perceive the connection between the behavior and the reinforcement. Thus, effective reinforcement generally occurs shortly following the behavior.

> **KEY FACT**
>
> Classical conditioning causes a previously neutral stimulus to produce a characteristic (and preexisting) response.
> Operant conditioning uses effective reinforcement and punishment to alter voluntary behavior.

> **KEY FACT**
>
> Intermittent reinforcement is more resistant to extinction than is continuous reinforcement.

TABLE 2-11. Mature Defense Mechanisms

DEFENSE MECHANISM	DEFINITION	EXAMPLE
Altruism	Guilty feelings relieved by generosity and personal sacrifice.	Mafia boss making a large donation to charity.
Humor	Appreciation of the amusing aspects of an anxiety-inducing setting.	Nervous medical student joking about the boards.
Sublimation	Redirecting unacceptable impulses into more acceptable actions.	Joining the military out of a desire to kill.
Suppression	Voluntarily keeping a thought away from consciousness.	Refusing to think about getting revenge on someone.

- **Fixed-ratio** schedule: Reinforcement occurs after a set number of behaviors. Example: Vending machines.
- **Variable-ratio** schedule: Reinforcement occurs after a varying number of behaviors. Example: Casino slot machines.
- **Fixed-interval** schedule: Reinforcement occurs after a set time interval (and a response on the part of the organism). Example: Timed pet feeders.
- **Variable-interval** schedule: Reinforcement occurs at varied times. Example: Pop quizzes.

EGO DEFENSE MECHANISMS

Anna Freud, Sigmund Freud's daughter and a renowned psychoanalyst in her own right, believed strongly in the importance of unconscious drives in determining behavior, but she also emphasized the importance of the ego, or executive decision making, in the functioning of the person. One aspect thereof is the **ego defense mechanism.** These mechanisms are automatic, unconscious, and act in response to psychological stress or threat. Some are mature (Table 2-11); others are immature (Table 2-12).

TABLE 2-12. Immature Defense Mechanisms

DEFENSE MECHANISM	DEFINITION	EXAMPLE
Acting out	Unacceptable thoughts and feelings are expressed through actions.	Temper tantrums. Person A has regular meetings w/ person B, and A hates B so A is regularly late to the meetings.
Dissociation	Avoidance of stress by a temporary drastic change in personality, memory, consciousness, or motor behavior.	In extreme cases, dissociative identity disorder can result in which the individual develops multiple identities ("multiple personality disorder" such as described in the book *The Strange Case of Dr. Jekyll and Mr. Hyde* by Robert Louis Stevenson).
Denial	Pretending, believing, and/or acting as though an undesirable reality is nonexistent.	Common response in patients newly diagnosed with cancer or AIDS.
Displacement	Feelings one wishes to avoid are directed at a neutral party.	Man arguing with his wife after being reprimanded by his boss.
Fixation	Partially remaining at an age-inappropriate level of development.	Functional adult nibbling on her nails.
Identification	Learning unacceptable behavior from a model.	Abused child becoming an abuser.
Intellectualization	Focusing on the intellectual aspects of a situation to avoid anxiety.	Doing vigorous research on one's terminal disease to distract oneself from distress.
Isolation	Separation of feelings from ideas and events.	Attending a loved one's funeral without emotion.
Projection	Attributing an unacceptable impulse to an outside source rather than to oneself.	Man who wants another woman thinking that his wife is cheating on him.

TABLE 2-12. Immature Defense Mechanisms (continued)

DEFENSE MECHANISM	DEFINITION	EXAMPLE
Rationalization	Creating a logical argument to avoid blaming oneself.	A woman who is passed over for a desirable promotion saying that her current position is better.
Reaction formation	To avoid anxiety, acting the extreme opposite of an unacceptable manner.	Behaving obsequiously toward in-laws one strongly dislikes.
Regression	Abandoning a normal maturity level and going back to an earlier one.	Previously toilet-trained child wetting the bed.
Repression	Keeping anxiety-provoking thoughts and feelings from consciousness.	Involuntary or unconscious burying of memories of child abuse.
Splitting	Perceiving people as either all good or all bad.	Patient saying that all nurses are cold, but all doctors are friendly.

NOTES

Biochemistry

KEY FACT

Effective carriers are molecules that are relatively stable as leaving groups. These include phosphoryl (ATP), electrons (NADH, NADPH, FADH$_2$), sugars (UDP glucose), methyl (SAM), 1 carbon (THF), CO$_2$ (biotin), and acyl (coenzyme A).

KEY FACT

Nucleotide = nucleoside + phosphate(s)

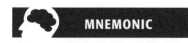

MNEMONIC

PURines: **PUR**e **A**s **G**old; **pY**rimidines: c**Y**tosine, th**Y**mine

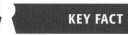

KEY FACT

Transition: Mutations that substitute a pyrimidine for a pyrimidine.
Transversion: Mutations that substitute a purine for a pyrimidine or vice versa.

KEY FACT

The more G-C rich a sequence is, the higher the temperature needed to denature it. This has important implications for the melting temperature of DNA sequences used in experimental settings (eg, polymerase chain reaction).

Molecular Biology

NUCLEOTIDES

General Structure

Nucleotides are composed of three subunits (Figure 3-1):

1. Pentose sugar
   - Ribose
   - Deoxyribose
2. Nitrogenous base
   - Purine
   - Pyrimidine
3. Phosphate group: Forms the linkages between nucleotides.

In contrast, a **nucleoside** is composed of only two units: a pentose sugar and a nitrogenous base. Nucleotides are linked by a **3′–5′ phosphodiester bond** (Figure 3-2). By convention, DNA sequences are written from the 5′ end to the 3′ end.

PENTOSE SUGAR

Can be either **ribose**, which is found in RNA, or **2-deoxyribose**, which is found in DNA (Figure 3-1). 2-Deoxyribose lacks a hydroxyl (−OH) group at the 2′ carbon (C2).

NITROGENOUS BASE

The two types differ by the number of rings composing the base.

PURINES VERSUS PYRIMIDINES

Each **purine** (adenine [A], guanine [G], xanthine, hypoxanthine, uric acid) is composed of two rings, whereas each **pyrimidine** (cytosine [C], uracil [U], thymine [T]) is composed of one ring (Figure 3-3). Note that **uracil** is found only in RNA, whereas **thymine** is found only in DNA. All other bases are found in both RNA and DNA (Table 3-1). The pyrimidines may be derived

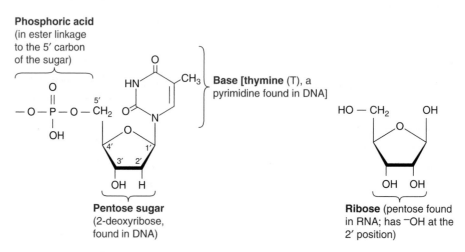

FIGURE 3-1. The general structure of nucleotides. Ribose and deoxyribose pentose sugars only differ at the 2′-carbon, in which deoxyribose lacks a hydroxyl (−OH) group.

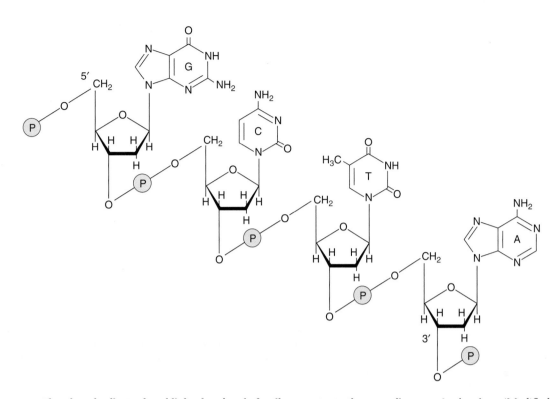

FIGURE 3-2. **The phosphodiester bond links the 3′ end of a ribose sugar to the preceding sugar's 5′ carbon.** (Modified with permission from Murray RK, et al. *Harper's Illustrated Biochemistry*, 26th ed. New York: McGraw-Hill, 2003.)

from one another: deaminating cytosine results in uracil. Adding a methyl group to uracil produces thymine.

- Substrates for DNA synthesis include: dATP, dGTP, dTTP, dCTP (d = deoxy).
- Substrates for RNA synthesis include: ATP, GTP, UTP, CTP.

BASE PAIRING

G-C bonds (3 H-bonds) are stronger than A-T bonds (2 H-bonds) (Figure 3-4). Increased G-C content increases the **melting temperature** (T_m), which is the temperature at which half of the DNA base-pair hydrogen bonds are broken. Chargaff's rule also dictates that the G content equals the C content, and the A content equals the T content.

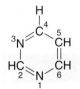

Purine

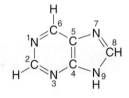

Pyrimidine

FIGURE 3-3. **Base structures of pyrimidines and purines.** (Modified with permission from Murray RK, Granner DK, Rodwell VW. *Harper's Illustrated Biochemistry*, 27th ed. New York: McGraw-Hill, 2006: 294.)

TABLE 3-1. **Purines Versus Pyrimidines**

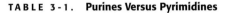

PURINES	PYRIMIDINES
Two rings	One ring.
Adenine	Cytosine.
Guanine	Thymine (found only in DNA).
Xanthine, hypoxanthine, uric acid	Uracil (found only in RNA).

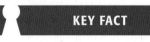

KEY FACT

Chargaff's rule: %A = %T and %G = %C.

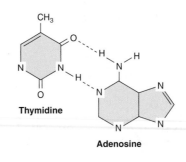

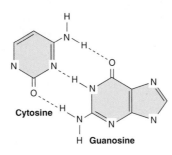

FIGURE 3-4. **Hydrogen bonding between base pairs.** (Modified with permission from Murray RK, Granner DK, Rodwell VW. *Harper's Illustrated Biochemistry*, 27th ed. New York: McGraw-Hill, 2006: 313.)

Nucleotide Synthesis

PURINE NUCLEOTIDE SYNTHESIS

Occurs through either the de novo or the salvage pathway. De novo synthesis utilizes elemental precursors and is used primarily for rapidly dividing cells. The salvage pathway recycles the nucleosides and nitrogenous bases that are released from degraded nucleic acids; it is considered the major route for synthesis in adults.

De Novo Synthesis

- Rate-limiting step by **glutamine PRPP (5-phosphoribosyl-1-pyrophosphate) amidotransferase.**
- PRPP amidotransferase is inhibited by downstream products (inosine monophosphate [IMP], guanosine monophosphate [GMP], adenosine monophosphate [AMP]) and purine analogs (allopurinol and 6-mercaptopurine).
- Required cofactors: tetrahydrofolate (THF), glutamine, glycine, aspartate.
- **Reciprocal substrate effect:** GTP and ATP are substrates in AMP and GMP synthesis, respectively. For example, ↓ GTP → ↓ AMP → ↓ ATP. This allows for balanced synthesis of adenine and guanine nucleotides.

Purine Salvage Pathway (Figure 3-5)

- Recycles ~90% of the preformed purines that are released when cells' nucleases degrade endogenous DNA and RNA and make new purine nucleotides.
- Catalyzed by hypoxanthine-guanine phosphoribosyltransferase (HGPRT), which is inhibited by IMP and GMP.
- Nitrogenous base (guanine, hypoxanthine) + PRPP → GMP/IMP + PP$_i$.

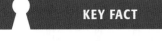

KEY FACT

A pyrimidine nucleotide always base pairs with a purine nucleotide (and vice versa).

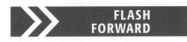

FLASH FORWARD

Allopurinol and 6-mercaptopurine are purine analogs that inhibit PRPP amidotransferase.

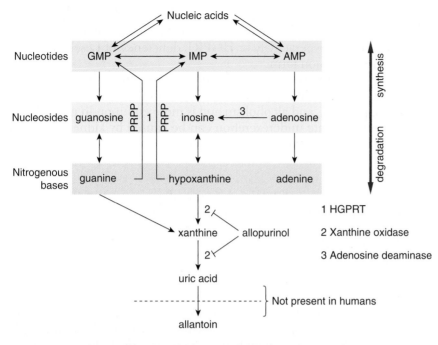

FIGURE 3-5. Purine salvage pathway and deficiencies. HGPRT = hypoxanthine phosphoribosyltransferase.

PURINE SALVAGE DEFICIENCIES

Lesch-Nyhan Syndrome

X-linked recessive disorder of failed purine salvage due to the **absence of HGPRT.** HGPRT converts hypoxanthine → IMP and guanine → GMP. The inability to salvage purines leads to excess purine synthesis and consequent excess uric acid production.

PRESENTATION

Retardation, cerebral palsy, self-mutilation, aggression, gout, choreoathetosis, arthritis, nephropathy.

DIAGNOSIS

Orange crystals in diaper, difficulty with movement, self-injury, **hyperuricemia.**

TREATMENT

Allopurinol, which inhibits xanthine oxidase. Treatment does not ameliorate neurologic symptoms.

PROGNOSIS

Urate nephropathy, death in the first decade, usually as a result of renal failure.

Gout

Disorder associated with **hyperuricemia,** due to either overproduction or underexcretion of uric acid. Uric acid is less soluble than hypoxanthine and xanthine, and, therefore, **sodium urate crystals** deposit in joints and soft tissues, leading to arthritis.

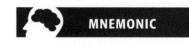

MNEMONIC

Lesch-Nyhan Syndrome
Lacks
Nucleotide
Salvage (purine)

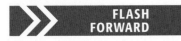

Differential diagnosis for increased uric acid and gout:
- Lesch-Nyhan
- Alcoholism
- G6P deficiency, hereditary fructose intolerance, galactose 1P uridyl transferase deficiency—all disorders with increased accumulation of phosphorylated sugars, increased degradation products (eg, AMP)

- **Primary gout:** Due to hyperuricemia without evident cause. Affected individuals may have a familial disposition. May occur in association with PRPP synthetase hyperactivity or HGPRT deficiency of Lesch-Nyhan syndrome; most common form.
- **Secondary (acquired) gout:** Uric acid overproduction can be caused by leukemia, myeloproliferative syndrome, multiple myeloma, hemolysis, neoplasia, psoriasis, and alcoholism and is more common in men. Secondary gout due to urate underexcretion can be caused by kidney disease and drugs such as aspirin, diuretics, and alcohol.

PRESENTATION

Monoarticular arthritis of distal joints (eg, **podagra**—gout of the great toe), often with history of hyperuricemia for > 20–30 years, precipitated by a sudden change in urate levels (eg, due to large meals, alcohol), eventually leads to nodular **tophi** (urate crystals surrounded by fibrous connective tissue) located around the joints and Achilles tendon.

DIAGNOSIS

Arthritis, hyperuricemia, detection of **negatively bifringent** crystals from articular tap. Negatively birefringent crystals will be **yeLLow** when **paraLLel** to polarized light, blue when perpendicular. Note: **positively birefringent** crystals are characteristically found in **pseudogout.**

TREATMENT

Normalize uric acid levels (allopurinol, probenecid for chronic gout), decrease pain and inflammation (colchicines, nonsteroidal anti-inflammatory drug for acute gout), avoid large meals and alcohol.

Severe Combined (T and B) Immunodeficiency (SCID)

Autosomal recessive disorder caused by a deficiency in **adenosine deaminase (ADA).** Excess ATP and dATP causes an imbalance in the nucleotide pool via inhibition of **ribonucleotide reductase** (catalyzes ribose → deoxyribose). This prevents DNA synthesis and decreases the lymphocyte count. It is not understood why the enzyme deficiency devastates lymphocytes in particular.

PRESENTATION

Children recurrently infected with bacterial, protozoan, and viral pathogens, especially *Candida* and *Pneumocystis jiroveci.*

DIAGNOSIS

No plasma cells or B or T lymphocytes on complete blood count (CBC), no thymus.

TREATMENT

Gene therapy, bone marrow transplantation.

PROGNOSIS

Poor.

PYRIMIDINE NUCLEOTIDE SYNTHESIS

Like purines, pyrimidine synthesis can occur through de novo synthesis or may be recycled through the salvage pathway. The salvage pathway relies on pyrimidine phosphoribosyl transferase enzyme, which is responsible for recycling orotic acid, uracil, and thymine, but not cytosine. De novo synthesis relies on a different set of enzymes.

Hereditary Orotic Aciduria

Deficiency in orotate phosphoribosyl transferase and/or OMP decarboxylase (pyrimidine metabolism).

PRESENTATION

Retarded growth, severe anemia.

DIAGNOSIS

Low serum iron, leukopenia, megaloblastosis, white precipitate in urine.

TREATMENT

Synthetic cytidine or uridine given to maintain pyrimidine nucleotide levels for DNA and RNA synthesis.

Nucleotide Degradation

Products of purine degradation include **uric acid**, which is excreted in urine. Pyrimidine degradation yields β-**amino acids, CO$_2$,** and **NH$_4$$^+$**. For example, thymine is degraded into β-aminoisobutyrate, CO$_2$, and NH$_4$$^+$. Since thymine degradation is the only source of β-aminoisobutyrate in urine, **urinary β-aminoisobutyrate levels** are often used as an **indicator of DNA turnover** (↑ in chemotherapy, radiation therapy).

DNA

DNA Synthesis

- Building blocks: Deoxyribonucleotides (dNTPs).
- **dADP, dGDP, dCDP, dUDP synthesis:** Depends on **ribonucleotide reductase** enzyme, which converts ADP, GDP, CDP, and UDP into dADP, dGDP, dCDP, and dUDP, respectively. **dATP,** an allosteric inhibitor, strictly regulates ribonucleotide reductase in order to control the overall supply of dNDPs.
- **dTDP synthesis: Thymidylate synthase** catalyzes the transfer of one carbon from N^5,N^{10}-methylene tetrahydrofolate (FH$_4$) to dUDP, yielding dTDP. The N^5,N^{10}-FH$_4$ coenzyme then must be regenerated by **dihydrofolate reductase,** which uses NADPH.

DNA Structure

The structure of DNA is characterized by its **polarity,** with a **5′ phosphate** end and a **3′ hydroxyl** end (Figure 3-6). It is composed of two polynucleotide strands that run **antiparallel** to each other (ie, in opposite directions). The two strands coil around a common axis to form a right-handed double helix (also called B-DNA). Rarely, there is also left-handed DNA, called Z-DNA. Nitrogenous bases sit inside the helix, whereas the phosphate and deoxyribose units sit outside. Each turn of the helix consists of 10 base pairs.

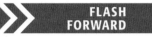

FLASH FORWARD

Chemotherapeutics exploit these pathways: Hydroxyurea inhibits ribonucleotide reductase; 5-fluorouracil (5-FU) inhibits thymidylate synthase; methotrexate and pyrimethamine inhibit dihydrofolate reductase.

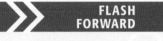

FLASH FORWARD

Bacterial dihydrofolate reductase is inhibited by the antimetabolite trimethoprim. It is often used in combination with sulfonamides (eg, sulfamethoxazole) to sequentially block folate synthesis.

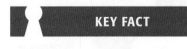

KEY FACT

Conditions that lead to denaturation of the DNA helix: Heat, alkaline pH, formamide, and urea.

Double-stranded DNA   DNA double helix

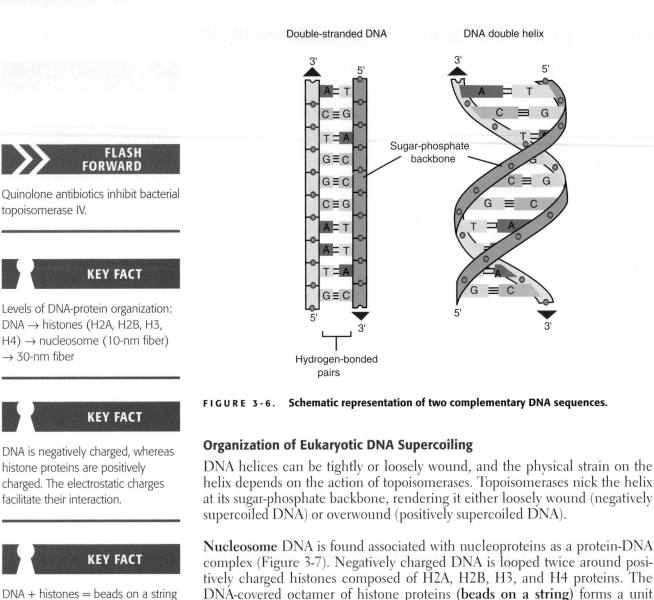

Sugar-phosphate backbone

Hydrogen-bonded pairs

FIGURE 3-6. Schematic representation of two complementary DNA sequences.

>> **FLASH FORWARD**

Quinolone antibiotics inhibit bacterial topoisomerase IV.

KEY FACT

Levels of DNA-protein organization: DNA → histones (H2A, H2B, H3, H4) → nucleosome (10-nm fiber) → 30-nm fiber

KEY FACT

DNA is negatively charged, whereas histone proteins are positively charged. The electrostatic charges facilitate their interaction.

KEY FACT

DNA + histones = beads on a string

MNEMONIC

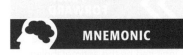

Eu = true, "truly transcribed"

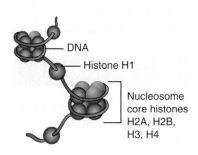

— DNA

— Histone H1

Nucleosome core histones H2A, H2B, H3, H4

FIGURE 3-7. Chromatin structure and related proteins.

Organization of Eukaryotic DNA Supercoiling

DNA helices can be tightly or loosely wound, and the physical strain on the helix depends on the action of topoisomerases. Topoisomerases nick the helix at its sugar-phosphate backbone, rendering it either loosely wound (negatively supercoiled DNA) or overwound (positively supercoiled DNA).

Nucleosome DNA is found associated with nucleoproteins as a protein-DNA complex (Figure 3-7). Negatively charged DNA is looped twice around positively charged histones composed of H2A, H2B, H3, and H4 proteins. The DNA-covered octamer of histone proteins (**beads on a string**) forms a unit called a **nucleosome** (also called 10-nm fibers). H1 histone and linker DNA tie one nucleosome to the next; the nucleosomes, in aggregate, condense further to form the 30-nm fiber. The 30-nm fibers associate and loop around scaffolding proteins. During mitosis, DNA condenses to form chromosomes.

HETEROCHROMATIN

- Condensed.
- Transcriptionally inactive.
- Found in mitosis as well as interphase.

EUCHROMATIN

- Less condensed.
- Transcriptionally active.
- Includes the 10-nm and 30-nm fibers.

CHROMATIN STRUCTURE

Influenced by both **DNA methylation** and **histone acetylation**. Usually, inactive genes have increased amounts of methylated DNA. Acetylation of histone loosens the chromatin structure. Loosened DNA is more accessible, and more genes can be transcribed.

DNA Replication in Prokaryotes

SEMICONSERVATIVE REPLICATION (FIGURE 3-8)

Each parent DNA strand serves as a template for the synthesis of one new daughter DNA strand. The resulting DNA molecule has one original parent strand and one newly synthesized strand.

SEPARATION OF TWO COMPLEMENTARY DNA STRANDS

Replication begins at a single, unique nucleotide sequence known as the **origin of replication**. A replication fork forms and marks a region of active synthesis. Replication is bidirectional with a leading and a discontinuous/lagging strand.

- Leading strand is replicated **in the direction** in which the replication fork is moving. Synthesized continuously.
- Lagging strand is copied **in the opposite direction** of the moving replication fork. Synthesized discontinuously. The short, discontinuous fragments are known as **Okazaki fragments.**
- Involves several other proteins (Table 3-2).

RNA PRIMER

Made by **primase**; necessary for DNA polymerase III to initiate replication.

CHAIN ELONGATION

Catalyzed by **DNA polymerase III,** which has both polymerase and proofreading functions.

- Elongates the DNA chain by adding deoxynucleotides (dNTPs) to the 3′-hydroxyl end of the RNA primer. Continues to add dNTPs from the **5′ → 3′ direction** until it reaches the primer of the preceding fragment.
- Proofreads each newly added nucleotide. Has **3′ → 5′ exonuclease activity.**

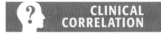
KEY FACT

Increased DNA methylation → *decreased* gene transcription
Increased histone acetylation → *increased* gene transcription

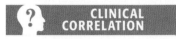
CLINICAL CORRELATION

Antibodies against the SS-A and/or SS-B antigens are often present in Sjögren syndrome.

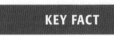
CLINICAL CORRELATION

Antihistone antibodies are found in patients with drug-induced lupus. Medications commonly associated with this condition include **H**ydralazine, **I**soniazid, **P**rocainamide, and **P**henytoin. (It's not **HIPP** to have lupus).

KEY FACT

DNA polymerase III has 5′ → 3′ polymerase activity and 3′ → 5′ exonuclease activity.

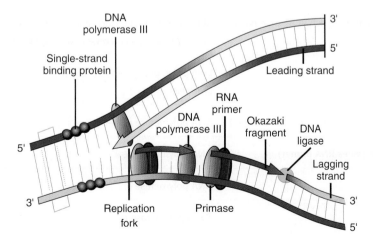

FIGURE 3-8. Prokaryotic DNA replication and DNA polymerases. DNA replication with the leading and lagging strands.

TABLE 3-2. **Other Important Proteins Involved With Prokaryotic DNA Replication**

PROTEIN	FUNCTION
DnaA protein	Binds to origin of replication and causes dsDNA to melt into a local region of ssDNA.
DNA helicase	Unwinds double helix. Requires energy (ATP).
Single-stranded DNA-binding (SS-B) protein	Binds and stabilizes ssDNA to prevent reannealing.
RNA primase	Synthesizes 10 nucleotide primer.
DNA topoisomerase	Creates a nick in the helix to relieve the supercoils/strain imposed by DNA unwinding.

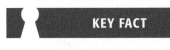

KEY FACT

DNA polymerase I excises RNA primer with 5′ → 3′ exonuclease.

KEY FACT

mRNA = largest type of RNA (massive = mRNA)
rRNA = most abundant type of RNA (rampant = rRNA)
tRNA = smallest type of RNA (tiny = tRNA)

DNA POLYMERASE I

Degrades RNA primer. Has 5′ → 3′ exonuclease activity.

DNA LIGASE

Seals the remaining nick by creating a phosphodiester linkage.

Overall, eukaryotic DNA replication is similar to that of prokaryotic DNA synthesis, with several notable exceptions (Table 3-3). Namely, replication begins at **consensus sequences** that are rich in A-T base pairs. Eukaryotic genome has multiple origins of replication. Eukaryotes have separate polymerases (α, β, γ, δ, ε) for synthesizing RNA primers, leading-strand DNA, lagging-strand

TABLE 3-3. **Prokaryotic Versus Eukaryotic DNA Replication**

	PROKARYOTES	EUKARYOTES
DNA	Circular, small	Linear, long
Sites of replication	Only one (origin of replication, rich in AT base pairs), bound by DnaA proteins	Multiple sites that include a short sequence that is rich in AT base pairs **(consensus sequence)**
Primer synthesis	RNA primase	DNA polymerase α—primase activity, initiates DNA synthesis
Leading strand synthesis	DNA polymerase III (chain elongation, proofreading)	DNA polymerase α, δ—DNA elongation
Lagging strand synthesis	DNA polymerase I (degrades RNA primer)	DNA polymerase α, δ
DNA repair		DNA polymerase β, ε
Proofreading	DNA polymerase III	?DNA polymerase α
Mitochondrial DNA	N/A	DNA polymerase γ—replicates mitochondrial DNA
RNA primer removal	DNA polymerase I	RNase H

TABLE 3-4. Comparison of the Three Types of RNA

RNA Type	Function	Abundance in Cell (% of Total RNA)	Notes
mRNA	Messenger—carries genetic information from nucleus to cytosol.	5	Largest type
rRNA	Ribosomal.	80	Most abundant type
tRNA	Transfer—serves as an adapter molecule that recognizes genetic code (the **codon**) that is carried by mRNA. A codon comprises three adjacent nucleotides that encodes one and only one amino acid. Carries and matches a specific amino acid that corresponds to the codon.	15	Smallest type

DNA, mitochondrial DNA, and DNA repair (mutations and DNA repair are discussed later in the chapter).

RNA

Building blocks are ribonucleotides connected by phosphodiester bonds.

RNA Versus DNA

RNA differs from DNA in the following ways:

- Smaller than DNA.
- Contains ribose sugar (deoxyribose in DNA).
- Contains uracil (thymine in DNA).
- Usually exists in single-strand form.

Types of RNA

There are three types of RNA involved in protein synthesis, each with a specific function and location in the cell (Table 3-4).

tRNA Structure

75–90 nucleotides in a cloverleaf form. Anticodon end is opposite the 3' aminoacyl end. All tRNAs, both eukaryotic and prokaryotic, have CCA at the 3' end, in addition to a high percentage of chemically modified bases. The amino acid is covalently bound to the 3' end of the tRNA (Figure 3-9). The anticodon of the tRNA is the same sequence as the DNA template strand (Figure 3-10).

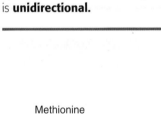
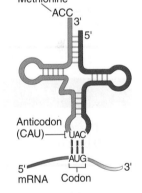

FIGURE 3-9. tRNA structure.

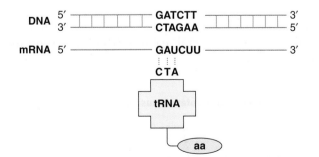

FIGURE 3-10. How the DNA template relates to mRNA and to the tRNA anticodon.

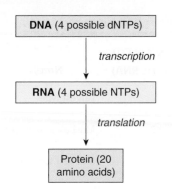

FIGURE 3-11.   **The central dogma.** RNA is made from DNA, and protein is made from RNA.

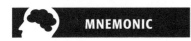

Stop codons—

UGA = U Go **A**way
UAA = U Are **A**way
UAG = U Are **G**one

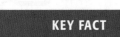

DNA and RNA are synthesized 5′ to 3′.
Protein is synthesized from N- to C-terminus.

DNA—A and **T** base pair
RNA—A and **U** base pair

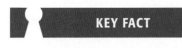

DNA polymerase has proofreading activity, but eukaryotic and prokaryotic RNA polymerases do not.

FEATURES OF THE GENETIC CODE

Central Dogma

The central dogma states that RNA is synthesized from a DNA template and protein is synthesized from an RNA template (Figure 3-11).

DNA and RNA sequences are read in triplets (a **codon**), in which each codon encodes either an amino acid (61 possible codons) or a "stop" signal (UGA, UAA, UAG). The **start codon** AUG (or rarely GUG) is the mRNA initiation codon. It fixes the reading frame and encodes slightly different amino acids in prokaryotes versus eukaryotes (Table 3-5). For both prokaryotes and eukaryotes, the genetic code is **unambiguous, redundant,** and **(almost) universal.**

Unambiguous

1 codon → 1 amino acid.

Degenerate/Redundant

More than 1 codon may code for the same amino acid (eg, three codons encode for the same stop signal).

Universal

Used by almost all known organisms with some exceptions (eg, mitochondria, Archaebacteria, mycoplasma, and some yeasts).

Direction of DNA, RNA, and Protein Synthesis

During DNA/RNA and protein synthesis, nucleotides and amino acids are always added in a set direction (Table 3-6).

TRANSCRIPTION

The DNA template is transcribed into RNA by RNA polymerase in a process similar to that of DNA replication/synthesis.

RNA is composed of uracil (U) instead of thymine (T) bases. Therefore, in RNA, adenine (A) pairs with a uracil (U) instead of thymine (T).

The RNA immediately produced by RNA polymerase (before it undergoes modification) is known as the **primary transcript** or heterogeneous nuclear RNA (hnRNA).

- Eukaryotes modify hnRNA, but prokaryotes do not (Table 3-7).
- Eukaryotes and prokaryotes possess different RNA polymerases.

Whereas prokaryotes have only one RNA polymerase that synthesizes all RNA types, eukaryotes have several, each of which is responsible for making mRNA, rRNA, and tRNA.

TABLE 3-5.   Start Codon in Prokaryotes Versus Eukaryotes

Prokaryotes	AUG → *formyl*-methionine (f-met).
Eukaryotes	AUG → methionine (may be removed before translation is completed).

TABLE 3-6. **Direction of DNA, RNA, and Protein Synthesis**

MOLECULE TYPE	DIRECTION OF SYNTHESIS	NOTES
DNA	5′ End of nucleotide added to	5′ Triphosphate group is the energy source for the phosphodiester bond.
RNA	3′-OH group of growing DNA/RNA ($5' \rightarrow 3'$).	
Protein	Amino acids linked N-terminus to C-terminus ($\mathbf{N} \rightarrow \mathbf{C}$).	

Transcription in Prokaryotes

In contrast to eukaryotes, prokaryotic RNA polymerase synthesizes all three types of RNA. It does not require a primer, and cannot proofread or correct mistakes. Structurally, it has two forms:

- **Core enzyme** composed of four subunits ($\alpha_2\beta\beta'$).
- **Holoenzyme,** a core enzyme with a sigma subunit that allows the enzyme to recognize promoter sequences.

Transcription occurs in three steps—initiation, elongation, and termination.

INITIATION

Sigma subunit of RNA polymerase recognizes promoter region of the sense strand of DNA, binds to DNA, and unwinds double helix. Upstream consensus sequences help the RNA polymerase find the promoter.

ELONGATION

RNA grows as a polynucleotide chain from the 5′ end to the 3′ end. Meanwhile, RNA polymerase moves along the DNA template from the 3′ end to the 5′ end (Figure 3-12).

TERMINATION

RNA polymerase and/or specific termination factors (eg, rho factor in *Escherichia coli*) recognize special DNA sequences that cause their dissociation from the DNA template.

- Termination can be rho-dependent or independent.
- Rho-dependent termination requires participation of a protein factor.

TABLE 3-7. **Factors That Affect Modification of the Primary Transcript[a]**

RNA TYPE	POST-TRANSCRIPTIONAL MODIFICATION	
	PROKARYOTES	EUKARYOTES
mRNA	No—identical with primary transcript	Yes
tRNA	Yes	Yes
rRNA	Yes	Yes

[a]Whether or not the primary transcript is modified depends on the RNA type (mRNA, tRNA, rRNA) and the organism (eukaryotes versus prokaryotes).

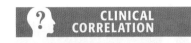

KEY FACT

Prokaryotes are unable to modify their primary transcript. One end of the mRNA can be translated, while the other end is still being transcribed!

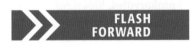

CLINICAL CORRELATION

The antibiotic rifampin, a drug commonly used in the treatment of tuberculosis, inhibits DNA-dependent RNA polymerase by binding the beta-subunit of the RNA polymerase, thereby preventing transcription of DNA to RNA. It is notably lipophilic and readily crosses the blood-brain barrier, making it a good candidate for treating CNS infections related to tuberculosis.

FLASH FORWARD

Rifampin and actinomycin D inhibit various parts of the transcriptional machinery.

- **Rifampin:** Binds β subunit of RNA polymerase and inhibits initiation of RNA synthesis.
- **Actinomycin D:** Binds DNA and prevents RNA polymerase from moving along template.

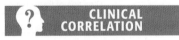

CLINICAL CORRELATION

Actinomycin D is a compound that binds DNA at the transcription initiation complex and prevents RNA polymerase-catalyzed elongation. It can also bind DNA duplexes, which makes it a good candidate drug for preventing DNA replication. Originally used as an antibiotic, it is now more commonly used as a chemotherapeutic agent used to treat gestational trophoblastic tumors, Wilms' tumor and rhabdomyosarcoma.

Prokaryotes have one RNA polymerase that makes *all* types of RNA.
Eukaryotes have several RNA polymerases for each RNA type.

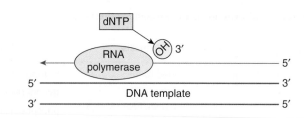

FIGURE 3-12. **Elongation step in transcription.** RNA synthesis occurs from 5′ to 3′, whereas the RNA polymerase moves along the DNA template in the 3′ to the 5′ direction.

Rho-independent termination requires a specific secondary structure (a hairpin loop followed by a string of Us) in the newly synthesized RNA (Figure 3-13).

The flow of genetic information: DNA → (replication) → DNA → (transcription) → mRNA, tRNA, rRNA → (translation) → protein.

Transcription in Eukaryotes

Transcription in eukaryotes involves both RNA polymerase and additional transcription factors that bind to DNA. Different RNA polymerases are required to synthesize different types of eukaryotic RNA (Table 3-8).

REGULATION OF GENE EXPRESSION AT THE LEVEL OF TRANSCRIPTION

Based on DNA sequences that may be located distant from, near, or within (eg, in an intron, which is not expressed) the gene being regulated (Figure 3-14). These DNA sequences include:

In **eukaryotes,** RNA processing occurs in the nucleus.
In **prokaryotes,** RNA is not processed. The primary transcript is translated as soon as it is made.

- **Promoters:** In eukaryotes, includes a TATA sequence (the **TATA box**) and/ or a CAAT sequence 25 and 70 base pairs, respectively, upstream of ATG start codon. Critical for initiation of transcription. Mutations may decrease the quantity of gene transcribed.
- **Enhancer:** Stretch of DNA that increases the rate of transcription when bound by transcription factors.
- **Silencer:** Stretch of DNA that decreases the rate of transcription when bound.

INtrons stay **IN** the nucleus, whereas **EX**ons **EX**it and are **EX**pressed.

TRANSCRIPTION

Follows the same steps as prokaryotes (initiation, elongation, and termination), but requires different RNA polymerase machinery.

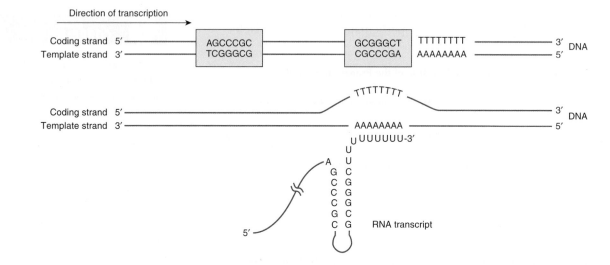

FIGURE 3-13. **Typical prokaryotic termination sequence.** (Modified with permission from Murray RK, Granner DK, Rodwell VW. *Harper's Illustrated Biochemistry*, 27th ed. New York: McGraw-Hill, 2006: 353.)

TABLE 3-8. **Eukaryotic RNA Polymerases and Their Function**

RNA POLYMERASE	RNA TYPE MADE	NOTES
RNA polymerase I	rRNA.	rRNA (28S, 18S, and 5.8S).
RNA polymerase II	mRNA.	Cannot initiate transcription by itself, requires transcription factors.
RNA polymerase III	tRNA.	tRNA, rRNA 5S.
Mitochondrial RNA polymerase	Transcribes RNA from mitochondrial genes.	Inhibited by rifampin, more closely resembles bacterial RNA polymerase than eukaryotic RNA polymerase.

RNA PROCESSING

Unlike in prokaryotic mRNA, the primary transcript (hnRNA) is both spliced and modified with a 5′-cap and a 3′-tail before leaving the nucleus (Table 3-9). The cap contains 7-methylguanine, which protects it against nuclear digestion and helps insure correct alignment of the RNA and ribosome for translation. The 3′ poly-A tail protects the mRNA from exonucleases, allows it to be exported from the nucleus, and is important for translation. Splicing prevents translation of introns. Once modified, the RNA is known as mRNA (Figure 3-15).

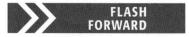
FLASH FORWARD

Defects in post-transcriptional RNA processing can cause pathology.

- Systemic lupus erythematosus is associated with the production of antibodies to host protein, including small nuclear ribonucleoprotein particles **(snRNPs).**
- Fifteen percent of genetic diseases result from defective RNA splicing (ie, incorrect splicing of β-globin mRNA is responsible for some cases of β-thalassemia).

TRANSLATION

Translation is the process by which mRNA base sequences are translated into an amino acid sequence and protein. It involves all three types of RNA; mRNA is the template for protein synthesis. tRNA contains a three-base anticodon that hydrogen bonds to complementary bases in mRNA. Each tRNA molecule carries an amino acid that corresponds to its anticodon. rRNA—along with other proteins—composes the ribosomes. Ribosomes coordinate the interactions among mRNA, tRNA, and the enzymes necessary for protein synthesis.

TABLE 3-9. **Types and Function of Post-transcriptional Modification**

POST-TRANSCRIPTIONAL MODIFICATION	DESCRIPTION	FUNCTION
5′ Capping	7-Methyl-guanosine added to 5′ end of RNA.	Prevents mRNA degradation, allows translation (protein synthesis) to begin.
Poly-A tail	40–200 adenine nucleotides added to 3′ end of RNA by polyadenylate polymerase.	Stabilizes mRNA, facilitates exit from nucleus. Note: not all mRNAs have a poly-A tail (eg, histone mRNAs).
RNA splicing	Performed by the spliceosome, which is composed of small nuclear ribonucleoprotein particles **(snRNP).** Binds the primary transcript at splice junctions flanked by GU-AG.	**Introns** (DNA sequences that do not code for protein) are removed and **exons** (coding sequences) are spliced together (see Figure 3-15). The excised intron is released as a lariat structure.

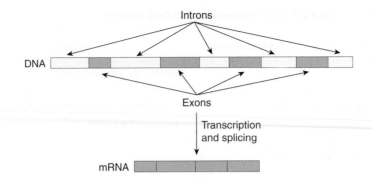

FIGURE 3-14.   **Schematic representation of introns versus exons.**

Ribosomes

The site of protein synthesis. Composed of rRNA and protein. Consist of two subunits—one large, one small. The subunits in prokaryotes and eukaryotes differ in size (S values are usually not additive); eukaryotic ribosomes are larger.

	(Small subunit)		(Large subunit)		
Prokaryote ribosome:	30S	+	50S	=	70S
Eukaryote ribosome:	40S	+	60S	=	80S

tRNA Structure

Distinct structure designed to "translate" the mRNA sequence into the corresponding amino acid sequence (Figure 3-10). tRNA is composed of 75–90 nucleotides in a cloverleaf form. The anticodon end is opposite the 3′ aminoacyl end and is antiparallel and complementary to the codon in mRNA (Figure 3-9). All tRNAs—both eukaryotic and prokaryotic—have CCA at the 3′ end, in addition to a high percentage of chemically modified bases. The amino acid is covalently bound to the 3′ end of the RNA.

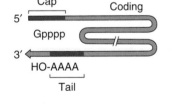

FIGURE 3-15.   **Structure of a typically processed mRNA in eukaryotes.**

tRNA Charging

Requires aminoacyl-tRNA synthetase, ATP, and tRNA. Each amino acid has a specific synthetase that transfers energy from 1 ATP to the bond between the amino acid and the 3′ hydroxyl (OH) group of the appropriate tRNA (Figure 3-16). This bond contains the energy that later forms the peptide bond when the amino acid is added to the growing peptide. If an amino acid is incorrectly paired with tRNA, aminoacyl-tRNA synthetase hydrolyzes the amino acid–tRNA bond.

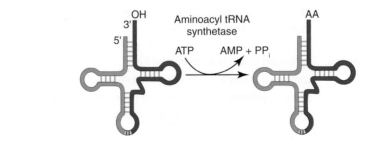

FIGURE 3-16.   **tRNA charging.**

TABLE 3-10.   **Prokaryotic Versus Eukaryotic Translation**

PROKARYOTE	EUKARYOTE
> 1 coding region **(polycistronic),** each of which is independently translated by ribosomes.	RNA encodes only 1 polypeptide chain **(monocistronic).**
Each region has its own initiation codon and produces a separate polypeptide. Thus, the mRNA may contain multiple proteins.	Each mRNA contains only 1 protein.

tRNA Wobble

The code for certain amino acids relies only on the base sequence of the first two nucleotides in the codon. As described earlier, often the same amino acid has multiple codons that differ in the third "wobble" position. Therefore, < 61 tRNAs are needed to translate all 61 codons.

Protein Synthesis

Proteins are assembled from the N- to the C-terminus, whereas the mRNA template is read from the 5′ to the 3′ end. The number of proteins that the mRNA can encode differs between prokaryotes and eukaryotes (Table 3-10). mRNA from eukaryotes encodes for only one protein, whereas prokaryotic mRNA can encode several different proteins. Protein synthesis occurs in three steps (**initiation, elongation,** and **termination**), which are followed by post-translational modifications.

Initiation

In prokaryotes, the complex formed for initiation of translation consists of 30S ribosomal subunit, mRNA, f-Met tRNA, and three initiation factors. The formation of the initiation complex differs between prokaryotes and eukaryotes, as summarized in Table 3-11.

Elongation

Three-step cycle in which tRNA delivers the appropriate amino acid to the ribosome, the amino acid forms a peptide bond to the growing peptide chain, and the ribosome shifts one codon so that the next codon can be translated (Figures 3-17 and 3-18).

> **KEY FACT**
>
> There are significant differences in gene expression between prokaryotes and eukaryotes. The use of different enzymes for protein synthesis allows for selective targeting of prokaryotic enzymes and organelles, with minimal effects on their eukaryotic counterparts.

> **CLINICAL CORRELATION**
>
> The differences in enzymes used for similar metabolic processes in eukaryotes and prokaryotes allows for selective targeting of prokaryotic enzymes by antibiotics and antivirals. As such, these drugs will selectively affect prokaryotic cells or viral infected eukaryotic cells, with minimal to no effects on healthy eukaryotic cells.

TABLE 3-11.   **Prokaryotic Versus Eukaryotic Translation**

	PROKARYOTES	EUKARYOTES
Ribosomal binding	30S ribosomal subunit binds Shine-Dalgarno sequence, which is 6–10 nucleotides upstream (toward 5′ end) of AUG codon.	No Shine-Dalgarno sequence, 40S ribosomal subunit binds 5′ cap and moves down mRNA until it encounters AUG codon.
Initiator tRNA	fMet (methionine with a formyl group attached).	Met (methionine only).
Assembly of initiation complex	Facilitated by initiation factors (IF-1, IF-2, IF-3), 50S ribosomal subunit binds to make 70S complex.	Initiation factors (eIF, and at least 10 other factors).

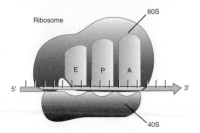

FIGURE 3-17. Schematic representation of eukaryotic ribosome and the sites involved in protein synthesis. P (peptidyl) site initially binds initiator tRNA, later binds growing peptide chain. A (aminoacyl) site binds incoming tRNA molecule with activated amino acid (ie, bound amino acid with high-energy bond). E site receives uncharged tRNA once amino acid has been added to polypeptide.

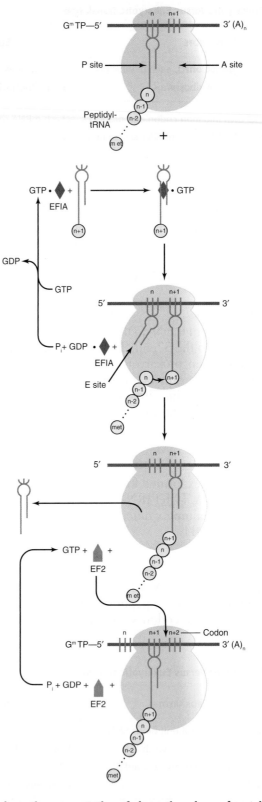

FIGURE 3-18. Schematic representation of elongation phase of protein synthesis. (Modified with permission from Murray RK, Granner DK, Rodwell VW. *Harper's Illustrated Biochemistry*, 27th ed. New York: McGraw-Hill, 2006: 375.)

- Aminoacyl-tRNA (charged tRNA) binds A site.
- Amino acid in A site forms peptide bond with peptide in P site. Reaction is catalyzed by peptidyl transferase and uses energy from the bond between the amino acid and tRNA. The peptide in the P site is effectively transferred to the amino acid–tRNA in the A site, leaving the tRNA in the P site empty.
- Ribosome translocates one codon (requires EF-2, GTP hydrolysis) toward the 3′ end of mRNA. Uncharged tRNA is now in the E site (where it exits), and tRNA with the growing peptide chain enters the P site.

TERMINATION

Occurs when one of three stop codons (**UGA, UAA, UAG**) is encountered. Peptide is released from ribosome via release factor (RF) protein and GTP.

POST-TRANSLATIONAL MODIFICATION

Modification may result in the removal of amino acids or addition of additional molecules to make protein active and/or properly tag the protein for proper transport to its final destination.

- **Trimming** removes portions of the peptide chain to make the protein active (ie, zymogen, an inactive precursor of a secreted enzyme).
- Protein may be covalently modified through **phosphorylation** and **glycosylation**. Phosphorylation turns the protein on or off. Proteins that will be secreted or reside in the plasma membrane or lysosomes will be glycosylated in the endoplasmic reticulum (ER) and Golgi apparatus.

Mutations and DNA Repair

DNA mutations and the intrinsic cellular mechanisms that act to minimize their occurrence play a very important role in health and disease. Not only do DNA mutations result in numerous pathologic conditions, they also form the basis for the evolution of novel traits in species.

DEFINITIONS

Mutation

A mutation is any change in the sequence of DNA base pairs that is permanent and arises by chance. To be considered a mutation, the change in the base-pair sequence must not be a result of recombination.

DNA Repair

Several molecular mechanisms exist to ensure that most changes in the DNA sequence are repaired and thus do not become permanent mutations. It is estimated that between 1000 and 1,000,000 DNA sequence damaging events occur in each cell every day. However, most of these are quickly corrected by one of the DNA repair mechanisms. Note that DNA repair is independent of the proofreading action of DNA polymerase during DNA replication.

FLASH FORWARD

Drugs selective for prokaryotic protein synthesis machinery.

Drug	Site of Action
Tetracycline	Prevents initiation since charged tRNA cannot bind ribosome.
Streptomycin	Prevents initiation since code is misread.
Erythromycin	Inhibits translocation.

FLASH FORWARD

Many proteins of the coagulation cascade and enzymes involved in digestion (eg, trypsinogen, pepsinogen) are zymogens.

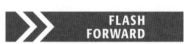

CLINICAL CORRELATION

In xeroderma pigmentosum, an autosome recessive disorder involving defective nucleotide excision repair genes, DNA repair is impaired, preventing the ability of the cell to repair damage caused by ultraviolet light. Susceptible individuals are more likely to develop basal cell carcinomas, melanoma and squamous cell carcinomas. XP is more common among Japanese people.

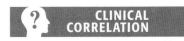
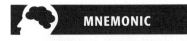
Types of Mutations

Mutated DNA includes DNA in which one nucleotide has changed (**point mutation**) and DNA in which one or more nucleotides have been added or removed. Since the DNA code is read in triplets (a **codon**, three consecutive nucleotides, encodes an amino acid), adding or removing one or two nucleotides will cause a **frame shift mutation.** Point mutations lead to one of three outcomes: the identity of the amino acid is unchanged (**silent mutation**); the amino acid is changed to another amino acid (**missense mutation**); or a stop signal is introduced (**nonsense mutation**).

POINT MUTATIONS

Point mutations occur when a single DNA nucleotide base is replaced by a different nucleotide. These are also known as **substitutions.** Occasionally, single nucleotide deletions or insertions are also considered point mutations, but they cause reading frame shifts.

There are three types of point mutations: missense mutations, nonsense mutations, and silent mutations.

- **Missense mutations:** The replacement of a single nucleotide base with a different one, resulting in a change in the codon so that it codes for a different amino acid (Figure 3-19B). These are common types of mutations and cause several genetic diseases.
- **Nonsense mutations:** Mutation causes premature introduction of a STOP codon (TAA, TAG, or TGA). This causes the translation of the mRNA to stop, resulting in a truncated protein (Figure 3-19C).
- **Silent mutations:** Mutation results in the same amino acid as the original. Because the genetic code is redundant (ie, several codons code for the same amino acid), in some cases a change in a single nucleotide base still codes for the same amino acid (Figure 3-19D). Most often, this results from a base change in the **third** position of the codon (**wobble position**). The resulting protein is identical to the wild-type protein.

With respect to their biochemical origin, point mutations can be one of five types: transition, transversion, tautomerism, depurination, or deamination.

- **Transition:** A mutation in which a pyrimidine is replaced by a pyrimidine, or a purine by a purine. For example, a replacement of a G-C pair by an A-T pair would result in a transition.
- **Transversion:** A purine replaced by a pyrimidine or vice versa. An A-T pair replaced by either a T-A or C-G pair would be a transversion.
- **Tautomerism:** The modification of a base caused by migration of a proton or a hydrogen bond, which results in switching of an adjacent single and a double bond.
- **Depurination:** Caused by a spontaneous hydrolysis of a purine base (A or G), in such a way that its deoxyribose-phosphate backbone remains intact.
- **Deamination:** A spontaneous reaction that can result in the conversion of cytosine into uracil (C to U), 5-methylcytosine into thymine, or adenine into hypoxanthine (A to HX). Of note, the deamination of C to U is the only of these that can be corrected, since uracil can be recognized, whereas thymine and hypoxanthine are not detected as errant.

Insertions

Insertions are mutations in which one or several base pairs are added to the DNA sequence. Most commonly, insertions of short DNA fragments called **transposons** (or transposable elements) are responsible. Insertions may result

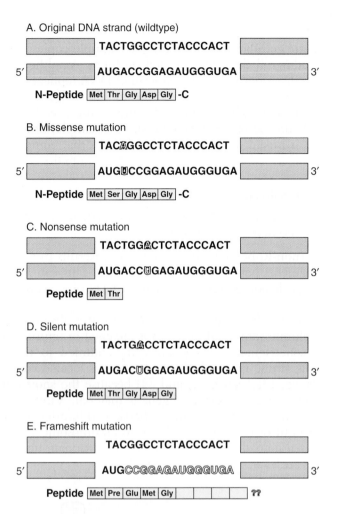

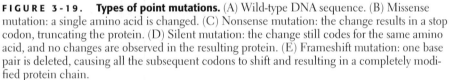

FIGURE 3-19. **Types of point mutations.** (A) Wild-type DNA sequence. (B) Missense mutation: a single amino acid is changed. (C) Nonsense mutation: the change results in a stop codon, truncating the protein. (D) Silent mutation: the change still codes for the same amino acid, and no changes are observed in the resulting protein. (E) Frameshift mutation: one base pair is deleted, causing all the subsequent codons to shift and resulting in a completely modified protein chain.

from errors in DNA replication of nucleotide repeats. Insertions can result in frameshift mutations and splice site mutations.

FRAMESHIFT MUTATIONS

Because codons are always read in triplets, adding or deleting any number of bases that is not a multiple of three shifts the reading frame during translation and greatly alters the amino acid sequence of the protein (Figure 3-19E).

SPLICE SITE MUTATIONS

At times, insertions of nucleotide bases in certain regions of a gene can alter the splicing of introns from the precursor mRNA. This results in mRNA that contains introns, resulting in significantly altered protein products.

Deletions

Deletions refer to the loss of one or several nucleotides from the DNA sequence. Much like insertions described above, they can result in frameshift mutations and splice site mutations. They are generally irreversible.

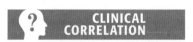

A splice site mutation in the β-globin gene is responsible for certain cases of β-thalassemia.

Amplifications

Amplifications are cellular events resulting in multiple copies of whole DNA segments, including all the genes located on them. Amplifications are usually caused by a disproportionately high level of DNA replication in a limited portion of the genome. In this manner, the multiplied genes are effectively amplified, leading to a higher number of copies of the encoded protein. This can alter the phenotype of the affected cell. For example, drug resistance in certain cancers is linked to amplifications of genes that confer resistance to chemotherapeutic agents by preventing their uptake into the cell.

Chromosomal Translocations

A chromosomal translocation is defined as an exchange of genetic material between two nonhomologous chromosomes.

- **Reciprocal (non-Robertsonian)** translocation: Results in a true exchange of DNA fragments between two chromosomes. This can lead to the formation of new fusion genes, or a changed level of expression of existing genes.
- **Robertsonian** translocation: A large fragment of a chromosome attaches to another chromosome, but no DNA is attached in return (Figure 3-20). Common Robertsonian translocations are confined to the acrocentric chromosomes (those in which the centromere is located very near to one of the ends, eg, 13, 14, 15, 21, and 22) because the short arms of these chromosomes contain no essential genetic material. A minority of cases of **Down syndrome** are caused by the Robertsonian translocation of approximately one third of chromosome 21 on to chromosome 14. The proportion of affected individuals due to trisomy, Robertsonian translocation and other causes are 95%, 3%, and 2%, respectively.

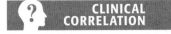

CLINICAL CORRELATION

The *bcr-abl* gene, associated with chronic myelogenous leukemia (CML), results from a translocation event between chromosomes 9 and 22 (Philadelphia chromosome). The chemotherapeutic imatinib mesylate (Gleevac) is a specific inhibitor of the tyrosine kinase domain in *abl* and c-kit and is a useful agent in the treatment of chronic myelogenous leukemia (CML) and gastrointestinal stromal tumors (GIST), respectively.

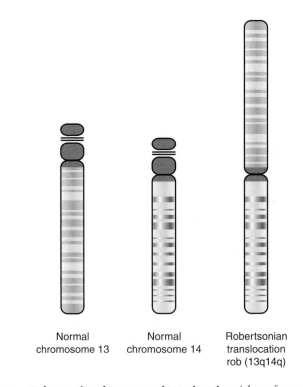

Normal
chromosome 13

Normal
chromosome 14

Robertsonian
translocation
rob (13q14q)

FIGURE 3-20.   Robertsonian chromosomal translocation. A large fragment of a chromosome attaches to another chromosome, but no DNA is attached in return, resulting in the loss of a small amount of genetic material.

Interstitial Deletions

Deletions of large DNA fragments on a single chromosome that results in the pairing of two genes that are not normally in sequence. Like chromosomal translocations, such events can lead to the formation of fusion oncogenes.

Chromosomal Inversions

Chromosomal inversions refer to a large segment of a single chromosome becoming reversed within the same chromosome, usually resulting from a rearrangement following chromosomal breakage. Similar to translocations and interstitial deletions, chromosomal inversions can create fusion genes.

ORIGINS OF MUTATIONS

Most mutations arise spontaneously, usually as a result either of errors in DNA replication (eg, point mutations and amplifications) or random cellular events (including chromosomal translocations and inversions). However, many mutations are directly caused by specific agents, collectively known as **mutagens.** Some mutagens are external, whereas some are formed as by-products of cellular metabolism (eg, reactive oxygen species [ROS]).

The type of cell in which a mutation arises is also important. When a mutation arises in a germ cell, it is termed a **germline mutation.** These mutations can be passed to the offspring. Conversely, a mutation in a somatic cell is termed a **somatic mutation** and cannot be passed on to offspring. However, somatic mutations are passed on to the somatic daughter cells of the organism (ie, cancers resulting from somatic mutations).

MUTAGENS

These are agents that directly cause or increase the likelihood of changes in the DNA sequence. Innumerable mutagens have been identified, and novel ones are continually discovered. Mutagens generally fall into two categories: **chemical agents** and **ionizing radiation.** Because mutations often give rise to cancer, they are often also **carcinogens.**

Chemical Agents

ALKYLATING AGENTS

Chemical agents that transfer alkyl groups to other molecules, including DNA. Specifically, they cross-link guanine nucleotides in DNA, thus causing damage to the DNA that can lead to mutations in both replicating and nonreplicating cells. However, some alkylating agents are used as anticancer drugs because of their unique ability to introduce sufficient DNA damage to render a cell unable to divide. Examples of these chemotherapeutics include **cisplatin** and **carboplatin.**

BASE ANALOGS

Chemical agents that are similar to one of the four nucleotide bases found in DNA and can thus be incorrectly incorporated into DNA during replication. However, they differ enough chemically that they cause mismatch during base pairing, thus introducing mutations in daughter DNA strands. An example of a base analog is bromodeoxyuridine (**BrdU**), which researchers often use to identify dividing cells because it is incorporated into the DNA during replication.

Do not confuse base analogs with antimetabolites, which also share similarity with regularly occurring nucleotides, but upon incorporation into DNA, inhibit further replication. As a result, they can be considered competitive inhibitors of DNA replication and are used as anticancer chemotherapeutics.

METHYLATING AGENTS

Methylating agents, such as ethyl methanesulfonate (EMS), that introduce mutations by transferring methyl groups to DNA nucleotide bases. These substances are typically not used as anticancer agents because do not cause cell death.

DNA INTERCALATING AGENTS

Cause DNA damage by inserting themselves between two nucleotide base pairs. This physically interferes with DNA transcription and replication, leading to mutation events. Examples include **ethidium bromide,** a fluorescent DNA dye commonly used in research laboratories, and **aflatoxin,** a carcinogen produced by a fungus from the genus *Aspergillus.* Some DNA intercalating agents, such as **doxorubicin** and **daunorubicin,** are used as cancer chemotherapeutics. **Thalidomide,** a teratogen associated with numerous cases of phocomelia (very short or absent long bones and flipper-like appearance of hands and/or feet) in the 1960s, is also a DNA intercalating agent. It is now only used as a last resort anti-inflammatory agent in the treatment of erythema nodosum leprosum and sarcoidosis and as a salvage chemotherapeutic agent in patients with multiple myeloma.

DNA CROSS-LINKING AGENTS

These chemical agents act as mutagens by forming covalent bonds between nucleotide bases in DNA, therefore interfering with replication and transcription. A typical example is **platinum,** a derivative of which, **cisplatin,** is a chemotherapeutic agent commonly used in cancers.

REACTIVE OXYGEN SPECIES

ROS are free radicals, molecular species which are rendered highly reactive by the presence of unpaired electrons. They damage DNA by "stealing" electrons from DNA to become more stable. Examples include **superoxide, hydrogen peroxide,** and **hydroxyl radicals.** These species are thought to be important in age-related cellular damage.

Ionizing Radiation

Ionizing radiation, produced by radioactive materials, is electromagnetic radiation with energy high enough to ionize a molecule or atom by removing an electron from its orbit. This process causes significant DNA damage, resulting in mutations and eventual cell death. Although potentially very dangerous, this type of radiation can be used in targeted cancer treatment and radiography (X-rays).

Ultraviolet Radiation

Ultraviolet (UV) radiation is a type of electromagnetic radiation with a shorter wavelength and higher energy than that of visible light. It causes DNA damage by inducing the formation of covalent bonds between adjacent thymine nucleotides, giving rise to bulky thymine dimers. This is the basis for increased risk of skin cancer resulting from sun overexposure (Figure 3-21). For example, DNA damage to melanocytes can result in loss of control mechanisms for

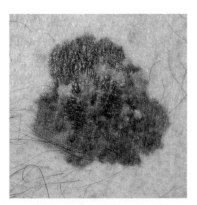

FIGURE 3-21. Skin cancer.
Clinical appearance of malignant melanoma, a skin cancer caused by UV radiation, often a consequence of sun overexposure. (Reproduced with permission from Wolff K, Goldsmith LA, Katz SI, et al. *Fitzpatrick's Dermatology in General Medicine,* 7th ed. New York: McGraw-Hill, 2008.)

cellular growth, creating uninhibited growth patterns seen in various types of melanomas.

DNA REPAIR

DNA repair mechanisms are responsible for minimizing the negative effects that DNA damage has on the cell. DNA damage occurs almost constantly in living cells. When DNA damage surpasses a certain threshold, either because there is too much accumulated damage or because DNA repair mechanisms are no longer effective, a cell can have one of the following three fates:

1. **Senescence:** A cell enters a dormant state that is irreversible, in which the main cellular processes and functions are suspended.
2. **Apoptosis:** A cell undergoes programmed cell death, or suicide, by activating specialized signal cascades.
3. **Cancer:** A cell starts undergoing unregulated cell division, resulting in neoplasia and tumor growth.

DNA repair is thus extremely important for proper functioning of cells and the organism as a whole. A number of specialized DNA repair mechanisms have evolved, and are discussed below (Figure 3-22 for an overview).

Direct Reversal

When specific DNA nucleotides are damaged by chemical modification, the resulting molecular species are specific to the nucleotide that was damaged. The cell can use this information to determine the original nucleotide and can directly reverse the damage using mechanisms specific to the type of damage. Examples include the repair of **UV light–induced thymine dimers.** Similarly, guanine bases that undergo methylation are repaired by methylguanine methyltransferase (**MGMT**). Certain cases of cytosine and adenine methylation are also repaired using direct reversal mechanisms.

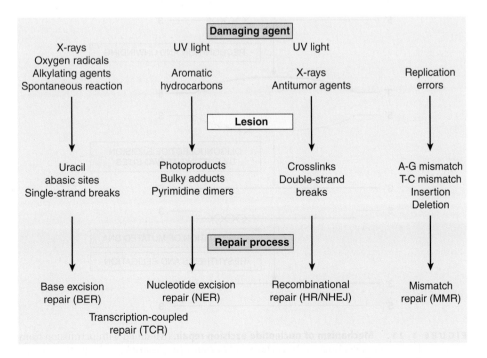

FIGURE 3-22.   DNA repair mechanisms. Different agents cause a wide variety of DNA damage. Specialized mechanisms have evolved to repair this damage.

Single-Strand Damage

When only one of the strands in the DNA double helix is damaged, the complementary base on the opposite strand can be used as a template for repair. Several DNA repair mechanisms rely on this principle.

BASE EXCISION REPAIR

When single nucleotides are damaged by alkylation, deamination, or oxidation reactions, two enzymes, **DNA glycosylase** and **AP** endonuclease remove and repair the damaged bases. Endonuclease nicks the phosphodiester bond next to the base, releases deoxyribose, and creates a gap. **DNA polymerase** then inserts the correct nucleotide in its place (based on the complementary base), and the nick is sealed by **DNA ligase.** The most common DNA damage is the deamination of cytosine to uracil.

NUCLEOTIDE EXCISION REPAIR (NER) (FIGURE 3-23)

A set of mechanisms similar to base excision repair, but used to excise and replace longer stretches of nucleotides (2–30 bases). UV-damaged DNA: dimers form between adjacent pyrimidines (eg, thymine), thus preventing DNA replication. **UV-specific endonuclease** (uvrABC excinuclease) recognizes the damaged base and makes a break several bases upstream (toward the 5′ side). Helicase removes the short stretch of nucleotides. The gap is filled in by DNA polymerase, and DNA ligase seals the nick.

MISMATCH REPAIR

Mismatch repair is used when there is an error in the pairing of nucleotides secondary to DNA replication or recombination. The base pair mismatch repair system detects errors that escaped proofreading during DNA replication.

> **KEY FACT**
>
> Defects in mismatch repair can lead to hereditary nonpolyposis colon cancer (HNPCC). Other diseases caused by genetic defects:
>
> | Genetic Defect | Disease |
> | --- | --- |
> | ATM | Ataxia-telangiectasia (AT) |
> | UVR ABC | Xeroderma pigmentosum (XP) |
> | MSH, MLH | Hereditary nonpolyposis colorectal cancer (HNPCC) |
> | Helicase | Wermer |
> | BRCA1 | Breast cancer |

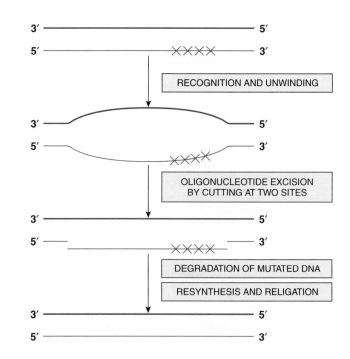

FIGURE 3-23. **Mechanism of nucleotide excision repair.** (Modified with permission from Murray RK, Granner DK, Rodwell VW. *Harper's Illustrated Biochemistry*, 27th ed. New York: McGraw-Hill, 2006: 345.)

- **Identify the mismatched strand:** In newly synthesized DNA, adenine residues in GATC sequence motifs have not yet been methylated. Thus, the DNA parent strand, but not the newly synthesized strand, is methylated.
- **Repair damaged DNA:** The mismatched strand is nicked with endonuclease and the mismatched base(s) is/are removed. The sister strand is used as a template, and DNA polymerase fills in the gap.

Double-Strand Breaks

The situation is distinctly different when both strands of the DNA double helix are broken. In this case, no direct template exists to guide the cell's repair process. Double-stranded breaks can be repaired by either homologous recombination (recombinatorial repair or crossing over) or nonhomologous end joining (NHEJ). In NHEJ, specific proteins bring the ends of two DNA fragments together. However, this is error prone and mutagenic.

NONHOMOLOGOUS END JOINING

When both strands of DNA are broken in a region that has not yet been replicated, there is truly no template for the cell to use to reconstruct the damaged DNA. However, because a complete break of the DNA double helix is highly deleterious for the cell, an attempt is made to fix the break using NHEJ. In this process, DNA ligase–containing complexes join the separated ends of the double helix, relying on microhomologies between the ends of the single-stranded fragments. However, by definition, NHEJ is always mutagenic.

RECOMBINATORIAL REPAIR

Sometimes a double-stranded break occurs during DNA replication. In this case, a fragment of the DNA has already been replicated and can serve as a template for the repair of the double-stranded break. Molecularly, the enzymatic complex involved in recombinatorial repair is similar to that involved in chromosomal crossover.

Translesion Synthesis

As a last resort, cells perform translesion synthesis as a means of continuing DNA replication. When DNA damage is extensive enough to prevent the replication machinery from advancing, special DNA polymerases repair the damaged DNA by inserting nucleotide bases. These nucleotide bases are not completely arbitrary, but they are also not based on a template. Therefore, translesion synthesis introduces mutations by necessity, but enables the cell to continue DNA replication.

CELL CYCLE CHECKPOINTS

When entering cell division or mitosis (M), the cell cycle enters the G_1 phase (growth phase 1). At this point, nonproliferating cells enter G_0, a quiescent phase, whereas active cells proceed to the synthesis (S) phase, which is characterized by DNA replication. Following the S phase is the G_2, or growth phase 2, a short period before the cell divides again (reenters the M phase).

Several checkpoints exist in the cell cycle for a damaged cell to prevent itself from proceeding to the next phase in the cycle (Figure 3-24).

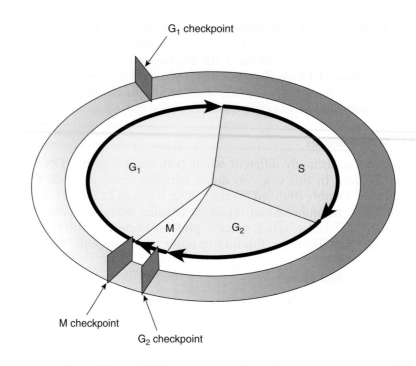

FIGURE 3-24. **Cell cycle checkpoints.** At several points during the cell cycle, a dividing cell ensures that multiple criteria are satisfied before proceeding with the cycle. Most notably, these include the G_1, G_2, and M (mitosis or anaphase) checkpoints.

G_1 Checkpoint

The first checkpoint takes place at the end of the G_1 phase. At this point, most eukaryotic cells decide whether to proceed with DNA replication (enter S phase) or become quiescent (enter the G_0 phase). The decision is made based on the availability of nutrients, the amount of DNA damage present, and surrounding conditions. This checkpoint is largely dependent on **p53** (a tumor suppressor protein), which can allow the cell to enter the S or the G_0 phases, or—if the amount of damage is too great—undergo apoptosis. Mutations in the *p53* gene are present in many cancers and are the basis for the **Li-Fraumeni syndrome.**

G_2 Checkpoint

The second crucial checkpoint occurs at the end of growth phase 2 (G_2) just before mitosis. This is the final checkpoint before the cell commits to division. Two crucial molecules, the maturation promoting factor (**MPF**) and a cyclindependent kinase (**CDK**), regulate this step.

M (Mitosis or Anaphase) Checkpoint

The final checkpoint in the cell cycle takes place in anaphase, when the action of CDK-1 triggers the destruction of **cyclins,** causing the cell to exit mitosis and initiate cytokinesis.

PATHOLOGY

Xeroderma Pigmentosum

CLINICAL FEATURES

Xeroderma pigmentosum (XP) is an autosomal recessive disorder caused by mutations that incapacitate the NER mechanism, rendering the cells unable to repair damage caused by UV radiation. Therefore, people with XP **cannot tolerate sunlight.**

Although patients are born with normal skin, the first signs of XP usually become apparent early in life (6 months of age) and include freckle-like increased pigmentation and diffuse erythema and scaling, especially in light-exposed areas. The second stage of disease usually involves the development of telangiectasias, skin atrophy, mottled irregular pigmentation, and other characteristics of poikiloderma. The final stage, which can occur in childhood, gives rise to malignancies, including malignant melanoma, squamous cell and basal cell carcinomas, and fibrosarcoma. In addition, patients exhibit generalized photosensitivity, photophobia, and conjunctivitis (80%). Neurologic problems are seen in approximately 20% of the patients and can include microcephaly, spasticity, hyporeflexia, ataxia, motor neuron signs, and mental retardation. These symptoms are related to the severity of the disease. Patients with XP are also more susceptible to infection.

CELLULAR CHARACTERISTICS

UV radiation causes DNA damage by inducing the formation of covalent bonds between adjacent thymine nucleotides, giving rise to bulky thymine dimers. Under normal circumstances, this damage is reversed by the **NER** mechanism. However, in XP, some of the proteins involved in NER are mutated, rendering the cell unable, or less able, to repair UV-induced damage. This leads to the accumulation of mutations and eventual development of skin cancers.

GENETICS

XP is an autosomal recessive disease caused by mutations in one of the seven identified XP repair genes (XPA through XPG). Seven subtypes of XP are recognized (XPA–XPG, respectively), and occur with different frequencies. Different subtypes differ in their severity and clinical manifestations. The overall incidence of the disease is about 1 in 250,000 except in Japan, where it is as high as 1 in 40,000.

TREATMENT AND PROGNOSIS

The only treatment for XP is the avoidance of sunlight. The main causes of mortality in XP are skin neoplasms, in particular, **malignant melanoma** and squamous cell carcinoma. Patients younger than 20 years have a 1000 times higher incidence of both melanoma and nonmelanoma, as compared to the general population. The average life span of a person with XP is reduced by about 40 years. Oral **retinoids** have been used to reduce the incidence of skin cancer, but they cause irreversible calcification of tendons and ligaments. **5-Fluorouracil** and topical **imiquimod** and **acitretin** have been used to treat keratoses. It has recently been discovered that topically applied bioengineered DNA repair enzymes lower the incidence of certain skin lesions during a year of treatment.

Fanconi Anemia

CLINICAL FEATURES

Fanconi anemia (FA) is an autosomal recessive disease characterized by **bone marrow failure and DNA repair defects.** Patients often develop pancytopenia as a consequence of **aplastic anemia,** leukemias, and solid tumors. In particular, liver, head and neck, esophageal, and vulvar cancers are very common. Newborns sometimes exhibit characteristic abnormalities, including genitourinary problems and poor growth. Pigmentation and **café-au-lait spots** are also often present. Symptoms of bone marrow failure include petechiae, bruises, pallor, fatigue, and infections.

CELLULAR CHARACTERISTICS

At least 11 genes are involved in the FA pathway. Mutations in any of these genes render cells more susceptible to damage by O_2-free radicals. These mutations also cause deficiencies in DNA repair mechanisms and interfere with cell cycle control. Hematopoietic cells are particularly affected, and the risk of malignancy is increased in many tissues.

GENETICS

FA is an autosomal recessive disorder that affects approximately 1 in 360,000 people worldwide; in Ashkenazi Jewish and Afrikaners populations, the incidence is approximately 10 times higher. The mutation can occur in any of the 11 genes involved in the pathway.

TREATMENT AND PROGNOSIS

There are no specific treatments for FA. The highest mortality and morbidity arise from bone marrow failure, leukemias, and solid cancers. Therefore, the treatments are focused on those specific clinical features.

Cockayne Syndrome

CLINICAL FEATURES

Cockayne syndrome (CS), like XP, is an autosomal recessive disorder caused by mutations that affect the **NER** mechanism, thus rendering the cells unable to repair damage caused by UV radiation. However, unlike XP, skin malignancies are uncommon. CS is characterized by birdlike facies, progressive retinopathy, dwarfism, and photosensitivity. Patients tend to have large ears, a thin nose, and microcephaly, with deeply set eyes, short stature, and long limbs. Skin hyperpigmentation, telangiectasia, and erythema are also common. They exhibit premature signs of aging and progressive neurologic deterioration.

CELLULAR CHARACTERISTICS

The faulty NER mechanism leads to the inability of cells to repair DNA damage caused by exposure to UV light. This results in the accumulation of mutations and overall **accelerated aging of the cells.**

GENETICS

Both of the main types of CS are autosomal recessive and are involved in NER. The incidence of the disorder is less than 1 in 250,000. It affects both genders and all races equally.

TREATMENT AND PROGNOSIS

There is no cure for CS, and treatment is largely supportive. It involves protecting the patients from sun exposure, using sunscreen, and treating neurologic deficiencies that arise, such as deafness. CS-1, or classic CS usually presents in childhood, followed by progressive neurologic deterioration, with death typically occurring by the third decade. In contrast, CS-2 is a much more severe form of the disease and usually presents shortly after birth, with patients generally surviving to six or seven years of age.

Trichothiodystrophy

CLINICAL FEATURES

Trichothiodystrophy (TTD) is the rarest disorder arising from deficiencies in the NER mechanism. It is a heterogeneous group of autosomal recessive disorders characterized by sulfur-rich brittle hair and nails; photosensitive, dry, thickened, scaly skin ("fishskin"); and both physical and mental retardation. Skin cancer is typically not associated with the disorder.

CELLULAR CHARACTERISTICS

As in XP and CS, deficiencies in numerous proteins involved in NER results in the accumulation of UV light-induced DNA damage.

GENETICS

TTD is an extremely rare disorder, with only over a dozen cases reported. The genetic abnormalities are heterogeneous, but all include genes involved in nucleotide exchange repair.

TREATMENT AND PROGNOSIS

No cure exists for TTD, and much like in other nucleotide exchange repair disorders, the treatment is largely supportive.

Ataxia-Telangiectasia

CLINICAL FEATURES

Ataxia-telangiectasia (AT) is a heterogeneous disease, typically characterized by progressive neurologic dysfunction, cerebellar ataxia, sinopulmonary infections, telangiectasias, increased risk of malignancy, and hypersensitivity to X-rays. Neurologically, it can progress to spinal muscular atrophy and peripheral neuropathies. Patients characteristically have dull, relaxed facies and oculomotor signs. About 30% of patients also have mild mental retardation. Skin and hair tend to show accelerated signs of aging.

CELLULAR CHARACTERISTICS

The protein affected by the AT mutation has been shown to be required for the maintenance of genome stability. Patients have higher frequencies of **chromosome and chromatid breaks and rearrangements,** disproportionately affecting chromosomes 7 and 14, which are responsible for T-cell receptor and immunoglobulin regulation.

GENETICS

Several genetic AT variants exist. The disease is inherited in an autosomal recessive pattern, and involves a mutation in the *ATM* gene (AT mutated), located on chromosome 11. It affects an estimated 1 in 100,000 people across all races and both sexes.

TREATMENT AND PROGNOSIS

The treatment in AT is aimed at controlling recurrent infections and malignancies. Supportive neurologic care is often required; the prognosis is very poor. Most patients survive until early or mid-adolescence, with the usual causes of death being bronchopulmonary infections and cancer.

Hereditary Nonpolyposis Colorectal Cancer (HNPCC)

CLINICAL FEATURES

Affected individuals have a significantly increased risk of developing colorectal cancer in addition to other malignancies, such as cancers of the endometrium, ovary, stomach, and brain. Also known as Lynch syndrome, patients affected by this disorder have an **80% lifetime likelihood of developing colorectal cancer.** Female patients have an estimated 30–50% chance of developing endometrial cancer.

CELLULAR CHARACTERISTICS

Several genes involved in the **mismatch DNA repair** pathway are involved in pathogenesis in HNPCC. This leads to significant **microsatellite instability** resulting in the accumulation of mutations that give rise to malignancies.

GENETICS

HNPCC is an **autosomal dominant** disorder. It is caused by mutations in a number of genes, most notably *MSH2*, *MLH1*, and *PMS2*. In addition, *ras* gene mutations can be detected in the stool. HNPCC is thought to account for about 5% of all colorectal cancers.

TREATMENT AND PROGNOSIS

Treatment is focused on the prevention and treatment of colorectal malignancies or other cancers. Some affected individuals elect to undergo prophylactic colectomy or hysterectomy. Common screening for cancers, including colonoscopy, pelvic exam, and urine cytology are recommended. According to the most recent guidelines, colonoscopy should be performed every two years beginning at age 25, or five years younger than the age of the earliest diagnosis in the family, whichever is earlier. Beginning at age 40, colonoscopy should be performed annually.

Hereditary Breast Cancer

CLINICAL FEATURES

Patients affected with hereditary breast cancer have a 60 to 80% lifetime risk of developing breast cancer (compared with an average 11% lifetime risk in American women). Characteristically, there is a strong family history of breast cancer, and the patients often develop cancer at an early age. They may also develop bilateral disease. The malignancies disproportionately include **serous adenocarcinomas.** Patients with *BRCA2* mutations also have a significantly higher risk of developing ovarian, prostate, and pancreatic cancers.

CELLULAR CHARACTERISTICS

The genes involved in typical cases of hereditary breast cancer involve the DNA repair machinery. A higher frequency of *p53* mutations is seen in affected patients.

GENETICS

Hereditary breast cancer is inherited as an **autosomal dominant** trait. It typically involves mutations of the *BRCA1* and *BRCA2* genes. Although it predominantly affects women, it is important to note that these mutations significantly increase the risk of breast tissue cancers in men as well. About 5% of all breast cancers are thought to be hereditary forms. Ashkenazi Jewish populations have increased frequencies of some common mutations in *BRCA1* and *BRCA2* genes.

TREATMENT AND PROGNOSIS

Primary interventions include breast cancer screening and mammography. Prophylactic mastectomy, oophorectomy, and chemoprevention remain controversial. The cancers are typically of higher histologic grade and are also more likely to be estrogen receptor and progesterone receptor negative, which carries implications in treatment and prognosis.

Bloom Syndrome

CLINICAL FEATURES

Bloom syndrome (BS) is a rare autosomal recessive disorder characterized by growth delay (usually of prenatal onset), a significantly increased risk of malignancy (approximately 300-fold), and recurrent respiratory and gastrointestinal infections due to compromised immunity. Telangiectatic erythema is often seen in a butterfly facial distribution. (In fact, the disease is also known as congenital telangiectatic erythema.)

CELLULAR CHARACTERISTICS

The mutation causing BS affects a gene coding for a protein with a helicase activity thought to be involved in the maintenance of genomic stability. A significantly higher frequency of sister chromatid exchanges and chromosomal instability is also seen and is thought to be due to consistent overproduction of superoxide radicals.

GENETICS

BS is an autosomal recessive disorder caused by a mutation in the *BLM* gene on chromosome 15. It is a very rare disorder (about 170 cases have been reported) that affects both sexes and all races, although it is somewhat more common in Ashkenazi Jews.

TREATMENT AND PROGNOSIS

Typically, there is no specific treatment for BS. Interventions are aimed at dealing with neoplasms, infection, and dermatologic manifestations. Sunscreen and sun avoidance are recommended. The highest risk of death is due to cancers, typically in the second and third decades of life.

Werner Syndrome

CLINICAL FEATURES

Werner syndrome (WS) is an autosomal recessive disease characterized by onset of accelerated aging, usually in the late teen years. The disease is also known as **progeria** of the adult. Affected individuals appear disproportionately aged, including thin, tight, scleroderma-like skin, muscle atrophy, wrinkling, hyperkeratosis, gray, thinning hair, and nail dystrophy. Cataracts, osteoporosis, neoplasias, diabetes mellitus, and arteriosclerosis are generally the sources of morbidity and mortality. Of note, development is typically normal in the first decade of life.

CELLULAR CHARACTERISTICS

The gene involved in WS codes for a DNA helicase involved in DNA repair mechanisms and general transcription and replication. WS particularly affects connective tissues, and overproduction of both collagen and collagenase has been reported. As in other diseases of this type, it is thought that the overall phenotype results from deficiencies in genome maintenance.

GENETICS

As noted, WS is a rare autosomal recessive disorder linked to a mutation in the WS gene, which codes for a helicase. It is estimated to affect 1 in 1,000,000 people. Even though no racial predilection is reported, more than 80% of the reported cases are found in Japan. It affects both men and women.

TREATMENT AND PROGNOSIS

There is no cure for WS, and the prognosis is grim. Treatments are aimed at conditions arising from the accelerated aging process, including cancers, diabetes mellitus, and arteriosclerotic complications. The mean survival for patients with WS is the middle of the fourth decade, with death usually resulting from malignancies and arteriosclerosis.

Enzymes

GENERAL

Enzymes are biologic polymers that catalyze chemical reactions, allowing them to proceed at rates that are compatible with life as we know it.

Nomenclature

The suffix "-ase" **always** indicates an enzyme (eg, DNA polymerase). Most enzyme names end with -ase.

Another common enzyme suffix is "-in" (eg, fibrin).

Function

Enzymes allow nutrients to be absorbed and used by the body in many ways, as shown in Figure 3-25.

Activity

Many enzymes are dependent on the presence of a cofactor. A **cofactor** is a small molecule that binds to an enzyme, affording that enzyme catalytic activity. Without the cofactor, the enzyme is inert (ie, it is an **apoenzyme**). All cofactors belong to one of two classes: metals (eg, Mg^{2+}, Zn^{2+}) or small organic molecules (eg, biotin, THF).

Many cofactors are derived from vitamins, for this reason, vitamin deficiencies can be devastating. However, not all symptoms of vitamin deficiencies result from the loss of enzymatic activity.

Vitamin deficiencies can lead to cofactor deficiencies. Once these cofactors are deficient, associated holoenzymes are left unformed, which subsequently results in an inability for certain cellular reactions to occur. This can lead to the phenotypic manifestations of vitamin deficiency disease states.

For example, vitamin B_1 (thiamine) deficiency → thiamine pyrophosphate (TPP) deficiency → pyruvate dehydrogenase, α-ketoglutarate dehydrogenase, and transketolase remain in their inactive, apoenzymatic forms → cells' ability to produce energy is drastically reduced → beriberi (neurologic dysfunction, cardiac dysfunction, weight loss).

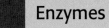

KEY FACT

Almost all enzymes are proteins. However, recent research has revealed that some RNA molecules can act as enzymes (known as ribozymes).

KEY FACT

Apoenzyme + cofactor = holoenzyme.

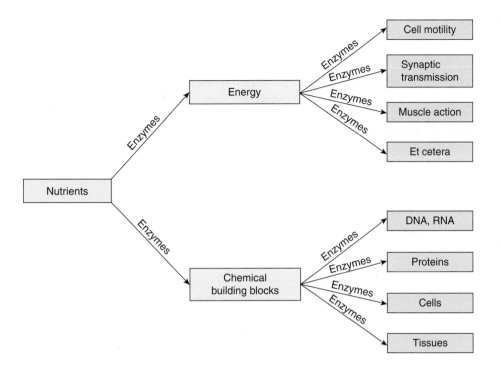

FIGURE 3-25.   Enzyme functions.

THERMODYNAMICS

Enzyme activity can be quantified by several variables, as described in Table 3-12.

GIBBS FREE ENERGY CHANGE

$$\Delta G = \Delta H - T\Delta S$$

ΔG represents the difference in free energy state between the products and the reactants in a reaction. Systems favor low-energy states. Thus, a reaction proceeds in the direction that decreases the system's free energy.

If the reaction, A + B → C + D, is characterized by **ΔG** = −3.0 kJ/mol, then by definition, the reverse reaction, C + D → A + B, is characterized by ΔG = +3.0 kJ/mol.

In this example, A + B → C + D is said to be **exergonic.** It proceeds spontaneously (ie, no energy input is required to drive the reaction).

The reverse reaction, C + D → A + B is said to be **endergonic.** It does not proceed spontaneously but will occur if sufficient energy is added to the system.

For the reaction, A + B $\underset{\leftarrow}{\rightarrow}$ C + D.

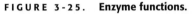

KEY FACT

Enzymes do *not* affect ΔG. Therefore, they do not affect the direction, extent, or spontaneity of a reaction.

TABLE 3-12.　**Thermodynamic Properties**

	ΔG	ΔG_{ACT}	ΔH	ΔS
Represents	Change in free energy.	Free energy of activation.	Change in enthalpy (heat content).	Change in entropy.
Information given	Direction and extent of a reaction.	Rate of reaction.	Whether heat is given off or absorbed.	Level of disorder in system.
Affect by enzymes	No.	Yes—they lower it, which increases the reaction rate.	No.	No.
If < 0	Exergonic reaction—will proceed spontaneously.	Does not occur.	Exothermic reaction—heat is given off.	Does not occur (except in isolated subsets of a system).
If it = 0	System is at equilibrium.	Does not occur.	No change in heat.	The components of the system have neither absorbed nor given off energy.
If > 0	Endergonic reaction— energy input necessary to drive reaction.	Energy of transition state— minimum energy required of reacting molecules for reaction to proceed.	Endothermic reaction— heat is absorbed.	Spontaneous reaction.

THE EQUILIBRIUM CONSTANT

$$\mathbf{K'_{eq}} = [C]\,[D]\,/\,[A]\,[B]$$

K'_{eq} represents the ratio of the concentration of products to reactants when the reaction is at equilibrium (the rates of the forward and reverse reactions are equal, and there is no net change in the amounts of products or reactants).

When $K'_{eq} > 1$, the equilibrium lies to the right, and favors formation of products.

When $K'_{eq} < 1$, the equilibrium lies to the left and favors formation of reactants.

ΔG and K'_{eq} are related by the expression:

$$\Delta G = \Delta G^{\circ\prime} + RT \ln K'_{eq}$$

$\Delta G^{\circ\prime}$ represents the **standard free-energy change,** or the change in free energy when the concentration of the reactants and products are each 1.0 M and the pH is 7. R is the gas constant (8.31 J/mol · K, but do *not* memorize it), and T is the absolute temperature.

KINETICS

Many enzymes' kinetic properties can be explained by the Michaelis-Menten model. For the purposes of Step 1, you can assume Michaelis-Menten kinetics unless stated otherwise.

The Michaelis-Menten model states that:

$$E + S \underset{k_{-1}}{\overset{k_1}{\rightleftharpoons}} ES \overset{k_2}{\rightarrow} E + P$$

- E (enzyme) + S (substrate) must combine to form an ES (enzyme-substrate complex), which then proceeds to E + P (product).
- k_1 represents the rate of complex formation, while k_{-1} represents the rate of dissociation of the complex *back* to reactant.
- k_2 represents the rate of formation of product from the complex.

The concentration of enzyme-substrate complex is dependent on the rates of its formation (k_1) and dissociation (k_1 and k_2).

$$ES \text{ formation} = k_1[E][S]$$

$$ES \text{ breakdown} = (k_{-1} + k_2)[ES]$$

Assuming steady-state conditions for the complex,

$$k_1[E][S] = (k_{-1} + k_2)[ES]$$

or

$$[E][S]/[ES] = (k_{-1} + k_2)/k_1$$

The familiar Michaelis-Menten constant, K_m, combines all of the rate terms.

$$K_m = (k_{-1} + k_2)/k_1$$

K_m compares the rate of breakdown of the complex with the rate of formation, thus representing the affinity that an enzyme and substrate have for each other.

The lower the K_m, the higher the affinity.

The higher the K_m, the lower the affinity.

The rate of the enzymatic reaction, V, is defined as the rate of formation of P.

$$V = k_2[ES]$$

V, therefore, is directly related to [ES], and inversely related to K_m.

These relationships are summarized in Table 3-13 and are represented graphically in Figure 3-26.

> **KEY FACT**
>
> Memorize the indications on these graphs (Figures 3-26 and 3-27). It will save you a lot of time during the exam.

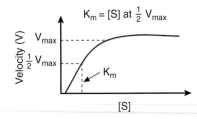

$K_m = [S]$ at $\frac{1}{2} V_{max}$

FIGURE 3-26.   Many functions of enzyme.

TABLE 3-13. K_m Relationships

K_m	INDICATES	IMPLICATION	V
Low	Low k_1 or k_2 *or* High k_{-1}	High enzyme-substrate affinity because ES state is preferred over E and S.	Fast
High	High k_1 or k_2 *or* Low k_{-1}	Low enzyme-substrate affinity because E and S are preferred over ES state.	Slow

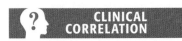

CLINICAL CORRELATION

Alcohol dehydrogenase catalyzes the conversion of methanol to formic acid and formaldehyde. The accumulation of these products causes blindness. The antidote for methanol poisoning is ethanol administration. Ethanol **competitively inhibits** alcohol dehydrogenase by binding to the enzyme's active site and preventing the enzyme from binding to methanol. Inhibition of methanol binding prevents further accumulation of formic acid and formaldehyde by promoting the conversion of ethanol of nontoxic acetaldehyde.

CLINICAL CORRELATION

Once ethanol is oxidized by alcohol dehydrogenase to acetylaldehyde, acetylaldehyde dehydrogenase further oxidizes the aldehyde to acetic acid. This conversion is inhibited by the medication disulfiram, which is used to treat chronic alcoholism by causing an acute illness upon ingestion of ethanol. A "disulfiram effect" can also be seen by a number of other medications including metronidazole, tolbutamide, cefoperazone, and cefotetan.

As the substrate concentration increases, the rate of the reaction, V, increases. The asymptotic V_{max} occurs at the substrate concentration that saturates the enzyme's active sites. At this [S], adding more substrate will not increase the rate of the reaction because there are no additional sites for the formation of the ES complex. Often, the relationship between V and S is plotted reciprocally as a **Lineweaver-Burk plot** to obtain a linear plot, as shown in Figure 3-27.

Inhibitors are molecules that bind to an enzyme and decrease its activity.

Competitive inhibitors **compete** for the active site. They bind at the same site as the substrate, thus preventing the substrate from binding.

Noncompetitive inhibitors bind at a site **distinct** from the active site. They reduce the enzyme's efficiency without affecting substrate binding. These differences are summarized in Table 3-14.

REGULATION

An enzyme's efficacy is regulated by many factors.

pH

The activity of enzymes is dependent on pH. Each enzyme has an optimal pH at which it is maximally active.

- The optimal pH varies by enzyme.
- The optimal pH often depends on the ionization state of the enzyme's side chain(s).
- The optimal pH often "makes sense" physiologically.
- Pepsin is an enzyme that breaks down protein in the stomach. Its optimal pH is about 2, which corresponds to the stomach's acidic environment.

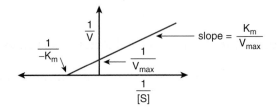

slope $= \dfrac{K_m}{V_{max}}$

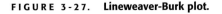

FIGURE 3-27.   Lineweaver-Burk plot.

TABLE 3-14.   Enzyme Inhibition

	COMPETITIVE INHIBITORS	WHY	NONCOMPETITIVE INHIBITORS	WHY
Resemble substrate	Yes	—	No	—
Overcome by increasing [S]	Yes	Greater probability that substrate, rather than inhibitor, will bind active site.	No	Inhibition is due to effect on enzyme alone, not enzyme-substrate interaction.
Bind active site	Yes	—	No	—
Effect on V_{max}	Unchanged	With maximal [S], inhibition is overcome.[a]	Down	Enzyme cannot function at maximal efficiency.
Effect on K_m	Up	Presence of inhibitor decreases the likelihood of enzyme-substrate binding (affinity of the enzyme for the substrate).	Unchanged	Inhibitor does not affect likelihood of enzyme-substrate binding since it binds to the enzyme at a separate site.

[a]Although V_{max} itself is unchanged, it occurs at a greater [S] than when no inhibitor is present.

Temperature

In general, as temperature increases, an enzyme's activity also increases (the heat increases the kinetic energy in the system). In biology lab, you probably incubated many enzymatic reactions at 37°C or higher. At these temperatures, the enzyme-catalyzed reactions occur much more rapidly than they would have occurred at room temperature (22°C).

- Above a certain temperature, enzymatic activity rapidly decreases. This is due to protein denaturation.
- Each enzyme has a different optimum temperature.

Concentration

- Increased enzyme concentration increases activity because more active sites are available for binding by reactants.
- Decreased enzyme concentration decreases activity because fewer active sites are available for binding by reactants.
- In the cell or the body, the concentration of any enzyme is determined by the relative rates of enzyme synthesis and enzyme degradation.
- Enzyme synthesis may be increased in the presence of an inducer or decreased in the presence of a repressor.
- Inducers and repressors act at the level of transcription by binding to DNA regulatory elements.
- Enzyme degradation is mediated by ubiquitination, which tags proteins for destruction by the proteasome.

Covalent Modification

An enzyme's activity can be altered by the attachment or removal of other molecules. Such additions or subtractions may change the enzyme's structure or other properties, resulting in a change in enzyme activity.

Phosphorylation and Dephosphorylation

Each of these processes can increase *or* decrease enzymatic activity, depending on the particular enzyme.

- Phosphorylation occurs at serine, threonine, and tyrosine residues.
- Kinases are enzymes that catalyze phosphorylation.
- Phosphatases are enzymes that catalyze dephosphorylation.
  - **Acetylation** and **dephosphorylation** (eg, COX-2)
  - γ-**Decarboxylation** (eg, thrombin)
  - **ADP-ribosylation** (eg, RNA polymerase)

Zymogens (Proenzymes)

Inactive precursors to enzymes that must be cleaved in some way to achieve their active form.

Example: The complement and coagulation cascades each consist of a chain of zymogens.

- Once activated, each zymogen cleaves and activates the next zymogen in the sequence.
- This mechanism allows large quantities of the complement and clotting proteins to be present at sites where they might be needed.
  - Because the factors are inactive, there is little risk of excessive immune response or thrombosis, respectively.
  - Because the factors are already synthesized and localized, the systems may be mobilized extremely quickly when needed.

Allosteric Regulation

An enzyme's activity can be modified by the binding of a ligand to an allosteric site (a site **distinct from** the active site).

- The modulator may increase or decrease the enzyme's activity.
- The modulator may be the reactant or product itself, or it may be a distinct molecule.
- In many cases, the product of a reaction binds to its enzyme at an allosteric site to decrease further formation. This is a common mechanism of **feedback inhibition.**

The Cell

CELLULAR ORGANELLES AND FUNCTION

The **plasma membrane** is composed of a **lipid bilayer,** which separates the cytosol from the extracellular environment, maintains the structural integrity of the cell, and serves as an **impermeable barrier to water-soluble molecules** (Figure 3-28). The lipid bilayer is a continuous double-sided membrane that is a dynamic, fluid structure. The membrane's fluidity allows movement of molecules laterally within a single membrane and can be influenced by the factors listed in Table 3-15.

There are two main functional groups within the lipid bilayer: **lipid molecules** and **membrane proteins.**

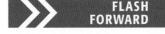

FLASH FORWARD

Trypsin is a digestive enzyme that plays a major role in protein degradation. Its activity is controlled by the enzyme **enterokinase** (only expressed in the small intestine), which cleaves the zymogen trypsinogen to active trypsin.

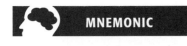

MNEMONIC

Allos = other. An **allosteric** site is one *other* than the active site.

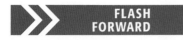

FLASH FORWARD

G_q protein signaling involves the cleavage of inositol phospholipids (phosphatidyl inositol 4,5 bisphosphate = PIP_2), which are present in the plasma membrane in smaller quantities than the four major phospholipids listed in Table 3-16.

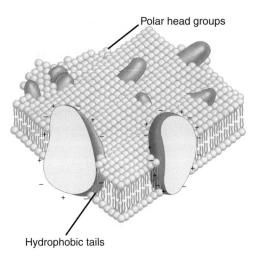

Polar head groups

Hydrophobic tails

FIGURE 3-28.   **Plasma membrane structure.**

Lipids

Membrane lipids fall into the following three classes:

1. **Phospholipids:** The most abundant lipid molecules. Phospholipids are **amphipathic,** having both a **hydrophilic (polar) head group** and typically two **hydrophobic (nonpolar) tails** (Figure 3-28). This amphipathic nature results in the spontaneous formation of a lipid bilayer when phospholipids are placed in an aqueous environment. There are four major phospholipids, arranged asymmetrically within the lipid bilayer (Table 3-16). This asymmetry has many important functional consequences for the cell and, if altered, can trigger inflammatory reactions in surrounding cells.
2. **Cholesterol:** Decreases the fluidity of the membrane (Table 3-15).
3. **Glycolipids:** Sugar-containing lipids found only on the outer membrane.

Proteins

The second major component of the lipid bilayer is proteins, which carry out most membrane functions. The plasma membrane contains two main types of proteins: peripheral membrane proteins and transmembrane proteins (Figure 3-28).

PERIPHERAL MEMBRANE PROTEINS

- Are **hydrophilic** only.
- Bind to either the inner or outer membrane via noncovalent interactions with other membrane proteins.
- Do **not** extend into the hydrophobic interior of the membrane.

KEY FACT

It requires **energy** to run **uphill** = **active transport**
It's **easy** to run **downhill** = no energy required for **passive transport**

TABLE 3-15.   **Factors That Affect Plasma Membrane Fluidity**

INCREASE MEMBRANE FLUIDITY	DECREASE MEMBRANE FLUIDITY
↑ Temperature.	↓ Temperature.
↑ Unsaturation of fatty acids (↑ no. of double bonds).	↓ Unsaturation of fatty acids (↓ no. of double bonds).
↓ Cholesterol content.	↑ Cholesterol content.

TABLE 3-16. Membrane Location of the Four Major Phospholipids

Outer Membrane	Inner Membrane
Phosphatidylcholine	Phosphatidylethanolamine
Sphingomyelin	Phosphatidylserine

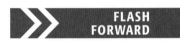

FLASH FORWARD

The Na⁺-K⁺ pump transports three positive ions out of the cell and only two positive ions into the cell, resulting in the creating of a relative negative charge inside the cell. This **electrical membrane potential** has many important functional consequences for the cell.

FLASH FORWARD

Ouabain and the **cardiac glycosides (digoxin and digitoxin)** both bind and inhibit the Na⁺-K⁺ ATPase by competing for sites with on the extracellular side of the pump. The binding of these inhibitors results in increased cardiac contractility (through a Ca^{2+}-dependent mechanism).

TRANSMEMBRANE PROTEINS

- Are **amphipathic** (have both hydrophobic and hydrophilic regions).
- Hydrophobic regions pass through the hydrophobic interior of the membrane and interact with the hydrophobic tails of the lipid molecules.
- Hydrophilic regions are exposed to water on both sides of the membrane.

Membrane proteins play many important roles in the plasma membrane, including functioning in transport and as receptors and enzymes.

TRANSPORT PROTEINS

Transmembrane proteins that allow small polar molecules (that would otherwise be inhibited by the hydrophobic interior of the plasma membrane) to cross the lipid bilayer. There are two main classes of transport proteins (Figure 3-29):

- **Carrier proteins (transporters):** Undergo **conformational changes** to move specific molecules across the membrane.
- **Channel proteins (ion channels):** Form a narrow **hydrophilic pore** to allow passage of small inorganic ions.

Transport across the membrane can either be **active,** in which the solute is pumped "uphill" against its electrochemical gradient in an energy-dependent manner, or **passive,** in which the transport of a solute is driven by its electro-

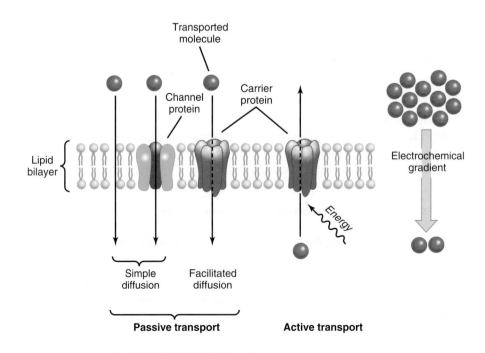

FIGURE 3-29.   Carrier proteins and channel proteins.

chemical gradient "**downhill**" (Figure 3-30). Active transport can be driven either by ATP hydrolysis or by harnessing energy from the downhill flow of another solute. Transport via carrier proteins can be either active or passive, whereas transport by channel proteins is always passive.

CARRIER PROTEINS (TRANSPORTERS)

There are three types of carrier proteins, most of which use active transport mechanisms (Figure 3-31):

- **Uniporters:** Transport a single solute from one side of the membrane to the other.
- **Symporters:** Transport two solutes across the membrane in the same direction.
- **Antiporters:** Transport two solutes across the membrane in opposite directions.

The most important carrier protein is the **Na^+-K^+ ATPase** or **Na^+-K^+ pump,** which is found in the basolateral membrane of nearly all cells. The Na^+-K^+ pump is an **antiporter** that utilizes the energy released from ATP hydrolysis to pump **three Na^+ ions out of the cell** and **two K^+ ions into the cell** with each cycle (Figure 3-32). The transport cycle depends on the phosphorylation and dephosphorylation of the Na^+-K^+ pump.

CHANNEL PROTEINS (ION CHANNELS)

Form **small, highly selective hydrophilic pores** that allow the **passive transport of specific inorganic ions** (primarily Na^+, K^+, Ca^+, or Cl^-) down their electrochemical gradients. Transport across ion channels (which do not need to undergo a conformational change) is much faster than transport via carrier proteins. Ion channels are selectively opened and closed in response to different stimuli, which determines the specific ion channel type:

- **Voltage stimulus** = voltage-gated ion channels
- **Mechanical stress stimulus** = mechanical-gated ion channels
- **Ligand binding stimulus** = ligand-gated ion channels

The activity of the majority of these channels is also regulated by protein phosphorylation and dephosphorylation.

The most common ion channels are the **K^+ leak channels,** which are found in the plasma membrane of almost all animal cells. K^+ leak channels are **open even when unstimulated or in a resting state,** which makes the plasma membrane much more permeable to K^+ than to other ions. This K^+-selective permeability plays a critical role in maintaining the membrane potential in nearly all cells.

G-PROTEIN COUPLED RECEPTORS

In addition to transporting small molecules, membrane proteins can also function as receptors. **G-protein coupled receptors,** the most important class of cell membrane receptors, are proteins that traverse the plasma membrane seven times (**seven-pass receptors**). They are **coupled to trimeric GTP-binding proteins (G proteins),** which are composed of **three subunits: α, β, and γ.** The G proteins are found on the cytosolic face of the membrane and serve as relay molecules. G-protein coupled receptors have extremely diverse functions and respond to a vast array of stimuli. However, all G-protein coupled receptor signaling is transduced via a similar mechanism (Figure 3-33).

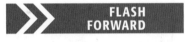

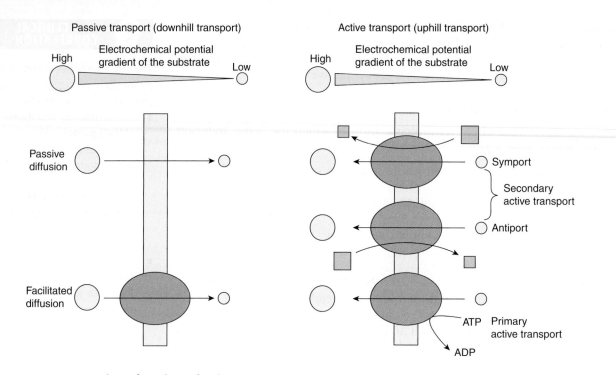

Passive transport (downhill transport)

Active transport (uphill transport)

Electrochemical potential gradient of the substrate

High — Low

Electrochemical potential gradient of the substrate

High — Low

Passive diffusion

Facilitated diffusion

Symport

Secondary active transport

Antiport

ATP   Primary active transport

ADP

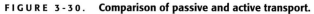

FIGURE 3-30. **Comparison of passive and active transport.**

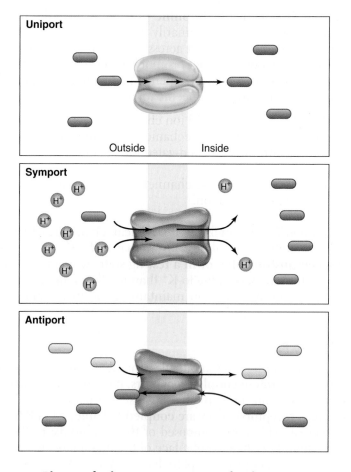

Uniport

Outside   Inside

Symport

H^+

Antiport

FIGURE 3-31. **Diagram of uniporters, symporters, and antiporters.**

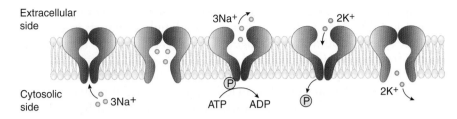

FIGURE 3-32.   The Na$^+$-K$^+$ pump transport cycle.

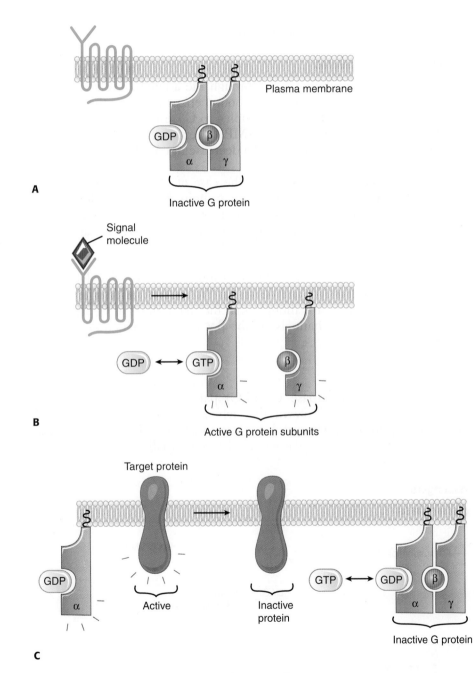

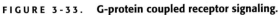

FIGURE 3-33.   G-protein coupled receptor signaling.

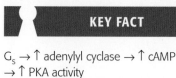

KEY FACT

$G_s \rightarrow \uparrow$ adenylyl cyclase $\rightarrow \uparrow$ cAMP $\rightarrow \uparrow$ PKA activity
$G_i \rightarrow \downarrow$ adenylyl cyclase $\rightarrow \downarrow$ cAMP $\rightarrow \downarrow$ PKA activity

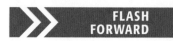

FLASH FORWARD

Autonomic receptor types:
Adrenergic: Q-I-S-S: $\alpha_1 \rightarrow G_q$, $\alpha_2 \rightarrow G_i$, $\beta_1 \rightarrow G_s$, $\beta_2 \rightarrow G_s$
Muscarinic: Q-I-Q: $M_1 \rightarrow G_q$, $M_2 \rightarrow G_i$, $M_3 \rightarrow G_q$

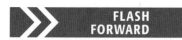

FLASH FORWARD

Cholera toxin is an enzyme that catalyzes **ADP ribosylation of the α_s subunit.** This blocks GTPase activity so it is continuously bound to GTP and therefore continuously active. The resulting activation of adenylyl cyclase causes large effluxes of Na^+ and water into the gut lumen, resulting in **severe diarrhea.**

When the receptor is **inactive,** the α subunit (active subunit) of the G protein is bound to **GDP.** When the receptor is **stimulated,** a change in conformation causes the α subunit to exchange GDP for **GTP,** thereby releasing itself from the $\beta\gamma$ complex. Once released, it binds and activates target proteins. α Subunit activity is short-lived, however, because the **GTPase** quickly hydrolyzes GTP to GDP, resulting in its inactivation. The target proteins activated by the α subunit vary, depending on which of the three main types of G protein is involved.

- Gs (stimulatory G protein) = $\uparrow$ cAMP levels
- Gi (inhibitory G protein) = $\downarrow$ cAMP levels
- Gq = activates phospholipase C (PLC)

G_s- AND G_i-PROTEIN SIGNALING

Both the G_s and G_i **proteins** signal through the **adenylyl cyclase pathway.** Adenylyl cyclase is a plasma-membrane-bound enzyme that synthesizes cyclic AMP (cAMP) from ATP. Receptors coupled to G_s result in the **activation of adenylyl cyclase** and an **increase in cAMP.** Receptors coupled to G_i result in the **inhibition of adenylyl cyclase** and a **decrease in cAMP.**

Increased concentrations of cAMP (in the case of G_s) results in the activation of cAMP-dependent protein kinase **protein kinase A (PKA),** which phosphorylates certain intracellular protein targets to cause a specific cellular response. A protein phosphatase dephosphorylates the protein targets, thus turning off their activity.

In G_i-protein signaling, the activated α_i subunit inhibits adenylyl cyclase, resulting in decreased cAMP and decreased PKA activity. Although this does elicit a cellular response, it is thought that the main effect of G_i signaling is the activation of K^+ ion channels via the $\beta_i\gamma_l$ complex, which allows K^+ to flow into the cell.

G_Q-PROTEIN SIGNALING

Occurs via the **phospholipase C (PLC) pathway.** Phospholipase C is a plasma membrane–bound enzyme that, when activated, cleaves the inositol phospholipid **phosphatidylinositol 4,5-bisphosphate (PIP$_2$),** which is present in the inner leaflet of the plasma membrane in small amounts (see discus-

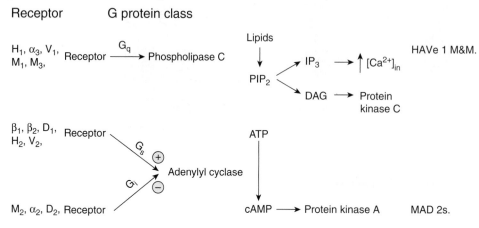

FIGURE 3-34. G-protein coupled receptor summary.

sion of plasma membranes earlier under The Cell). This cleavage results in the formation of **inositol 1,4,5-triphosphate (IP_3)** and **diacylglycerol (DAG)**. IP_3 causes **Ca^{2+} release from the ER,** which activates the **Ca^{2+}/calmodulin-dependent protein kinase (or cAM-kinase).** cAM-kinase then phosphorylates certain intracellular proteins, resulting in a specific cellular response. DAG activates **protein kinase C (PKC)** directly, which also phosphorylates certain intracellular proteins, resulting in a specific cellular response (Figure 3-34).

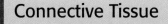

Connective Tissue

CLASSIFICATION

One of the four basic tissue types, connective tissue serves as the structural support and internal framework of the body. There are many types of connective tissue (ie, bone, ligaments, tendons, cartilage, adipose tissue, and aponeuroses), but they all contain the same basic structural components: **few cells** and a large amount of **extracellular matrix (ECM)** that includes **ground substance and fibers.** Adult connective tissue can be classified based on the composition and function of each tissue type.

Composition

- **Loose connective tissue:** Loosely arranged fibers, abundant cells, and ground substance (ie, lamina propria).
- **Dense irregular connective tissue:** Irregularly arranged collagen fibers and few cells (ie, reticular layer of the dermis).
- **Dense regular connective tissue:** Densely packed parallel fibers with few cells packed in between (ie, tendons, ligaments, aponeuroses).

Function

- **Structural:** Forms capsules around organs or adipose tissue that fills the spaces between organs.
- **Support:** Hard connective tissue with fibrous components arranged in parallel arrays (ie, bone, cartilage).
- **Nutrition:** Helps facilitate uptake of nutrients from extracellular space.
- **Defense:** The presence of phagocytic cells (ie, macrophages) and immunocompetent cells (ie, plasma cells and eosinophils) in the ECM are part of the body's defense mechanism against foreign objects.

GROUND SUBSTANCE

Ground substance is a viscous, clear substance that occupies the space between the cells and fibers within connective tissue. Ground substance contains three main types of macromolecules:

- Proteogylcans
- Glycoproteins
- Fibrous proteins

The fibrous proteins and glycoproteins are embedded in a proteoglycan gel, where they form an extensive **ECM** that serves both structural and adhesive functions.

FLASH FORWARD

Pertussis toxin is an enzyme that catalyzes the **ADP ribosylation of the α_i subunit,** blocking its dissociation from the $\beta_i\gamma_i$ complex so it is unable to inhibit adenylyl cyclase. Thus, adenylyl cyclase is permanently activated resulting in **whooping cough.**

KEY FACT

$G_q \rightarrow \uparrow$ PLC activity $\rightarrow PIP_2 \rightarrow IP_3$ + DAG

$IP_3 \rightarrow \uparrow Ca^{2+} \rightarrow \uparrow$ CaM-kinase activity

DAG $\rightarrow \uparrow$ PKC activity

Proteoglycans

These macromolecules consist of a **core protein** that is covalently attached to approximately 100 **glycosaminoglycan (GAG)** molecules and a **linker protein,** which binds hyaluronic acid (HA) and strengthens its interaction with the proteoglycan molecule (Figure 3-35). Proteoglycans are very large, highly negatively charged macromolecules that attract water into the ground substance, giving it a gel-like consistency. This highly hydrated gel is able to resist compressive forces while allowing diffusion of O_2 and nutrients between the blood and tissue cells.

Glycosaminoglycans (GAGs)

GAGs are long polysaccharide chains composed of repeating disaccharide units. One of the disaccharide units is always an **amino sugar** (N-acetylglucosamine or N-acetylgalactosamine), which is most often **sulfated (SO_4^{2-}).** The second sugar is usually an **uronic acid** (glucuronic or iduronic). GAGs are the most negatively charged molecules produced by animal cells because of the sulfate and carboxyl groups present on most of their sugars. These highly negatively charged molecules are essential for maintaining the high water content present in ground substance. Five types of GAGs are found in the human body (Table 3-17).

Glycoproteins

Glycoproteins are large, multidomain proteins that help organize the ECM and attach it to surrounding cells. There are two main glycoproteins: **fibronectin** and **laminin,** both of which are present in the **basal lamina** of cells.

BASAL LAMINA (BASEMENT MEMBRANE)

Basal lamina is specialized ECM that underlies all epithelial cells and surrounds individual muscle, fat, and Schwann cells. It separates the cells from the underlying connective tissue, serves as a filter in the renal glomerulus, and functions as a scaffold during tissue regeneration/wound healing. The basal

> **FLASH FORWARD**

Alport syndrome results from a **mutation** in the α_5 **chain of type IV collagen,** which destroys the ability of the glomerular basement membrane to properly filter blood in the kidney. Patients with Alport syndrome suffer from **kidney failure, nerve deafness,** and **ocular disorders** (all organ sites where the α_5 chain of type IV collagen are found).

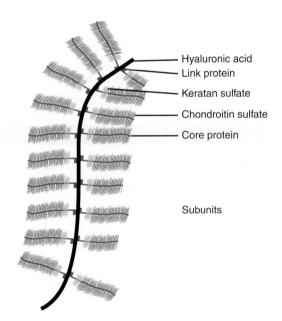

Hyaluronic acid
Link protein
Keratan sulfate
Chondroitin sulfate
Core protein

Subunits

FIGURE 3-35. Proteoglycan structure.

TABLE 3-17. Glycosaminoglycans

GAG	LOCATION
Hyaluronic acid	Most connective tissues bind to the link protein of many proteoglycans to form proteoglycan aggregates.
Chondroitin sulfate	Cartilage and bone; heart valves.
Keratan sulfate	Cartilage, bone, cornea, and intervertebral disk.
Dermatan sulfate	Dermis of skin, blood vessels, and heart valves.
Heparan sulfate	Basal lamina, lung, and liver.

lamina is synthesized by the cells that rest on it and contains the following elements:

- Fibronectin
- Laminin
- Heparan sulfate
- Type IV collagen

FIBRONECTIN

Fibronectin is a dimer composed of two large subunits bound together by disulfide bridges that each contain domains specialized for binding a specific molecule (ie, integrins, collagen, or heparan) or cells. Fibronectin helps cells attach to the extracellular matrix via its different binding domains.

LAMININ

Laminin is composed of three long polypeptide chains (α, β, γ) arranged in the shape of an asymmetrical cross. Individual laminin molecules self-assemble and form extensive networks that bind to type IV collagen and form the major structural framework of basement membranes. Laminin also contains many functional domains that bind other ECM components and cell surface receptors, thus linking cells with the ECM.

FIBERS

Fibers are present in varying amounts based on the structural and functional needs of the connective tissue type. **All fibers are produced by fibroblasts** present in the connective tissue and are composed of long peptide chains. There are three types of connective tissue fibers:

- Collagen fibers
- Reticular fibers
- Elastic fibers

Collagen Fibers

Composed of collagen, the most abundant protein in the human body. Collagen fibers are flexible and provide high tensile strength to tissues. Collagen consists of **three polypeptide chains (α chains) wound around each other to** form a long, stiff **triple helical structure** (Figure 3-36). Collagen is **glycine**

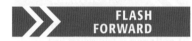

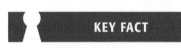

KEY FACT

Collagen amino acid sequence = **Gly-X-Y (X and Y commonly proline or hydroxyproline, respectively)**

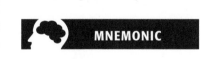

MNEMONIC

Type **I: B**one
Type **II: Car**two**l**age
Type **IV:** Under the **floor** (basement membrane)

Amino acid sequence   — Gly — X — Y — Gly — X — Y — Gly — X — Y —

Secondary structure

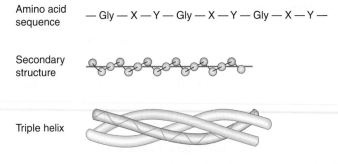

Triple helix

FIGURE 3-36.   Structure of a collagen molecule. (Modified with permission from Murray RK, Granner DK, Rodwell VW. *Harper's Illustrated Biochemistry*, 27th ed. New York, NY: McGraw-Hill; 2006: 39.)

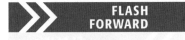

FLASH FORWARD

During **wound healing, type III collagen** is laid down first in **granulation tissue.** As healing progresses, fibroblasts secrete **type I collagen,** which **eventually replaces type III collagen in late wound repair.**

KEY FACT

**Wound healing: Type III →
Type I**

Three: owie (just scraped your
    knee).
One: it's all done.

and **proline rich,** with glycine present as every third amino acid. The repeating amino acid sequence found in collagen is thus **gly-X-Y,** in which X and Y can be any amino acid (but X is commonly proline and Y is commonly hydroxyproline). One-third of the collagen amino acid structure is glycine; proline or hydroxyproline typically constitute one-sixth of the amino acid content of collagen. This sequence is absolutely critical for triple-helix formation.

The α chains in each collagen molecule are not the same. They range in size from 600 to 3000 amino acids. At present, at least 42 types of α chains encoded by different genes have been identified, and 27 different types of collagen have been categorized based on their distinct α chain compositions. Depending on the specific type of collagen molecule, it may consist of three identical α chains (homotrimeric) or consist of two or three genetically distinct α chains (heterotrimeric). The most important collagen types are described in Table 3-18.

TABLE 3-18.   Collagen Types, Composition, and Location

TYPE	COMPOSITION[a]	LOCATION
I	$[\alpha_1(I)]_2, \alpha_2(I)$	Most abundant (90%). **Bone,** tendon, skin, dentin, fascia, cornea, late wound repair.
II	$[\alpha_1(II)]_3$	**Cartilage,** vitreous body, nucleus pulposus.
III (reticulin)	$[\alpha_1(III)]_3$	Skin, **blood vessels,** uterus, fetal tissue, **granulation tissue.**
IV	$[\alpha_1(IV)]_2, [\alpha_2(IV)]$	**Basal lamina** (basement membrane); kidney, glomeruli, lens capsule.
X	$[\alpha_1(X)]_3$	Epiphyseal plate.

[a]The Roman numerals simply indicate the chronological order of discovery and that each α chain has a unique structure that differs from the α chains with different numerals.

COLLAGEN SYNTHESIS

Connective tissue cells or fibroblasts produce the majority of the collagen fibers. The biosynthesis process involves a series of both intra- and extracellular events (Figure 3-37).

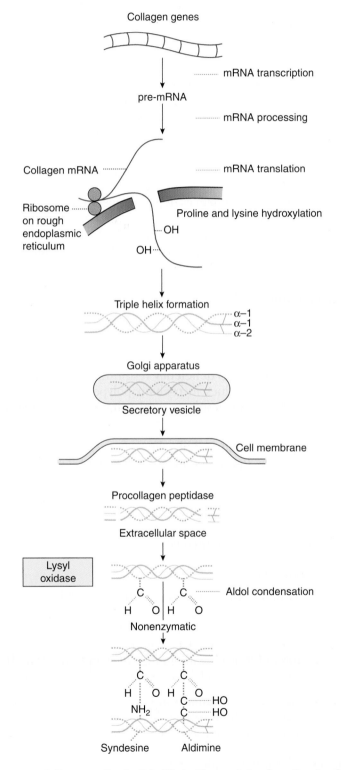

FIGURE 3-37. **Collagen synthesis.** (Modified with permission from Brunicardi FC, Andersen DK, Billiar TR, et al. *Schwartz's Principles of Surgery*, 8th ed. New York: McGraw-Hill, 2007: 227.)

INTRACELLULAR EVENTS

- Uptake of amino acids (proline, lysine, etc.) by endocytosis.
- Formation of α chains (preprocollagen) mRNA in nucleus.
- Nuclear export of preprocollagen mRNA followed by entry into the rough ER (RER).
- Synthesis of preprocollagen α chains with registration sequences by ribosomes within the RER.
- Hydroxylation of proline and lysine within the RER catalyzed by peptidyl proline hydroxylase and peptidyl lysine hydroxylase. *This step requires vitamin C.*
- Glycosylation of hydroxylysine residues within the RER.
- Formation of α chain triple helix (procollagen) within the RER.
- Addition of carbohydrates within the Golgi network.
- Packaging into vesicles and movement to the plasma membrane.
- Exocytosis of procollagen.

EXTRACELLULAR EVENTS

- Cleavage of registration sequences of procollagen to form tropocollagen by procollagen peptidases.
- Self-assembly of tropocollagen into fibrils.
- Cross-linking of adjacent tropocollagen molecules catalyzed by lysyl oxidase.

Clinical Considerations

Many disorders are associated with defects in collagen synthesis.

SCURVY

Scurvy is caused by vitamin C deficiency resulting in the inability to hydroxylate proline and lysine residues in α-chain polypeptides of collagen molecules (see step 5 above). This results in **weakening of the capillaries** and the following complications:

- Ulceration of gums and gingival bleeding.
- Loose teeth (due to loss of periodontal ligaments, which are collagen rich).
- Tissue hemorrhage.
- Anemia.
- Poor wound healing.
- Impaired bone formation (in infants).

OSTEOGENESIS IMPERFECTA (OI)

Primarily an **autosomal dominant** disorder, OI is caused by a **variety of gene defects** leading to either **less collagen or less functional collagen** than normal (with the same amount of collagen present). Both conditions result in **weak or brittle bones.** The incidence is approximately 1:10,000 individuals. There are four types of OI, each with a range of symptoms. Type II is fatal in utero or in the neonatal period. The most common characteristics are:

- **Multiple fractures with minimal trauma** (may occur during the birthing process and is often confused with child abuse).
- **Blue sclerae** (due to the translucency of the connective tissue over the choroids).
- **Hearing loss** (abnormal middle ear bones).
- **Dental imperfections** (defects in enamel synthesis = amelogenesis imperfecta).

KEY FACT

Defect in collagen synthesis:
- Collagen has three polypeptide chains that form a triple helix. Chains are made up of glycine-X-Y repeats.
- Point mutation in glycine prevents the formation of a triple helix.

EHLERS-DANLOS SYNDROME

Ehlers-Danlos syndrome is actually a group of rare genetic disorders resulting in **defective collagen synthesis.** There are over 10 types, with disease severity ranging from mild to life-threatening, depending on the specific mutation. The most common symptoms are:

- Hyperextensible skin.
- Bleeding tendency (easy bruising), associated with berry aneurysms.
- Hypermobile joints.

Reticular Fibers

Type III collagen fibrils arranged in a mesh-like pattern provide a supporting framework for cells in various tissues and organs. Reticular fibers contain a higher content of sugar groups (6–12% compared with 1% in collagen fibers) and are easily identified by the periodic acid–Schiff (PAS) stain. They are also recognized with silver stains and are thus termed **argyrophilic** (silver-loving) (Figure 3-38). Networks of reticular fibers are found in loose connective tissue in the space between the epithelia and connective tissue, as well as around adipocytes, small blood vessels, nerves, and muscle cells. Reticular fibers are also found in the stroma of hemopoietic, lymphatic, and endocrine tissues.

Elastic Fibers

Elastic fibers, which allow tissues to stretch and distend, are found in skin, vertebral ligaments (ligamenta flava of the vertebral column and ligamentum nuchae of the neck), the vocal folds of the larynx, and elastic arteries.

Elastic fibers consist of two structural components: elastin and surrounding fibrillin microfibrils.

ELASTIN

This highly hydrophobic protein, like collagen, is rich in proline and glycine. However, unlike collagen, elastin is poor in hydroxyproline and lacks hydroxylysine. The glycine molecules are randomly distributed, allowing for random coiling of its fibers. Elastin is produced by fibroblasts and smooth muscle cells, and its synthesis parallels collagen production. In fact, both processes

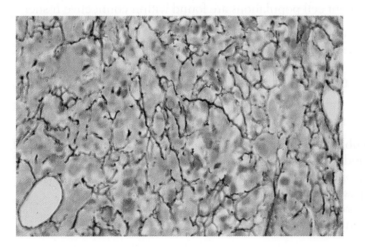

FIGURE 3-38. **Reticular fibers (silver stain).** (Reproduced with permission from Lichtman MA, Beutler E, Kipps TJ, et al. *Williams Hematology*, 7th ed. New York: McGraw-Hill, 2007: Plate XIV-12.)

can occur simultaneously within the same cell. Elastin synthesis entails two main steps:

- **Secretion of tropoelastin** (elastin precursor).
- **Cross-linking of tropoelastin** molecules via their two unique amino acids—**desmosine and isodesmosine**—to form extensive networks of elastin fibers and sheets.

Single elastin polypeptides adopt a loose "random coil" conformation when relaxed. When individual elastin proteins are cross-linked into an elastic fiber network, their collective random coil properties allow the network to stretch and recoil like a rubber band.

FIBRILLIN-I

Fibrillin-I is a glycoprotein that forms fine microfibrils. Its microfibrils are formed first during elastic fiber genesis; elastin is then deposited on to the surface of the microfibrils. Elastin-associated fibrillin microfibrils play a major role in organizing elastin into fibers.

MARFAN SYNDROME

Marfan syndrome is a relatively common (1:3–5000) **autosomal dominant** connective tissue disorder caused by a **mutation in the fibrillin gene (FBN1)**. In individuals with Marfan syndrome elastin-associated fibrillin microfibrils are absent, resulting in the formation of **abnormal elastic tissue.** The severity of the disease varies; affected individuals may die young or live essentially normal lives. Common symptoms include:

- **Bone elongation** (tall individuals with long, thin limbs).
- **Spider-like fingers** (arachnodactyly).
- **Hypermobile joints.**
- **Lens dislocation** (glaucoma and retinal detachment also common).
- **Cardiac abnormalities** (mitral valve prolapse is common).
- **Aortic rupture—most common cause of death** (due to loss of elastic fibers in tunica media).

CELLS

Two different cell populations are found within connective tissue:

- Resident cells
- Transient cells

Resident Cells

Relatively stable, permanent residents of connective tissue. These cells remain in the connective tissue and include:

- **Fibroblasts and myofibroblasts** (primary cells involved in collagen and ground substance secretion).
- **Macrophages** (arise from migrating monocytes).
- **Adipose cells.**
- **Mast cells** (arise from stem cells in the bone marrow).
- **Mesenchymal cells.**

Transient Cells

Wandering cells that have migrated into the connective tissue from the blood in response to specific stimuli (usually during inflammation). This population is not normally found in connective tissue and is composed of cells involved in the immune response:

- Lymphocytes
- Plasma cells
- Neutrophils
- Eosinophils
- Basophils
- Monocytes

Homeostasis and Metabolism

Various processes contribute to maintaining the energy, structure, and waste removal needs of living cell. These systems are intricate and interdependent, as summarized in Figure 3-39.

Metabolism converts four classes of substrate into energy or other usable products. These substrates include:

- Carbohydrates
- Lipids and fatty acids
- Proteins and amino acids
- Nucleotides

CARBOHYDRATE METABOLISM

A process by which carbohydrates are broken down into water and carbon dioxide, accompanied by the generation of energy, mainly in the form of **adenosine triphosphate (ATP)**. The overall reaction is relatively simple.

$$C_6H_{12}O_6 + 6O_2 \rightarrow 6H_2O + 6CO_2$$

However, the process is complicated by its relation to other metabolic cycles, namely, the fatty acid cycle, the urea cycle, Kreb cycle (tricarboxylic acid, TCA cycle), and the hexose monophosphate (HMP) shunt.

Intake and Absorption

Digestion of carbohydrates begins in the mouth and ends in the small intestine with absorption of the breakdown products. **Polysaccharides** (starch) and **oligosaccharides** (sucrose and lactose) are converted into **disaccharides** and **monosaccharides.**

- The monosaccharides are absorbed via transporters and carried to the liver through the portal vein.
- Ultimately, these are oxidized, stored as glycogen, transformed to fat (triglycerides), or transported as glucose via the circulation.

Glycolysis

FUNCTION

Initial step in the metabolism of glucose to produce energy for the cell. Glycolysis usually occurs under aerobic environments, but can occur under anaerobic conditions.

LOCATION

Cytoplasm of all cells that utilize glucose.

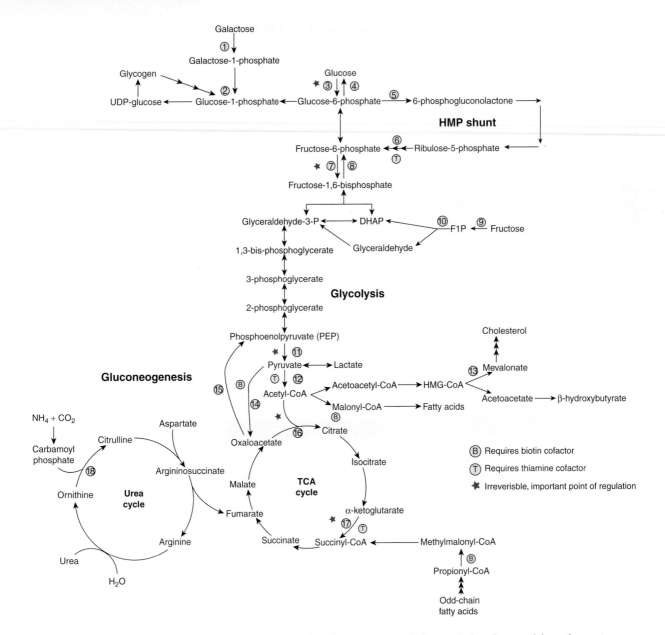

FIGURE 3-39. **Metabolic pathways.** (1) Galactokinase (mild galactosemia); (2) Galactose-1-phosphate uridyltransferase; (severe galactosemia); (3) Hexokinase/glucokinase; (4) Glucose-6-phosphatase (von Gierke); (5) Glucose-6-phosphate dehydrogenase (G6PD); (6) Transketolase; (7) Phosphofructokinase; (8) Fructose-1,6-bisphosphatase; (9) Fructokinase (essential fructosuria); (10) Aldolase B (fructose intolerance); (11) Pyruvate kinase; (12) Pyruvate dehydrogenase; (13) HMG-CoA reductase; (14) Pyruvate carboxylase; (15) phosphoenolpyruvate (PEP) carboxykinase; (16) Citrate synthase; (17) α-Ketoglutarate dehydrogenase; (18) Ornithine transcarbamylase.

REACTANTS

One molecule of glucose.

PRODUCTS

Aerobic glycolysis: Two molecules of pyruvate, two ATP, two NADH. Anaerobic glycolysis: Two molecules of lactic acid (from pyruvate), two ATP, two NADH.

CYCLE

See Figure 3-40.

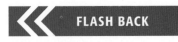

FLASH BACK

A kinase is an enzyme that phosphorylates a substrate.

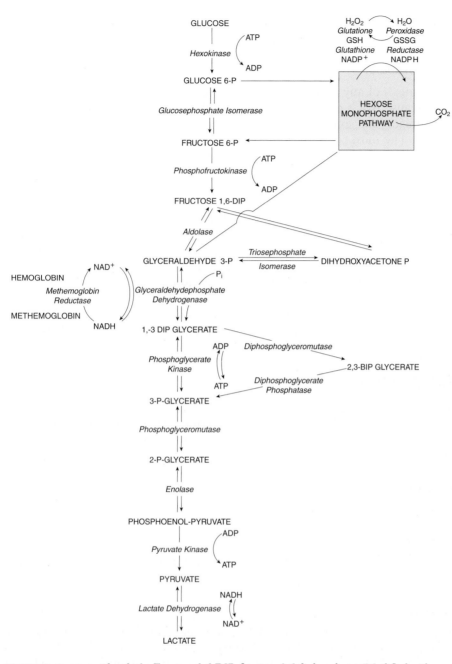

FIGURE 3-40. **Glycolysis.** Fructose 1,6-DIP, fructose 1,6-diphosphate. (Modified with permission from Lichtman MA, Beutler E, Kipps TJ, et al. *Williams Hematology*, 7th ed. New York: McGraw-Hill, 2006: 605.)

REGULATION

Phosphorylation of glucose to glucose-6-phosphate (G6P) blocks its ability to diffuse across the cell membrane, **trapping** it within the cell. Two kinases in the cytosol are involved. The process consumes one molecule of ATP per molecule of glucose phosphorylated.

- **Hexokinase:** Ubiquitous, nonspecific (phosphorylates many different six-carbon sugars), low K_m (easily saturable), feedback inhibited by G6P.
- **Glucokinase:** Mainly in the liver, very specific for glucose, high K_m (not easily saturable), feedback inhibited by fructose-6-phosphate (F6P, the product of the subsequent step in glycolysis).

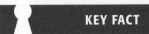

■ **Pyruvate dehydrogenase:** Converts pyruvate to acetyl-CoA, which enters the Kreb cycle, an irreversible and important regulatory step.

PATHOPHYSIOLOGY

Deficiencies of any of the glycolytic enzymes can lead to episodes of hemolysis because RBCs depend solely on glycolysis for their energy needs. These deficiencies are exacerbated by certain drugs (sulfa drugs, antimalarial agents). The most common such disorder is glucose-6-phosphate dehydrogenase (**G6PD**) deficiency. In this disorder, RBCs cannot phosphorylate glucose and, thus, cannot carry out glycolysis. This step is illustrated in Figures 3-41 and 3-42.

G6PD deficiency is especially prominent in the African-American community, although variants are also seen in Mediterranean and Asian populations. The RBC is protected from oxidative stress by glutathione (GSH). Since the regeneration of GSH depends on NADPH production and thus the HMP shunt, G6PD leads to denaturation of hemoglobin, resulting in the formation of Heinz bodies in the RBCs of affected individuals. **Favism** is a similar condition seen in individuals of Mediterranean origin. G6PD deficiency is exacerbated by consumption of fava beans (common in Mediterranean diets), usually within 24–48 hours after consumption.

Kreb (TCA) Cycle

FUNCTION

The Kreb cycle produces high-energy electron carriers (NADH, FADH$_2$) for ATP generation in the mitochondria and completes the metabolism of glucose (final common pathway).

LOCATION

Mitochondria (inner matrix).

REACTANTS

Pyruvate is the chief substrate. Proteins and fats enter the cycle after being converted to acetyl-CoA.

PRODUCTS

Three NADH, one FADH$_2$, two CO$_2$, and one GTP. Each NADH molecule ultimately yields three ATP. Each FADH$_2$ is worth one ATP. The GTP is converted into ATP in a reaction that does not require energy. Each acetyl-CoA molecule yields 12 ATP molecules.

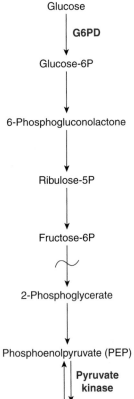

FIGURE 3-42. Glycolysis flow chart highlighting deficiencies and diseases. G6PD = glucose-6-phosphate dehydrogenase.

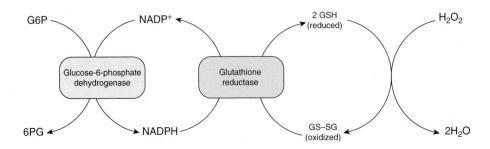

FIGURE 3-41. Role of glucose-6-phosphate dehydrogenase. 6GP = 6-phosphogluconate; G6P = glucose-6-phosphate; NADP = nicotinamide adenine dinucleotide phosphate; NADPH = reduced form of nicotinamide adenine dinucleotide phosphate.

CYCLE

Summarized in Figure 3-43.

REGULATION

The cycle is controlled at three major steps:

- Acetyl-CoA + oxaloacetate (OAA) → citrate, catalyzed by citrate synthase (allosterically inhibited by ATP).
- Isocitrate → α-ketoglutarate, controlled by isocitrate dehydrogenase (activated by ADP and inhibited by ATP and NADH).
- α-Ketoglutarate → succinyl-CoA, controlled by α-ketoglutarate dehydrogenase (inhibited by succinyl-CoA and NADH).

Electron Transport Chain and Oxidative Phosphorylation

FUNCTION

High-energy electrons from NADH and $FADH_2$ are transduced to ATP.

LOCATION

Mitochondria (inner membrane).

REACTANTS

High-energy electrons from NADH and $FADH_2$, O_2. As electrons are transported down the electron transport chain, they release energy that allows these complexes to pump protons across the mitochondrial membrane. This creates a concentration and charge gradient across the membrane. Protons eventually travel down this gradient via ATP synthase, providing the energy needed to convert ADP into ATP.

Since NADH and $FADH_2$ cannot physically cross the mitochondrial membrane, the electrons are shuttled into mitochondria by organ-specific shuttles.

- **Glycerol phosphate shuttle** → ubiquitous; transfers NADH electrons to mitochondrial $FADH_2$.
- **Malate-aspartate shuttle** → found in muscle, liver, and heart; transfers NADH electrons to mitochondrial NADH.

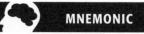

MNEMONIC

TCA intermediates—

Can I Keep Selling Sex For Money, Officer?

Citrate
Isocitrate
α-**K**etoglutarate
Succinyl-CoA
Succinate
Fumarate
Malate
Oxaloacetate

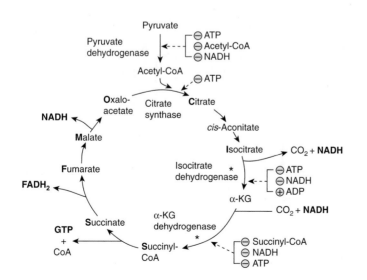

FIGURE 3-43. **Kreb (TCA) cycle.** Steps with * indicate regulatory steps. α-KG, α-ketoglutarate.

KEY FACT

Uncoupling of the electron transport chain leads to leakiness of the inner mitochondrial membrane, resulting in slow dissipation of the proton gradient, and ATP production to slow and eventually cease. Heat is released. 2,4-Dinitrophenol increases the permeability of the mitochondrial membrane → dissipation of the hydrogen gradient. Brown fat: uncoupling of electron transport chain via protein called thermogenin → allows protons to cross the mitochondrial membrane, bypassing active transport → release of heat.

PRODUCTS

ATP and H_2O.

CYCLE

Summarized in Figure 3-44.

Pentose Phosphate Pathway (HMP Shunt)

FUNCTION

Shunts G6P to form ribulose-5-phosphate for nucleotide synthesis. Generates NADPH as a reducing equivalent for GSH/GSSG (the premier antioxidant system in the cell) and NADPH for steroid and fatty acid biosynthesis.

LOCATION

Cytoplasm of all cells.

REACTANTS

G6P.

PRODUCTS

NADPH, which is used in steroid and fatty acid biosynthesis and regeneration of GSH in the GSH/GSSG antioxidant system. Ribose-5-phosphate, CO_2.

CYCLE

Summarized in Figures 3-45 and 3-46.

REGULATION

The reaction consists of two parts:

- The first irreversible step is catalyzed by G6PD to produce NADPH from G6P (this step is oxidative).
- The second, reversible, step isomerizes the sugars so they can reenter glycolysis. This step is nonoxidative.

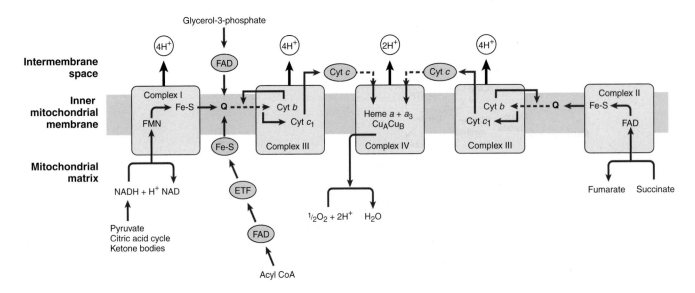

FIGURE 3-44.   Electron transport chain and oxidative phosphorylation. ADP = adenosine diphosphate; ATP = adenosine triphosphate; CoQ = coenzyme Q; NADP = nicotinamide adenine dinucleotide phosphate; NADPH = reduced form of nicotinamide adenine dinucleotide phosphate; P_i = inorganic phosphate. (Reproduced with permission from Murray RK, et al. *Harper's Illustrated Biochemistry*, 28th ed. New York: McGraw-Hill, 2009: Figure 13-5.)

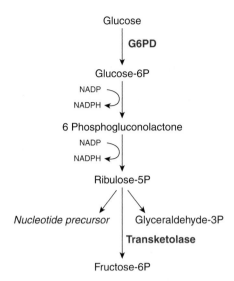

FIGURE 3-45. **Pentose phosphate pathway (HMP shunt).** G6PD = glucose-6-phosphate dehydrogenase; NADP = nicotinamide adenine dinucleotide phosphate; NADPH = reduced form of nicotinamide adenine dinucleotide phosphate.

PATHOPHYSIOLOGY

G6PD deficiency has a high prevalence among African-Americans. Please see discussion under Glycolysis.

Fructose Metabolism

FUNCTION

Converts dietary fructose into a substrate for glycolysis.

LOCATION

Muscle, kidney, and liver.

REACTANTS

Fructose and ATP.

PRODUCTS

Glyceraldehyde-3-phosphate.

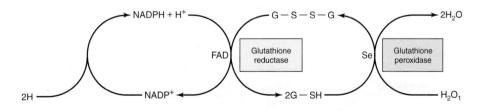
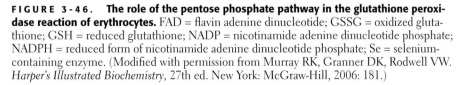

FIGURE 3-46. **The role of the pentose phosphate pathway in the glutathione peroxidase reaction of erythrocytes.** FAD = flavin adenine dinucleotide; GSSG = oxidized glutathione; GSH = reduced glutathione; NADP = nicotinamide adenine dinucleotide phosphate; NADPH = reduced form of nicotinamide adenine dinucleotide phosphate; Se = selenium-containing enzyme. (Modified with permission from Murray RK, Granner DK, Rodwell VW. *Harper's Illustrated Biochemistry*, 27th ed. New York: McGraw-Hill, 2006: 181.)

CYCLE

See Figure 3-47.

- Dietary sucrose is broken down by sucrase in the small intestine to fructose and glucose.
- Fructose is phosphorylated by hexokinase to fructose-6-phoshate in muscle and kidney.
- In the liver, fructose is converted to fructose-1-phosphate by fructokinase.
- Fructose-1-phosphate aldolase converts fructose-1-phosphate to dihydroxyacetone phosphate (DHAP) and glyceraldehyde. DHAP can be combined with glyceraldehyde and converted to glyceraldehyde-3-phosphate, which can enter glycolysis.

PATHOPHYSIOLOGY

- Deficiencies in fructokinase are benign, leading to **fructosuria** (essential fructosuria).
- Fructose-1-phosphate aldolase deficiency leads to **hereditary fructose intolerance,** characterized by severe hypoglycemia upon sucrose or fructose ingestion).

Galactose Metabolism

FUNCTION

Converts dietary galactose (from lactose) to a form that can enter glycolysis.

LOCATION

Kidney, liver, and brain.

REACTANTS

Galactose and ATP.

PRODUCTS

Glucose-1-phosphate.

CYCLE

See Figure 3-48.

- Dietary lactose is broken down in the small intestine by lactase to galactose and glucose.
- Galactose is phosphorylated by galactokinase to galactose-1-phosphate.
- Galactose-1-phosphate is converted by galactose-1-phosphate uridyl transferase to glucose-1-phosphate.

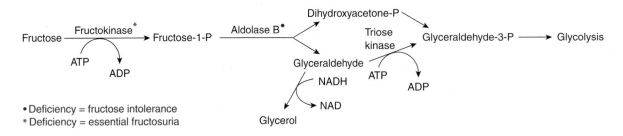

FIGURE 3-47. Fructose metabolism in the liver. ADP = adenosine diphosphate; ATP = adenosine triphosphate; NADP = nicotinamide adenine dinucleotide phosphate; NADPH = reduced form of nicotinamide adenine dinucleotide phosphate.

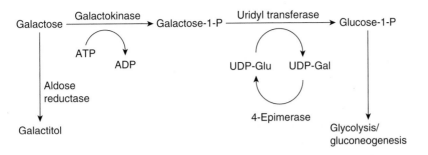

FIGURE 3-48. **Galactose metabolism.** ADP = adenosine diphosphate; ATP = adenosine triphosphate; Gal = galactose; Glu = glucose; UDP = uridine diphosphate.

Pathophysiology

- Deficiencies in galactokinase lead to **galactosemia** and early cataract formation.
- Deficiencies in galactose-1-phosphate uridyl transferase lead to severe galactosemia with growth and mental retardation and possibly early death.

Anaerobic Metabolism and Cori Cycle

Function

Shuttles lactate from muscle into the liver, allowing muscle to function anaerobically when energy requirements exceed oxygen consumption.

Location

Muscle and liver.

Reactants

Anaerobic metabolism uses glucose. The Cori cycle begins with lactate and consumes six ATP.

Products

Anaerobic metabolism produces two net ATP and two pyruvates per glucose molecule. Lactate is converted to glucose in the Cori cycle.

Cycle

See Figure 3-49.

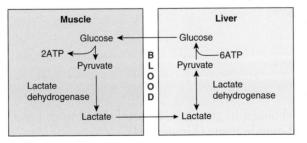

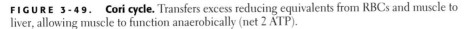

FIGURE 3-49. **Cori cycle.** Transfers excess reducing equivalents from RBCs and muscle to liver, allowing muscle to function anaerobically (net 2 ATP).

Gluconeogenesis

FUNCTION

Generates glucose from glycolysis, fatty acid, or TCA (Kreb's) cycle intermediates.

LOCATION

Cytoplasm and mitochondria of kidney, liver, and intestinal epithelium.

REACTANTS

Pyruvate.

PRODUCTS

Glucose.

CYCLE

See Figure 3-50.

REGULATION

Although some of the steps in glycolysis and the TCA cycle are irreversible, they can be bypassed by the use of ATP or GTP and four enzymes, found only in the kidney, liver, and intestinal epithelium.

- Pyruvate carboxylase converts pyruvate → OAA.
- PEP (phosphoenolpyruvate) carboxykinase converts OAA → PEP.
- Fructose-1,6-bisphosphatase converts fructose-1,6-bisphoshate → fructose-6-phosphate.
- Glucose-6-phosphatase converts glucose-6-phosphatase → glucose.

Glycogen Metabolism

FUNCTION

Helps maintain glucose homeostasis by forming (**glycogenesis**) or breaking down (**glycogenolysis**) glycogen. Crucial for the storage of energy derived from carbohydrate metabolism.

LOCATION

Glycogenesis—liver and muscle. Glycogen*olysis*—heart, liver, and muscle.

REACTANTS

Glucose/glycogen.

PRODUCTS

Glycogen/glucose.

GLYCOGENESIS

Glucose is catabolized to glycogen, its insoluble storage form. Mainly stored in the liver and muscle tissue (Figure 3-51).

GLYCOGENOLYSIS

Release of glucose from glycogen stores. See Figure 3-51.

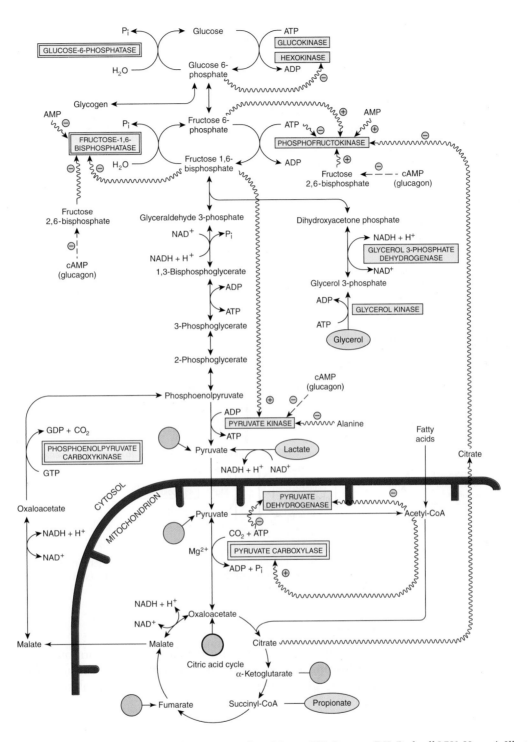

FIGURE 3-50. **Gluconeogenesis.** (Modified with permission from Murray RK, Granner DK, Rodwell VW. *Harper's Illustrated Biochemistry*, 27th ed. New York: McGraw-Hill, 2006: 168.)

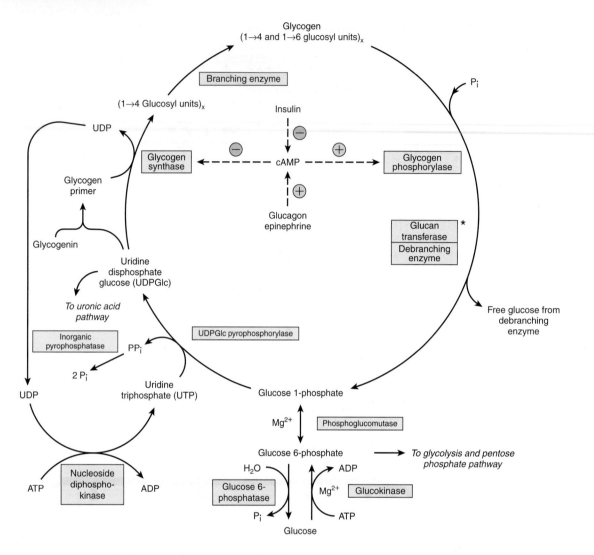

FIGURE 3-51. Glycogenesis. Pathways of glycogenesis and of glycogenolysis in the liver. (≈, Stimulation; ∅, inhibition.) *Glucan transferase and debranching enzyme appear to be two separate activities of the same enzyme. (Reproduced with permission from Murray RK, Bender DA, Botham KM, et al. *Harper's Illustrated Biochemistry*, 28th ed. New York: McGraw-Hill, 2009: Fig. 19-1.)

REGULATION

These opposing processes are regulated by the hormones insulin and glucagon. **Insulin** promotes the removal of glucose from the bloodstream, thereby increasing **glycogenesis** and decreasing glycogenolysis. Glucagon does the opposite.

PATHOPHYSIOLOGY

There are 12 types of glycogen storage diseases. All result in abnormal glycogen metabolism and an accumulation of glycogen within cells. See Table 3-19 for the most common types and Table 3-20 for a summary of the metabolic cycles and pathways.

TABLE 3-19. Glycogen Storage Diseases

Type	Disease	Enzyme	Tissue	Clinical Features
I	Von Gierke disease	Glucose-6-phosphatase.	Liver and kidney.	Severe fasting hypoglycemia. Lactic acidosis. Hepatomegaly (100%). Short stature (90%). Delayed puberty. Bleeding diathesis (especially epistaxis). Hepatic adenomas (75%), renal failure and gout in 20s and 30s.
II	Pompe disease	α-1,4-Glucosidase (acid maltase).	All organs (enzyme is in lysosomes).	Progressive muscle weakness. Breathing and feeding difficulties. Hyporeflexia or areflexia due to glycogen accumulation in spinal motor neurons. Cardiomegaly leading to congestive heart failure and death before the age of 2.
III	Cori disease	Debranching enzyme (α-1,6-glucosidase).	Muscle and liver.	Similar to type I without lactic acidosis. ■ Hypoglycemia. ■ Hepatomegaly. ■ Delayed (ultimately normal) growth. Symptoms, including hepatomegaly, usually regress in adulthood.
V	McArdle disease	Myophosphorylase.	Muscle.	Muscle weakness and cramps after exercise. Myoglobinuria (burgundy urine) after exercise.

Urea Cycle

FUNCTION

Excretion of NH_4^+ from amino acid metabolism; accounts for 90% of nitrogen in urine.

LOCATION

Mitochondria and cytoplasm.

REACTANTS

CO_2 and NH_4^+.

REGULATION

Carbamyl phosphate synthase catalyzes the formation of carbamoyl phosphate from CO_2 and NH_4^+. This enzyme, in turn, is activated by N-acetylglutamic acid.

PRODUCTS

Urea and fumarate (fumarate enters the TCA).

CYCLE

See Figure 3-52.

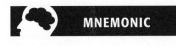

MNEMONIC

Urea cycle–

Ordinarily, Careless Crappers Are Also Frivolous About Urination

Ornithine
Carbamoyl phosphate
Citrulline
Aspartate
Argininosuccinate
Fumarate
Arginine
Urea

TABLE 3-20. Summary of Metabolic Cycles and Pathways

CYCLE/PATHWAY	FUNCTION	LOCATION	REACTANTS	PRODUCTS
Glycolysis	Breakdown of sugars for Kreb's cycle.	Cytoplasm of cells that use glucose.	Glucose.	2 Pyruvate, 2 ATP, and 2 NADH.
Kreb cycle (TCA cycle)	Production of high-energy electron carriers for the ATP generation mitochondria.	Mitochondria.	Pyruvate (alternatively, fats and proteins after conversion to acetyl-CoA).	3 NADH, 1 $FADH_2$, 2 CO_2, 1 GTP. All equivalent to 12 ATP per acetyl-CoA.
Electron transport chain/oxidative phosphorylation	Transduction of high-energy e^- from NADH and $FADH_2$ to ATP.	Mitochondria.	NADH, $FADH_2$, and O_2 as the final electron acceptor.	ATP and H_2O.
Pentose phosphate pathway (HMP shunt)	1. Shunts G6P to form ribulose-5—for nucleotide synthesis. 2. Generation of NADPH for: 　▪ Regeneration of GSH in the GSH/GSSG antioxidant system vi. 　▪ Steroid and fatty acid biosynthesis.	Cytoplasm.	G6P.	Ribulose-5-phosphate, NADPH, and CO_2.
Fructose pathway	Converts fructose to substrate for glycolysis.	Muscle, kidney, and liver.	Fructose.	Glyceraldehyde-3-phosphate.
Galactose pathway	Converts galactose to substrate for glycolysis.	Kidney, liver, and brain.	Galactose and ATP.	
Cori cycle/anaerobic metabolism	Cori cycle shuttles lactate from anaerobic metabolism in muscle to liver.	Shuttles lactate from muscle to liver.	Lactate and 6 ATP.	Glucose.
Gluconeogenesis	Generates glucose from glycolysis intermediates, fatty acid or TCA cycle.	Cytoplasm and mitochondria of kidney and liver, interstitial epithelium.	All substrates end up as pyruvate/phosphoenolpyruvate → converted to glucose.	Glucose.
Glycogen metabolism	Maintains glucose homeostasis.	Glycogenesis (muscle and liver), glycogenolysis (heart, muscle, and liver).	Glycogen/glucose.	Glycogen/glucose.
Urea cycle	Excretion of NH_4^+ from amino acid metabolism.	Partly in the mitochondria and partly in the cytoplasm.	CO_2 and NH_4^+.	Urea and fumarate (enters TCA).

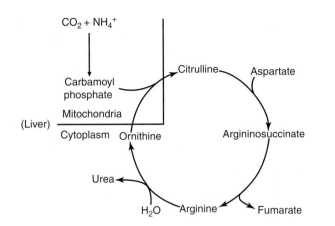

FIGURE 3-52. **Urea cycle.**

Amino Acids

AMINO ACID METABOLISM

Metabolism is a key process in the human body as it provides the energy required to maintain the body's organization. Metabolism utilizes various chemical reactions to extract energy and building blocks from food. Amino acids are extensively used in the synthesis of new proteins (eg, enzymes, hormones, growth factors) and can also be used as an energy source.

AMINO ACID STRUCTURE

Amino acids consist of a carboxylic acid, an amine group, and a characteristic functional side group (Figure 3-53).

Acidic Amino Acids

Aspartic acid and glutamic acid contain an additional carboxylic acid group and are negatively charged at physiologic pH (7.4).

Basic Amino Acids

Arginine, lysine, and histidine are polar and very hydrophilic. At physiologic pH (7.4), arginine and lysine are positively charged, whereas histidine has no net charge. Arginine is the most basic amino acid and is found in high concentrations along with lysine bound to negatively charged DNA in histones, the major component of chromatin.

THE AMINO ACID POOL

Amino acids are continually being used to synthesize proteins, and proteins are continually being broken down into amino acids. This dynamic pool of amino acids is in equilibrium with tissue protein.

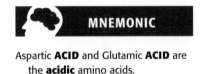

MNEMONIC

Aspartic **ACID** and Glutamic **ACID** are the **acidic** amino acids.

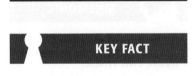

KEY FACT

All acidic and basic amino acids are polar, but not all polar amino acids are acidic or basic.

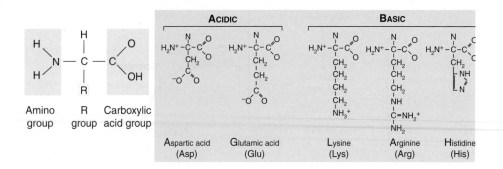

FIGURE 3-53. **Amino acid structure.** An amino acid consists of three main groups (1) an amine group, (2) a functional side group, and (3) a carboxylic acid group. At physiologic pH, acidic amino acids are negatively charged, whereas basic amino acids, with the exception of the histidine, have a net positive charge.

Replenishment

Takes place through:

- De novo synthesis
- Dietary supply
- Protein degradation

Depletion

Occurs through:

- Protein synthesis
- Oxidation of excess amino acids

Any amino acid not immediately used must be converted to glycogen or fat stores, as protein cannot be stored.

ESSENTIAL AMINO ACIDS

Of the 20 amino acids in the body, 10 cannot be synthesized de novo in adequate amounts and must be consumed in the diet. These essential amino acids include:

- Phenylalanine (Phe)
- Valine (Val)
- Threonine (Thr)
- Tryptophan (Trp)
- Isoleucine (Ile)
- Methionine (Met)
- Histidine (His)
- Arginine (Arg)
- Leucine (Leu)
- Lysine (Lys)

Histidine and arginine are essential only for periods when cell growth demands exceed production, such as during childhood.

MNEMONIC

All essential amino acids–

PriVaTe TIM HALL:

Phe
Val
Thr
Trp
Ile
Met
His
Arg
Leu
Lys

NONESSENTIAL AMINO ACIDS

The remaining amino acids can be synthesized using the TCA cycle and other metabolic intermediates in reactions that are discussed later.

- Tyrosine (Tyr)
- Glycine (Gly)
- Alanine (Ala)
- Cysteine (Cys)
- Serine (Ser)
- Aspartate (Asp)
- Asparagine (Asn)
- Glutamate (Glu)
- Glutamine (Gln)
- Proline (Pro)

METABOLIC REACTIONS

Two simple reactions are the key to understanding amino acid metabolism: **transamination** and **oxidative deamination**.

Transamination

DEFINITION

Transfers an α-amino group to an α-keto acid group, creating a new amino acid (Figure 3-54).

- Transfer agent is an **aminotransferase/transaminase** (eg, aspartate transaminase [AST], alanine aminotransferase [ALT]).
- Acceptor (usually α-ketoglutarate, can be pyruvate, oxaloacetate) becomes a new amino acid.
- Donor becomes a new α-keto acid.
- Reaction important for both synthesis and breakdown of amino acids.

SITE

Cytosol and mitochondria.

> **FLASH FORWARD**
>
> Aminotransferases are important liver enzymes used in diagnostic testing.

> **KEY FACT**
>
> Vitamin B_6 and niacin deficiencies affect the functioning of transaminases.

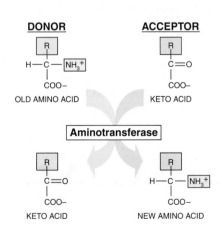

FIGURE 3-54.   Transamination reaction. In this reaction, an α-amino group is transferred from the donor amino acid to the acceptor keto acid, creating a new amino acid. In essence, the α-amino group is being transferred from one carbon skeleton to another.

COFACTORS

All aminotransferases require the vitamin B_6 derivative **pyridoxal phosphate (PLP)**.

Oxidative Deamination

DEFINITION

Removes an α-amino group, leaving a carbon skeleton (Figure 3-55).

- Ammonia released enters urea cycle.
- Carbon skeletons used as glycolytic and TCA cycle intermediates.
- **Glutamate,** with the assistance of glutamate dehydrogenase, is the only amino acid that **undergoes rapid oxidative deamination.**

SITE

Mitochondria.

CONTROL

Reversible reaction driven by need for TCA intermediates.

- **Low energy (GDP, ADP) activates.**
- **High energy (GTP, ATP) inhibits.**

NONESSENTIAL AMINO ACID BIOSYNTHESIS

Nonessential amino acids can be synthesized in adequate amounts from essential amino acids and from intermediates of glycolysis and the TCA cycle (Figure 3-62).

Tyrosine

PRECURSOR

Phenylalanine.

SYNTHESIS

Irreversible hydroxylation catalyzed by **phenylalanine hydroxylase** and its required cofactor **tetrahydrobiopterin** (Figure 3-56).

SIGNIFICANCE

Tyrosine is the precursor for catecholamines (eg, dopamine, adrenaline, noradrenaline), melanin, and thyroxine. A genetic deficiency of phenylalanine hydroxylase causes **phenylketonuria (PKU)** (discussed later), which results in the buildup of phenylalanine and an inability to produce tyrosine.

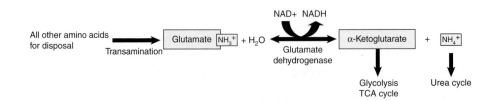

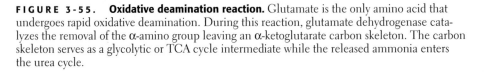

FIGURE 3-55.   Oxidative deamination reaction. Glutamate is the only amino acid that undergoes rapid oxidative deamination. During this reaction, glutamate dehydrogenase catalyzes the removal of the α-amino group leaving an α-ketoglutarate carbon skeleton. The carbon skeleton serves as a glycolytic or TCA cycle intermediate while the released ammonia enters the urea cycle.

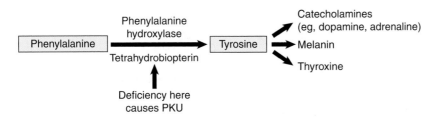

FIGURE 3-56.   Tyrosine synthesis. Hydroxylation of phenylalanine by phenylalanine hydroxylase results in the formation of tyrosine. Tyrosine can then be used for the synthesis of other compounds. Deficiencies in either phenylalanine or its required cofactor tetrahydrobiopterin cause the disease phenylketonuria.

Serine, Glycine, Cysteine

PRECURSORS

Glycolysis intermediates. Serine can act as precursor for glycine and cysteine. Cysteine synthesis from serine also requires the essential amino acid methionine.

SYNTHESIS

- **Serine:** Mainly a three-step process from glycolytic intermediates in the cytosol. Can also be synthesized in a reversible reaction by transfer of a hydroxymethyl group from glycine in the mitochondria (Figure 3-57).
- **Glycine:** Mainly from CO_2, NH_4^+, and N_5N_{10}-methylene **tetrahydrofolate** in mitochondria. Can also be synthesized by the reverse of the serine synthesis reaction in the mitochondria (Figure 3-57).
- **Cysteine:** Synthesis is a multistep process with four main steps (Figure 3-58):
    1. Methionine activation.
    2. Homocysteine formation.
    3. Homocysteine and serine condensation to cystathionine.
    4. Cystathionine hydrolysis to cysteine and homoserine.

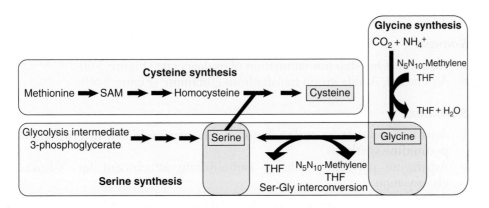

FIGURE 3-57.   Serine, glycine, cysteine synthesis. Serine (Ser) is mainly synthesized in a three-step process from the glycolytic intermediate 3-phosphoglycerate. Alternatively, serine can be formed from glycine (gly) by transfer of a hydromethyl carbon group. Glycine, in turn, can be synthesized from serine in a reversal of the previous reaction. However, it is mainly synthesized from CO_2, NH_4^+, and N^5N^{10}-methylene tetrahydrofolate. Cysteine synthesis requires methionine and serine. SAM, S-adenosyl methionine; THF, tetrahydrofolate.

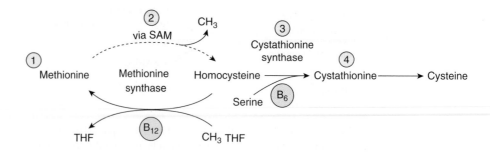

FIGURE 3-58. Cysteine synthesis. Synthesis of cysteine from serine occurs in the cytosol and requires the essential amino acid methionine. The key steps are (1) activation of methionine, (2) formation of homocysteine, (3) condensation of serine and homocysteine to from cystathionine, and (4) hydrolysis of cystathionine to form cysteine. SAM, S-adenosyl methionine; THF, tetrahydrofolate.

SIGNIFICANCE

- Glycine is notably a component of **collagen** and an inhibitory **neurotransmitter.** It is also used in the antioxidant glutathione (along with glutamate and cysteine), creatine, porphyrins, and purines.
- Cysteine synthesis interruption can lead to a buildup of homocysteine in the urine known as **homocystinuria** (discussed later).

Alanine

PRECURSOR

Pyruvate.

SYNTHESIS

One-step transamination of pyruvate (Figure 3-59).

Aspartate, Asparagine

PRECURSOR

TCA cycle intermediate oxaloacetate.

SYNTHESIS

- Aspartate: One-step transamination of oxaloacetate (Figure 3-60).
- Asparagine: Amide group transfer from glutamine (Figure 3-60).

SIGNIFICANCE

- Aspartate serves as an amino donor in the **urea cycle** and in **purine and pyrimidine synthesis.**
- Asparagine provides a site of carbohydrate attachment for N-linked glycosylation.

Glutamate, Glutamine, Proline, Arginine

PRECURSOR

α-Ketoglutarate. Glutamate also serves as a precursor to glutamine, proline, and arginine.

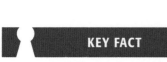
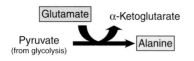

FIGURE 3-59. Alanine synthesis. Alanine is synthesized from the glycolytic intermediate pyruvate by a one-step transamination.

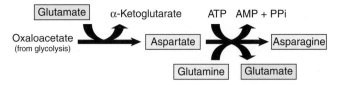

FIGURE 3-60. **Aspartate and asparagine synthesis.** Aspartate is formed in a one-step transamination from the TCA cycle intermediate oxaloacetate. Asparagine is then formed by amidation of aspartate. AMP, adenosine monophosphate; ATP, adenosine triphosphate; PPi, pyrophosphate.

SYNTHESIS (FIGURE 3-61)

- **Glutamate:** Reductive amination of α-ketoglutarate. Also commonly from transamination of most other amino acids.
- **Glutamine:** Amidation (the addition of an amide group) of glutamate.
- **Proline:** Three-step synthesis from glutamate involving reduction, spontaneous cyclization, and another reduction.
- **Arginine:** Two-step synthesis from glutamate involving reduction and transamination to ornithine. Ornithine is then sent to the urea cycle where it is metabolized to arginine.

Although the details of these synthetic pathways can seem overwhelming, it is important to have a familiarity with the overall picture of nonessential amino acid synthesis and from where in the TCA cycle the precursors are obtained (Figure 3-62).

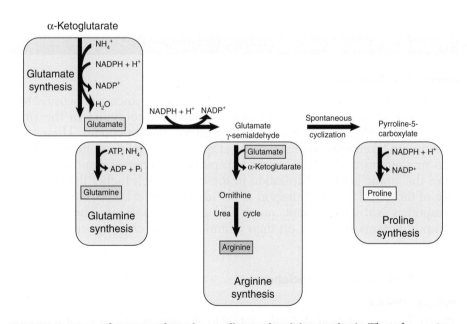

FIGURE 3-61. **Glutamate, glutamine, proline, and arginine synthesis.** These four amino acids are formed from α-ketoglutarate. (1) Glutamate is formed from a direct reductive amination. (2) Glutamine can then be formed from glutamate by amidation. At this branch point, either (3) proline can be formed in three steps or (4) ornithine can be formed in two and sent to the urea cycle, where it is metabolized to arginine. ADP, adenosine diphosphate; ATP, adenosine triphosphate; NADP, nicotinamide adenine dinucleotide phosphate; NADPH, reduced form of nicotinamide adenine dinucleotide phosphate.

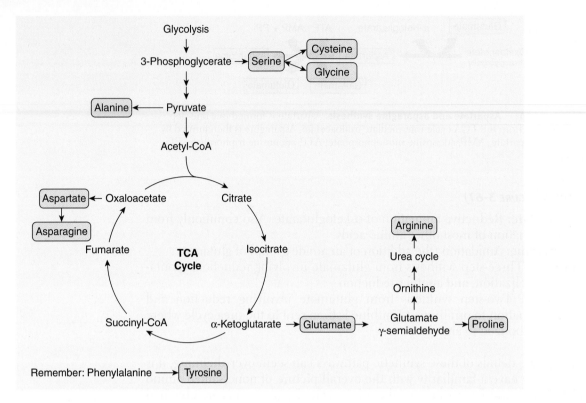

FIGURE 3-62. **Biosynthesis of nonessential amino acids.** This overview highlights the precursors and pathways used in nonessential amino acid synthesis. TCA, tricarboxylic acid.

AMINO ACID TISSUE METABOLISM

Amino Acid Transport

Protein digestion begins in the stomach, where gastric juice and pepsin break down proteins to form large peptides. Degradation continues in the small intestine to produce free amino acids, dipeptides, and tripeptides. These components are taken into epithelial cells via specific transporters and hydrolyzed into free amino acids. Amino acid transport is an energy-requiring process, since the amino acid concentration in the cell is much higher than that outside of the cell. Luminal transport is Na⁺-dependent, whereas contraluminal transport is Na⁺-independent, much like glucose transport. The four main transport systems are based on their amino acid side chain specificity (Table 3-21).

Amino Acid Transport Deficiency

HARTNUP DISEASE

This is a rare autosomal recessive defect in the intestinal and renal transporters for **neutral amino acids.** The symptoms are due to a **loss of tryptophan,** which is a nicotinamide precursor. Thus, many aspects of the presentation **mimic niacin (vitamin B₃) deficiency** (pellagra).

PRESENTATION

Patients exhibit pellagra-like skin lesions and neurologic manifestations ranging from ataxia to frank delirium.

TABLE 3-21. **Important Amino Acid Transport Systems**

Amino Acid Specificity	Amino Acids Transported	Diseases Resulting from Defective Carrier System
Small, aliphatic	Alanine, serine, threonine.	Nonspecific
Large, aliphatic, aromatic	Isoleucine, leucine, valine, tyrosine, tryptophan, phenylalanine.	Hartnup disease
Basic	Arginine, lysine, cysteine, ornithine.	Cystinuria
Acidic	Glutamate, aspartate.	Nonspecific

DIAGNOSIS

Diagnosis is made by detection of neutral aminoaciduria, which is not present in pellagra.

TREATMENT

Management is targeted at replacing niacin and providing a high-protein diet with nicotinamide supplements.

CYSTINURIA

Autosomal recessive defect in kidney tubular reabsorption of the **basic amino acids** resulting in high levels of their excretion. The low solubility of cysteine leads to precipitation and **kidney stone** formation.

PRESENTATION

Most of the symptoms are due to stone formation.

DIAGNOSIS

Quantitative urinary amino acid analysis confirms the diagnosis.

TREATMENT

Management strives to eliminate precipitation and stone formation by increasing urine volume (high daily fluid ingestion) and urinary alkalization.

ABSORPTIVE STATE METABOLISM

Once amino acids are absorbed, most are transaminated to **alanine, the main amino acid secreted by the gut,** and released into the portal vein destined for the liver (Figure 3-63). In the liver, amino acids meet a use-it-or-lose-it fate. They can either be used for protein synthesis or transaminated to glutamate for rapid oxidative deamination and urea excretion. Excess amino acids must either be used directly for energy or converted to glycogen or fat stores. They **cannot be stored as protein.**

AMINO ACID DERIVATIVES

Amino acids serve as precursors to synthesize many important compounds. Three simple reactions are the key to understanding amino acid derivatives: decarboxylation, hydroxylation, and methylation.

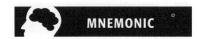

MNEMONIC

Amino acid transport deficiency in cystinuria—

COLA
Cysteine
Ornithine
Lysine
Arginine

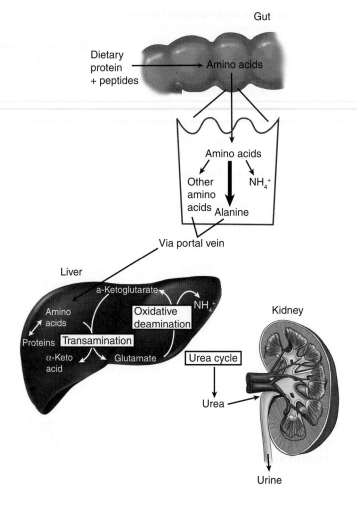

FIGURE 3-63. Absorptive state amino acid metabolism. When digested, protein is broken down into amino acids, most of which are converted to alanine and shuttled via the portal vein to the liver. The liver can use the amino acids for protein synthesis or lose the amino acids via entry to the urea cycle and excretion from the kidney.

- **Decarboxylation:** Removal of a carboxyl group (–COOH) from a compound.
- **Hydroxylation:** Addition of a hydroxyl group (–OH) to a compound, thus oxidizing it.
- **Methylation:** Addition of a methyl group (–CH$_3$) to a compound.

Methionine Derivative

S-ADENOSYLMETHIONINE (SAM)

Main biosynthetic reaction methyl donor.

- **Synthesis location:** All living cells.
- **Synthesis reaction:** Methionine and ATP.

Tyrosine Derivatives

THYROID HORMONES

Control the body's metabolic rate.

- **Synthesis location:** Thyroid follicle cells.
- **Synthesis reaction:** See Figure 3-64.
  - Tyrosine converted to the glycoprotein thyroglobulin.

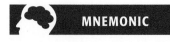

KEY FACT

Much like the amino acid pool, there exists a dynamic one-carbon pool. These one-carbon units are used for molecular synthesis and elongation, but require activation by a carrier (usually SAM or folate) to enable their transfer.

MNEMONIC

SAM is the methyl donor man.

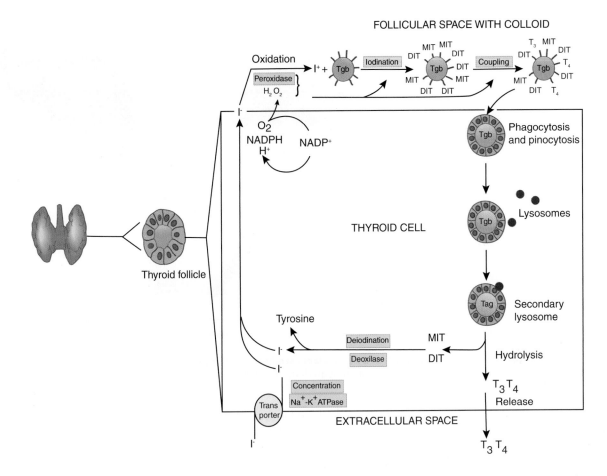

FOLLICULAR SPACE WITH COLLOID

FIGURE 3-64. **Thyroid hormone synthesis.** Thyroglobulin (Tgb), which is rich in tyrosine, is transported to the lumen, where its tyrosine residues are iodinated. The various forms of thyroid hormones (triiodothyronine, T_3, thyroxine, T_4) produced can then be released in a regulated manner. DIT, diiodotyrosine; MIT, monoiodotyrosine.

- Iodide oxidized to iodine (I_2) and incorporated into the tyrosine side chains of the thyroglobulin. (*Note:* Thyroid hormone also contains the 21st amino acid, selenocysteine.)
- Tyrosine + one I_2 = monoiodinated tyrosine (MIT).
- Tyrosine + two I_2 = diiodinated tyrosine (DIT).
- DIT + DIT = thyroxine (T_4).
- MIT + DIT = triiodothyroxine (T_3, active form).

MELANIN

Provides pigmentation, forms cap over keratinocytes for protection from UV rays.

- **Synthesis location:** Hair and skin melanocytes.
- **Synthesis reaction:** See Figure 3-65.
  - Tyrosine hydroxylation at two sites.
  - Catalyzed by **tyrosinase.**
  - Requires cofactors copper and ascorbate.
  - Reactive molecules variably polymerize to form different melanins.

CATECHOLAMINES

Control body's stress responses acting as neurotransmitters or hormones.

- **Synthesis location:** Central nervous system, adrenal medulla.
- **Synthesis reaction:** See Figure 3-66.

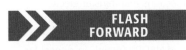

FLASH FORWARD

This would be good time to review the regulation of thyroid hormone synthesis.

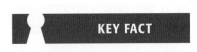

KEY FACT

Tyrosinase, also known as tyrosine hydroxylase, deficiency is one cause of albinism.

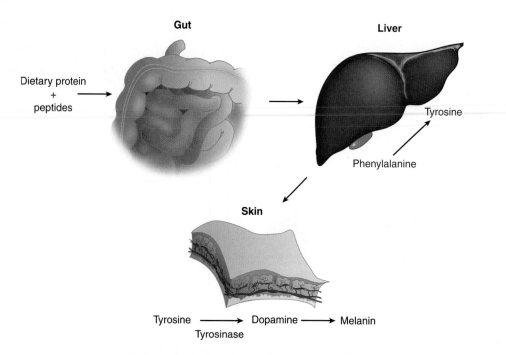

FIGURE 3-65. Melanin synthesis. Tyrosine can be converted by the enzyme tyrosine hydroxylase to a more active form that polymerizes to four different melanins.

- Tyrosine hydroxylation and decarboxylation to **dopamine.**
- Dopamine hydroxylation to **norepinephrine.**
- Norepinephrine methylation to **epinephrine** using the methyl donor SAM.
- Metabolism occurs through the enzymes **catecholamine O-methyltransferase (COMT)** and **monoamine oxidase (MAO).**

Tryptophan Derivatives

NIACIN (VITAMIN B₃)

Forms essential redox reaction cofactors NAD^+, $NADP^+$.

- **Synthesis location:** Liver.
- **Synthesis reaction:**
  - Tryptophan five-membered aromatic ring cleaved and rearranged to six-membered ring using its α-amino group.
  - Reaction very slow and requires cofactors pyridoxine (vitamin B_6), riboflavin (vitamin B_2), and thiamine (vitamin B_1).

SEROTONIN

- **Synthesis location:** CNS serotonergic neurons, GI tract enterochromaffin cells.
- **Synthesis reaction:** Tryptophan aromatic ring hydroxylation and then decarboxylation (Figure 3-67).

Serotonin is also present in high levels in platelets, but is taken up rather than synthesized.

KEY FACT

The body derives energy from the many redox (oxidation-reduction) reactions that transfer electrons. NAD^+ (mainly in mitochondria for oxidative, catabolic reactions) and $NADP^+$ (mainly in cytosol for reductive, anabolic reactions) act to accept and donate these electrons.

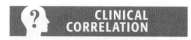

CLINICAL CORRELATION

Serotonin levels can be diminished in patients with depression. For this reason, selective serotonin reuptake inhibitors (SSRIs) are widely used.

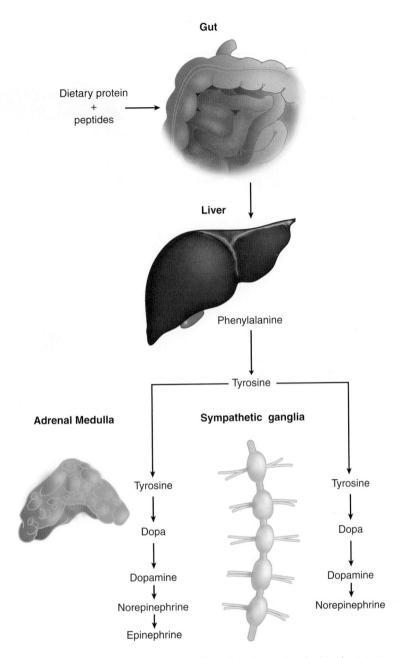

FIGURE 3-66. Catecholamine synthesis. Phenylalanine is absorbed in the intestine and converted to tyrosine in the liver. Tyrosine can then be converted to dopamine in the substantia nigra or further processed to norepinephrine in sympathetic ganglion neurons or to epinephrine in the adrenal medulla.

MELATONIN

Controls circadian rhythm functions.

- **Synthesis location:** Pineal gland pinealocytes.
- **Synthesis reaction:** See Figure 3-67.
    - Tryptophan conversion to serotonin (see earlier discussion).
    - Serotonin acetylation and methylation.

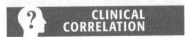

CLINICAL CORRELATION

Pharmacologically, melatonin has been used to treat circadian rhythm disorders such as jet lag.

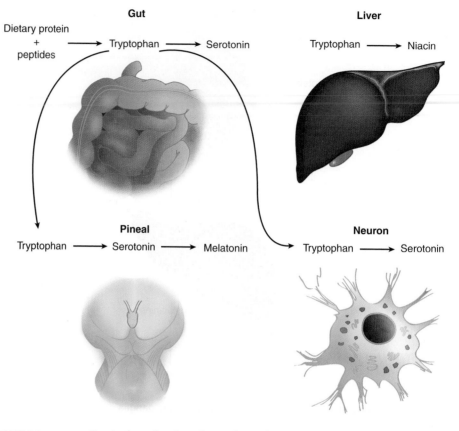

FIGURE 3-67. **Serotonin and melatonin synthesis.** Serotonin is derived from tryptophan via hydroxylation and decarboxylation of the aromatic ring. Melatonin can then be derived from serotonin via acetylation and methylation.

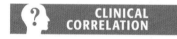

CLINICAL CORRELATION

Histidine can be metabolized to histamine, which is rapidly deactivated or stored in the granules of mast cells. These cells are degranulated when exposed to an allergen.

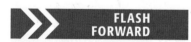

FLASH FORWARD

Enzyme deficiencies can inhibit various steps in the synthesis of heme, resulting in a group of diseases known as the porphyrias. Synthesis can be inhibited by lead.

Histidine Derivative

HISTAMINE

Mediates inflammatory responses, acts as neurotransmitter, stimulates gastric acid secretion.

- **Synthesis location:** Connective tissue mast cells, GI tract enterochromaffin cells.
- **Synthesis reaction:** Histidine decarboxylation.

Glycine Derivative

HEME

Electron carrier in cytochromes and enzymes, O_2 carrier in hemoglobin and myoglobin.

- **Synthesis location:** Mitochondria and cytosol of bone marrow erythroid cells (for hemoglobin), liver hepatocytes (for cytochromes).
- **Synthesis reaction:** See Figure 3-68.
  - Eight-step reaction with first three and last three occurring in the mitochondria.
  - Δ-Aminolevulinic acid (ALA) synthesis—irreversible, rate-limiting step.
    - Glycine and succinyl-CoA condensation.
    - Catalyzed by ALA synthase, requires PLP cofactor.
  - Porphobilinogen (PBG) formation—dehydration of two ALA molecules.

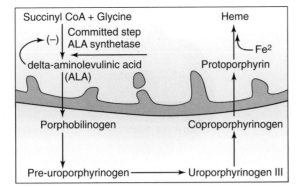

FIGURE 3-68. **Heme synthesis.** Glycine and succinyl-CoA combine to form protoporphyrin IX, which is used to form aminolevulinic acid (ALA). Two ALA molecules then condense to form porphobilinogen (PBG). Four molecules of PBG then condense to form pre-uroporphyrinogen. The remaining reactions alter side chains and the degree of porphyrin unsaturation.

- Uroporphyrinogen I (UROgen I) formation—condensation of four PBG molecules (inactive).
- Uroporphyrinogen III (UROgen III) formation—produces an active molecule.
- Coproporphyrinogen III formation, protoporphyrin IX formation, which alters side chains and porphyrin unsaturation degree.
- Heme formation—insertion of Fe^{2+}.

Arginine Derivatives

CREATINE

High-energy phosphate storage.

- **Synthesis location:** Liver, precursor formed in kidney.
- **Synthesis reaction:** See Figure 3-69.
    - Arginine and glycine formation of guanidoacetate in kidney.
    - Guanidoacetate methylation using SAM as methyl donor.

For storage, phosphate of ATP can be transferred to creatine, forming creatine phosphate. Phosphate transfer can be reversed in energy-depleted muscle, generating creatine and ATP. Creatine and creatine phosphate spontaneously cyclize, creating creatinine for excretion in urine.

UREA

Nontoxic disposable form of ammonia that is generated during amino acid turnover.

- **Synthesis location:** Liver.
- **Synthesis reaction:** Arginine cleavage to urea and ornithine in the urea cycle.
    - Urea travels via the blood to the kidneys, where it is excreted in the urine.

NITRIC OXIDE

Positively regulates vessel dilation through smooth muscle relaxation.

- **Synthesis location:** Small-vessel endothelial cells.
- **Synthesis reaction:** Arginine oxidation.

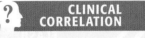

CLINICAL CORRELATION

Creatine phosphokinase is released into the circulation if muscle or brain is injured. This includes damage to heart muscle as well as skeletal muscle. Measurement of cardiac-specific creatine phosphokinase is important in the diagnosis of myocardial infarction.

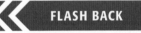

FLASH BACK

The urea cycle prevents ammonia toxicity.

CLINICAL CORRELATION

During erection, nitric oxide (NO) is released in the corpus cavernosum of the penis, leading to smooth muscle relaxation. Sildenafil citrate, also known as Viagra, is a selective inhibitor of the phosphodiesterase that prolongs the effects of NO.

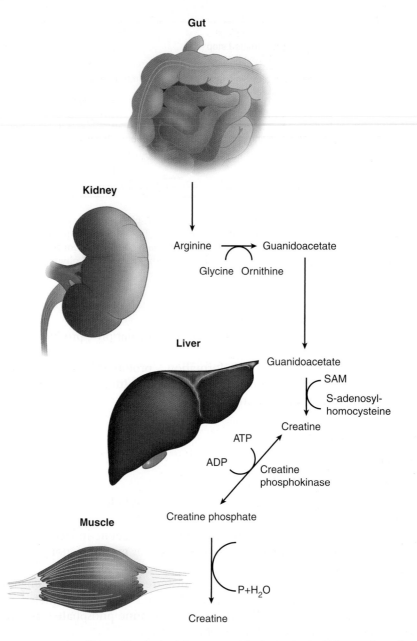

FIGURE 3-69. Creatine synthesis. Arginine reacts with glycine in the kidney to form the precursor guanidoacetate. Guanidoacetate is then methylated, using SAM, in the liver forming creatine. A high-energy phosphate group from ATP can then be transferred creating creatine phosphate. In muscle, when energy demand is high, the high-energy phosphate can be removed and creatine phosphate is converted back to creatine.

Glutamate Derivative

γ-AMINOBUTYRIC ACID (GABA)

Acts as an inhibitory neurotransmitter.

- **Synthesis location:** Central nervous system.
- **Synthesis reaction:** Glutamate decarboxylation.

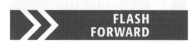

FLASH FORWARD

GABA analogs, such as gabapentin, were initially designed for use as anticonvulsants.

Review of Amino Acid Derivatives

Amino Acid	Derivative(s)
Methionine	SAM
Tyrosine	Thyroid hormones, melanin, catecholamines
Tryptophan	Niacin, serotonin, melatonin
Histidine	Histamine
Glycine	Heme
Arginine	Creatine, urea, nitric oxide
Glutamate	GABA

AMINO ACID BREAKDOWN

Excess amino acids and used amino acids must be degraded and eliminated from the body. This process can be thought of as consisting of two steps: disposal of the α-amino group and disposal of the carbon skeleton.

Disposal of the α-Amino Group

The α-amino group can be disposed of by two possible routes, both of which begin with transamination to create a common pool of glutamate (Figure 3-70). In the first route, glutamate undergoes oxidative deamination in the mitochondria, and the amino group is sent to the urea cycle for disposal. In the second route, the glutamate is transaminated a second time with a transfer of the α-amino group to oxaloacetate to form aspartate. This occurs mainly in the liver and is catalyzed by AST. The aspartate can then enter the urea cycle via condensation with citrulline and the amino group is again disposed of.

Alanine-Glucose Cycle

During amino acid catabolism the ammonium accumulated in skeletal muscle must be transported to the liver for disposal. However, ammonium is a toxic molecule (the reason we have the urea cycle), so alanine is used as a carrier in the circulation (Figure 3-71). In muscle, a common pool of glutamate is again created via transamination. Glutamate is transaminated a second time, transferring the α-amino group to pyruvate, which forms alanine. This reaction is catalyzed by ALT. Alanine is released into the circulation, as occurs during amino acid absorption. The alanine is taken up by the liver and the reaction is reversed, adding the glutamate from the muscle to the common pool in the liver which is processed as described earlier.

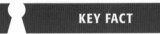

KEY FACT

Amino acids are converted to alanine for circulation and glutamate for rapid oxidative deamination and disposal.

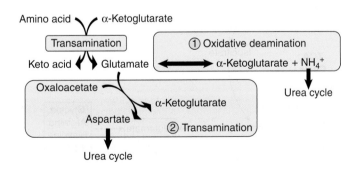

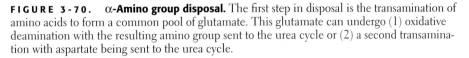

FIGURE 3-70. α-Amino group disposal. The first step in disposal is the transamination of amino acids to form a common pool of glutamate. This glutamate can undergo (1) oxidative deamination with the resulting amino group sent to the urea cycle or (2) a second transamination with aspartate being sent to the urea cycle.

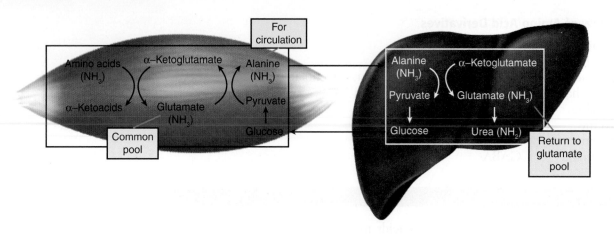

FIGURE 3-71. **Alanine-glucose cycle.** Alanine is used as a carrier to transport α-amino acid groups from the skeletal muscle to the liver for disposal via the urea cycle. This cycle allows carbon skeletons to be converted between protein and glucose.

Disposal of the Carbon Skeleton

The remaining carbon skeleton can then be salvaged as TCA cycle and glycolytic intermediates. All 20 amino acids break down to seven common products: acetyl-CoA, acetoacetyl-CoA, pyruvate, oxaloacetate, fumarate, succinyl-CoA, and α-ketoglutarate (Figure 3-72). Ketogenic amino acids are those that are broken down into the **ketone body formers acetyl-CoA and acetoacetyl-CoA.** Glucogenic amino acids are those that are broken down to **pyruvate or TCA intermediates** that can be channeled into gluconeogenesis. Only leucine and lysine are considered to be purely ketogenic. **Isoleucine, phenylalanine, tyrosine, and tryptophan are both ketogenic and glucogenic.** All other amino acids are purely glucogenic.

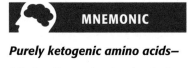

MNEMONIC

Purely ketogenic amino acids—

JKL: Just **K**etogenic = **L**eucine, **L**ysine

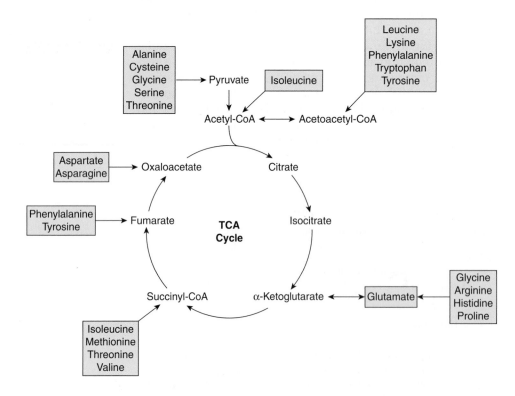

FIGURE 3-72. **Amino acid carbon skeleton recycling.** The 20 amino acids can be broken down to seven common carbon skeletons, which can be feed into the tricarboxylic acid (TCA) cycle. Depending on the energy needs of the cell, these products can also be used to synthesize fat or glycogen.

AMINO ACID DEFICIENCIES

Phenylketonuria (PKU)

Autosomal recessive deficiency of **phenylalanine hydroxylase** or in some cases its cofactor tetrahydrobiopterin (Figure 3-73). The lack of this enzyme causes a **buildup of phenylalanine** and an **inability to produce tyrosine.** Excess phenylalanine is converted into the phenylketones: phenylpyruvate, phenyllactate, and phenylacetate.

INCIDENCE

PKU is one of the most common amino acid deficiencies, with an incidence of 1 in 13,500–19,000 live births.

PRESENTATION

If untreated, infants present at 6–12 months with CNS symptoms of developmental delay, seizures, and failure to thrive. Patients also exhibit characteristics of hypopigmentation such as fair hair, blue eyes, and pale skin. Hypopigmentation occurs because tyrosine, a derivative of phenylalaline, is the precursor for melanin.

DIAGNOSIS

In the United States all neonates are screened for raised blood levels of phenylalanine.

TREATMENT

Classically, management of the condition is accomplished by **restriction of dietary phenylalanine,** which is contained in aspartame (eg, NutraSweet), and an increase in dietary tyrosine along with monitoring of blood phenylalanine levels. However, new treatments are in development and in use.

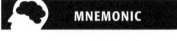

MNEMONIC

PKU: Disorder of **aromatic** amino acid metabolism—musty body **odor.**

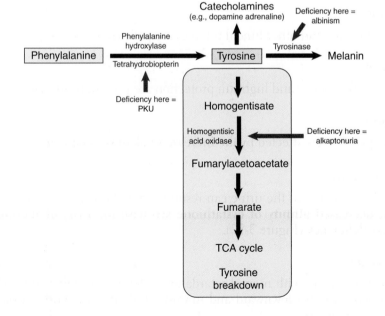

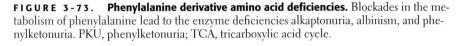

FIGURE 3-73. **Phenylalanine derivative amino acid deficiencies.** Blockades in the metabolism of phenylalanine lead to the enzyme deficiencies alkaptonuria, albinism, and phenylketonuria. PKU, phenylketonuria; TCA, tricarboxylic acid cycle.

Alkaptonuria

Congenital deficiency of **homogentisic acid oxidase,** an enzyme used in the degradation of tyrosine (Figure 3-73). This deficiency results in a buildup of homogentisate that polymerizes to a black-brown pigment. This pigment deposits in connective tissue, including cartilage.

PRESENTATION

Alkaptonuria is one of the few inborn errors of metabolism that does not manifest until **adulthood.** In this disease, joint damage and arthritis become apparent at presentation. However, it may be detected at an earlier age, since **urine and sweat may turn black** upon standing, owing to the formation of alkapton.

DIAGNOSIS

This condition may be diagnosed by allowing the patient's urine to stand and monitoring for colorimetric change. The results can be confirmed quantitatively with a measurement of homogentisate in the urine.

TREATMENT

There is no specific treatment for alkaptonuria, and the clinical effects of dietary restriction are limited.

Albinism

Deficiency of the enzyme **tyrosinase,** which catalyzes conversion to melanin, or defective **tyrosine transporters.** The disorder can also result from lack of migration of neural crest cells.

PRESENTATION

Neonates present with amelanosis (whitish hair, pale skin, gray-blue eyes), nystagmus, and photophobia (low pigment in iris and retina leads to failure to develop fixation reflex).

DIAGNOSIS

Iris translucency and other fundal findings are pathognomonic signs.

TREATMENT

Tinted contact lenses and high sun protection are important in management.

PROGNOSIS

Disease prognosis is affected by the **increased risk of skin cancer.**

Homocystinuria

Excess homocystine in the urine can result from **cystathionine synthase deficiency, decreased affinity of cystathione synthase for PLP, or methionine synthase deficiency** (Figure 3-57).

PRESENTATION

Patients can present with mental retardation, osteoporosis, tall stature, kyphosis, lens sublaxation (downward and inward), and atherosclerosis (stroke and myocardial infarction).

DIAGNOSIS

Diagnosis consists of measuring excess homocystine in the urine of a patient without vitamin B_{12} deficiency.

TREATMENT

The management depends on the underlying cause of the homocystinuria. For cystathionine synthase deficiency, treatment is a dietary decrease in methionine and increase in cysteine. For decreased affinity of PLP, treatment is increased vitamin B_6.

Maple Syrup Urine Disease

Deficiency of the enzyme α-keto acid dehydrogenase, which catalyzes degradation of the branched-chain amino acids (**isoleucine, valine, leucine**). This leads to an increase of α-keto acids in the blood, especially leucine.

PRESENTATION

Affected infants are normal at birth but develop a characteristic odor, lethargy, feeding difficulties, coma, and seizures. If untreated, this leads to CNS defects, mental retardation, and death.

DIAGNOSIS

High levels of branched-chain amino acids in the urine and blood are used for diagnosis.

TREATMENT

Dietary restriction of branched-chain amino acids.

PROGNOSIS

If untreated, the infant dies in the first month of life.

Nutrition

VITAMINS

Vitamins are ubiquitous to enzymatic processes. Both anabolic (formation) and catabolic (breakdown) reactions require vitamins.

Vitamins are divided into those that are **soluble in water** and those that are **soluble in fat.**

Water-soluble vitamins are readily absorbed from the gut directly into the bloodstream, where they are maintained until they are excreted by the kidney in urine (with a few exceptions). Water-soluble vitamins are less likely to achieve toxic levels because they are readily excreted in the urine. Patients are more likely to be deficient in them as there is limited storage in the body for water-soluble vitamins.

Fat-soluble vitamins dissolve in dietary fats and migrate through the lymphatic system before entering the blood bound to protein carriers such as albumin. These vitamins are stored in adipose and other fatty tissues and accumulate, making it possible to reach toxic levels. Patients are less likely to be deficient in fat-soluble vitamins because of their ability to accumulate in lipid. However, in patients with malabsorptive diseases, such as celiac disease, cystic fibrosis, and pancreatic insufficiency, deficiency in fat-soluble vitamins is possible.

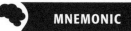

MNEMONIC

Branched-chain amino acids blocked in maple syrup urine disease—

I Love Vermont maple syrup:

Isoleucine
Leucine
Valine

KEY FACT

Amino acid deficiencies are autosomal recessive disorders, present in the neonatal period (except for alkaptonuria) and are usually treated with dietary restrictions.

KEY FACT

Water-Soluble Vitamins
Vitamin B_1 (thiamine)
Vitamin B_2 (riboflavin)
Vitamin B_3 (niacin)
Vitamin B_5 (pantothenic acid)
Vitamin B_6 (pyridoxine)
Vitamin B_{12} (cyanocobalamin)
Folic acid
Biotin
Vitamin C (ascorbic acid)

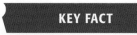

KEY FACT

Fat-Soluble Vitamins
Vitamin A (retinols)
Vitamin D, vitamin D_2 (ergocalciferol), vitamin D_3 (cholecalciferol)
Vitamin E (α-tocopherol)
Vitamin K (phylloquinone)

Water-Soluble Vitamins

VITAMIN B₁—THIAMINE

Thiamine is a water-soluble vitamin, found in grains, meats, and legumes, used as a coenzyme in many biochemical reactions involving **carbohydrate metabolism.** The biologically active form, thiamine pyrophosphate (TPP, also called thiamine diphosphate), is found in liver, kidneys, and leukocytes.

TPP, as its name implies, is formed from the transfer of ATP to thiamine. Once formed, it is used in the cell as a coenzyme for:

- Transketolation reactions found in the pentose phosphate pathway.
- Conversion of pyruvate to acetyl-CoA.
- Conversion of α-ketoglutarate to succinyl-CoA.
- Creation of branched-chain amino acids leucine, isoleucine, and valine.

In the United States, thiamine deficiency is most commonly due to chronic alcoholism. Absence of thiamine decreases the amount of acetyl-CoA available to enter the TCA cycle and increases the amount of pyruvate available for anaerobic oxidation. This leads to increased lactic acid production.

Clinically, signs of thiamine deficiency include:

- Muscle cramps
- Paresthesias
- Irritability
- Beriberi (wet or dry)

Beriberi is divided into wet and dry. Wet beriberi involves the cardiovascular system, whereas dry beriberi involves the nervous system (dry beriberi with Wernicke-Korsakoff syndrome).

Wet beriberi is characterized by neuropathy as well as heart failure, which may be high output, and includes a **triad of peripheral vasodilation, biventricular failure,** and **edema.** It is often brought on by physical exertion and increased carbohydrate intake.

Dry beriberi occurs with little physical exertion and decreased caloric intake and may affect peripheral nerves (motor and sensory neuropathy). **Wernicke-Korsakoff syndrome** occurs in chronic alcoholics with thiamine deficiency. **Wernicke's** encephalopathy consists of the triad: **ophthalmoplegia** (and nystagmus), **truncal ataxia,** and **confusion.** Untreated encephalopathy progresses to **Korsakoff** syndrome. Korsakoff syndrome consists of **impaired short-term memory** and **confabulation,** with otherwise grossly normal cognition.

VITAMIN B₂—RIBOFLAVIN

Riboflavin, used as a cofactor in the oxidation and reduction of various substrates, is found in milk and other dairy products. It serves as a precursor to the **coenzymes flavin mononucleotide (FMN)** and **flavin adenine dinucleotide (FAD).**

In the formation of both FMN and FAD, riboflavin reacts with ATP. In the formation of FMN, riboflavin reacts with a single ATP, yielding FMN and ADP as a by-product. In the formation of FAD, FMN reacts with a second ATP molecule, yielding FAD and pyrophosphate (PPi) as a by-product.

KEY FACT

It is traditional to give thiamine before glucose in alcoholic patients to avoid precipitating Wernicke's encephalopathy (although thiamine is taken up by cells more slowly than glucose).

Because of their ability to add/subtract two hydrogen atoms, FMN and FAD are favored in **fatty acid oxidation, amino acid oxidation,** and the **TCA cycle.** Riboflavin is also important for **erythrocyte integrity,** through erythrocyte glutathione reductase, and also for the conversion of **tryptophan to niacin.**

Deficiencies in riboflavin, leading to deficiencies in FMN and FAD, clinically cause **glossitis, cheilosis, and corneal vascularization.** It may also cause angular stomatitis, seborrheic dermatitis, and weakness. Because erythrocyte glutathione reductase depends on riboflavin, patients may also have anemia secondary to **red blood cell lysis.**

KEY FACT

Absence of vitamin B_2 causes the two **C**'s:
Cheilosis
Corneal vascularization

VITAMIN B_3—NIACIN

Niacin, found in liver, milk, and unrefined grains, is another coenzyme used in oxidation and reduction reactions. Niacin appears in the diet as tryptophan, **nicotinamide adenine dinucleotide (NAD)** or its phosphorylated form, **nicotinamide adenine dinucleotide phosphate (NADP),** both forms are hydrolyzed by intestinal enzymes to form nicotinamide. Intestinal flora convert NAD and NADP to nicotinic acid. The body is also capable of converting tryptophan to niacin.

Pharmacologically, nicotinic acid can be a treatment option to decrease total and LDL cholesterol (and has some effects to raise HDL). Its side effects include flushing, pruritus (both of which are treated with aspirin), hives, nausea, and vomiting.

Pellagra is the name of niacin deficiency. Patients can get pellagra from lack of dietary niacin, isoniazid use, Hartnup disease, or malignant carcinoid syndrome. Pellagra is characterized by **diarrhea, dermatitis,** and **dementia** (Figure 3-74). If untreated, pellagra can be fatal. Dietary replacement of both tryptophan and niacin is the treatment.

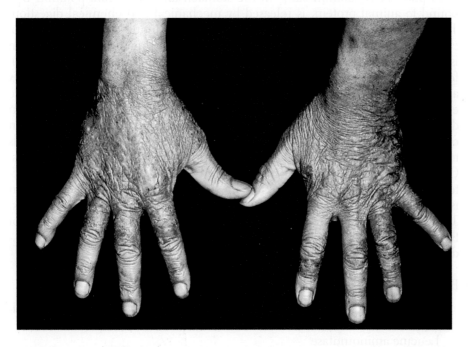

FIGURE 3-74. **Pellagra.** Signs of pellagra include hyperpigmented, brittle, cracked, and scaly skin. (Reproduced with permission from Wolf K, Johnson RA, Suurmond D. *Fitzpatrick's Color Atlas & Synopsis of Clinical Dermatology,* 5th ed. New York: McGraw-Hill, 2005: 457.)

Hartnup disease is a genetic defect in tryptophan membrane transport that causes intestinal malabsorption and poor renal resorption. Therefore, simple replacement therapy is insufficient. Similarly, in **malignant carcinoid syndrome,** tryptophan is used for excessive 5-hydroxytryptamine (5-HT) production and is less available for NAD synthesis, causing pellagra that is nonresponsive to therapy.

VITAMIN B$_5$—PANTOTHENIC ACID

Pantothenic acid is the major constituent of CoA, and it is found in most foods. It is a cofactor for acyl transfers (pantothen-A is in the CoA complex). These reactions take place in the TCA cycle, fatty acid oxidation, acetylations, and cholesterol synthesis. Deficiency of vitamin B$_5$ is rare in humans, but may result in paresthesias or dysesthesias, and gastrointestinal distress.

VITAMIN B$_6$—PYRIDOXINE

A pyridine derivative, pyridoxine, along with pyridoxal and pyridoxamine, serve as building blocks for **PLP,** which is the coenzyme involved in **amino acid metabolism** (eg, conversion of serine to glycine). These molecules are found in wheat, egg yolk, and meats. The coenzyme is responsible for numerous processes including transamination, deamination, decarboxylation, and condensation and creation of the liver enzymes **AST** and **ALT.**

Although clinical manifestations are rare, a deficiency of vitamin B$_6$ can result in **convulsions** as well as **hyperirritability.** Decreased concentrations of vitamin B$_6$ deficiency may occur after use of oral contraceptives, isoniazid, cycloserine, and penicillamine. Too much vitamin B$_6$ can cause sensory neuropathy that is unrelieved when toxicity is corrected.

VITAMIN B$_{12}$—COBALAMIN

Animal products (meat or dairy) are the only dietary source of vitamin B$_{12}$. Absorption of cobalamin starts in the stomach after ingestion. Vitamin B$_{12}$, bound to animal protein, is released by mechanical and chemical digestion. The parietal cells, located primarily at the gastric fundus, secrete both hydrochloric acid and **intrinsic factor** in response to the meal. As the cobalamin is released from the animal protein, it is bound by **R protein (haptocorrin),** forming a stable complex in the low pH. The R protein–cobalamin complex and the secreted intrinsic factor move into the duodenum, where pancreatic enzymes degrade R protein. The R protein–cobalamin complex is broken down and allows intrinsic factor to bind B$_{12}$. **The intrinsic factor–cobalamin complex** formed in the duodenum moves toward the distal ileum and binds to the **intrinsic factor–cobalamin receptor** expressed on the enterocytes. Once bound, the entire unit is internalized by the enterocyte. Intrinsic factor is degraded in the enterocyte, freeing cobalamin. The available cobalamin is bound to plasma **transcobalamin II** (TCII), forming yet another complex. The TCII/cobalamin complex then migrates through the basolateral side of the enterocyte into circulation, stored in the liver, and made available for B$_{12}$-dependent enzymes.

B$_{12}$-dependent enzymes:

- Methylmalonyl-CoA mutase (converts propionyl-CoA to methylmalonyl-CoA and then to succinyl-CoA)
- Leucine aminomutase
- Methionine synthase

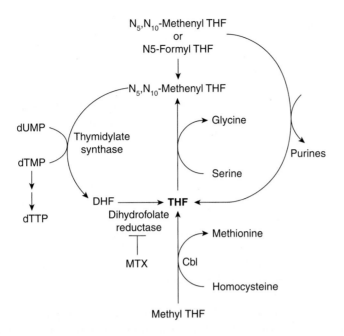

FIGURE 3-75. **Tetrahydrofolate metabolism.** Cbl = cobalamin; DHF = dihydrofolate; dTMP = deoxythymidine monophosphate; dTTP = deoxythymine triphosphate; dUMP = deoxyuridine monophosphate; MTX = methotrexate; THF = tetrahydrofolate. (Modified with permission from Kasper DL, Braunwald E, Fauci AS, et al. *Harrison's Principles of Internal Medicine*, 16th ed. New York: McGraw-Hill, 2005: 602.)

Cobalamin is used as a cofactor for **methionine synthase** and **methylmalonyl-CoA synthase.** Methionine synthase catalyzes homocysteine to methionine via a one-carbon transfer from methyl-THF to create THF (Figure 3-75). These one-carbon transfers are necessary for **de novo synthesis of purines** and require folate as a cofactor. Deficiency in cobalamin causes a buildup of methyl-THF (unconjugated form), which eventually leaves the cell and can lead to a corresponding folate deficiency.

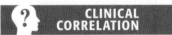

Vitamin B$_{12}$ deficiency can lead to megaloblastic anemia, just like folate deficiency. A hallmark finding in megaloblastic anemia is hypersegmented neutrophils on peripheral smear (Figure 3-76).

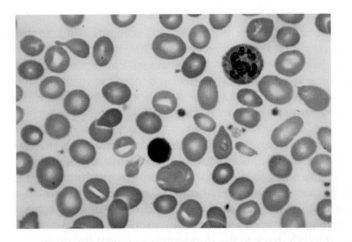

FIGURE 3-76. **Hypersegmented neutrophil.** (Reproduced with permission from Lichtman MA, Shafer MS, Felgar RE, Wang, N. *Lichtman's Atlas of Hematology*. New York: McGraw-Hill, 2007: Figure I.C.97.)

Vitamin B$_{12}$ deficiency can be caused by a myriad of disorders. **Dietary deficiency** is rare, because the liver stores large quantities of vitamin B$_{12}$. **Pernicious anemia** is a common cause of megaloblastic anemia (mean corpuscular volume [MCV] > 100 fL). It is typically caused by an autoimmune attack on gastric parietal cells, which leads to decreased production of intrinsic factor (accompanied by achlorhydria and atrophic gastritis). **Gastrectomy** (and similarly gastric bypass surgery) disrupts secretion of intrinsic factor by gastric parietal cells, leading to decreased absorption of vitamin B$_{12}$. **Infectious** causes include *Helicobacter pylori*, which causes chronic gastritis; *Diphyllobothrium latum*, in which the fish tapeworm competes for vitamin B$_{12}$ absorption in the intestine; and blind loop syndrome, in which bacterial overgrowth also competes for vitamin B$_{12}$ absorption in the intestine. **Structural abnormalities of the terminal ileum** (Crohn disease, surgical resection) can cause decreased absorption of vitamin B$_{12}$. **Pancreatic insufficiency** leads to a decrease in enzymes necessary to break down the R protein–cobalamin complex, preventing cobalamin from binding with intrinsic factor. Finally, **deficiency of transcobalamin II** prevents cobalamin from entering systemic circulation.

Clinical signs of vitamin B$_{12}$ deficiency include a neuropathy characterized by defective myelin formation and consequent subacute degeneration of the posterior and lateral spinal columns. This results in symmetrical paresthesias and ataxia, loss of proprioception and vibration senses, and, in severe cases, spasticity, clonus, paraplegia, and fecal and urinary incontinence. The mechanism for this defect is uncertain, but it may be that lack of vitamin B$_{12}$ causes decreased folate, which in turn decreases methionine levels and leads to impaired myelin production.

The most evident sign of vitamin B$_{12}$ deficiency, however, is megaloblastic change of the red blood cells (seen on a peripheral blood smear) and mean cell volume (MCV). **Elevated MCV** (> 110 fL) and **hypersegmented neutrophils** (lobe count ≥ 4) indicate deficiency. The megaloblastic changes due to vitamin B$_{12}$ deficiency are indistinguishable from those due to folate deficiency; however, **only vitamin B$_{12}$ deficiency causes neuropathy.**

FOLIC ACID

Present in fruits and vegetables, folic acid is required for erythropoiesis and one-carbon transfers. It is responsible for the conversion of homocysteine to methionine (where vitamin B$_{12}$ is a cofactor), conversion of serine to glycine (where B$_6$ is a cofactor), and conversion of deoxyuridylate to thymidylate for DNA synthesis, and it is indirectly responsible for purine ring formation (through its derivatives) (Figure 3-75).

Folate is maintained in the body via the **folate enterohepatic cycle.** Dietary folate (available as polyglutamates) undergoes hydrolysis and reduction from enzymes on mucosal cell membranes to form monoglutamate. **Dihydrofolate reductase** found in the duodenal mucosa methylates the folate and allows it to be absorbed by enterocytes in the jejunum. Folate then joins with plasma-binding proteins and travels systemically or to the liver, where it is converted and secreted in bile back to the duodenum to repeat the cycle.

Causes of folate deficiency include **inadequate dietary intake, malabsorptive diseases, liver dysfunction, medications,** and states of **increased folate consumption.** Inadequate dietary intake is seen in alcoholics or persons who do not consume a lot of raw vegetables. Malabsorptive diseases that affect the jejunum, celiac sprue, and biliary diseases alter the folate enterohepatic cycle. Liver dysfunction, seen in alcoholic cirrhotics, also interfere with the enterohepatic cycle and may interfere with production of plasma-binding proteins. Medications such as **methotrexate** and **trimethoprim** inhibit dihydrofolate reductase and decrease absorption of dietary folate. Other medications (phenytoin) can also interfere with absorption. Finally, pregnancy, hemolytic anemias, and other states that require a large amount of folate can simply deplete the available stores of folate and create a relative deficiency because of increased demand.

Clinical symptoms of folic acid deficiency consist of megaloblastic anemia (with mucosal changes). However, there are no neurologic sequelae from folic acid deficiency in adults. (in contrast to what occurs with vitamin B_{12} deficiency, which consists of a megaloblastic anemia and neurologic symptoms). Note that folic acid deficiency in pregnant women is associated with increased rate of neural tube defects.

BIOTIN

Biotin is a water-soluble vitamin found in peanuts, cashews, almonds, and other foods. Intestinal flora also synthesize biotin. Raw egg whites contain **avidin,** which binds to biotin, forming a nonabsorbable complex. The biotin coenzyme **carries carboxylate** and is involved in carboxylation reactions important for carbohydrate and lipid metabolism. Biotin participates in several key reactions, including conversion of **pyruvate to oxaloacetate** (by pyruvate carboxylase in the TCA cycle) and conversion of **propionyl-CoA to methylmalonyl-CoA** (by propionyl-CoA carboxylase, in synthesis of odd-chain fatty acids).

VITAMIN C—ASCORBIC ACID

Vitamin C or ascorbic acid is found in citrus fruits. Dietary vitamin C is taken up in the ileum. It provides reducing equivalents for several enzymatic reactions, particularly those catalyzed by **copper- and iron-containing enzymes,** and is linked to increased iron absorption in the intestine. Vitamin C is necessary for proper hydroxylation of proline and lysine used in **collagen synthesis.** It also serves as an antioxidant and facilitates iron absorption by keeping iron in its reduced state. Many copper-containing or iron-containing hydroxylases require ascorbic acid to maintain normal metabolism. **Dopamine β-hydroxylase,** involved in the conversion of tyrosine to norepinephrine and epinephrine, requires ascorbate to reduce copper after it has been oxidized in the reaction. Likewise, **proline and lysine hydroxylase** are required for the posttranslational modification of procollagen to form collagen, because hydroxylated residues are required for the formation of stable triple helices and for cross-linking of collagen molecules to form fibrils.

Scurvy results from vitamin C deficiency. Swollen gums, bruising, anemia, and poor wound healing are signs of scurvy and are due in part to impaired collagen formation (Figure 3-77).

Fat-Soluble Vitamins

VITAMIN A—RETINOIDS

Vitamin A (eg, retinol, retinaldehyde, retinoic acid) is found in fish oils, meats, dairy products, and eggs. β-Carotene, a precursor of vitamin A that is

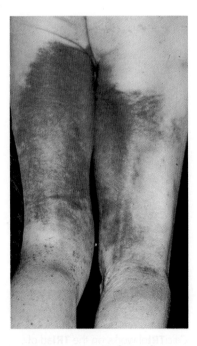

> **KEY FACT**
>
> Folate deficiency leads to hyperhomocysteinemia (elevated levels of homocysteine), which leads to atherosclerosis.

> **KEY FACT**
>
> Genetic disorders of collagen synthesis include osteogenesis imperfecta and Ehlers-Danlos syndrome.

FIGURE 3-77. Ecchymosis secondary to vitamin C deficiency. (Reproduced with permission from Wolff K, Johnson RA, Suurmond D. *Fitzpatrick's Color Atlas and Synopsis of Clinical Dermatology,* 5th ed. New York: McGraw-Hill, 2005: 453.)

metabolized by intestinal mucosal cells into retinaldehyde, is found in green vegetables. Vitamin A in the form of retinol is absorbed into the **intestinal mucosal cells** and is transported **to the liver via chylomicrons.** Vitamin A is delivered to the rest of the body via prealbumin and retinol-binding protein.

Vitamin A combines with opsin in the eye to form rhodopsin in the rod cells of the retina. A similar reaction produces iodopsin in cone cells. These proteins play a crucial role in sensing light in the retina and are essential for vision. Vitamin A also has a role in the differentiation and proliferation of epithelial cells in the respiratory tract, skin, cornea, conjunctiva, and other tissues.

Deficiency of vitamin A, therefore, causes vision problems, disorders of epithelial cell differentiation and proliferation, and impaired immune response. Symptoms may include headaches, skin changes, sore throat, and alopecia. Progression of visual symptoms for vitamin A deficiency include loss of green light sensitivity, poor adaptation to dim light, night blindness (loss of retinol in rod cells). **Xerophthalmia** (squamous epithelial thickening), **Bitot spots** (squamous metaplasia), and **keratomalacia** (softening of the cornea) also occur in vitamin A deficiency. Metaplasia of respiratory epithelia is seen (often common in cystic fibrosis due to failure of fat-soluble vitamin absorption) as well as frequent respiratory infections (secondary to respiratory epithelial defects).

Because vitamin A is stored in the liver and is lipophilic, the body can store large amounts of the vitamin. Toxicity can occur acutely, chronically, or as a teratogenic effect. Acute toxicity can be caused from a large, single dose of vitamin A and results in nausea, vertigo, and blurry vision. Chronic toxicity can manifest as ataxia, alopecia, hyperlipidemia, or hepatotoxicity. In the first trimester of pregnancy, excess vitamin A can be very teratogenic and can lead to fetal loss.

VITAMIN D—CHOLECALCIFEROL

Vitamin D plays an important role in bone metabolism by regulating plasma calcium concentrations. Vitamin D is absorbed from dietary sources and is also synthesized in the skin. Vitamin D absorption is regulated by serum calcium concentrations.

In the presence of UV light, 7-dehydrocholesterol present in the skin is converted to previtamin D. Once previtamin D is formed, it is converted to cholecalciferol, which enters the circulation. Activation of cholecalciferol takes place in the liver and the kidney. The **liver** converts cholecalciferol to **25-hydroxy derivative.** The **kidney** converts the 25-hydroxy derivative into **1,25-hydroxy vitamin D (1,25 OHD, calcitriol),** its active metabolite. The kidney also converts 25-hydroxy derivative into 24,25-hydroxyvitamin D, an inactive metabolite (Figure 3-78). Vitamin D–binding globulin stores vitamin D and is also responsible for its systemic transport in the circulation.

Vitamin D maintains the plasma calcium concentration by increasing intestinal absorption of calcium, minimizing calcium excretion in the distal renal tubules, mobilizing bone mineral in bones. It also stimulates osteoblasts and improves calcification of bone matrix (and, hence, bone formation).

Activated vitamin D, binds to a nuclear receptor in cells of interest (intestinal cells, renal cells, and osteoblasts) and induces gene expression. It is regulated

KEY FACT

Calci**TRI**ol works on the **TRI**ad of intestines, kidneys, and bone to maintain plasma calcium levels.

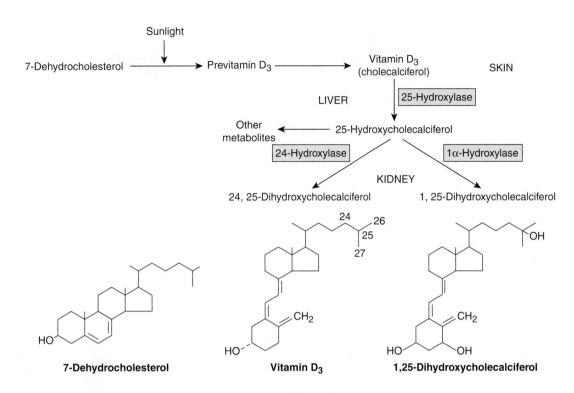

FIGURE 3-78. **Various pathways of vitamin D formation.** (Modified with permission from Ganong WF. *Review of Medical Physiology,* 22nd ed. New York: McGraw-Hill, 2005: 388.)

by a series of feedback mechanisms involving PTH (parathyroid hormone), calcium, and phosphate. Low levels of calcium stimulate PTH synthesis and secretion, which in turn prompt the conversion of 25-hydroxy derivative to 1,25-dihydroxyvitamin D (calcitriol). In turn, calcitriol has a negative feedback effect on its own production and PTH production. In excess, calcitriol also promotes the production of 24,25-dihydroxyvitamin D.

In the presence of excess calcitriol and thus calcium from either bone or intestinal absorption, high levels of calcium act to decrease PTH production, and high levels of phosphate act to decrease conversion of 25-hydroxy derivative to 1,25-dihydroxyvitamin D by blocking the 1α-hydroxylase enzyme involved in the activation of the 25-hydroxy derivative (Figures 3-79 and 3-80).

Deficiency of vitamin D leads to **rickets** in children and **osteomalacia** in adults, the differences being open (in children) or closed (in adults) epiphyseal plates. Rickets results from not receiving enough calcium and phosphate going to the sites where bone mineralization is taking place.

Clinically, children with rickets show signs of hypocalcemia, bowing of the lower extremities, and poor dentition. The treatment for vitamin D–deficient rickets and osteomalacia is vitamin D therapy. In vitamin D–resistant rickets, vitamin D repletion does not treat the syndrome, and a genetic abnormality may be present.

- **Type I vitamin D–resistant rickets** occurs when there is a genetic mutation of 1α-hydroxylase. This can be treated with 1,25-dihydroxyvitamin D bypassing the conversion of 25-hydroxy derivative in the kidney. If supplementation of 1,25-dihydroxyvitamin D does not treat the underlying problem, then the patient has **type II vitamin D–resistant rickets.**

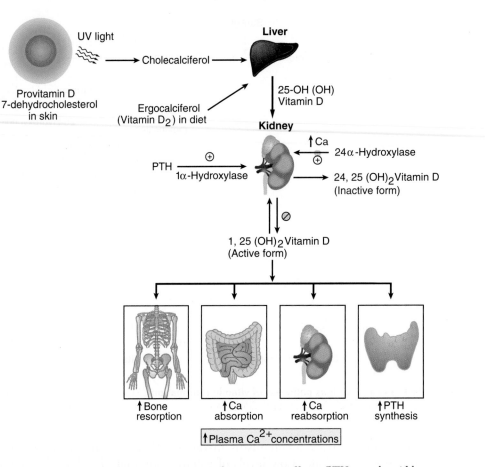

FIGURE 3-79. Vitamin D target organs and consequent effects. PTH, parathyroid hormone. (Modified with permission from Molina PE. *Endocrine Physiology*, 2nd ed. New York: McGraw-Hill, 2006: 110.)

- Type II vitamin D–resistant rickets occurs when the 1,25-dihydroxyvitamin D receptor is mutated and therefore unresponsive to both vitamin D and calcitriol.
- **X-linked rickets** is entirely due to renal phosphate wasting. In this condition, 1,25-OHD levels are elevated.

Excess vitamin D leads to hypercalcemia and all of the sequelae associated with it (eg, kidney stones, dementia, constipation, abdominal pain, depression). Sarcoidosis can lead to excess vitamin D since pulmonary macrophages can produce calcitriol. Similarly, lymphoma can produce calcitriol.

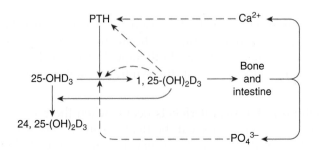

FIGURE 3-80. Vitamin D regulation. Solid lines indicate stimulation. Dashed lines indicate inhibitory. PTH, parathyroid hormone. (Modified with permission from Ganong WF. *Review of Medical Physiology*, 22nd ed. New York: McGraw-Hill, 2005: 389.)

VITAMIN E—α-TOCOPHEROL

Vitamin E is a lipid-soluble antioxidant found in sunflower oil, corn oil, soybeans, meats, fruits, and vegetables. It can be found in cell membranes and serves as an antioxidant like glutathione and vitamin C. It is used to react to the radicals formed by peroxidation of fatty acids. Like other fat-soluble vitamins, vitamin E is absorbed in the intestine and travels to the liver via chylomicrons to the liver. Fat malabsorption diseases (cystic fibrosis, liver disease) decrease the amount of vitamin E available. Deficiency of vitamin E is uncommon, but can cause hemolytic anemia, peripheral neuropathy, and ophthalmoplegia. In excess, vitamin E can interfere with vitamin K metabolism.

VITAMIN K—PHYLLOQUINONE

Vitamin K is found in either vegetable or animal sources (phylloquinone) or through bacterial flora (menaquinone). It is used by the liver in clotting proteins for the carboxylation of glutamate residues. It forms **γ-carboxyglutamate** in the postsynthetic modification of clotting proteins. Prothrombin and coagulation factors VII, IX, and X, and the antithrombotic proteins C and S all have these residues (Figure 3-81). They are essential because γ-carboxyglutamate acts as a chelator, trapping calcium ions. This allows the clotting proteins to bind to negatively charged phospholipids at the surface of platelets and to function at these membranes.

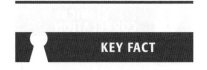

KEY FACT

Vitamin K–dependent coagulation factors are factors II (prothrombin), VII, IX, and X as well as protein C and protein S.

KEY FACT

Supratherapeutic levels of warfarin lead to bleeding (intracranial, GI, intraperitoneal), ecchymoses, and skin necrosis.

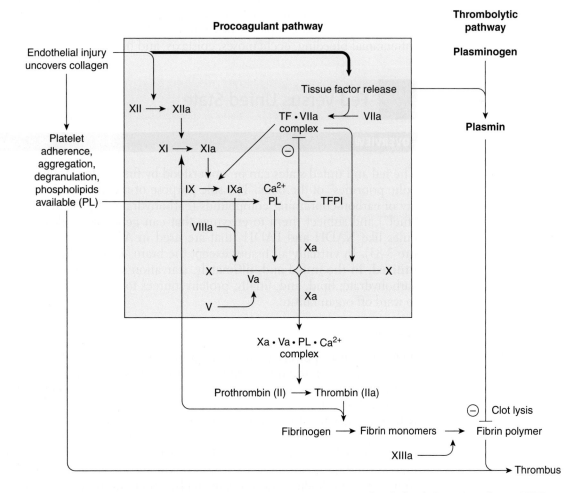

FIGURE 3-81.   Procoagulation and thrombolytic coagulation pathways. PL = phospholipid; TF = tissue factor; TPFI = tissue plasminogen pathway inhibitor. (Modified with permission from McPhee SJ, Ganong WF. *Pathophysiology of Disease: An Introduction to Clinical Medicine,* 5th ed. New York: McGraw-Hill, 2006: 120.)

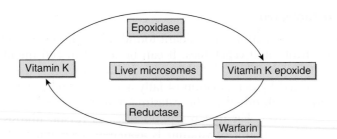

FIGURE 3-82. **Warfarin prevents conversion of vitamin K epoxide to vitamin K.** (Modified with permission from Kasper DL, Braunwald E, Fauci AS, et al. *Harrison's Principles of Internal Medicine*, 16th ed. New York: McGraw-Hill, 2005: 683.)

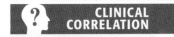

CLINICAL CORRELATION

Rat poison is a type of "superwarfarin" and causes severe coagulopathy. Treatment for ingestions is with high doses of vitamin K.

The reduced form of vitamin K is oxidized by γ-glutamyl carboxylase (and epoxidase) to form the γ-carboxyglutamate (Gla) in the postsynthetic modification. The oxidized form of vitamin K, or **vitamin K epoxide,** needs to be converted back to the reduced form to be used again. **Warfarin** blocks the use of the **2,3-epoxide reductase** in its reaction with **vitamin K epoxide and NADH** (Figure 3-82). The resulting vitamin K epoxide is soluble in water and excreted from the body. The overall effect is anticoagulation, reducing the total amount of biologically active coagulation factors.

Vitamin K deficiency is rare in otherwise healthy adults. Symptoms of vitamin K deficiency are similar to those of warfarin toxicity in that both have an apparent lack of vitamin K, resulting in a decrease of coagulation factor function. Signs and symptoms of vitamin K deficiency include GI bleeding, intracranial bleeding, ecchymoses, epistaxis, and hematuria.

Fed Versus Unfed State

OVERVIEW

The fed and unfed states can be understood by first understanding the "metabolic priorities" of the body. The sole purpose of metabolism is to take a variety of carbon-containing compounds (carbohydrates, lipids, and peptides, or "fuel") and subject them to enzymes that can generate ATP or other molecules like NADH and $FADH_2$ that are used in ATP-forming reactions (Figure 3-83). In virtually all tissues except the brain, **insulin directs how fuel is utilized.** In the unfed and, ultimately, starvation states, the body catabolizes carbohydrate, lipid, and, finally, protein sources to generate the ATP required to ward off organ failure.

The Brain

ATP, of course, powers virtually all important cellular and molecular processes. The most important ATP-consuming processes, however, are those occurring in the brain. The body does everything possible to ensure the brain receives the carbon-containing compounds it needs to function. The brain is highly specialized for its job and is not equipped to store **fats as triglycerides** or **glucose as glycogen** as other tissues do. It therefore requires a constant source of fuel from the blood (which is why "strokes," a cessation of blood flow to the brain, can be so damaging). Glucose is the brain's preferred fuel source. Ketone bodies (but not fatty acids, which are bound to albumin) can traverse the blood-brain barrier and be used as fuel too.

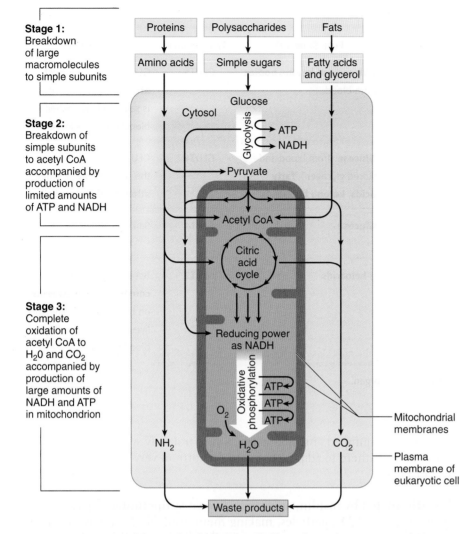

FIGURE 3-83. **Breakdown of carbohydrates, lipids, and proteins generates ATP or ATP equivalents.** The body has evolved enzymatic processes that are capable of producing ATP from a variety of carbon-containing compounds.

Conceptually, the body can be divided into three metabolic parts: muscle tissue, adipose tissue, and the liver. Each is discussed briefly.

Muscle Tissue

Skeletal muscle tissue is the most versatile catabolizer: it contains all the enzymes needed to catabolize glucose, fatty acids, and ketones to produce ATP. **When insulin levels are high,** a glucose transporter known as GLUT4 is displayed on the cell membrane, allowing myocytes to take up glucose from the blood (Table 3-22). **When insulin levels are low,** myocytes breakdown stored glycogen to generate glucose. In fact, the majority of glycogen in the body is made and stored by muscle tissue (the liver being responsible for the rest).

Adipose Tissue

If skeletal muscle is considered versatile, adipose is somewhat dull. It uses glucose for fuel. Although it is the main storage site for fatty acids in the form of triacylglycerides, it is an unimportant source of fatty acid synthesis. The liver,

TABLE 3-22. The Four "Metabolic" Organs and Their Features

Organ	Fuel Storage	Effect of Insulin	Fuel Sources[a]	Transporter	Comments
Brain	None	None.	**Glucose** and **ketone bodies** from blood.	GLUT3	GLUT3 has the **highest affinity** for glucose (it is saturated even when blood glucose is low).
Muscle	Glycogen	Glucose uptake by GLUT4; glycogen synthesis.	**Glucose** (from blood and stored glycogen), **fatty acids, ketone bodies.**	GLUT4	GLUT4 is only present on the cell membrane **when stimulated by insulin.**
Adipose	Triacylglyceride	Glucose uptake by GLUT4; triacylglyceride synthesis.	**Glucose.**	GLUT4	Same as above.
Liver	Glycogen	Glycogen synthesis; fatty acid synthesis.	α-Ketoacids.	GLUT2	Because GLUT2 is **constitutively expressed** on the cell membrane, the liver is always "monitoring" blood glucose.

[a]Fuel sources are listed from most to least preferred for each organ.

GLUT = glucose transporter.

a much better equipped "metabolic machine," not only synthesizes fatty acids but also delivers them to adipose tissue in the form of very low density lipoproteins (VLDLs).

When stimulated by insulin, an enzyme known as **lipoprotein lipase** releases fatty acids from VLDL particles, making them available for uptake by adipocytes. At the same time, insulin promotes the display of GLUT4 transporters on the adipocyte membrane, permitting the entry of glucose. Glucose is then converted into glycerol-3-phosphate and combined with fatty acids to form triacylglycerides (Figure 3-84). **In the absence of insulin,** an intracellular enzyme known as **hormone-sensitive lipase** mediates the breakdown of stored fats into fatty acids that can be released into the blood.

The Liver

The liver is the most impressive metabolic machine. It contains enzymes capable of metabolizing the three major fuel sources:

- **Carbohydrates:** Glucose can be synthesized into glycogen; glycogen can be broken down into glucose; glucose may either be catabolized via glycolysis or, more commonly, released into the blood.
- **Lipids:** Fats obtained from the diet can either be synthesized into triglycerides and packaged into VLDLs (if the body is in a fed state) or catabolized to ketone bodies (if the body is in an unfed state); the liver also uses fats to synthesize cholesterol and bile acids.
- **Proteins:** Amino acids are a "last resort" carbon source because they form the structural (cytoskeletal) and functional (enzymatic) basis of all cells; when amino acid catabolism does occur, the α-amino group is removed and excreted as **urea.**

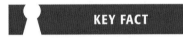

KEY FACT

Both lipoprotein lipase and hormone-sensitive lipase are produced by adipocytes. Whereas hormone-sensitive lipase remains **within the cell,** lipoprotein lipase is released and associates with **capillary endothelial cells.** This allows it to act on VLDL particles floating in the blood.

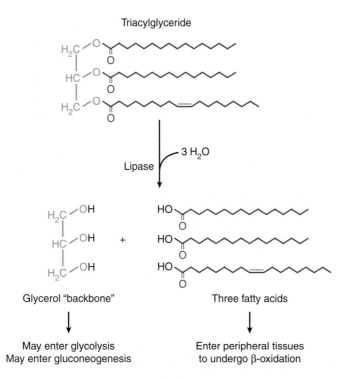

Triacylglyceride

Lipase — 3 H$_2$O

Glycerol "backbone"   Three fatty acids

May enter glycolysis   Enter peripheral tissues
May enter gluconeogenesis   to undergo β-oxidation

FIGURE 3-84. **Components of triacylglyceride.** A triacylglyceride is composed of a glycerol backbone (green) and three "acyl" of fatty acid tails (red). Cells that use triacylglycerides as fuel can catabolize glycerol using glycolysis or, in the liver, glycerol can be used to generate glucose via gluconeogenesis. Each fatty acid may undergo β-oxidation to generate reduced form of nicotinamide adenine dinucleotide (NADH), reduced form of flavin adenine dinucleotide (FADH$_2$), and acetyl CoA, which in turn are used to produce ATP.

Since a primary function of the liver is to generate fuel sources for other tissues, it tends not to use glucose or fatty acids for its own metabolic needs. Instead it relies on α-**ketoacids** created when amino groups are removed from amino acids.

INSULIN AND THE FED STATE

Insulin is an anabolic hormone used by the body to **maximize the storage of dietary glucose in the well-fed state.** Its actions serve to decrease serum glucose levels. It targets tissues responsible for glucose storage and utilization, such as the liver, muscle, and adipose tissues (Figure 3-85).

In the **liver,** insulin:

- Inhibits gluconeogenesis
- Inhibits breakdown of glycogen
- Promotes glycogen synthesis

In **muscle** cells, insulin:

- Promotes glycogen synthesis
- Increases glucose entry into cells (mediated by GLUT4)
- Stimulates the entry of amino acids (desirable for protein synthesis)

KEY FACT

In adipocytes, insulin regulates the entry and metabolism of glucose. Once it enters the fat cell, glucose is converted to glycerol-3-phosphate, the substrate used for triacylglycerol synthesis.

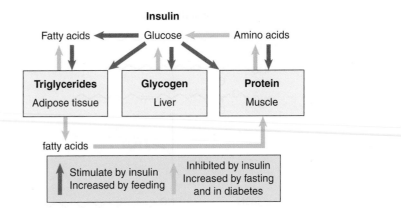

FIGURE 3-85. Targets of insulin. Pathways in blue indicate targets that are stimulated by insulin. Pathways in red indicate targets that are inhibited by insulin. The blue pathways are increased by feeding, whereas the red pathways are increased by fasting. (Modified with permission from Brunton LL, Lazo JS, Parker KL. *Goodman and Gilman's The Pharmacological Basis of Therapeutics*, 11th ed. New York: McGraw-Hill, 2006: 1621.)

In **adipose** tissue, insulin:

- Increases glucose uptake into cells (mediated by GLUT4)
- Increases triacylglycerol synthesis
- Decreases triacylglycerol degradation
- Inhibits activity of hormone-sensitive lipase
- Increases lipoprotein lipase activity

STAGES OF STARVATION

When thinking about starvation, it is useful to consider the "four metabolic organs": the brain, muscle tissue, adipose tissue, and liver. Starvation is discussed for each organ in the following sections.

Early Starvation

Homeostasis functions to prevent blood glucose levels from becoming too high (by releasing insulin) and from falling too low (by releasing glucagon). When blood glucose drops below 70 mg/dL, glucagon begins to be released from the α-cells of the pancreas. If blood glucose gets too low (< 50 mg/dL roughly), the brain will not have enough fuel to generate the ATP it needs, and permanent damage can occur.

The main target of glucagon is the liver, where it **promotes the release of glucose** into the blood by:

- Inhibiting **glycogen synthase,** which synthesizes glycogen, and activating **glycogen phosphorylase,** which breaks glycogen down
- Promoting gluconeogenesis
- Increasing uptake of amino acids, thereby providing additional carbon skeletons for **gluconeogenesis**
- Promoting ketone body formation

In the muscle, glucagon **has no effect** on glycogen stores.

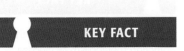

KEY FACT

Epinephrine activates *muscle* glycogen phosphorylase.
Glucagon activates *liver* glycogen phosphorylase.

In adipose tissue, glucagon inhibits fatty acid synthesis by inhibiting the action of **acetyl CoA carboxylase,** the enzyme that mediates the first committed step.

Glucagon mediates each of the previously mentioned effects by stimulating the production of **cAMP,** which then activates **protein kinase A.**

Because glucagon and insulin oppose one another, when glucagon is high, insulin is low. In the absence of insulin, neither muscle nor fat displays the GLUT4 transporter, the net effect being **maximum delivery of glucose to the brain.**

As the liver's glycogen stores are depleted, it must begin to supply the brain with the other source of fuel that neurons can utilize: **ketone bodies** (Table 3-23). Recall, when insulin levels are low, **lipoprotein lipase** is not active; when glucagon levels are high, **hormone-sensitive lipase** is active. The net result is **the release of fatty acids into the blood,** which can be converted into ketone bodies by the liver.

Late Starvation

With prolonged starvation, the body's ability to produce adequate glucose for the brain diminishes. Though muscle continues to store glycogen, it is unable to contribute to the glucose pool because muscle tissue (unlike the liver) does not contain **glucose-6-phosphatase,** the enzyme that dephosphorylates G6P to form glucose, which can freely leave the cell.

Once glucose precursor stores are depleted, the liver begins to produce ketone bodies from fatty acids. In time, fatty acid stores are also depleted, and the liver begins to rely on proteins as a source of carbon. This compromises the integrity of tissues and ultimately, leads to organ failure and death.

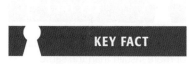
KEY FACT

Phosphorylation of glucose to G6P by **hexokinase** (or **glucokinase** in the liver) is the first step of glycolysis and effectively **"traps" glucose** within cells. This occurs because phosphorylated glucose is too polar and too bulky to pass through glucose transporter channels.

KEY FACT

Because the body relies on fatty acid stores before it draws on protein sources, the amount of fat a person has largely determines how long he or she can survive during starvation.

ENDOCRINE PANCREAS

The pancreas contains both exocrine and endocrine functions. The **exocrine** function of the pancreas is to secrete **digestive enzymes** and bicarbonate-rich fluids into the duodenum. The **endocrine** function of the pancreas is to release **insulin, glucagon,** and **somatostatin.**

TABLE 3-23. **Summary of Action of Insulin and Glucagon**

	LIVER	ADIPOSE TISSUE	MUSCLE
Increased by insulin	Fatty acid synthesis Glycogen synthesis Protein synthesis	**Glucose** uptake Fatty acid synthesis	**Glucose** uptake Glycogen synthesis Protein synthesis
Decreased by insulin	Ketogenesis Gluconeogenesis	Lipolysis	
Increased by **glucagon**	Glycogenolysis Gluconeogenesis Ketogenesis	Lipolysis	

(Reproduced with permission from Murray RK, Granner DK, Rodwell VW. *Harper's Illustrated Biochemistry*, 27th ed. New York: McGraw-Hill, 2000: 174.)

Multiple endocrine neoplasia (MEN) type 1, or **Wermer syndrome,** consists of parathyroid, pituitary, and enteropancreatic tumors. Among the pancreatic tumors are **insulinomas** (causing fasting hypoglycemia), **glucagonomas** (causing migratory necrolytic erythema and symptoms similar to diabetes mellitus), and **somatostatinomas** (also causing a diabetes-like condition, steatorrhea, and cholelithiasis).

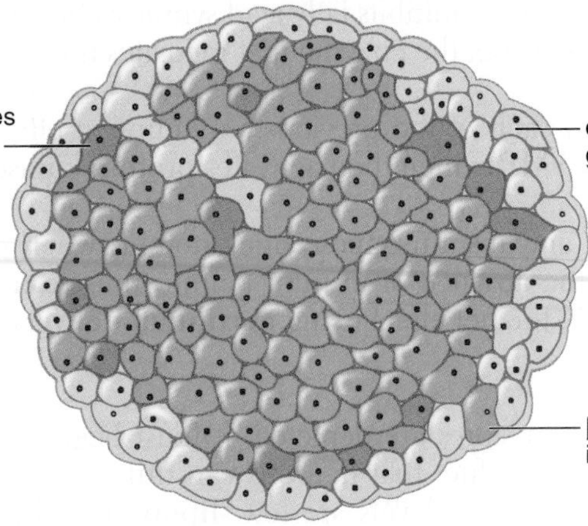

δ-cell (secretes somatostatin)

α-cell (secretes gluc-α-gon)

β-cell (secretes insulin)

FIGURE 3-86. **Schematic drawing of an islet of Langerhans.** Note that β-cells predominate and are located centrally. Alpha-cells are the next most prevalent cell type and form the periphery of the islet. Delta-cells are the least represented.

Oral glucose stimulates the release of more insulin than the same amount of IV glucose. This is because enteral meals cause the release of **incretins** from the GI tract. Incretins are polypeptides that potentiate glucose-stimulated release of insulin.

Insulin is an anabolic polypeptide hormone (ie, it induces growth of muscle, fat, and other tissues) produced by the β-cells of the **islets of Langerhans** (Figure 3-86). The **α-cells** secrete glucagon. Finally, **δ-cells** secrete somatostatin. The β-cells are typically located centrally with α-cells and δ-cells located around them, allowing for **paracrine regulation.**

Insulin

The hormone insulin is actually derived from a much larger polypeptide that undergoes several cleavage steps. Figure 3-87 explains these steps in detail. Although not part of the "mature hormone," these cleaved segments allow insulin to fold properly (Figure 3-88).

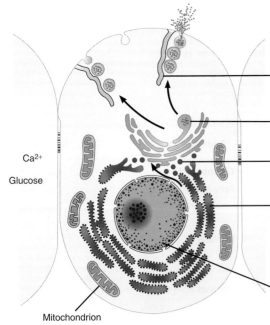

5. After a meal, entry of glucose into β-cells results in calcium influx, which causes secretory vesicles to fuse with the cell membrane and release their contents (insulin and C peptide) into the bloodstream.

4. In the **Golgi apparatus,** enzymes cleave proinsulin to produce **insulin** and **C peptide,** which bud from the Golgi as secretory vesicles.

3. Small vesicles containing proinsulin bud from the ER and travel toward the Golgi apparatus.

2. The mRNA is delivered to the cytosol, where translation begins, but because the developing polypeptide contains an N-terminal signal sequence, the entire mRNA-ribosome-polypeptide complex is shuttled to the endoplasmic reticulum. There, the remainder of the polypeptide **(preproinsulin)** is produced and is "threaded" into the ER lumen. The N-terminal signal sequence is snipped off to produce **proinsulin.**

1. In the nucleus, the gene encoding insulin is transcribed to produce mRNA.

Ca^{2+}

Glucose

Mitochondrion

FIGURE 3-87. **Formation and secretion of insulin.**

Insulin secretion is **stimulated** by ingestion of carbohydrates, proteins, and (less potently) fats. It is **inhibited** by epinephrine, norepinephrine, and glucocorticoids (all hormones that are known for increasing blood glucose levels), as well as growth hormone.

INSULIN SECRETION

Insulin secretion starts with glucose entering the β-islet cells through the **GLUT2 transporter.** Glucose is then phosphorylated by glucokinase and is trapped in the β-cells. The glucose molecule is used to form ATP, which inhibits the ATP-sensitive potassium channels that are used to pump potassium out of the cell. Retention of intracellular potassium causes the cell membrane to depolarize, which causes an influx of extracellular calcium through voltage-sensitive calcium channels. The rise in intracellular calcium triggers the release of vesicles containing insulin and C-peptide (Figure 3-89).

MECHANISM OF ACTION OF INSULIN

Insulin binds to the insulin receptor, a tyrosine kinase. Once insulin binds to the external part of the receptor, tyrosine residues on the internal part of the receptor become autophosphorylated. Once activated, the tyrosine kinase phosphorylates insulin receptor substrate (IRS) proteins. The newly activated IRS proteins in turn, activate cellular kinases and phosphatases that vary depending on the type of cell. After insulin binds to its receptor, both are taken up into the cell. Although insulin is then degraded, its receptor may return to the cell membrane.

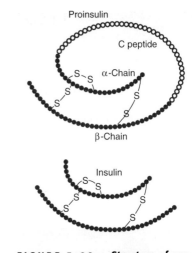

FIGURE 3-88. Structure of proinsulin and insulin. Proinsulin contains the "C peptide" segment, which links the insulin α- and β-chains and allows the protein to fold properly during its formation. (Modified with permission from Molina PE, *Endocrine Physiology*, 2nd ed. New York: McGraw-Hill, 2006: 159.)

>> **FLASH FORWARD**

Exenatide is an **incretin mimetic** approved by the FDA in 2005 to improve glycemic control in patients already using insulin for the treatment of type 2 diabetes.

KEY FACT

Cells that **do not** require insulin for the uptake of glucose:
- Hepatocytes
- Erythrocytes
- Cells of the nervous system
- Intestinal mucosa
- Renal tubules
- Cornea

Seconds to minutes: Transports glucose into cells.

Minutes to hours: Induces changes in enzymatic activity.

Hours to days: Increases glucokinase, phosphofructokinase, and pyruvate kinase.

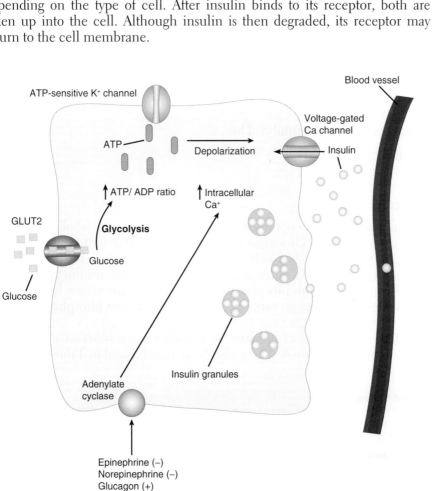

FIGURE 3-89. Pancreatic β-cell insulin secretion. ADP, adenosine diphosphate; ATP, adenosine triphosphate; GLUT-2, glucose transporter 2.

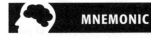
INSULIN AND HYPERKALEMIA

Insulin is used to treat **hyperkalemia** (serum $K^+ > 5.5$ mEq/L), a serious electrolyte abnormality that results in muscle paralysis. When serum K^+ levels are too high, the electrochemical gradient that usually drives K^+ out of cells is reduced. More K^+ remains within the cell, which causes a slight baseline depolarization in the **resting membrane potential**. The slightly more positive membrane potential prevents voltage-gated Na^+ channels from completely resetting, which results in an effective "cellular paralysis." Clinically, the following tissues are most affected:

- Skeletal muscle and nerves (fatigue, weakness, and, ultimately, paralysis)
- Cardiac muscle (loss of coordinated contractions causing arrhythmias and death)
- Smooth muscle (especially in the GI tract, resulting in paralysis or "ileus")

Because insulin **stimulates K^+ entry into cells, it can be used to treat severe hyperkalemia. Glucose, however, must be given simultaneously to avoid hypoglycemia.**

Glucagon

Glucagon is a polypeptide hormone secreted by **α-cells of the pancreatic islets**. Glucagon regulates the actions of insulin and **maintains serum glucose levels**. It does so by activation of hepatic glycogenolysis and gluconeogenesis.

Stimuli for glucagon release include:

- Hypoglycemia (primary stimulus)
- Amino acids
- Epinephrine

Release of glucagon is inhibited by:

- Insulin
- Hyperglycemia

Molecular Pathways

Insulin and glucagon oppose one another in glycogen metabolism by acting on two key enzymes. **Glucagon synthase** is responsible for forming glycogen. **Phosphorylase kinase** breaks it down. Since insulin signals the well-fed state, glucose is preferentially stored as glycogen. As expected, insulin **activates** glucagon synthase and **inhibits** phosphorylase kinase. This occurs because insulin initiates a transduction pathway that relies on **protein phosphatase 1**.

Glucagon does the exact opposite by initiating a transduction pathway that relies on **protein kinase A**. These effects are summarized in Table 3-24.

TABLE 3-24. **Molecular Effects of Insulin and Glucagon**

	TRANSDUCTION PATHWAY	GLUCAGON SYNTHASE	PHOSPHORYLASE KINASE	OVERALL EFFECT
Insulin	Protein phosphatase 1 (removes phosphate groups).	**Activated** by dephosphorylation.	**Inhibited** by dephosphorylation.	Production of glycogen
Glucagon	Protein kinase A (adds phosphate groups).	**Inhibited** by phosphorylation.	**Activated** by phosphorylation.	Glycogen breakdown

Fatty Acid Metabolism

Fatty acids are the precursors for a variety of physiologically important molecules. As **phospholipids** and **glycolipids** they are components of the cell membrane. They are employed as **hormones,** and, as **ecosanoids,** they serve as mediators of inflammation. Finally, they can be catabolized **to generate ATP** for the body.

The steps of fatty acid synthesis and oxidation can be tedious. A few points are worth understanding before diving into the details. The first is that triacylglycerides are an **extremely efficient way to store carbon skeletons** that can be used to generate ATP. Because fats exclude water, much space is saved. Glycogen, in contrast, attracts a huge number of water molecules because of its many hydroxyl groups. (If humans used glycogen as their sole storage source, the average man would weigh nearly double, or about 350 pounds!)

Second, **the catabolism of a triacylglyceride yields a very large number of ATP equivalents.** This is in part due to the sheer number of carbon atoms in a triacylglyceride molecule and in part due to the fact that no component of the triacylglyceride—the glycerol "backbone" nor the fatty acid constituents—goes unused (Figure 3-84). Glycerol can enter **glycolysis** or **gluconeogenesis.** Each of the three fatty acid tails may undergo **β-oxidation.** In fact, the complete oxidation of **palmitate,** a common 16-carbon fatty acid, generates enough acetyl CoA, FADH$_2$, and NADH to produce the equivalent of 106 ATP molecules!

FATTY ACID SYNTHESIS

Fatty acid synthesis occurs in the brain, liver, kidney, lung, and adipose tissue. Though it appears complicated, synthesis of a fatty acid occurs by repetition of the steps shown in Figure 3-90. The most important features of fatty acid synthesis are as follows:

- *Activation:* The enzyme **acetyl CoA carboxylase** adds carbon dioxide to **acetyl CoA** (a 2-carbon molecule) to form **malonyl CoA** (a 3-carbon molecule).
- *Elongation:* Each step of elongation uses the 3-carbon malonyl CoA molecule. **Two carbons are added to the growing fatty acid and one carbon is lost as carbon dioxide.**
- *Termination:* Malonyl CoA donates 2 carbons to the growing fatty acid chain until the chain is 16 carbons in length (**palmitate**). Sixteen is common stopping point because the enzyme **thioesterase recognizes and cleaves 16-carbon fatty acids.** Addition of more carbon units, or the introduction of double bonds, is carried out by enzymes associated with the ER.

FATTY ACID SYNTHASE

All the reactions involved in elongation and termination are carried out by a single 260-kilodalton polypeptide known as **fatty acid synthase.** Fatty acid synthase has multiple enzymatic domains in proximity, allowing for coordination between the many synthetic steps.

The exact chemical reactions are less important than understanding how the domains of fatty acid synthase interact with one another. In Figure 3-90, the domain marked as "1" can be thought of as a "placeholder." The domain

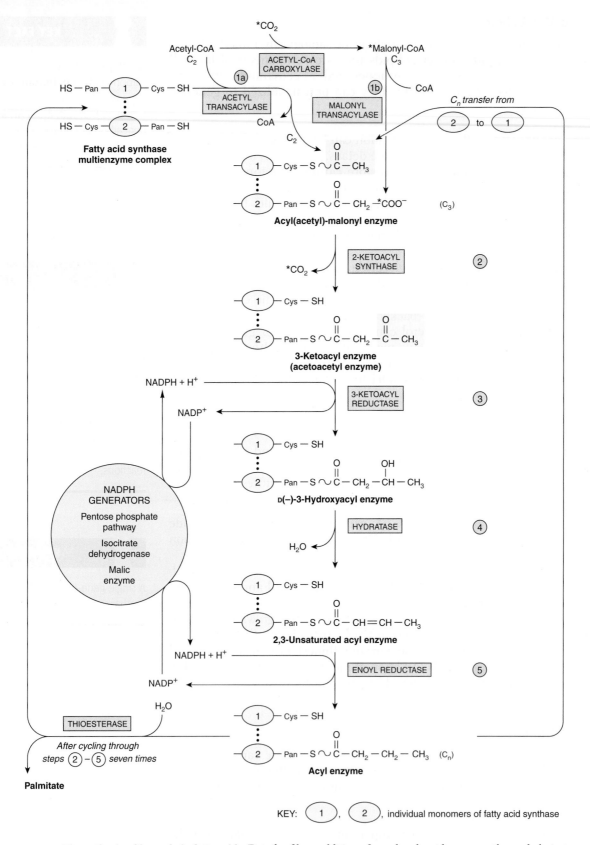

FIGURE 3-90. **Biosynthesis of long-chain fatty acids.** Details of how addition of a malonyl residue causes the acyl chain to grow by two carbon atoms. Cys = cysteine residue; Pan = 4′-phosphopantetheine. (Modified with permission from Murray RK, Granner DK, Rodwell VW. *Harper's Illustrated Biochemistry*, 27th ed. New York: McGraw-Hill, 2006: 198.)

marked as "2" is the "business end" where the reactions that create the long fatty acid chain take place. The steps summarized here refer to Figure 3-90:

- Domain 1 is "loaded" with acetyl CoA (step 1a), and domain 2 is "loaded" with malonyl CoA (Step 1b).
- The acetyl group of domain 1 is transferred to domain 2 (step 2), and CO_2 is released from the malonyl group, resulting in a 4-carbon chain.
- The 4-carbon chain undergoes a series of chemical reactions (steps 3, 4, and 5) carried out by domain 2 to produce a "mature" 4-carbon fatty acid.
- The fatty acid is then transferred from domain 2 to domain 1 so that domain 2 can be "reloaded" with another malonyl group in preparation for the next cycle.

Note that in the second cycle, domain 1 no longer accepts an acetyl group as illustrated by step 1a. This is because domain 1 is now "holding" the growing fatty acid chain. The fatty acid on domain 1 is transferred to domain 2, CO_2 is released, and this time the result is a 6-carbon chain.

Fatty Acid Oxidation

The enzymes involved in fatty acid oxidation are found in the **mitochondrial matrix,** whereas enzymes of fatty acid synthesis are in the **cytosol.** This separation ensures that fatty acids are not consumed by the cell as soon as they are created. But how do fatty acids enter the mitochondria when needed? The answer is the **carnitine translocase** or **carnitine transport system (CTS).**

The outer mitochondrial membrane is relatively permeable, but the inner mitochondrial membrane is not. The CTS is essentially a channel for fatty acids that employs **carnitine,** an ammonium compound, to handle large molecules like fatty acids.

Once inside the matrix, the fatty acid chain is broken at the bond between the α and β carbons and is appropriately titled β-oxidation (Figure 3-91). The process of β-oxidation removes two carbon units as acetyl CoA per cycle. A 16-carbon fatty acid like palmitate yields a total of eight acetyl CoA molecules following complete β-oxidation.

In addition, the $FADH_2$ and NADH formed from β-oxidation are used in the **electron transport chain** for the generation of ATP. As mentioned in the beginning of this section, the complete β-oxidation of palmitate into acetyl CoA, $FADH_2$ and NADH produces 106 ATP equivalents.

KETONES

The body is unable to convert free fatty acids (FFA) into glucose (the brain's favorite food). Therefore, **the liver must convert fatty acids (and ketogenic amino acids) into ketone bodies, which can be utilized by the brain** (Figure 3-92).

The two ketone bodies made by the liver are **acetoacetate** and **β-hydroxybutyrate.**

Anabolism

Low insulin/glucagon ratio stimulates the ketogenic pathway:

- All the material for ketone body synthesis comes from acetyl-CoA, the breakdown product of most fatty acids and ketogenic amino acids (Figure 3-93).

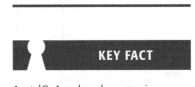

KEY FACT

Propionyl CoA (3-carbons), not acetyl CoA (2-carbons), acts as the substrate for long-chain fatty acids containing an odd number of carbons.

KEY FACT

AcetylCoA carboxylase requires NADPH, ATP, Mn^{2+}, biotin, and carbonate.

KEY FACT

Stearyl-CoA is used in the brain during myelination for sphingolipids.

KEY FACT

Fatty acids with an odd number of carbon atoms that undergo β-oxidation produce acetyl CoA, until they are shortened to **propionyl CoA** (3 carbons). Propionyl CoA can be converted to succinyl CoA to enter the TCA cycle.

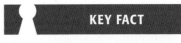

KEY FACT

Ketone bodies are best thought of as "acid bodies."

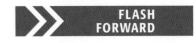

FLASH FORWARD

Statins block HMG-CoA reductase, the committed step in cholesterol synthesis.

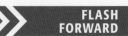

FLASH FORWARD

Ethanol is metabolized to acetaldehyde and then acetate by **alcohol dehydrogenase** and **aldehyde dehydrogenase,** respectively (Figure 3-94). Both steps consume NAD^+ and generate NADH. The increase in NADH favors the conversion of pyruvate to lactate (since NADH serves as a reactant). This depletes the pool of pyruvate available for the TCA cycle and, consequently, oxidative phosphorylation. This effectively places the alcoholic into a **constant state of anaerobic glycolysis,** seriously impairing his or her ability to generate ATP. This, compounded by general malnutrition, may explain why alcoholics are far more vulnerable to metabolic derangements in times of stress and illness.

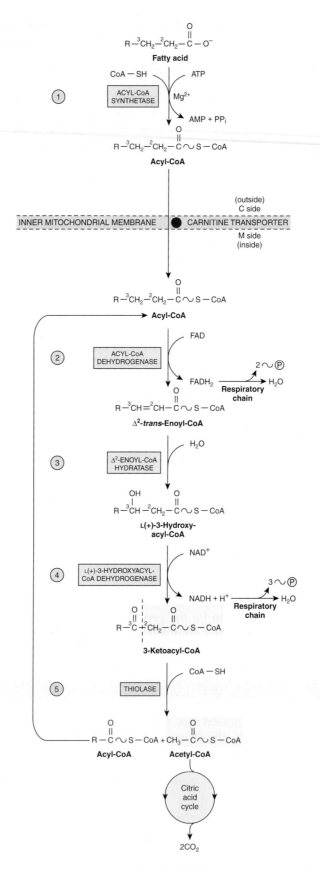

FIGURE 3-91. **Fatty acid oxidation.** β-Oxidation of fatty acids. Long-chain acyl-CoA is cycled through reactions 2–5, acetyl-CoA being split off, each cycle, by thiolase (reaction 5). When the acyl radical is only four carbon atoms in length, two acetyl-CoA molecules are formed in reaction 5. (Modified with permission from Murray RK, Granner DK, Rodwell VW. *Harper's Illustrated Biochemistry,* 27th ed. New York: McGraw-Hill, 2006: 189.)

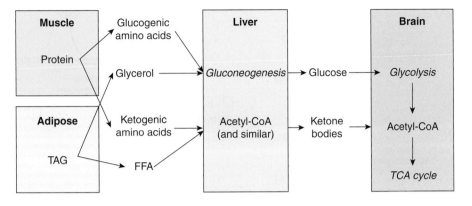

FIGURE 3-92. **Brain energy supply in the prolonged fasting state.** FFA, free fatty acid; TAG, triacylglycerol; TCA, tricarboxylic acid.

- Two molecules of acetyl-CoA unite with the help of β-ketothiolase, forming acetoacetyl-CoA.
- There is no hydrolase to split this molecule into acetoacetate and CoA, so a two-step detour must be taken:
  1. A synthase enzyme combines acetoacetate-CoA with another molecule of acetyl-CoA, forming β-hydroxy-β-methylglutaryl-CoA (HMG-CoA), and a subsequent cleavage by HMG-CoA lyase yields the ketone body acetoacetate.
  2. Reduction with NADH-dependent β-hydroxybutyrate dehydrogenase provides the second ketone body, β-hydroxybutyrate.

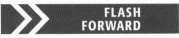

FLASH FORWARD

The conversion of acetaldehyde to acetate by aldehyde dehydrogenase is inhibited by **disulfiram.** The antibiotic metronidazole is thought to have some disulfiram-like activity. Patients on metronidazole must refrain from drinking alcohol because the inability to clear acetaldehyde from the body can result in **nausea, flushing, and respiratory difficulties.** This is the basis for prescribing disulfiram to recovering alcoholics: the nausea is meant to deter relapse. Of course, this requires the patient to take the drug as prescribed in the first place!

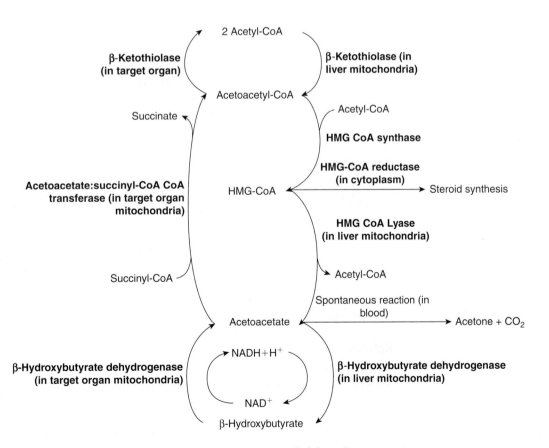

FIGURE 3-93. **Ketone body synthesis.** HMG CoA = 3-hydroxy-3-methylglutaryl coenzyme A.

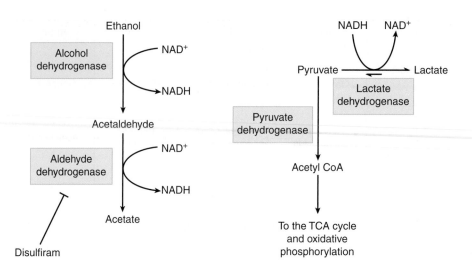

FIGURE 3-94. **Production of NADH during ethanol metabolism drives the conversion of pyruvate to lactate.** NAD = nicotinamide adenine dinucleotide; NADH = reduced form of nicotinamide adenine dinucleotide.

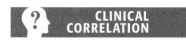

CLINICAL CORRELATION

Diabetes mellitus (DM) type 1 is an autoimmune disease in which β-cells in the pancreas are attacked. There is virtually no insulin produced.

In type 2 DM, the pancreas often produces more insulin than is normal, but peripheral tissues are relatively resistant to insulin action.

Notice that HMG-CoA is also a precursor for **sterol synthesis.** The difference is that all ketone body synthesis takes place in liver mitochondria, whereas sterols are produced in the cytosol. Formation of β-hydroxybutyrate requires NADH. Hence, the ratio of [β-hydroxybutyrate]/[acetoacetate] in the blood reflects the ratio of [NADH]/[NAD$^+$] in the mitochondria.

- Blood tests are the most reliable gauge of ketone levels because urine tests (using nitroprusside strips) only detect acetoacetate. Routine tests do not typically screen for β-hydroxybutyrate.
- Alcohol (ethanol) consumption leads to NADH accumulation, which drives the conversion of acetoacetate to β-hydroxybutyrate. Hence, ketone levels in alcoholics may be underestimated if nitroprusside strips are used.
- High ketone concentrations often manifest a fruity smelling breath; acetoacetate decomposes into acetone, which has a low vapor pressure and is therefore largely cleared by the lungs.

Catabolism

- Once β-hydroxybutyrate and acetoacetate reach the mitochondria of the target organ, the former is converted to the latter by β-hydroxybutyrate dehydrogenase.
- Acetoacetate: Succinyl-CoA transferase subsequently attaches coenzyme A to acetoacetate, making it a ready substrate for β-ketothiolase.
- Thus, each ketone body delivers two units of acetyl-CoA to the target organ; β-hydroxybutyrate also provides an NADH. Note that synthesis and subsequent degradation of one acetoacetate molecule results in net energy loss due to cleavage of one succinyl-CoA molecule.

Ketosis

Fasting ketosis refers to an increase in the concentration of ketone bodies when liver glycogen is diminished. An overnight fast or high-intensity exercise is enough to result in ketosis, which becomes more prominent if the subject is on a low-carbohydrate diet and thus has low liver glycogen stores. Ketosis alone is not a pathologic process, and a glass of juice (ie, sugar) is the fastest remedy.

Alcoholic ketoacidosis manifests in chronic alcoholics following episodes of binge drinking. The hypoglycemia resulting from depleted glycogen and lack of gluconeogenesis (blocked by **high NADH/NAD$^+$**) causes mobilization of fat stores and their conversion to ketones. The resulting acidosis is usually not life-threatening, but may result in further complications.

Diabetic ketoacidosis (DKA) is a life-threatening condition, which may occur in type 1 diabetics with poorly controlled blood glucose. With insufficient insulin available, glucagon and other stress hormones are unopposed and begin to rise, despite high blood glucose levels. The liver produces exceptional amounts of ketone bodies, which make the blood more acidic. As acidemia worsens (and, by definition, protons in the blood increase), cells of the body begin to exchange one cation for another: protons are taken up from the blood and K$^+$ is released, resulting in **hyperkalemia.**

Typical causes of DKA include not taking insulin (common in teenagers with DM), infection, and other physiologic stressors that raise cortisol and consequently blood sugar in type 1 diabetics. Treatment includes:

- Isotonic IV saline
- Insulin
- K$^+$ replacement (high blood [K$^+$], but low total body K$^+$ due to diuresis)

Patients often present with increased respiratory rate and tidal volumes (**Kussmaul** respirations). As with all metabolic acidoses, a high respiratory rate is the primary respiratory compensation.

DKA is rare in type 2 diabetics. The best (though not universally accepted) explanation is that enough insulin is present in type 2 DM to oppose the effects of glucagon. Thus, glucagon levels never rise to the point of permitting ketones to accumulate.

Patients with type 2 DM, however, do suffer from **hyperglycemic hyperosmolar nonketotic coma** (HHNC). In this condition, serum glucose levels frequently exceed 1000 mg/dL (normal is about 100 mg/dL!). Patients in DKA rarely exceed 800 mg/dL. What explains this difference? Patients with DKA come to the attention of doctors sooner because **ketoacidosis** produces significant symptoms (shortness of breath and abdominal pain, for unclear reasons). The presenting symptoms of HHNC, on the other hand, are caused by **the gradual increase of blood glucose**, leading to blood hyperosmolarity:

- Excessive urination (**polyuria**) occurs because excess glucose spills into the kidney, drawing in water by osmosis
- Increasing thirst (**polydipsia**) to replace water volume being lost in the urine
- **Weight loss**

If hyperglycemia continues, the high osmolarity of the blood draws away intracellular fluid, most notably from the brain. The accompanying "cellular shrinking" disrupts normal brain function as manifested by neurologic deficits (as would be seen during a stroke), lethargy, and ultimately coma and death.

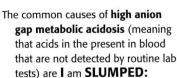

MNEMONIC

The common causes of **high anion gap metabolic acidosis** (meaning that acids in the present in blood that are not detected by routine lab tests) are **I** am **SLUMPED:**

Isopropyl alcohol
Salicylates
Lactate
Uremia
Methanol
Paraldehyde (paint sniffing)
Ethylene glycol (antifreeze)
Diabetic ketoacidosis

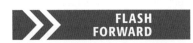

FLASH FORWARD

Intravenous fluids are the first-line treatment for many acute disorders and should be administered even before starting an "actual medication." Extra caution is warranted in patients with heart conditions, however, since the blood volume ejected with each contraction may be much lower than normal. The excess fluid can "back up" into the lungs (impairing gas exchange) and stretch the heart too much (causing arrhythmias and death).

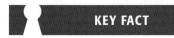

KEY FACT

Lipid + apolipoprotein = lipoprotein. Note that apolipoprotein alone does not contain any lipid.

KEY FACT

Without **ApoB-48,** chylomicrons cannot be released into the blood from intestinal cells. **ApoE** is recognized by hepatocytes and allows the liver to remove **chylomicron remnants** from the blood.

KEY FACT

Although LPL is produced by peripheral tissues, it is found on the apical membranes of the blood vessel **endothelium.** LPL, therefore, has access to chylomicrons in the blood.

CLINICAL CORRELATION

Familial hypercholesterolemia results from dysfunctional LDL receptors. LDL cannot be removed, cholesterol levels spike, and patients suffer from premature atherosclerosis.

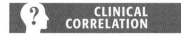

LIPOPROTEINS

Function and Structure

Because fat is hydrophobic and does not dissolve in blood, lipids require carrier molecules to enter the circulation.

- **Albumin** can carry fat in the form of free fatty acids from adipose tissue. Fatty acids are "free" in that they are not covalently attached to glycerol, but they are noncovalently bound to albumin in blood.
- Dietary fat from the intestine and fat from the liver associates with specialized amphiphilic (detergent-like) proteins, called **apolipoproteins.** Together with various lipids (cholesterol, cholesterol esters [CE], triglycerides [TG]), and phospholipids [PL]), the apolipoproteins form **lipoproteins.**
- Lipoproteins are spherical. Like a cell, their shell is formed by PL, cholesterol, and protein, whereas the core is composed of the more hydrophobic lipids.

Most lipoproteins are named according to their density. From low to high density: **Chylomicrons < VLDL < IDL < LDL < HDL.**

In general, higher density implies more protein, more cholesterol, more CE content, less TG, and smaller particle size. HDL is an exception in that its cholesterol content is only moderately high.

CHYLOMICRONS AND REMNANTS

- The dietary lipids (mostly TG, some cholesterol) in the cytoplasm of enterocytes enter the ER, where they assemble along with a freshly translated, large apolipoprotein, called **ApoB-48,** and a smaller protein **ApoA-1.** The resulting lipoprotein is called a **chylomicron.** "Chylo-," because these particles enter the lymphatic (chyle) vessels and the thoracic duct before actually reaching blood (Figure 3-95).
- When a chylomicron meets an HDL particle, they exchange ApoA-1 for **ApoC-2** (Figure 3-95).
- ApoC-2 is a cofactor for lipoprotein lipase **(LPL),** so that when chylomicrons reach **muscle** and **adipose tissue,** LPL cleaves the TG content (Figure 3-95). The resulting fatty acids are taken up by muscle or adipose cells then either stored or β-oxidized. Donation of ApoC-2 to chylomicrons can be regarded as an "activation step" since without it LPL would not act and chylomicrons would continue to float in the blood unchanged.
- As TG, but not PL leave the lipoprotein, a relative buildup of PL results in a large amount of surface shell and a small core. To avoid rupture of an enzyme, phospholipid transfer protein **(PLTP)** moves PL from chylomicrons to HDL.
- In addition, blood contains cholesterol ester transfer protein **(CETP),** which moves TG from chylomicrons to HDL, and CE in the opposite direction.
- Once most TGs have been removed by LPL, the chylomicron returns ApoC2 to an HDL particle, so that no further cleavage takes place. In exchange, HDL provides yet another apolipoprotein, called **ApoE.** The resulting shrunken, TG-depleted, CE-enriched, ApoE-labeled lipoprotein is known as the **chylomicron remnant** (Figure 3-95).

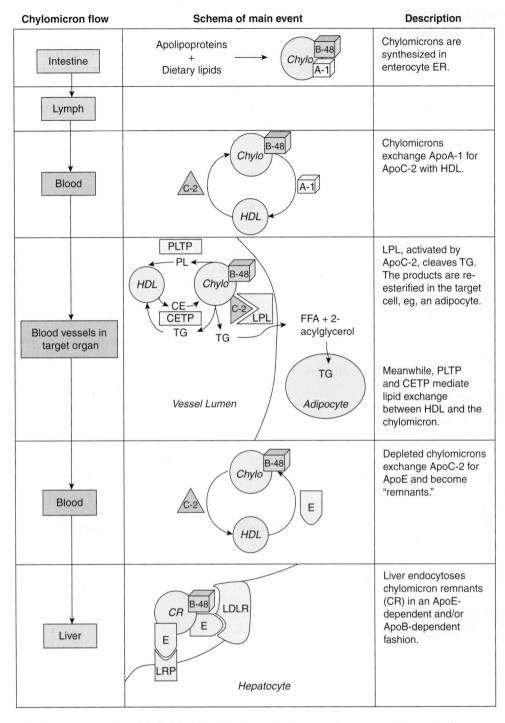

FIGURE 3-95. **Chylomicrons and important events in their life cycle.** Apo = apolipoprotein; ER = endoplasmic reticulum; CE = cholesterol ester = CETP = cholesterol ester transfer protein; Chylo = chylomicron; CR = chylomicron remnant; FFA = free fatty acid; HDL = high-density lipoproteins; LDLR = low-density lipoprotein receptor; LPL = lipoprotein lipase; LRP = low-density lipoprotein-related protein; PL = phospholipids; PLTP = phospholipid transfer protein; TG = triglyceride.

- The remnants are ready to leave the circulation by entering the liver (Figure 3-95). Hepatocytes have two receptors for chylomicrons. **The LDL receptor** requires both ApoE and ApoB-48 (or B-100) to bind. The low-density lipoprotein-related protein (**LRP**) receptor is specific for ApoE-labeled chylomicrons. So even when LDL receptors are not functional, as in familial hypercholesterolemia, chylomicron remnants do not accumulate, because of sufficient LRP activity.

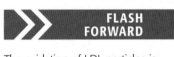
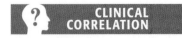
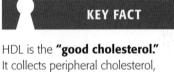
VLDL, IDL, AND LDL

Like the intestine, the liver packages all of its would-be secreted lipids into lipoproteins, called very-low-density lipoproteins (**VLDL**). VLDL is the hepatocyte's analog to the enterocyte's chylomicrons, with a few differences:

- The main VLDL apolipoprotein is the larger ApoB-100 (not ApoB-48).
- Although VLDL still contains more TG than cholesterol, it has a higher cholesterol content than do chylomicrons.
- The lipids packaged into VLDL are synthesized in the liver. This contrasts with the lipids in chylomicrons, which are from the diet.
- The VLDL remnants are called intermediate-density lipoproteins (**IDL**).
- Although IDL can be taken up by the liver, it often loses some of its ApoE and shrinks even further, resulting in **LDL.**
- Liver's LDL receptors can still recognize LDL. However, LDL also tends to cross the endothelium into various tissues. In capillaries, this is not a problem, but in large arteries, LDL can get trapped and oxidized in the vessel intima. Oxidation of LDL renders it recognizable by macrophages, resulting in endocytosis and formation of foam cells. Thus begins **atherosclerosis.**

HDL

High-density lipoproteins (HDLs) differ from the other lipoproteins in that HDL contains no large apolipoprotein (eg, ApoB-48 or B-100). ApoA-1 is the most characteristic protein.

HDL, commonly referred to as the "good cholesterol," has multiple functions (Figure 3-96):

- **Cholesterol collection:** Cells secrete cholesterol using a pump called **ABC1.** HDL then collects this peripheral cholesterol, using the plasma enzyme lecithin-cholesterol acyl transferase (**LCAT**).

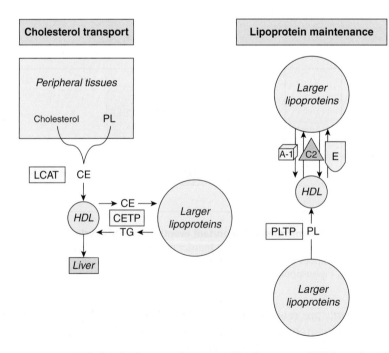

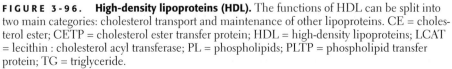

FIGURE 3-96.   High-density lipoproteins (HDL). The functions of HDL can be split into two main categories: cholesterol transport and maintenance of other lipoproteins. CE = cholesterol ester; CETP = cholesterol ester transfer protein; HDL = high-density lipoproteins; LCAT = lecithin : cholesterol acyl transferase; PL = phospholipids; PLTP = phospholipid transfer protein; TG = triglyceride.

- **LPL activation:** HDL supplies ApoC-2 to chylomicrons and VLDL in exchange for ApoA-1. Hence, the TGs in these large lipoproteins can be digested by LPL.
- **Lipoprotein size control:** Takes up excess phospholipids from other lipoproteins via phospholipid transfer protein.
- **Refills lipoproteins with CE:** HDL supplies CE to other lipoproteins in exchange for TG via CETP.
- **Provides the "exit" signal:** HDL supplies ApoE to depleted chylomicrons and VLDL in exchange for ApoC-2. Hence, the remnant lipoproteins (chylomicron remnants and IDL) can leave circulation because ApoE is recognized and taken up by hepatocytes.

Because a portion of HDL particles are degraded and endocytosed by the liver, there is a net flow of cholesterol from peripheral tissues into the liver. This is referred to as **"reverse cholesterol transport."** Notice that the enzyme CETP "short-circuits" this transport, by feeding the HDL cholesterol back into the tissue targeted lipoproteins. Consequently, drugs inhibiting CETP can be expected to lower peripheral cholesterol and are currently in clinical trials.

LIPASES

Lingual and gastric lipases only partially digest dietary TG. Their primary purpose is to emulsify the lipids for further digestion.

Pancreatic lipase, present in the small intestine, cleaves TG at positions 1 and 3, giving rise to FFA and 2-monoacylglycerol. These products then enter the enterocyte and re-esterify into a TG that can be exported in a chylomicron.

Lipoprotein lipase (LPL) mediates the same reaction as pancreatic lipase. However:

- LPL is present on the vascular endothelium of adipose and muscle.
- It requires ApoC-2 as a cofactor.
- LPL activity increases when insulin levels rise.
- The TG substrate comes from VLDL and chylomicrons.

Once again, the products of LPL digestion (FFA and 2-acylglycerol, which then become FFA and glycerol) enter the target cells. The myocytes use the FFA to fuel their β-oxidation, whereas adipocytes re-esterify them back to TG for storage. During re-esterification, the adipocyte uses endogenously synthesized glycerol phosphate from adipocyte carbohydrate metabolism. The glycerol from the LPL cleavage actually travels back to the liver.

Hormone-sensitive lipase is an intracellular enzyme, mainly present in adipocytes.

- It is induced in response to stress hormones such as glucagon, adrenocorticotropic hormone (ACTH), epinephrine, and norepinephrine.
- These hormones raise intracellular cAMP concentrations, and hence PKA activity.
- PKA phosphorylates hormone-sensitive lipase, thus activating the cleavage of stored TG into FFA and glycerol. These then enter the bloodstream and, mostly attached to albumin, travel back to the liver.
- Insulin inhibits this activation by favoring dephosphorylation of the enzyme.

Hepatic TG lipase degrades TG from IDL and chylomicron remnants previously endocytosed by the liver.

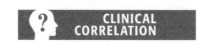
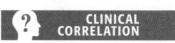
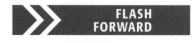

TABLE 3-25.   Key Proteins Involved in Lipoprotein Turnover

PROTEIN	LOCATION	FUNCTION
ApoB-48	Chylomicrons	Structural, chylomicron transport from small intestine → lymph → blood to bind LDLR.
ApoB-100	VLDL, IDL, LDL	Structural, transports liver apoliprotein (VLDL) → peripheral LDLR.
ApoA-1	HDL	Cholesterol collection and activation of LCAT.
ApoC-2	VLDL, chylomicrons	Lipoprotein lipase cofactor, release FA/glycerol from chylomicrons, VLDL, LDL.
ApoE	IDL, chylomicron remnants	Binds to LDLR, helps lipoproteins exit blood into liver.
PLTP	Blood	Moves phospholipids from large lipoproteins to HDL.
CETP	Blood	Exchanges CE for TG between HDL and large lipoproteins.
LCAT	Blood	Allows HDL to collect cholesterol.
ABC1	Cellular membrane	Secretion of cholesterol by tissues.

CE = cholesterol esters; HDL = high-density lipoproteins; IDL = intermediate-density lipoproteins; LCAT = lecithin-cholesterol acyl transferase; LDL = low-density lipoproteins; LDLR = low-density lipoprotein receptor; TG = triglycerides; VLDL = very-low-density lipoproteins.

Note that LPL and hormone-sensitive lipase both respond to insulin, though in opposite ways. However, their roles in diabetes are still being elucidated (Tables 3-25 and 3-26).

Dyslipidemias

A standard lipid profile measures LDLc (LDL cholesterol), HDLc (HDL cholesterol), total cholesterol, and TG in blood. Any significant difference from normal values constitutes a **dyslipidemia.**

- High LDLc and low HDLc are well-established risk factors for atherosclerosis and coronary artery disease. High TG is probably less important.
- Very high LDLc may also cause cholesterol to be deposited in skin or tendons (xanthomas), eyelids (xanthelasma), and cornea (arcus senilis).
- In most dyslipidemias, LDLc, HDLc, and TG are altered simultaneously. Isolated changes in one lipid are less common and are usually indicative of familial dyslipidemias.

TABLE 3-26.   Important Lipases

Lingual, gastric lipases	Saliva, stomach	Fat emulsification.
Pancreatic lipase	Pancreatic juice	Fat absorption by intestine.
Lipoprotein lipase	Endothelium	Fat absorption by muscle and adipose.
Hormone-sensitive lipase	Adipocyte cytoplasm	Release of fat during fast.
Hepatic TG lipase	Hepatocyte cytoplasm	Remnant TG IDL digestion.

IDL = intermediate-density lipoproteins; TG = triglycerides.

Primary causes of elevated blood lipids:

- Polygenic hypercholesterolemia (ie, family history)
- Familial dyslipidemias (often present with isolated lipid elevations)
- Gender (male > female) and age (increase with age)

Secondary causes of elevated blood lipids:

- Saturated fat, *trans* fat, cholesterol, and carbohydrates in diet
- Lack of exercise (low HDLc)
- High body mass index (BMI)
- Metabolic syndrome and diabetes (low HDLc, high TG, LDLc usually normal)
- AIDS (high TG owing to HIV infection *and* to treatment)
- Smoking (low HDLc)
- Hypothyroidism (due to reduced LDL receptors)
- Nephrotic syndrome
- Anorexia nervosa and stress

Causes of decreased lipid levels are:

- Infections, malignancies, hematologic disorders
- Liver disease
- Hyperthyroidism
- Genetic disorders (Tangier disease and abetalipoproteinemia)

Selected pathologic states are discussed later.

Diabetes (types 1 and 2) can cause hyperglycemia, which in turn causes:

- Increased VLDL synthesis, and impaired VLDL and chylomicron removal. Thus, TG accumulates in the plasma.
- Decreased turnover of lipoproteins causes HDLc levels to decrease.
- LDLc usually stays normal.
- First treat diabetes. If that fails to correct lipid levels, start lipid-lowering drugs.

See Table 3-27 for a summary of familial hyperlipidemias.

Familial hyperchylomicronemia (type I) is a rare disease.

- Lack of LPL or its cofactor, ApoC-2, prevents the breakdown of chylomicrons and their TG content, in particular. Hence, TG accumulates in blood.
- Since no treatment is available, patients must avoid fatty food for life.
- Acute pancreatitis and eruptive xanthomas are major complications, whereas atherosclerosis is usually **not** a problem.

Familial hypercholesterolemia (type IIa) is an autosomal dominant disease.

- Usually results from a defective LDL receptor (or ApoB-100). The cholesterol-laden LDL particles cannot be reclaimed by the liver (unlike chylomicron remnants, which are still recognized by the LRP receptor).
- Not only does LDL accumulate in the blood, but liver cholesterol synthesis is deprived of negative feedback, which further contributes to high cholesterol levels.

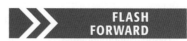

FLASH FORWARD

Smoking may cause a decrease in HDLc, which is a risk factor for coronary artery disease. However, smoking also causes damage to vessel walls, which is an **independent risk factor** for coronary artery disease.

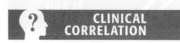

CLINICAL CORRELATION

Xanthomas are accumulations of lipid-laden macrophages in tissues.
Eruptive xanthoma = high TG
Tendinous xanthoma = high cholesterol
Palmar xanthoma = dysbetalipoproteinemia

KEY FACT

LDL receptor mutations are either **null** (complete absence of the gene product) or affect receptor **trafficking** (either to or from the membrane). The actual affinity for LDL tends not to be affected.

TABLE 3-27. Characteristics of Familial Dyslipidemias

FAMILIAL DYSLIPIDEMIA	LIPOPROTEINS ELEVATED	LIPIDS ELEVATED	PATHOPHYSIOLOGY	MAIN COMPLICATION
Type I: Hyperchylomicronemia	Chylomicrons	Cholesterol: + TG: +++	ApoC-2 or LPL deficiency	Pancreatitis, no atherosclerosis
Type IIa: Hypercholesterolemia	LDL	Cholesterol: +++ TG: no change	LDL receptor deficiency	Atherosclerosis
Type IIb: Combined hyperlipidemia	VLDL, IDL	Cholesterol: +++ TG: +++	VLDL overproduction	Atherosclerosis
Type III: Dysbetalipoproteinemia	IDL, chylomicron remnants	Cholesterol: ++ TG: ++	ApoE deficiency	Atherosclerosis
Type IV: Hypertriglyceridemia	VLDL	Cholesterol: + TG: +++	VLDL overproduction	Atherosclerosis
Type V: Mixed hypertriglyceridemia	VLDL, chylomicrons	Cholesterol: + TG: +++	VLDL overproduction	Pancreatitis, no atherosclerosis

FA = fatty acids; IDL = intermediate-density lipoproteins; LDL = low-density lipoproteins; LPL = lipoprotein lipase; TG = triglycerides; VLDL = very-low-density lipoproteins.

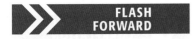

FLASH FORWARD

There are three types of lipid-lowering drugs:

Drugs that lower cholesterol: **Resins** and **ezetimibe**

Drugs that lower TG: **Fibrates**

Drugs that lower cholesterol *and* TG: **Niacin** and **statins** (especially atorvastatin)

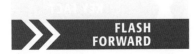

FLASH FORWARD

Think of **niacin** as the opposite of hyperlipidemia type IIb. This drug lowers TG and cholesterol by **inhibiting VLDL secretion.**

- **Homozygous** patients have extreme levels of blood LDL cholesterol (LDLc > 600 mg/dL) and suffer from severe premature atherosclerosis and coronary artery disease, which tends to be the cause of death before age 30 (without treatment).
- **Heterozygotes** have a slightly better prognosis, with LDLc of 200–400 mg/dL.
- Tendon xanthomas, particularly on Achilles tendon, are fairly pathognomonic.
- Treatment consists of:
  - Healthy diet
  - Cholesterol-lowering drugs (statins, niacin, cholestyramine but not fibrates)
  - LDL apheresis (a weekly plasmapheresis, used in homozygous patients)
  - Portocaval anastomosis (mechanism unknown)
  - Liver transplantation (the ultimate measure)

Familial combined hyperlipidemia (type IIb) is a fairly common autosomal dominant disease.

- Liver overproduces VLDL. Consequently, VLDL, LDL, or both accumulate in blood.
- As a result, TG, cholesterol, or both can be elevated.
- As with type Ia, patients can get atherosclerosis and coronary artery disease.
- Likewise, the treatment consists of diet, exercise, and lipid-lowering drugs, which may include fibrates to lower TG (unlike with type IIa, for which their application is of little usefulness).

Dysbetalipoproteinemia (type III) is an autosomal recessive disease.

- It is also known as **remnant removal disease** because lipoproteins lack functional ApoE and cannot "exit" the bloodstream.
- This is not sufficient to cause any pathology, but a concomitant condition (eg, obesity) can cause dysbetalipoproteinemia to manifest itself.
- Both blood TG and cholesterol become high, since chylomicron remnants and VLDL remnants (ie, IDL) accumulate.
- Patients present with palmar xanthomas (fairly pathognomonic) and atherosclerosis.
- Exercise, diet modification, and lipid-lowering drugs reduce the risk of atherosclerosis.

Familial hypertriglyceridemia (type IV) is a common autosomal dominant disorder.

- As in type IIb, there is an elevation in VLDL production, but TG accumulates in preference to cholesterol.
- There is some association with insulin resistance.
- Risk for ischemic heart disease (IHD) and atherosclerosis can be reduced with TG-lowering drugs, diet change, and exercise.

Familial mixed hypertriglyceridemia (type V) is an uncommon mixture of types I and IV familial dyslipidemias.

- VLDL and chylomicrons are elevated, probably as a result of overproduction. TG levels are high, whereas cholesterol concentration increases only moderately.
- Like type I, but unlike type IV, there is no major risk of atherosclerosis, so that pancreatitis and eruptive xanthomas remain the main complications.

Tangier disease is a rare autosomal recessive disorder.

- Tangier disease is due to lack of *ABC1* cholesterol transporter gene.
- Cholesterol accumulates inside cells.
- Blood HDL and cholesterol are low.
- The disease is characterized by atherosclerosis (compare with other dyslipidemias), hepatosplenomegaly, polyneuropathy (compare with metabolic storage diseases), and pathognomonic **orange tonsils.**
- No specific treatment. Enlarged organs are sometimes excised.

Abetalipoproteinemia is a rare autosomal recessive disease.

- Cells are unable to make functional ApoB-48 and ApoB-100, resulting in a deficiency of most lipoproteins.
- Lipids and lipid-soluble vitamins (especially **A** and **E**) are poorly absorbed **(steatorrhea).**
- CNS disease—vitamin deficiency causes progressive neurologic and optic degeneration.
- Hemolytic anemia—lipid imbalance causes RBC membranes to pucker **(acanthosis).**
- No treatment other than vigorous vitamin supplementation.

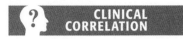

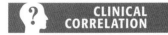

SPECIAL LIPIDS

Cholesterol

The highly lipophilic core of cholesterol contains four carbon rings and very few polar hydroxyl substituents; hence, it is poorly soluble in water. Cholesterol is found in:

- Plasma in the core of VLDL and LDL. It is mostly esterified to a fatty acid.
- In all plasma membranes, conferring rigidity (lipid rafts).
- In bile, where it is solubilized by phospholipids and bile salts.

Although all cells can synthesize cholesterol, some cells are able to further process it to:

- **Steroids** (adrenal cortex, ovary/testes, placenta)
- **Vitamin D** (skin, then liver and kidney)
- **Bile acids** (liver, then intestinal bacteria)

ANABOLISM

Cholesterol synthesis can be characterized by a few major enzymatic conversions (Figure 3-97):

- Cholesterol synthesis begins with conversion of three molecules of **acetyl-CoA** into **HMG-CoA**. The reactions are the same as in ketone body synthesis except that they occur in the **cytoplasm.**
- **HMG-CoA reductase,** the **rate-limiting** enzyme in cholesterol synthesis, converts HMG-CoA to **mevalonic acid.** This enzyme is anchored to the ER and utilizes two molecules of NADPH per reduction.
- Mevalonic acid then gives rise to either isopentenyl pyrophosphate (IPP) or dimethylallyl pyrophosphate (DPP). IPP and DPP are known as **activated isoprene units.**
- IPP and DPP combine, forming geranyl pyrophosphate (GPP).

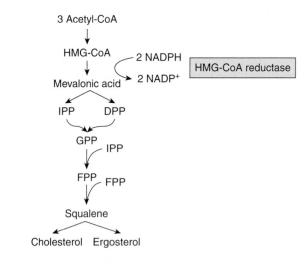

FIGURE 3-97. Cholesterol synthesis. DPP = dimethylallyl pyrophosphate; FPP = farnesyl pyrophosphate; GPP = geranyl pyrophosphate; HMG CoA = 3-hydroxy-3-methylglutaryl coenzyme A; IPP = isopentenyl pyrophosphate; NADP = nicotinamide adenine dinucleotide phosphate; NADPH = reduced form of nicotinamide adenine dinucleotide phosphate.

- GPP and IPP combine, forming farnesyl pyrophosphate (FPP).
- Two FPP molecules combine, forming **squalene.**
- Squalene then cyclizes, forming **lanosterol.**
- Finally, lanosterol is converted (via several steps) into cholesterol.

Plants and fungi convert lanosterol to **ergosterol,** a cholesterol analog.

CHOLESTEROL DERIVATIVES

Most cholesterol in the body actually exists in the form of **CE.** These are usually formed with a fatty acid.

Steroid hormones are derivatives of cholesterol (Figure 3-98). The main adrenal cortical hormones are **dehydroepiandrosterone** and its sulfate (DHEA and DHEA-S, respectively), **cortisol,** and **aldosterone. Androstenedione** and **testosterone** are produced by theca and Leydig cells. In women, granulosa cells along with several extraovarian tissues use aromatase to convert these androgens to **estrogens.** Similarly, in men, Sertoli cells convert testosterone to **dihydrotestosterone** (DHT).

Additional steroid hormones, especially **estriol** (E3) are produced by the placenta, which uses fetal DHEA as its substrate.

Deficiencies in 11β-hydroxylase, 17α-hydroxylase, and 21β-hydroxylase result in characteristic clinical signs that can be predicted from the relative excess or deficiency of the steroids they normally produce. Figure 3-99 provides a useful mnemonic for recalling the expected pathologic changes.

Another cholesterol derivative, **7-dehydrocholesterol,** is converted to **cholecalciferol** (vitamin D$_3$) in skin on exposure to UV light. Subsequent hydroxylations in liver and kidney produce the biologically active 1,25-dihydroxy-cholecalciferol, known as **calcitriol** (Figure 3-100). Note that irradiation of

> **? CLINICAL CORRELATION**
>
> The **triple screen** (an assay of blood α-fetoprotein, β-human chorionic gonadotropin, and estriol) detects congenital abnormalities in a second-trimester fetus.
>
> **Estriol** can also be detected in urine during third-trimester gestation and indicates general well-being of the fetus. A low E3 level can indicate serious congenital diseases, including Down syndrome.

> **? CLINICAL CORRELATION**
>
> Congenital deficiency in any of the "numbered" enzymes in Figure 3-98 leads to serious disease. Missing enzymes 3, 11, 17, or (most commonly) 21 manifest as the various forms of **congenital adrenal hyperplasia** (CAH). **5α-Reductase deficiency** in genetic males results in ambiguous genitalia that virilize during puberty.

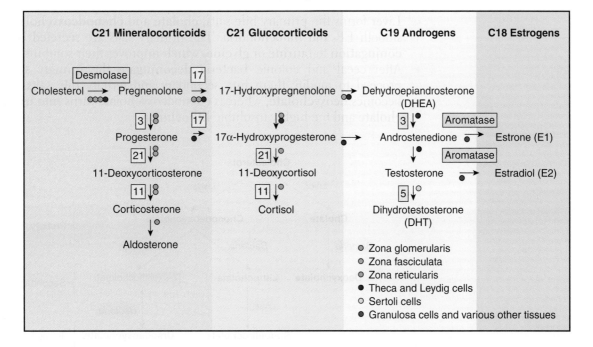

FIGURE 3-98. **Steroid hormone synthesis.** 3 = 3β-Hydroxysteroid dehydrogenase; 5 = 5α-reductase; 11 = 11β-hydroxylase; 17 = 17β-hydroxylase; 21 = 21β-hydroxylase.

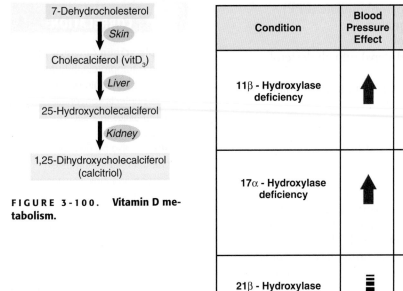

7-Dehydrocholesterol

↓ *Skin*

Cholecalciferol (vitD₃)

↓ *Liver*

25-Hydroxycholecalciferol

↓ *Kidney*

1,25-Dihydroxycholecalciferol
(calcitriol)

FIGURE 3-100. **Vitamin D metabolism.**

Condition	Blood Pressure Effect	Secondary Sex Effect	Clinical Description
11β - Hydroxylase deficiency	⬆	🧍	**Hypertension** (11-deoxycorticosterone has mineralocorticoid activity). "Androgenization" of females (clitoris which resembles a penis) and precocious puberty in males due to androgen excess.
17α - Hydroxylase deficiency	⬆	🧍	**Hypertension** (due to 11-deoxycorticosterone excess). Minimal androgen and estrogen levels lead to underdeveloped or absent external male genitalia (in males) and the absence of pubertal changes (in females).
21β - Hydroxylase deficiency	⬇	🧍	**Hypotension** (mineralocorticoid compunds are produced). "Androgenization" of females (clitoris which resembles penis) and precocious puberty in males due to androgen excess.

FIGURE 3-99. **Hydroxylase deficiency mnemonic.**

the plant lipid **ergosterol** produces vitamin D₂, which can undergo the same set of hydroxylations, but displays lower activity than vitamin D₃.

The liver also converts cholesterol into **bile salts** (Figure 3-101). These detergents are secreted into the intestine (in bile) and render dietary fat more absorbable. Although the intestine reclaims most bile salts (enterohepatic circulation), some are excreted. Therefore, bile excretion is one of the body's ways of reducing cholesterol load.

- **Liver** forms the primary bile salts, **cholate** and **chenodeoxycholate,** in its smooth ER and mitochondria. The primary salts are secreted only after **conjugation** to **taurine** or **glycine,** which improves their solubility.
- After cecal and colonic **bacteria deconjugate** the primary salts, they proceed to modify them into secondary and tertiary bile salts. Cholate becomes **deoxycholate,** whereas chenodeoxycholate turns into **ursodeoxycholate** and the highly insoluble **lithocholate.**

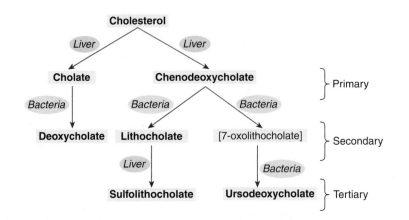

FIGURE 3-101. **Bile salts.**

- Most bile salts are reclaimed and **reconjugated** by the liver. In addition, sulfation of lithocholate also occurs in hepatocytes. The resulting **sulfolithocholate** is not reclaimed by the intestine, thus constituting an important "leak" in enterohepatic circulation.

Glycerophospholipids and Sphingolipids

STRUCTURE AND FUNCTION

Glycerophospholipids and sphingolipids can be thought of as substituted glycerol molecules. Fatty acids usually attach to two of the glycerol carbons, leaving the third carbon with a polar group. Therefore, most of these lipids are amphiphilic and consequently ideal constituents of lipid bilayers. See Figure 3-102 for a summary of their structures.

GLYCEROPHOSPHOLIPIDS

- C_2 and C_3 carry **esterified fatty acids.**
- C_1 carries a **polar head group,** consisting of a phosphate coupled to a polar molecule such as choline, ethanolamine, serine, or inositol. The resulting phospholipids are named accordingly: phosphatidylcholine, phosphatidylethanolamine, and so on.
- The synthetic pathways vary depending on the phospholipid. Note that the phosphate group is often derived from cytidine triphosphate (**CTP**) (rather than ATP).

SPHINGOLIPIDS

- C_3 carries a **carbon chain** (attached directly, not as an ester).
- The alcohol group on C_2 is changed into an **amine.** In some sphingolipids, this amine condenses with a fatty acid, thus becoming an **amide.**
- A glycerol molecule with the above modifications (carbon chain on C_3 and C_2 alcohol changed to amine) is called **sphingosine.**

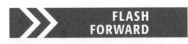

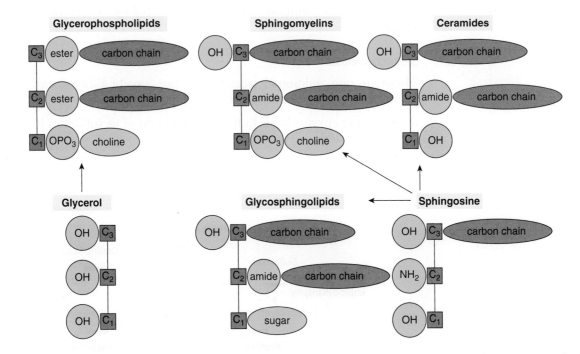

FIGURE 3-102. Glycerophospholipids, sphingolipids, and their backbone molecules. Choline is used here as an example of a polar head group component and can be replaced by several others, such as ethanolamine, inositol, and serine. Polar groups are blue, and lipophilic groups are brown.

> **?** CLINICAL CORRELATION

Ursodeoxycholate (Ursodiol) is used in treatment of radiolucent gallstones. It not only solubilizes cholesterol, but also inhibits its production. However, cholecystectomy is usually the preferred treatment, so ursodiol is reserved mostly for poor surgical candidates.

> **»** FLASH FORWARD

PIP$_2$ is an important membrane phospholipid, cleaved by **PLC** into **IP$_3$** and **DAG.** PLC responds to **G$_q$,** a G-protein subunit activated by: muscarinic, angiotensin, α_1-adrenergic, 5-HT$_{1c}$, 5-HT$_2$, TRH, and vasopressin V$_1$ receptors.

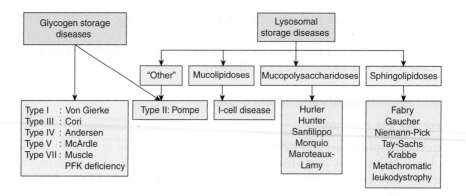

FIGURE 3-103.   **The storage diseases.** Pompe disease can be classified as both a glycogen and a lysosomal storage disease.

- C_1 carries a polar head group, which varies widely among the different sphingolipids:
  - **Ceramides** use a plain alcohol group as their polar heads.
  - Just like glycerophospholipids, **sphingomyelins** use a phosphate coupled to another polar molecule, including choline, ethanolamine, and others.
  - **Glycosphingolipids** carry a sugar on their C_1 and are subdivided into **cerebrosides** and **gangliosides.**

LYSOSOMAL STORAGE DISEASES

These diseases include **sphingolipidoses, mucopolysaccharidoses, mucolipidoses,** and the **type II glycogen storage disease** (Pompe disease). Their "taxonomy" is summarized in Figure 3-103.

Note that only the sphingolipidoses result from defects in lipid metabolism. We include other main lysosomal storage diseases in this chapter because of their clinical similarity; however, their etiology is not related to lipid metabolism.

SPHINGOLIPIDOSES

These are rare, autosomal recessive diseases (except Fabry disease, which is X-linked recessive). They share the following characteristics:

- A missing enzyme leads to the accumulation of its substrates in lysosomes (Figure 3-104).

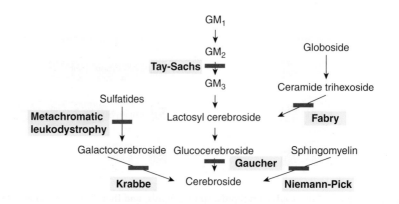

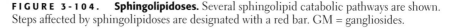

FIGURE 3-104.   **Sphingolipidoses.** Several sphingolipid catabolic pathways are shown. Steps affected by sphingolipidoses are designated with a red bar. GM = gangliosides.

- As with many autosomal recessive diseases, the incidence is higher in certain ethnic groups (eg, Tay-Sachs disease among Ashkenazi Jews).
- Each disease has many subtypes, usually organized by age of onset. Gaucher and Fabry diseases often present in adulthood, whereas most other sphingolipidoses are diagnosed in early infancy.
- Variable expressivity is often present (especially Gaucher disease). The early-onset diseases often include neurodegeneration.
- There is usually no effective treatment for the sphingolipidoses, and individuals who have early-onset disease die early.

Table 3-28 summarizes the sphingolipidoses.

The syndromes associated with these diseases tend to be complex and variable, with no "typical presentation." We include hypothetical presentations only to differentiate between the different sphingolipidoses:

- **Fabry:** A young man presents with a stroke. History reveals recurring pain in his hands and feet. Physical exam is significant for raised dark-red lesions all over his body and mitral valve prolapse.
- **Gaucher:** A girl of Ashkenazi Jewish heritage presents with chronic fatigue due to anemia. History reveals painful bone crises and pathologic fractures. Physical exam shows massively enlarged spleen and liver.
- **Niemann-Pick:** A 3-month-old infant presents with hepatosplenomegaly. Initially hypotonic, the infant later becomes spastic, rigid, and eventually unresponsive. He fails to meet developmental milestones and dies at age 2.
- **Tay-Sachs:** A 6-month-old infant becomes unresponsive and paralyzed and dies at age 3. Autopsy reveals microcephaly.
- **Christensen-Krabbe:** A 3-month-old infant will not feed and is irritable. He gradually becomes hypertonic, suffers from seizures, and assumes decerebrate posture. Eventually, he stops responding to all stimuli and dies.
- **Metachromatic leukodystrophy:** A 6-year-old girl's performance in school is declining. She becomes clumsy and unable to walk. She dies at age 16.

Mucopolysaccharidoses

Table 3-29 summarizes a subset of lysosomal storage diseases, called **mucopolysaccharidoses** (MPS). These result from lysosomal enzyme defects that lead to accumulation of GAGs, the principal glycopeptide components of ECM in connective tissue.

The four most important GAGs are heparan sulfate, dermatan sulfate, chondroitin sulfate, and keratan sulfate.

- In general, accumulation of GAGs causes **skeletal deformities** (usually leading to coarse facial features), **corneal clouding, cardiovascular disease** (especially valvulopathies), and **excessive hair.**
- Heparan sulfate accumulation is particularly deleterious to the nervous tissue, causing **cognitive defects.**
- Keratan sulfate accumulation damages mostly corneal and cartilaginous tissues, while sparing the brain.

Note the following:

- Morquio and Maroteaux-Lamy syndromes are the only MPS listed that spare cognitive function.
- All the listed MPS are autosomal recessive except **Hunter** syndrome.
- Multiple subtypes exist for each disease.

FLASH FORWARD

The two layers of a plasma membrane bilayer have distinct phospholipid composition. The inner layer consists primarily of negatively charged phospholipids (eg, phosphatidylserine), whereas the outer face contains phospholipids with no net charge (eg, phosphatidylcholine). In cells undergoing **apoptosis,** this polarization is lost; the negatively charged phospholipids displayed on the exterior of the cell serve as a "kill me" signal for leukocytes.

MNEMONIC

A **Hunter's** arrow **IS** aiming for the "X" = **Hunter syndrome,** caused by the absence of **I**duronate **S**ulfatase, is an **X**-linked disease.

A **Hurler's** stone can be used as a **cover** or a **lid** = **Hurler syndrome** results in **corneal clouding** ("cover") and is caused by the absence of α-**L-id**uronidase ("a lid").

A Hurler's massive stone wreaks more havoc than a Hunter's measly arrow = Hurler syndrome is a more aggressive and damaging disease.

KEY FACT

Sanfilippo disease is associated with severe mental retardation but little somatic symptoms. Morquio and Maroteaux-Lamy syndromes are the opposite.

MUCOLIPIDOSES

I-cell disease is an autosomal recessive disease.

▪ Caused by defective phosphotransferase. This Golgi enzyme targets newly synthesized enzymes to the lysosome by "labeling" them with mannose-6-phosphate. With a defective targeting system, these enzymes never reach the lysosome, thus preventing the organelle from working properly.

TABLE 3-28. Sphingolipidoses

Disease	Description	Deficient Enzyme, Accumulated Substrate, and Treatment if Possible
Fabry disease	▪ **Peripheral neuropathy of hands/feet.** ▪ X-linked recessive; heterozygous females display mild phenotype. ▪ Angiokeratomas (small, raised purple spots on skin). ▪ Cardiovascular/renal disease and strokes. ▪ Cataracts. ▪ Usually survive till adulthood—die with kidney and heart failure.	▪ α-Galactosidase A missing. ▪ Ceramide trihexoside accumulates.
Gaucher disease	▪ **Bone involvement: aseptic necrosis of femur, bone crises.** ▪ Several types, affect different ages. ▪ 1:1000 incidence among Ashkenazi Jews. ▪ Hepatosplenomegaly. ▪ Can present late in adulthood—expressivity varies. ▪ Anemia, thrombocytopenia. ▪ Mental retardation in some types. ▪ Gaucher cells (macrophages); "crinkled tissue paper cells" because of their large, foamy cytoplasm.	▪ δ-Glucocerebrosidase missing. ▪ Glucocerebroside accumulates. ▪ β-Glucocerebrosidase IV for treatment.
Niemann-Pick disease	▪ Types A and B; type A patients die by age 2–3; type B patients live longer. ▪ Progressive neurodegeneration, esp. in type A. ▪ Hepatosplenomegaly. ▪ Cherry-red spot (on macula). ▪ Foam macrophages in bone marrow.	▪ Sphingomyelinase missing. ▪ Sphingomyelin accumulates.
Tay-Sachs disease	▪ Multiple types, most common is infantile (death by 3 years). ▪ Ashkenazi Jews at increased risk. ▪ Progressive neurodegeneration, developmental delay, microcephaly. ▪ Cherry-red spot. ▪ Lysozymes with onion skin.	▪ Hexosaminidase A missing. ▪ GM_2 ganglioside accumulates.
Christensen-Krabbe disease	▪ Peripheral neuropathy. ▪ Developmental delay. ▪ Optic atrophy. ▪ Decerebrate posture. ▪ Death by 2 years. ▪ Globoid macrophages full of galactocerebroside, stain PAS⁺. ▪ Reported successful treatment with bone marrow transplantations.	▪ β-Galactosidase missing. ▪ Galactocerebroside and psychosine (which is the main toxin killing oligodendroglia) accumulate.
Metachromatic leukodystrophy	▪ Multiple types, but disease rarely manifests before 6 months. ▪ Central and peripheral demyelination with ataxia, dementia.	▪ Arylsulfatase A missing. ▪ Cerebroside sulfate accumulates.

TABLE 3-29. **Some Major Mucopolysaccharidoses**

Disease	Description	Deficient Enzyme and Accumulated Substrate
Hurler syndrome	▪ Most common. ▪ Onset age is 1 year, death by age 14. ▪ Starts with developmental delay, and coarse facial features with enlarged forehead (gargoylism). ▪ Corneal clouding, enlarged tongue, airway obstruction.	▪ α-L-Iduronidase missing. ▪ Heparan sulfate and dermatan sulfate accumulate.
Hunter syndrome	▪ X-linked recessive. ▪ Like Hurler, but milder, with longer survival. ▪ No corneal clouding. ▪ Type B has a very mild phenotype.	▪ Iduronate sulfatase missing. ▪ Heparan sulfate and dermatan sulfate accumulate.
Sanfilippo syndrome	▪ Developmental delay, with severe mental retardation. ▪ Onset in preschool children, death in midteens. ▪ Relatively little somatic change.	▪ Heparan-N-sulfatase (or others) missing. ▪ Heparan sulfate accumulates.
Morquio syndrome	▪ Diagnosis by age 2. ▪ Skeletal deformities, corneal clouding. ▪ No mental abnormalities. ▪ Death due to atlantoaxial instability (minor trauma can cause injury to spinal cord).	▪ N-acetyl-alactosamine-6-sulfate sulfatase missing. ▪ Keratan sulfate accumulates.
Maroteaux-Lamy syndrome	▪ Multisystemic disease, but spares the CNS.	▪ N-acetylhexosamine-4-sulfatase missing. ▪ Dermatan sulfate accumulates.

▪ Similar presentation to Hurler syndrome.
▪ Pathology significant for many membrane-bound inclusion bodies in fibroblasts.

OTHER LYSOSOMAL STORAGE DISEASES

Pompe disease is an autosomal recessive disorder that can also be classified as a type II glycogen storage disease. It has several subtypes (here we discuss the infantile form).

▪ It is caused by defective lysosomal α-1,4-glucosidase, a glycogen-breakdown enzyme.
▪ Unlike most other glycogen storage diseases, Pompe disease does not severely violate the cell's energy economy. This is because the main glycogenolytic pathway (eg, phosphorylase) is intact to break down most of the glycogen. However, the accumulation of glycogen in the lysosomes causes pathology (the glycogen storage diseases associated with energy economy are most frequently defects in the synthesis or degradation of glycogen granules in liver and muscle cytosol).
▪ Death occurs by 8 months of age.
▪ Pompe disease is characterized by cardiomegaly, hepatomegaly, macroglossia, hypotonia, and other systemic findings.
▪ As in most systemic diseases, several blood lab values tend to be abnormal. However, glucose, lipids, and ketones tend to be normal (in contrast to other glycogen storage diseases).

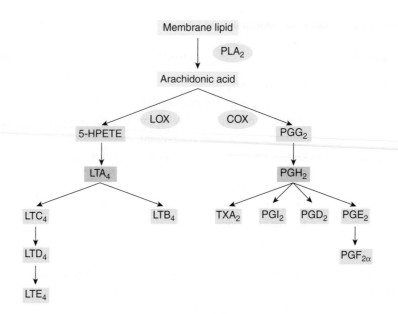

FIGURE 3-105. **Eicosanoid synthesis.** COX = cyclooxygenase; 5-HPETE = 5-hydroperoxyeicosatetraenoic acid; LOX = lipoxygenase; LT = leukotrienes; PG = prostaglandins; PLA$_2$ = phospholipase A$_2$; TXA$_2$ = thromboxanes A$_2$.

Eicosanoids

Eicosanoids are derivatives of polyunsaturated long-chain fatty acids, most notably **arachidonic acid.** Whereas steroid hormones play the role of systemic, long-term messengers, eicosanoids are involved in **local (autocrine or paracrine) signaling.**

They include:

- Prostaglandins
- Thromboxanes
- Leukotrienes

Arachidonic acid resides in membranes as part of phospholipids, and is released by the action of **phospholipase A$_2$ (PLA$_2$).**

Arachidonic acid is then modified by several different pathways:

- **Cyclooxygenase (COX)** 1 and 2 lead to the production of prostaglandin G$_2$ (PGG$_2$) and subsequently PGH$_2$, from which most other prostaglandins, prostacyclin (PGI$_2$), and thromboxane A$_2$ (TXA$_2$) are synthesized.
- **Lipoxygenase (LOX)** converts arachidonic acid into 5-hydroperoxyeicosatetraenoic acid (5-HPETE) and is later transformed into leukotrienes.

The main synthetic pathways of the arachidonic acid–derived eicosanoids are summarized in Figure 3-105. Note that not all eicosanoids are derived from arachidonic acid. For example, TXA$_3$, a thromboxane that prevents platelet aggregation, is a derivative of **omega-3 fatty acids.** For this reason, consuming fish oil (high in omega-3 fatty acids) is thought to reduce one's risk of **coronary artery disease.**

The important eicosanoids and their functions are summarized in Table 3-30. Synthetic analogs of several prostaglandins are employed in clinical medicine.

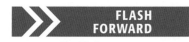

FLASH FORWARD

Corticosteroids block PLA$_2$ and interrupt COX synthesis.
NSAIDs, acetaminophen, and coxibs block COX-1, 2, or both.
Zileuton blocks lipoxygenase.
Zafirlukast and montelukast block leukotriene receptors.

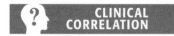

CLINICAL CORRELATION

To keep the patent ductus arteriosus (PDA) open in a neonate, use PGE$_2$ (or PGI$_2$). To promote closure of a PDA, use a COX inhibitor, such as indomethacin.

TABLE 3-30. Eicosanoids and Their Function

EICOSANOID	FUNCTION	MAIN SOURCE
LTA$_4$	Very little (only a transient compound).	Neutrophils
LTB$_4$	Neutrophil chemotactic factor.	Neutrophils, macrophages
LTC$_4$, LTD$_4$, LTE$_4$	Bronchoconstriction, vasoconstriction, smooth muscle contraction, and increased vascular permeability. Known as slow-reacting substance of anaphylaxis (SRS-A).	Mast cells
PGG$_2$, PGH$_2$	Precursors of PGI$_2$, PGD$_2$, PGE$_2$ (and PGF$_2\alpha$), and TXA$_2$.	Any cell that produces prostaglandins
PGE$_1$	Smooth muscle relaxant, vasodilator. Keeps PDA open and beneficial in male erectile dysfunction (available as **alprostadil** for these purposes). Inhibits platelet aggregation. **Misoprostol** is a synthetic analog. Used in prevention of NSAID-induced peptic ulcers and (in combination with mifepristone) as an abortifacient.	Various
PGE$_2$	Similar to PGE$_1$. Uterine contraction (**dinoprostone** can be used clinically to induce labor or abortion), bronchodilation. Keeps PDA patent.	Various
PGF$_2$	Like PGE$_2$ it causes uterine contractions and is used to induce labor or abortion. Increases outflow of aqueous humor (**latanoprost** is an analog available for treatment of open-angle glaucoma). Bronchoconstrictor.	Various
PGI$_2$ (prostacyclin)	Vasodilator and inhibitor of platelet aggregation. Bronchodilator and uterine relaxant. Keeps PDA open.	Endothelial cell
TXA$_2$	Opposite to prostacyclin (platelet aggregator, vasoconstrictor, bronchoconstrictor).	Platelets

LT = leukotriene; PDA = patent ductus arteriosus; PG = prostaglandin; TX = thromboxane.

HEME

Structure

Many proteins use the cofactor **heme** as a prosthetic group. Heme is not a peptide. It is the combination of an aromatic ring (known as **protoporphyrin IX**) and a **ferrous ion** (ie, Fe in its +2 state).

Heme Proteins

Heme is found in **hemoglobin** and **myoglobin** (heme plus "globin" peptides), where it tightly binds and carries O$_2$. The globin chains hold the heme in place with two histidine residues. The proximal histidine binds Fe^{2+}, and the distal histidine associates with O$_2$ to form something of a "heme sandwich" (Figure 3-106).

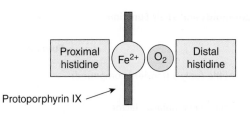

FIGURE 3-106.   Heme in hemoglobin (or myoglobin). In this figure, the flat aromatic ring of protoporphyrin IX ring is seen from the side.

Although best known as part of myoglobin and hemoglobin, heme's function is not limited to **O₂ storage and transport.** Because heme is an excellent means of transporting electrons, it is seen in a variety of biological reactions. It is found in **peroxidase,** in the mitochondrial electron transport system as part of **cytochrome c,** and in detoxification reactions it is part of the **cytochrome P450** system.

Heme Synthesis

- Given the preceding list of heme-containing proteins, it is not surprising that most heme synthesis occurs in **erythroid** and **liver** cells.
- The building blocks of heme are **succinyl-CoA** and **glycine.** The **Fe²⁺** is introduced at the very end of the pathway (once the large porphyrin ring is ready to "catch it").
- Knowing that succinyl-CoA is a product of the TCA cycle, it is easy to remember that heme synthesis begins in the mitochondrion. It also ends there, but several intermediate steps occur in the cytosol.

Table 3-31 summarizes the pathway.

Since ALA synthase catalyzes the first committed step, it is also the main site of regulation of heme synthesis in the liver. This enzyme is feedback-inhibited by:

- Its own product (**ALA**).
- The final pathway product (**heme**).
- Oxidized heme (**hematin,** which is heme carrying Fe^{3+} rather than Fe^{2+}).

In erythroid cells, this regulation is absent, so that all primordial RBCs produce heme without inhibition.

Porphyrias and Lead Poisoning

Porphyrias are diseases resulting from defects in heme synthesis.

Since heme is generally made in the blood and liver, porphyrias tend to affect these two systems (although virtually every organ suffers damage). In children, porphyrias often present as **encephalopathy** (confusion, inability to maintain attention, behavioral changes).

- In addition, the various synthetic precursors of heme are large aromatic rings that absorb light; their accumulation in skin thus causes a **photosensitivity rash** in many porphyrias.
- The inheritable forms of each disease are generally autosomal dominant, except erythropoietic porphyria, which is recessive.

TABLE 3-31. Heme Synthesis

CHEMICAL STEPS	ENZYME	DISEASE ASSOCIATED WITH ENZYME DEFECT	DESCRIPTION
Succinyl-CoA + glycine = ALA	ALA synthase		**ALA synthase** requires **vitamin B$_6$** as a cofactor; this reaction is the rate-limiting step.
ALA + ALA = PBG	ALA dehydrogenase		**ALA dehydrogenase** requires **zinc (Zn^{2+})**; it is inhibited by **lead (Pb^{2+}).**
Four PBGs = uroporphyrinogen I	Uroporphyrinogen I synthase	Acute intermittent porphyria	
Uroporphyrinogen I → uroporphyrinogen III	Uroporphyrinogen III synthase	Erythropoietic porphyria	In this reaction, the familiar porphyrin ring is formed.
Uroporphyrinogen III → coproporphyrinogen III	Uroporphyrinogen III decarboxylase	Porphyria cutanea tarda	Carboxy groups are removed in this step.
Coproporphyrinogen III → protoporphyrinogen IX	Coprophyrinogen III oxidase	Coproporphyria	
Protoporphyrinogen IX → protoporphyrin IX	Protoporphyrinogen oxidase		
Protoporphyrin IX → heme	Ferrochelatase		Ferrochelatase is inhibited by **lead (Pb^{2+}).**

Blue shading indicates reactions that occur in the mitochondrion. Orange shading indicates reactions occurring in the cytosol. ALA = Δ-aminolevulinic acid; PBG = porphobilinogen.

- The intermittent, or sporadic, nature of some porphyrias may complicate their diagnosis. In general, symptoms of porphyrias are triggered by events that increase heme synthesis.
- Because many of the enzymes of the P450 system employ the heme molecule, any medication or substance that up-regulates the production of P450 enzymes also stimulates the production of heme and heme precursors. This, in turn, can precipitate a porphyria attack.
- Although not a true porphyria, we include lead poisoning in the list, because it has major effects on heme synthesis.

Tables 3-32 and 3-33 describe and compare the porphyrias.

LEAD POISONING

Lead poisoning occurs both in children (**GI exposure** via chewing on objects with lead-based paint or working in a battery factory) and adults (plumbers **inhale** lead dust). Although best known as a heme synthesis inhibitor, lead poisons physiologic processes and can affect virtually every organ.

- Lead is chemically similar to calcium and zinc. This has two main consequences:
  - Lead is better absorbed when calcium or zinc are lacking in the diet. For this reason, it is especially important for children's diet to be replete in calcium and zinc.

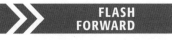

FLASH FORWARD

The most commonly known "P450-inducer" drugs are:
- Carbamazepine (antiseizure)
- Phenytoin (antiseizure)
- Barbiturates (antiseizure)
- Alcohol
- Griseofulvin (antifungal)
- Rifampin (antibacterial)

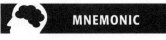

MNEMONIC

Porphyria cutanea **tarda** (PCT) is **"tardy"** compared with acute intermittent porphyria (AIP). (The enzyme defective in AIP precedes the enzyme defective in PCT in the synthetic pathway.)

TABLE 3-32.   **Acute Intermittent Porphyria Versus Coproporphyria**

	ACUTE INTERMITTENT PORPHYRIA (AIP)	**COPROPORPHYRIA**
Inheritance	**Autosomal dominant.**	**Autosomal dominant.**
Defective enzyme	**Uroporphyrinogen I synthase.**	Coprophyrinogen III oxidase.
Clinical presentation	Triad: GI problems (abdominal colic, nausea, constipation), peripheral motor neuropathy (can mimic Guillain-Barré), CNS symptoms (psychosis, depression, seizures); Unlike most other porphyrias, there is no skin rash.	Triad: GI problems (abdominal colic, nausea, constipation), peripheral motor neuropathy (can mimic Guillain-Barré), CNS symptoms (psychosis, depression, seizures); photosensitive skin rash and blisters.
Description	Affects patients < 40; attacks precipitated by **fasting** or anything that stimulates heme synthesis.	
Diagnosis	Elevated **PBG in urine (Watson-Schwartz test).**	Elevated porphyrins in the **stool** (better sensitivity than in urine).
Treatment	**Carbohydrates** (in diet or as IV glucose) or **heme arginate** (to inhibit ALA synthase).	Same as AIP.
Notes	If misdiagnosed, use of barbiturates to "treat" psychosis can exacerbate attack.	Best remembered as AIP with the rash of PCT.

ALA = Δ-aminolevulinic acid; PBG = porphobilinogen; PCT = porphyria cutanea tarda.

TABLE 3-33.   **Porphyria Cutanea Tarda Versus Erythropoietic Porphyria**

	PORPHYRIA CUTANEA TARDA (PCT)	**ERYTHROPOIETIC PORPHYRIA**
Inheritance	**Autosomal dominant or acquired.**	**Autosomal recessive.**
Defective enzyme	**Uroporphyrinogen III decarboxylase.**	**Uroporphyrinogen III synthase.**
Clinical presentation	**Photosensitivity rash and blisters,** which leave pigmented scars on healing.	Severe **photosensitivity rash, hemolytic anemia** and **port-wine urine.**
Description	Affects patients > 40; usually presents after exposure to medications (P450 inducers), **fasting, viral infection** (HepC or HIV) or hepatocellular **carcinoma.**	
Diagnosis	Elevated porphyrin in urine; tea-colored urine that turns pink on **Woods' lamp** illumination (PBG levels are normal).	Elevated porphyrin in urine by **Watson-Schwartz test**; blood smear may reveal hemolytic anemia.
Treatment	Treat underlying cause.	Prevention consists of total avoidance of sun exposure; in severe cases, blood transfusion and possibly bone marrow transplantation.
Notes	Most common porphyria in the United States; most commonly caused by HepC.	Very rare.

HepC = hepatitis C; PBG = porphobilinogen.

- Lead inhibits zinc-dependent enzymes and deposits in bone (replaces calcium) and may affect brain physiology (again, replacing calcium, which is important for neurotransmitter release).
- Lead **inhibits ferrochelatase** in the heme pathway so that protoporphyrin IX accumulates.
- Lead inhibits PBG synthase (because it relies on zinc), resulting in the accumulation of ALA. ALA chemically resembles γ-aminobutyric acid (GABA), which may explain the psychosis manifested in acute lead poisoning.
- Chronically, lead accumulates in kidneys, causing interstitial nephritis and eventually renal failure.

Clinically, lead poisoning can be subdivided into three categories:

1. In utero exposure even at very low concentrations has primarily neurologic consequences. It is an independent risk factor for spontaneous abortion.
2. Days or weeks after acute lead exposure, patients may develop the symptomatic triad of **abdominal colic, CNS symptoms (with cerebral edema),** and **sideroblastic anemia.** CNS symptoms can range from nonspecific cognitive problems and headache to frank **encephalopathy** with seizures.
3. **Chronic lead poisoning** (Figure 3-107) can present with the same symptoms, but is less clear-cut. In addition, patients can also present with **renal insufficiency,** gout, and (in children) **growth retardation.** Peripheral motor neuropathy may be present with characteristic **wrist drop.** Heart disease and **hypertension** can also occur.

Diagnosis of lead poisoning is established directly by measuring elevated lead levels in blood. Bone X-ray fluorescence can demonstrate chronic lead exposure (X-ray shows "lead lines" on epiphyseal bones).

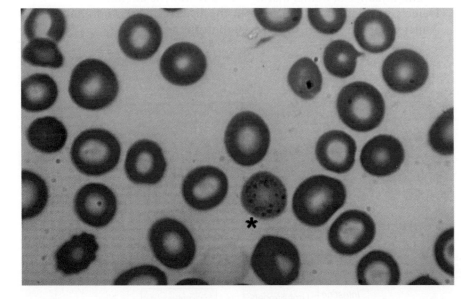

FIGURE 3-107. Basophilic stippling of red blood cell. The asterisk indicates coarse stippling characteristic of lead poisoning. (Reprinted with permission from Lichtman MA, Schafer JA, Felgar RE, Wang N. *Lichtman's Atlas of Hematology.* New York: McGraw-Hill, 2007: Figure I.C.78.)

CLINICAL CORRELATION

In the liver, the P450 system is responsible for the clearance of many drugs. When a P450-inducer drug is first administered to a patient, other medications the patient is taking may be metabolized and cleared more rapidly. In many cases, medication dosages will need to be increased in order to restore "therapeutic levels" while the patient is taking the P450-inducer drug. (This is also why alcohol consumption is discouraged while taking certain medications!)

FLASH FORWARD

When RNA precipitates in RBCs, it appears as blue dots in the cytosol (on a stained blood smear). Although this **basophilic stippling** (see Figure 3-107) can be seen in several other anemias (eg, the thalassemias), it remains very specific to lead poisoning.

Dimercaprol requires intramuscular injection, which is often painful. Succimer is a water-soluble form of dimercaprol that can be given by mouth. This makes it the preferred drug, particularly when treating children (unless lead poisoning is very severe).

FLASH BACK

Most chelating drugs are not selective for the metal they chelate. In addition to toxins other than lead (eg, mercury, arsenic), they may also remove useful physiologic ions (eg, zinc), resulting in deficiency.

CLINICAL CORRELATION

Causes of sideroblastic anemias include alcohol abuse, lead poisoning, and myelodysplastic syndrome. In all cases, the developing RBC is unable to insert iron into hemoglobin. Free iron accumulates in mitochondria, causing them to stain as blue dots around the nucleus. Remember that these **ringed sideroblasts** are seen only on bone marrow smears, in contrast to **basophilic stippling,** which appears on regular peripheral blood smears and represents ribosomal RNA.

CLINICAL CORRELATION

Carbon monoxide (CO) is released as heme is converted to biliverdin; this is the only biologic reaction that produces CO, which is therefore a highly specific marker for the amount of heme catabolism.

Blood tests show **sideroblastic anemia** (microcytic, hypochromic RBCs), and **basophilic stippling** of RBCs. Erythrocyte protoporphyrin IX is increased.

Severe symptoms (eg, encephalopathy) should be treated with ethylenediaminetetraacetic acid (**EDTA**) **calcium disodium, dimercaprol,** and **succimer.** Mild symptoms and prophylaxis may only require succimer.

Heme Catabolism

PATHWAY (FIGURE 3-108)

- When RBCs age, they are collected by the spleen, where their heme is released and degraded to **biliverdin** and subsequently **indirect bilirubin,** a linearized molecule devoid of iron.
- Indirect bilirubin is poorly water-soluble, but it attaches to albumin and is transported to the liver, where it is conjugated to glucuronic acid molecules. The resulting **direct bilirubin** is water-soluble.
- Conjugated bilirubin then enters the intestine via bile.
- Colonic bacteria deconjugate bilirubin and convert it to urobilinogen, which subsequently turns into **urobilin.** Urobilin contributes to the characteristic color of stool.
- Small portion of urobilinogen is reabsorbed, enters the blood, and is filtered into urine. The resulting urobilin also lends its color to urine.
- Note that in jaundice, bilirubin (not urobilin) causes yellow skin discoloration.

CAUSES OF ELEVATED BILIRUBIN

Elevated **indirect (unconjugated) bilirubin** is caused by defects of heme catabolism prior to and including conjugation:

- Overabundance of heme: mainly due to hemolytic anemia
- Defects in bilirubin conjugation in the liver (Gilbert syndrome, Crigler-Najjar syndrome, and neonatal hyperbilirubinemia)

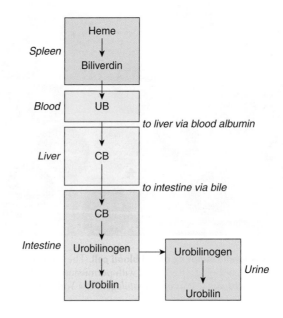

FIGURE 3-108. **Heme catabolism.** CB = conjugated bilirubin; UB = unconjugated bilirubin.

Direct (conjugated) bilirubin elevation results from dysfunctional steps down the excretion pathway:

- Defects of bilirubin secretion from the liver (Dubin-Johnson and Rotor syndromes)
- Obstruction of the biliary pathway (variety of hepatic and biliary disorders, including hepatitis, cirrhosis, or choledocholithiasis)

Hemoglobin

STRUCTURE

Hemoglobin is the chief O_2-binding protein in RBCs. In adults, it exists as a **tetramer,** mostly consisting of two α and two β subunits ($\alpha_2\beta_2$). Each subunit contains one heme molecule, each of which may bind one O_2 atom.

With no O_2 bound, the tetramer remains in a taut (T) conformation, notable for its low O_2 affinity. Once an O_2 molecule binds to one of the subunits, the entire tetramer twists into a relaxed (R) conformation, which is more willing to accommodate second, third, and fourth O_2 molecules. In other words, the more O_2 is around, the more likely the transition from T to R, and the higher the O_2 affinity of hemoglobin.

- This is an example of **cooperative binding,** in which affinity of a protein increases as more ligand is bound.
- Cooperative binding is a subtype of **allostery,** a more general concept, in which binding of one molecule to a protein somehow affects the binding of another molecule (may or may not be identical with the former).

Cooperative binding results in a sigmoidal hemoglobin binding curve (Figure 3-109). At low partial pressures of O_2 (Po_2), such as in peripheral tissues, the affinity of hemoglobin for O_2 is low. This allows hemoglobin to release its cargo O_2 to supply tissues. Conversely, at high Po_2 (as in the lungs), O_2 binding is enhanced.

Compare this with **myoglobin,** the O_2-binding protein in muscles. The amino acid sequence of myoglobin is similar to that of a hemoglobin subunit, except it does not form tetramers. As a result, the monomeric protein does not show allosteric binding, and its binding curve is therefore hyperbolic.

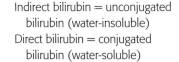
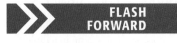
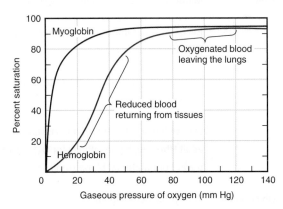

FIGURE 3-109. Hemoglobin binding curve. Myoglobin curve is included for comparison. (Modified with permission from Scriver CR, et al. *The Molecular and Metabolic Basis of Inherited Disease,* 7th ed. New York: McGraw-Hill, 1995.)

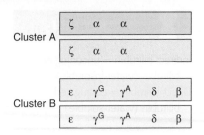

FIGURE 3-110. Hemoglobin genes. Clusters are shown in duplicates to emphasize the availability of two copies of each gene in a diploid cell. Only the most relevant genes are included.

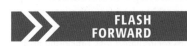

FLASH FORWARD

One of the major complications in thalassemias is iron overload. Hence, pharmacologic treatment includes iron chelation with **deferoxamine.** Sickle cell disease can be managed with **hydroxyurea,** which moderately augments HbF levels.

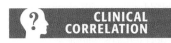

CLINICAL CORRELATION

Since hemoglobin becomes glycosylated in proportion to blood glucose concentration and HbA_{1c} has a long half-life, its levels reflect how well blood sugars have been managed for the previous **6–8 weeks.** In the treatment of diabetes mellitus, the goal is to keep HbA_{1c} < 7%.

HEMOGLOBIN ISOTYPES

Two gene clusters encode hemoglobin subunits: A and B (Figure 3-110). Ideally, two chains from cluster A and two chains from cluster B form the hemoglobin tetramer. For example, the major adult hemoglobin isotype (called HbA_1) comes in the form $\alpha_2\beta_2$, in which α chains come from cluster A and β chains come from cluster B.

Tables 3-34 and 3-35 describe some normal and pathologic hemoglobin isotypes, respectively.

ALLOSTERIC EFFECTORS

Several molecules may bind to hemoglobin (at a site distinct from O_2), either increasing or decreasing the stability of the R conformation. This results in changes in the net affinity of hemoglobin for O_2, visualized as horizontal shifts in the sigmoidal binding curve. Molecules that stabilize the R conformation increase O_2 affinity and therefore cause a **left shift.** As a result, the partial pressure at which 50% hemoglobin capacity is saturated (P_{50}) **decreases.** Conversely, stabilization of the T conformation results in lower affinity, **right shift** of the binding curve, and **higher P_{50}** (Figure 3-111).

Allosteric effectors producing a **left shift** in the O_2-binding curve include:

- Low partial pressure of CO_2 (P_{CO_2})
- Low temperature
- Alkaline environment (low H^+ concentration, high pH)
- Low 2,3-bisphosphoglycerate (2,3-BPG)
- Carbon monoxide poisoning
- Fetal hemoglobin (HbF; note that HbF is a hemoglobin variant, not an allosteric effector, its binding curve is left-shifted compared with the adult variant)

TABLE 3-34. Normal Hemoglobin (Hb) Isotypes

COMPOSITION	NAME	COMMENTS
$\alpha_2\beta_2$	HbA$_1$	Comprises vast majority of adult hemoglobin.
$\alpha_2\delta_2$	HbA$_2$	Minor component of adult hemoglobin. Unknown function.
		Becomes more important in β-chain deficiencies (eg, β-thalassemia).
$\alpha_2\gamma_2$	HbF	The major hemoglobin in the fetus. Low in adult, unless pathology present.
		Low affinity for 2,3-BPG. In effect, HbF has a lower P$_{50}$ than adult HbA$_1$ (ie, higher affinity for O$_2$). This allows O$_2$ to travel from maternal blood (umbilical veins) to fetal blood.
$\zeta_2\varepsilon_2$	Hb Gower-1	Embryonic hemoglobin.
$\zeta_2\gamma_2$	Hb Portland	Embryonic hemoglobin.

2,3-BPG = 2,3-bisphosphoglycerate.

TABLE 3-35. Blood Dyscrasias and Abnormal Hemoglobin Isotypes

	DISEASE	GENOTYPE	HEMOGLOBIN EXPRESSED
α-Thalassemia	Hydrops fetalis	All four α genes deleted.	HbH (δ_4) and Hb Barts (γ_4). Death in utero.
	HbH disease	Three α genes deleted.	HbH and Hb Barts, some HbA_2. Death by age 8.
	Thalassemia trait	Two α genes deleted.	HbA_2 and Hb Barts early in life. Mild phenotype.
	Carrier	One α gene deleted.	Normal HbA_1 content. Silent phenotype.
β-Thalassemia	Thalassemia major	Both β genes affected by a severe mutation (so that no or little β produced).	HbF and HbA_2 are the main isotypes available. HbA_1 reduced or absent.
	Thalassemia intermedia	Both β genes affected by a mild mutation.	As in thalassemia major, but more HbA_1.
	Thalassemia trait	Only one β gene affected by a mutation (mild or severe).	Normal HbA_1, but increased HbA_2.
Sickle cell anemia		Both β genes have a mutation at position 6 (glutamate → valine).	HbSS present, no HbA_1. HbF increased.
Sickle cell anemia carrier		One β gene with the above mutation.	HBSS present along with HbA_1.
Diabetes		Normal hemoglobin genes.	Normal hemoglobin pattern in addition to HbA_{1c}, a glycated form of HbA_1.

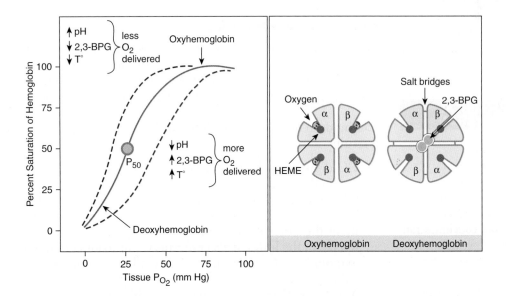

FIGURE 3-111. Hemoglobin allostery. 2,3-BPG = 2,3-bisphosphoglycerate. (Modified with permission from Kasper DL, Braunwald E, Fauci FS, et al. *Harrison's Internal Medicine*, 16th ed. New York: McGraw-Hill, 2005: 593.)

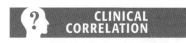

CLINICAL CORRELATION

2,3-BPG (made via a biochemical shunt in an RBC's glycolytic pathway) stabilizes the T conformation of adult hemoglobin. It has dual physiologic function:

- It becomes abundant in the face of O_2 shortage (eg, in patients with chronic obstructive pulmonary disease, but also in normal subjects living at high altitude). This leads to more effective O_2 release in peripheral tissues.
- It affects HbF less than maternal HbA_1. Hence, HbF has effectively higher O_2 affinity, thus aiding fetal blood oxygenation.

CLINICAL CORRELATION

An infant fed formula made with nitrate-contaminated water is particularly prone to developing methemoglobinemia (known as the **blue baby syndrome**). The abundant GI flora in a newborn can convert the nitrate contaminant into nitrite, a potent oxidant.

CLINICAL CORRELATION

Cyanosis, a blue skin discoloration, appears when blood deoxyhemoglobin concentration exceeds 5 g/dL; that is, it depends on the **absolute deoxyhemoglobin concentration** and not percent O_2 saturation. As a result, an anemic patient is less likely to be cyanotic, even if his or her blood is largely deoxygenated. Conversely, a patient with polycythemia rubra vera can appear cyanotic, despite a near-adequate SaO_2.

Allosteric effectors producing a **right shift** in the O_2-binding curve include:

- High P_{CO_2}
- High temperature
- Acidic environment (high $[H^+]$, low pH)
- High 2,3-BPG

METHEMOGLOBINEMIA

In methemoglobinemia, an unusually high percentage of hemoglobin contains iron in the ferric (Fe^{3+}) rather than ferrous (Fe^{2+}) state, thus preventing O_2 from binding. Normally, the methemoglobin reductase system is responsible for restoration of the Fe^{2+} state.

- In the uncommon, congenital forms of methemoglobinemia, methemoglobin reductase is faulty or there is a defect in hemoglobin itself that makes the reductase less effective.
- More commonly, methemoglobinemia is **acquired** by exposure to strong oxidants that overwhelm the reductase system. Such oxidants include **nitrates** (typically from fertilizer-contaminated water, wells, and so on), **aniline** dyes, **naphthalene** (in mothballs), **local anesthetics** (lidocaine), **vasodilators** (nitric oxide, nitroprusside), **antimalarials** (chloroquine, primaquine), **sulfonamides, dapsone,** and others.
- Laboratory tests usually show normal partial arterial pressure of oxygen (PaO_2), but decreased saturated level of oxygen in hemoglobin (SaO_2). Direct tests for methemoglobin detection are available.
- Cyanosis is usually the chief sign. Blood is dark and "chocolate-colored" and does not turn bright red on exposure to O_2.
- Treatment consists of removal of the offending toxin by using **methylene blue,** and sometimes **ascorbic acid.**
- Because methylene blue utilizes NADPH which is formed by G6PD in the pentose phosphate pathway, it is ineffective (and may even precipitate hemolysis) in patients with G6PD deficiency.

Carbon Monoxide Poisoning

Carbon monoxide (CO) is a colorless, odorless gas. Intoxication occurs either directly by inhalation of fumes from incompletely combusted fuel (car exhaust, heaters) or by inhalation of certain organic solvents (methylene chloride, a paint stripper), which are metabolized to CO in the liver.

CO binds to heme in hemoglobin with much higher affinity than does O_2. As a result:

- CO diminishes the O_2 carrying capacity of hemoglobin by competing for the binding sites.
- CO shifts the O_2-binding curve of hemoglobin to the left. In other words, binding of a CO molecule to one hemoglobin subunit increases the affinity of the other three subunits for O_2. Although this results in better O_2 uptake in the lungs, it also prevents O_2 unloading in the tissues.
- Symptoms of CO poisoning are usually very **nonspecific.** Cherry-red discoloration of skin is specific but not sensitive (pale skin is more common).
- As with methemoglobinemia, arterial blood gas tests show normal PaO_2 but diminished SaO_2. Direct CO detection tests are available. Note that smokers often present with values indicative of mild CO poisoning as a result of the CO in inhaled cigarette smoke.
- Treatment consists of 100% O_2 supplementation. Patients with severe cases may require hyperbaric O_2.

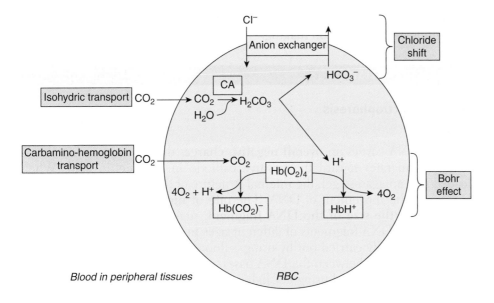

FIGURE 3-112. **O$_2$/CO$_2$ exchange in peripheral tissues.** CA = carbonic anhydrase; Hb = hemoglobin.

Carbon Dioxide

Although hemoglobin is primarily known for its O$_2$-carrying capacity, it is also an important transporter for CO$_2$. There are two main mechanisms by which this occurs (Figure 3-112):

- **Isohydric transport** accounts for 80% of CO$_2$ movement. As CO$_2$ diffuses into an RBC, the enzyme **carbonic anhydrase** combines it with water, yielding carbonic acid (H$_2$CO$_3$). As the word *acid* implies, H$_2$CO$_3$ tends to lose a proton, leaving behind the bicarbonate ion (HCO$_3^-$). The proton can bind to several **histidine** residues on hemoglobin, whereas HCO$_3^-$ leaves the RBC in exchange for chloride ion (Cl$^-$) (the chloride shift). Note that in isohydric transport, the CO$_2$ is not directly carried by hemoglobin.
- In **carbamino-hemoglobin transport**, which carries up to 20% of CO$_2$, the CO$_2$ molecule reacts directly with amino groups on hemoglobin. This reaction produces one free proton.

The reactions involved here are reversible, so the opposite processes take place in the lungs, where CO$_2$ is unloaded.

Recall that CO$_2$ and H$^+$ are allosteric effectors of hemoglobin, both causing an increase in P$_{50}$ and thus lower affinity for and increased release of O$_2$. In other words, the presence of CO$_2$ and protons is a signal for the hemoglobin molecule that it has reached the periphery and that its time to release its O$_2$ cargo. This is called the **Bohr effect.** Conversely, as blood returns to the lungs it faces high Po$_2$, which prompts the release of protons and CO$_2$. This is the **Haldane effect.**

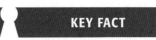

Laboratory Tests and Techniques

Hospital laboratories often use basic techniques of molecular biology and biochemistry to analyze clinical samples from patients. Although these tests are

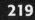

CLINICAL CORRELATION

Patients suffering from methemoglobinemia or CO poisoning display normal Pao$_2$, but have low Sao$_2$. Because the heme of patients with methemoglobinemia cannot bind *any* gas, their blood is dark red. On the other hand, the heme of CO poisoning victims avidly binds CO, and their blood may turn bright red.

KEY FACT

Hemoglobin's ability to bind and release O$_2$ at appropriate locations is caused by two main and distinct phenomena: cooperative binding of O$_2$ and the Bohr-Haldane effect.

often developed and used in basic science research, they aid in diagnosis and help guide clinical decision making.

DNA-BASED LAB TESTS

DNA Gel Electrophoresis

PRINCIPLE

Because DNA carries an **overall negative charge** (due to its phosphate backbone), it migrates toward the positive cathode in an electric field. When loaded into an agarose gel, the internal structure of the gel provides a physical barrier for the movement of DNA. The **rate of movement is inversely proportional to the size of the DNA fragment,** making it possible to separate and visualize DNA fragments of different sizes from a clinical sample. Visualization is typically carried out by using a fluorescent dye, ethidium bromide, which intercalates between the DNA bases, making it possible to detect DNA fragments within the gel using UV light.

USE

DNA electrophoresis is one of several techniques for analyzing DNA samples. The ability to separate DNA fragments based on their size is critical in polymerase chain reaction (PCR), DNA sequencing, DNA restriction digestion, and Southern blotting, all of which provide important information about the genetic makeup of clinical samples.

DNA Sequencing

PRINCIPLE

A single-stranded DNA fragment from a clinical sample is used as a template in the presence of DNA polymerase, a short primer, four standard deoxynucleotide bases (A, T, G, C), and a small amount of radiolabeled or fluorescently labeled dideoxynucleotide base. Although these bases are otherwise identical to the standard A, T, G, and C nucleotides, they terminate the growth of the DNA chain when they are incorporated into a growing DNA molecule because they lack a second O_2 atom (**dideoxy** nucleotide). This makes it impossible for the chain to accept and chemically react with the base that would follow.

At a certain point in chain synthesis, one of the dideoxynucleotide bases gets incorporated. This causes that particular growing DNA molecule to stop elongating. Statistically, this random incorporation of the dideoxynucleotides produces a sample with DNA fragments of different sizes, corresponding to each of the positions of a particular nucleotide in the DNA chain. Repeating this process for each of the four bases and separating the resulting fragments using DNA gel electrophoresis makes it possible to determine the sequence of bases in the DNA sample fragment because the relative positions of the fragments on the DNA gel reveal the order of the bases in the DNA molecule (Figure 3-113).

USE

DNA sequencing is used to confirm or exclude known sequence variants (genotyping) or to fully characterize a defined DNA region. It is most commonly used to detect specific mutations in diagnosis of genetic diseases.

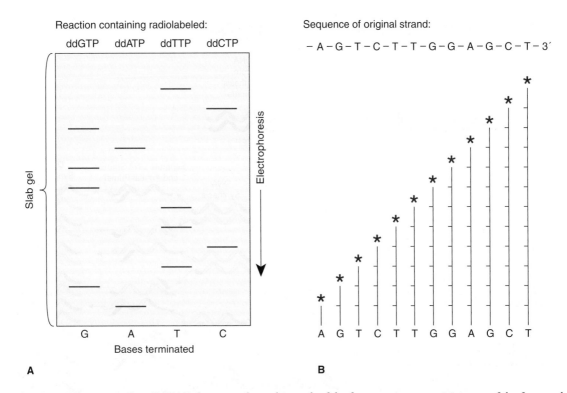

FIGURE 3-113.   DNA sequencing. (A) DNA fragments formed in each of the four reactions containing one of the four nucleotides are run on a DNA gel and separated by size. (B) Radiolabel (* asterisk) allows for the visualization of the DNA fragments containing dideoxynucleotides, which makes it possible to deduce the order of individual bases. dd = dideoxynucleotides. (Modified with permission from Murray RK, Granner DK, Rodwell VW. *Harper's Illustrated Biochemistry*, 27th ed. New York: McGraw-Hill, 2006: 411.)

CLINICAL EXAMPLES

In patients with a clinical diagnosis of **osteogenesis imperfecta,** a blood sample can be analyzed for mutations in *COL1A1* or *COL1A2* genes. Similarly, DNA of patients with **Ehlers-Danlos syndrome (EDL)** is analyzed for mutations in *COL3A1*. Genotyping is also used to diagnose **cystic fibrosis, β-thalassemia, muscular dystrophies,** and **sickle cell anemia.**

Polymerase Chain Reaction

PRINCIPLE

Polymerase chain reaction (PCR) is an important method for amplifying DNA, making it possible to increase the amount of DNA available for analysis from a small clinical sample. The original double-stranded DNA serves as a template. This reaction also requires a thermally stable DNA polymerase, primers flanking the region that needs to be amplified, and nucleotides. The mixture then undergoes the following procedure in an automated cycle (Figure 3-114). Of note, the polymerase usually used is Taq polymerase, which was first isolated from ***Thermus aquaticus,*** a bacterium found in **hot springs.**

- **Denaturing:** Heating to approximately 95°C separates the double-stranded DNA.
- **Annealing:** Cooling to approximately 45°C causes the primers to attach to single strands of DNA in complementary regions.
- **Elongation:** Heating to approximately 72°C causes Taq polymerase to synthesize a complementary DNA strand, starting at the primer.

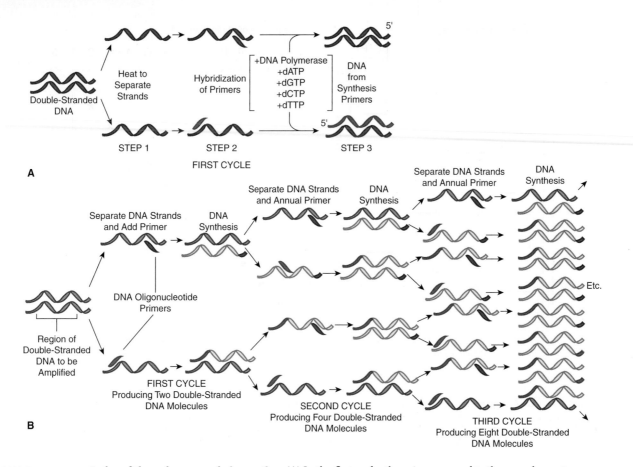

FIGURE 3-114. **Cycles of the polymerase chain reaction.** (A) In the first cycle, the primers anneal to the complementary sequences on the DNA in the sample, and the polymerase extends the strands in either the 3′ or the 5′ direction. (B) In each of the subsequent cycles, the newly synthesized strands are separated from the template, the primers reanneal, and the steps are repeated. The result is an exponential rise in the number of DNA fragments synthesized between the positions of the two original primers. Typically, about 30 cycles are conducted. d = deoxynucleotides.

This cycle is usually repeated approximately 30 times, resulting in an exponential increase in the number of synthesized copies of the original DNA fragment. The DNA is then available for further analysis.

USE

PCR is used to genotype specific mutations, detect hereditary diseases, diagnose viral diseases, and in genetic fingerprinting and paternity testing. It is now also used in clinical microbiology to identify pathogenic microorganisms.

CLINICAL EXAMPLES

PCR is used in early detection of hepatitis B virus (**HBV**), **HCV**, **HIV**, varicella-zoster virus (**VZV**), herpes simplex virus (**HSV**), cytomegalovirus (**CMV**), Epstein-Barr virus (**EBV**), **parvovirus B19**, and **influenza** viruses—often following initial antibody-based approaches. PCR detects the actual presence of the virus by amplifying viral DNA, even in the absence of the host's antibody response. **Group A streptococci**, *Legionella* **spp**, *Bordetella pertussis*, and vancomycin-resistant enterococcus (**VRE**) are examples of bacterial infections often identified using PCR. PCR is most widely used for identification of microbial pathogens, but it is also used for detection of tumor factors, profiling of cytokines, expression of various genes, and as an integral part of many approaches used in human genetic testing.

DNA Restriction Digest

PRINCIPLE

DNA restriction digest refers to a technique in which a **DNA sample is cut into pieces using restriction enzymes** (also known as restriction endonucleases). Each restriction enzyme cleaves double-stranded DNA within a certain base sequence (recognition sequence), and does so consistently (Figure 3-115). Therefore, a specific DNA sample that is fragmented using a known combination of restriction enzymes always results in a reproducible and unique pattern of DNA fragments. These fragments can then be visualized using DNA gel electrophoresis.

USE

DNA restriction is often part of **restriction fragment length polymorphism (RFLP) analysis.** This method relies on the fact that random mutations sometimes introduce or eliminate a restriction site. It is one of the methods used for DNA fingerprinting, in which different patterns of polymorphisms (variations in a population's DNA) in individuals are used as a basis for identification. More commonly, it is used in **single-nucleotide polymorphism (SNP) analysis,** in which changes in single nucleotides within a restriction enzyme recognition sequence are present in certain alleles and are correlated with genetic diseases. It is important to note that these are not disease-causing mutations; they are normal variations occurring within a population (alleles) that are **correlated** with certain genetic diseases.

CLINICAL EXAMPLES

The gene coding for **apolipoprotein E (ApoE),** which is associated with **Alzheimer disease,** contains two SNPs that result in three potential alleles for the *ApoE* gene, called E2, E3, and E4. It has been shown that people with at least one E4 allele have a greater chance of developing Alzheimer's, whereas the presence of the E2 allele seems to have a protective effect.

Fluorescence In Situ Hybridization (FISH)

PRINCIPLE

In the cytogenetic technique known as fluorescence in situ hybridization (FISH), a **fluorescently labeled DNA probe** is used to determine not just the **presence or absence of a particular DNA sequence in a sample,** but also to **visualize its location on the chromosome** (Figure 3-116).

- Single-stranded DNA that has been tagged with a fluorophore, antibody epitope, or biotin is added to a preparation of nuclear DNA, either in intact nuclei (interphase FISH) or chromosomes arranged on a slide (fiber FISH).
- After binding to the complementary sequence in the sample, the excess unbound probe is washed away.
- The sample is then imaged using fluorescence microscopy.

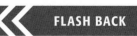

FLASH BACK

In DNA gel electrophoresis, the **rate of movement is inversely proportional to the size of the DNA fragment,** making it possible to separate and visualize DNA fragments of different sizes from a sample.

FLASH FORWARD

Cri du chat—partial deletion of the **short arm of chromosome 5,** which may be visualized by FISH → characteristic **cry similar to the mewing of kittens.** Patients exhibit failure to thrive and severe cognitive and motor delays, but typically are able to communicate socially. Often present are microcephaly and coarsening of facial features.

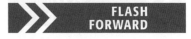

*Eco*RI

```
5'- - -TACT G AATTC ACG- - -3'
3'- - -ATGA CTTAA G TGC- - -5'
```

FIGURE 3-115. Typical endonuclease recognition site. This is an example of a specific sequence recognized by the *Eco*RI restriction endonuclease. *Eco*RI always recognizes this specific site and cleaves the DNA chain at the positions marked by the arrows.

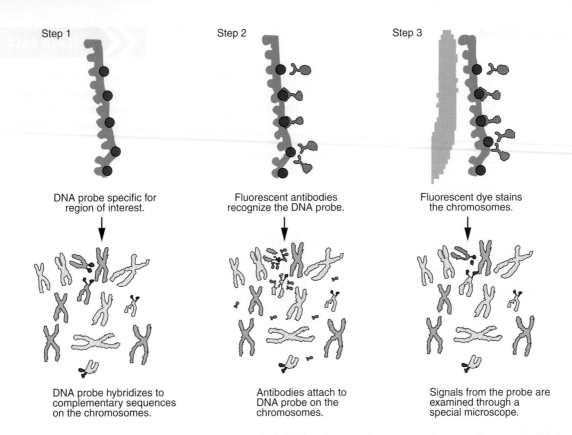

Step 1 — DNA probe specific for region of interest.

DNA probe hybridizes to complementary sequences on the chromosomes.

Step 2 — Fluorescent antibodies recognize the DNA probe.

Antibodies attach to DNA probe on the chromosomes.

Step 3 — Fluorescent dye stains the chromosomes.

Signals from the probe are examined through a special microscope.

FIGURE 3-116. **Fluorescence in situ hybridization.** Step 1: A DNA probe complementary to the gene of interest is added to the chromosomal preparation. Step 2: A fluorescent antibody against the epitope that was used to tag the DNA probe is added, and it binds to the DNA probe. Step 3: Chromosomes are counterstained with a fluorescent dye of a color different from that of the antibody. This enables clear visualization of the regions of interest under a fluorescent microscope.

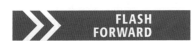

FLASH FORWARD

Angelman syndrome (AS)—loss of **maternal 15q11** (both copies of paternal origin) → mental retardation, seizures, **inappropriate outbursts of laughter.**

Prader-Willi syndrome (PWS)—loss of **paternal 15q11** (both copies of maternal origin) → mental retardation, obesity, hypotonia, weak cry.

AS and PWS are examples of **genomic imprinting,** in which the expression of a particular allele and the associated phenotype are exclusively determined by which parent contributed it.

USE

FISH is used to map specific DNA sequences such as genes or rearrangements to a particular position on a chromosome. It plays a particular role in detecting chromosomal abnormalities such as inversions or translocations. When using labeled primers for the 16S rRNA region of specific bacteria as probes, it can also determine the presence of microorganisms in clinical samples.

CLINICAL EXAMPLES

FISH is often used for detection of **aneuploidies** (eg, trisomy 21, 18, 13), including **sex chromosome number abnormalities** (eg, Klinefelter, Turner, and triple X syndromes). It can be used on tissue samples, as well as amniotic fluid. It is also used in the diagnosis of certain **cancers,** such as the Philadelphia chromosome (ie, *BCR-ABL* t(9,22) translocation) in chronic myelogenous leukemia (CML). Furthermore, it can be used for detection of **microdeletions,** such as 5p– in cri du chat, and 15q11.2–q13 in Prader-Willi and Angelman syndromes.

Southern Blot

PRINCIPLE

Southern blotting refers to a technique whereby a **DNA sample is separated according to fragment size** using gel electrophoresis and is then transferred on to a nitrocellulose or nylon membrane, where it is fixed in place. Much like FISH, a single-stranded DNA probe, usually labeled with a radioactive isotope, is allowed to incubate with the membrane containing the sample. This **radioactive DNA probe binds to complementary sequences** in the DNA sample. After the nonbound probe has been washed away, X-ray film is placed on top of the membrane. The radioactivity from the bound probe exposes the X-ray film in the exact position of the radiolabeled probe. This indicates the presence, and the position of the sequence of interest, within a particular DNA fragment from the original sample (Figure 3-117).

USE

Southern blotting is used in diagnosis of genetic disorders, especially those involving nucleotide expansions. It is also used in detection of viral and bacterial pathogens, as well as for certain forensic applications.

CLINICAL EXAMPLES

Southern blots are often used to detect trinucleotide expansion in **fragile X syndrome, Friedreich's ataxia,** and **myotonic dystrophy,** as well as **methylation or deletion of the SNRPN locus in Prader-Willi/Angelman syndromes.** Southern blotting has also been used to directly detect malaria parasites (*Plasmodium* spp.) in the blood of patients.

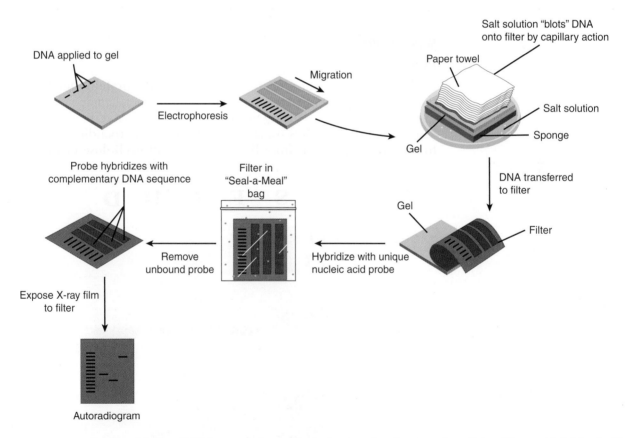

FIGURE 3-117. Southern blotting. DNA is separated according to size, transferred on to a nitrocellulose filter, and hybridized with radiolabeled probes specific for the sequence of interest. Exposure of the X-ray film reveals the position and size of the DNA fragments that contain the sequence of interest.

PROTEIN-BASED LAB TESTS

Protein Gel Electrophoresis

PRINCIPLE

Sodium dodecyl sulfate-polyacrylamide gel electrophoresis, or SDS-PAGE, as it is almost exclusively known, is a fundamental technique for **separating proteins based on size.** It is the protein counterpart to DNA agarose gel electrophoresis. Proteins are denatured using SDS detergent and then loaded on to a polyacrylamide gel. The buffer used in this technique gives the denatured proteins an **overall negative charge.** Therefore, when placed into an electric field, the proteins move through the gel matrix toward the positive electrode. Because the internal gel structure serves as a barrier for the movement of proteins, their migration toward the positive electrode is indirectly proportional to the size of the protein, with the **smallest proteins migrating farthest** (closest to the positive electrode). A standard mix of proteins of known sizes (ladder) is also run on the gel for comparison (Figure 3-118).

USE

Much like DNA gel electrophoresis, SDS-PAGE is a basic technique used in conjunction with other methods to analyze clinical samples. One of the most common uses is as part of Western blot analysis for detection of pathogens.

Western Blot

PRINCIPLE

In Western blotting (or protein immunoblotting), a **protein** sample is denatured using the SDS detergent and run on a polyacrylamide gel to separate the proteins present according to their size (see SDS-PAGE in preceding text). The second step involves using an **electrical field perpendicular to the gel to transfer the proteins from the gel on to a nitrocellulose membrane.** To

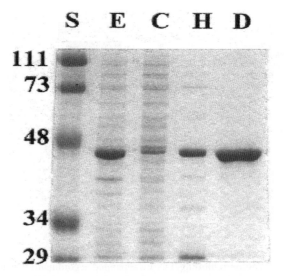

FIGURE 3-118.   Example of an SDS-PAGE (sodium dodecyl sulfate-polyacrylamide gel electrophoresis) gel. Photo of a protein electrophoresis gel, in which the protein was stained using Coomassie blue dye. Lane S contains protein standards of known molecular weights for comparison (numbers represent the size in kDa). Other lanes contain samples with different amounts of a particular protein (around 45 kDa in size). (Reproduced with permission from Murray RK, Granner DK, Rodwell VW. *Harper's Illustrated Biochemistry,* 27th ed. New York: McGraw-Hill, 2006: 25.)

prevent nonspecific antibody binding to the membrane, it is **blocked** by incubating in a solution of bovine serum albumin (BSA) or nonfat dry milk. The membrane is then incubated with a **primary antibody** specific for the protein of interest. After washing off the excess unbound primary antibody, a **secondary antibody** is added. This secondary antibody is conjugated to an enzyme; it is also specific for the primary antibody that was used in the previous step. Subsequent addition of a **substrate** for the enzyme causes a colorimetric reaction in the bands containing the protein of interest (Figure 3-119).

USE

Western blotting is used to detect the presence of a protein in a clinical sample, indicating an infection with a specific agent. This may refer to both antigens native to the pathogen (eg, in the case of **bovine spongiform encephalopathy** or **BSE**) or to the actual host antibodies that have developed in response to the infection (eg, **HIV** and **Lyme disease** [*Borrelia burgdorferi*]). Note that Western blots can also be used for relative quantification of the amount of protein present.

CLINICAL EXAMPLES

Western blotting is a confirmatory test performed when the results of an ELISA (see below) test are positive for HIV antibodies.

Enzyme-Linked Immunosorbent Assay (ELISA)

PRINCIPLE

ELISA is an immunologic technique widely used for the detection of antigens and antibodies in clinical samples. There are two types of assay:

- **Indirect ELISA**
- A known amount of an **antigen is fixed to a surface.**

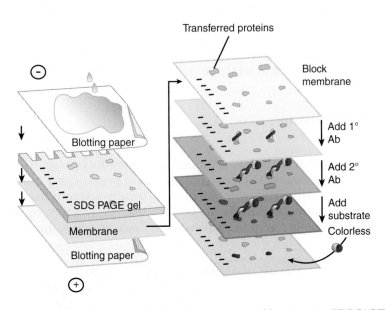

FIGURE 3-119. **Western blotting.** After they are separated by size using SDS-PAGE (sodium dodecyl sulfate-polyacrylamide gel electrophoresis), the proteins are transferred on to a membrane with the aid of an electric field. The membrane is then blocked and incubated with the primary and the secondary antibodies. Using a substrate, a color signal is produced showing the fragments that contain the protein of interest. 1° Ab, primary antibody; 2° Ab, secondary antibody.

- A clinical sample (usually the patient's serum) is then added on to the surface.
- If the sample contains antibodies against the antigen, the **antibodies bind the antigen** and remain attached to the surface.
- The surface is washed to remove any unbound (nonspecific) antibody.
- A **secondary, enzyme-linked antibody,** specific for the Fc portion of the human IgG, is then added to the reaction.
- This **secondary antibody binds the primary antibodies** present from the patient's serum.
- A substrate is then added, which results in a **colorimetric reaction catalyzed by the enzyme linked to the secondary antibody.**
- The color change can be quantified using a spectrophotometer and related to the amount of the antibody present in the clinical sample.
- **Direct, or "sandwich," ELISA** (Figure 3-120).
- The **antibody** specific for the antigen of interest is first **fixed to a surface** (1).
- A sample potentially containing the antigen of interest is added to the reaction.
- If the **antigen** is present in the sample, it **will bind to the fixed antibodies,** while the rest is washed away (2).
- A **second "layer" of the antibody** is then added, "sandwiching" the bound antigen (3).
- As in the indirect ELISA, an **enzyme-linked secondary antibody** and the substrate are then added, and the **colorimetric reaction** is read in a spectrophotometer (4 and 5).

ELISA is used for the detection of antibodies against many pathogens, as a means of establishing present or past infection with the pathogen. It is also sometimes used by the food industry to detect the presence of certain common allergens.

CLINICAL EXAMPLES

ELISA is the most *sensitive* screening test for HIV in individuals at risk for infection. A positive result is followed up by the more *specific* Western blot assay. ELISA is also used to screen for other viral pathogens, such as the West Nile virus.

Immunohistochemistry

PRINCIPLE

Similar to ELISA and Western blotting, immunohistochemistry (IHC) is a general technique that relies on visual detection of proteins in a sample using antibodies. The main difference is that IHC usually refers to the detection of antigens in **tissue samples.** Some authors refer to a variant of this technique under the term "immunocytochemistry," which differs from immuno-

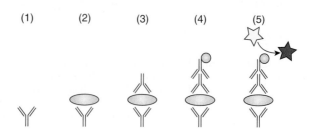

FIGURE 3-120.   ELISA. See text for a step-by-step explanation.

histochemistry in that immunocytochemistry uses cells grown in laboratory culture.

In both techniques, an antibody raised against the protein of interest is incubated with the tissue sample; the tissue is subsequently washed to remove unbound primary antibody. If the antigen is present in the tissue, bound antibodies stay attached. A secondary, enzyme-conjugated or fluorophore-conjugated antibody against the primary antibody is added to the reaction. Finally, the addition of the substrate causes a color change in the locations that contain the antigen of interest. These can be directly observed using a microscope. In the case of a fluorophore-labeled antibody, a fluorescent microscope is used for visualization, eliminating the need for the substrate-enzyme reaction (Figure 3-121).

USE

In the clinical setting, IHC is commonly used in histopathology, often to detect a specific cancer antigen in a tissue sample, thus confirming the tumor type. Tissue can come from diagnostic biopsies or tumor samples following resection.

CLINICAL EXAMPLES

Immunohistochemical techniques are used to detect the presence of markers such as the **carcinoembryonic antigen (CEA)** in adenocarcinomas, **CD15** and **CD30** in Hodgkin disease, **α-fetoprotein** in yolk sac tumors and hepatocellular carcinoma, **CD117** in gastrointestinal stromal tumors (GIST), and **prostate-specific antigen (PSA)** in prostate cancer.

Radioimmunoassay

PRINCIPLE

Radioimmunoassay (RIA) is used to measure small amounts of antigen in clinical samples. The protein of interest is first **labeled with a radioactive isotope** and allowed to bind to the antibody against that protein until the point of saturation. The clinical sample is then added to the mix, **causing any antigen in the sample to displace the radioactively labeled one from the antibodies.** This free radiolabeled antigen is then measured in the solution, making it possible to calculate the amount of the antigen in the original sample.

USE

RIA is used most commonly to measure various hormone levels in patients. It is also sometimes used to measure the amounts of vitamins, enzymes, and drugs in clinical samples.

CLINICAL EXAMPLES

RIA is routinely used to measure the levels of thyroid-stimulating hormone (TSH), T_3, and T_4 as part of a thyroid disease workup, as well as **insulin** levels in patients with suspected diabetes mellitus or insulinomas.

RNA-BASED LAB TESTS

Northern Blot

PRINCIPLE

Northern blotting is similar to Southern and Western blotting, except that the substance being analyzed is **RNA,** rather than DNA or protein. In Northern

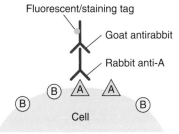

FIGURE 3-121. Immunohistochemical detection. An antibody specific to the protein of interest is incubated with a clinical sample and allowed to bind to it. Then a secondary antibody is used to provide a visual signal, which identifies and localizes the protein of interest if it is present in the sample.

blotting, a sample of RNA is run on an agarose gel and is then transferred to a nitrocellulose membrane. A radiolabeled RNA or single-stranded DNA is used as a probe. Finally, an X-ray film is exposed to the membrane, revealing the location of the RNA sequences of interest (Figure 3-122).

USE

Northern blotting is usually used in special laboratory studies to detect the levels of expression of a certain gene in clinical samples, as indicated by the amount of mRNA present.

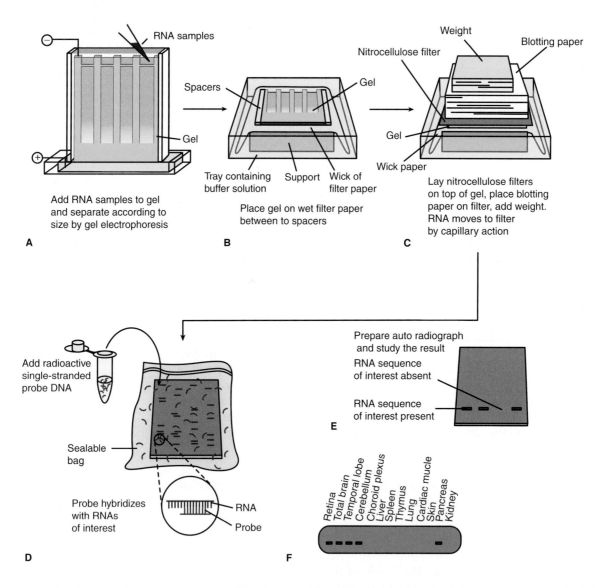

FIGURE 3-122. Northern blotting. (A–E) RNA is separated according to size, transferred on to a nitrocellulose filter, and hybridized with radiolabeled probes specific for the sequence of interest. Exposure of the X-ray film reveals the position and size of the RNA fragments that contain the sequence of interest. (F) The presence or absence of a particular RNA fragment can be determined and compared in several clinical samples, such as from different patients or different organs from the same patient.

Genetics

HARDY-WEINBERG GENETICS

Humans carry two copies of each gene in every somatic cell (one inherited from each parent). These copies, known as alleles, each can be dominant or recessive. **Hardy-Weinberg genetics** are used to describe the frequency of these alleles in large populations.

The percentage of each of the two alleles (p and q) in the population must total 100%.

$$p + q = 1.00$$

EXAMPLE

In a sample population, there are only two eye colors: brown and blue. If 90% of the alleles in the population are for brown eyes ($p = 0.90$), then the other 10% must be for blue eyes ($q = 0.10$).

To determine the number of people with each combination of alleles:

$$p^2 + 2pq + q^2 = 1.00$$

where p^2 and q^2 are the fractions of the population homozygous for p and q, respectively, and $2pq$ is the fraction heterozygous for p and q.

Using the previous example of eye color, if $p = 0.90$ and $q = 0.10$, then:

$p^2 = 0.90^2 = 0.81$ 81% homozygous for brown eyes
$2pq = 2 \times 0.90 \times 0.10 = 0.18$ 18% heterozygous for eye color
$q^2 = 0.10^2 = 0.01$ 1% homozygous for blue eyes

Disease inheritance depends on the number of copies of the mutant gene required to produce the condition and on which chromosome the gene is located.

Non–Sex Chromosome Diseases

Autosomal dominant and **autosomal recessive** diseases are caused by genes carried on chromosomes other than the X and Y sex chromosomes.

- **Autosomal dominant** diseases require the presence of only one mutant gene (or allele). These individuals are termed heterozygotes. Affected persons may be of both sexes and appear in most generations (Figure 3-123A).
- **Autosomal recessive** diseases require the presence of two mutant genes (homozygous). Affected persons are of both sexes, but autosomal recessive diseases appear sporadically and infrequently throughout a family tree (Figure 3-123B).

Sex Chromosome Diseases

X-linked recessive diseases affect males because they carry one X chromosome that is always inherited from the mother. Because they have only one

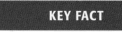

KEY FACT

When making calculations, remember that each person has **two** alleles. p and q refer to the number of alleles, not the number of people!

KEY FACT

Autosomal dominant diseases tend to cause death after puberty. Autosomal recessive diseases tend to manifest themselves earlier and cause death before puberty.

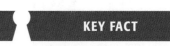

KEY FACT

Autosomal dominant inheritance: The affected person has **at least one affected parent.**
Autosomal recessive inheritance: The affected person is usually **born to unaffected parents;** there is an increased incidence of **parental consanguinity.**

KEY FACT

X-linked recessive inheritance: Affects mainly males; affected males are usually **born to unaffected parents;** the mother is an **asymptomatic carrier** but may have **affected male relatives.**
X-linked dominant inheritance: Affects more females than males; females are **often more mildly and more variably affected** than males due to random inactivation of one X chromosome (**"lyonization"**).

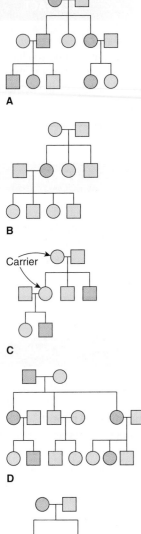

A

B

Carrier

C

D

E

FIGURE 3-123. **(A) Autosomal dominant inheritance. (B) Autosomal recessive inheritance. (C) X-linked recessive inheritance. (D) X-linked dominant inheritance. (E) Mitochondrial inheritance.**

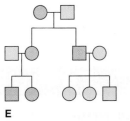

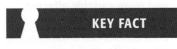

KEY FACT

Mitochondrial inheritance: Can affect both sexes, but is passed on by affected mothers only.

---

allele for each gene on the X-chromosome, the recessive mutant gene is always expressed (there can be no second, dominant allele to disguise the recessive allele) (Figure 3-123C).

X-linked dominant diseases affect both sexes. An affected male has only one X chromosome and thus always passes the disease to daughters. Affected mothers have a 50% chance of passing on the disease to offspring of either sex (Figure 3-123D).

MITOCHONDRIAL DISEASES

Mitochondria carry their own DNA, which is inherited from the mother. (Only the oocyte contributes mitochondria to the zygote; the sperm neck and tail, which carry mitochondria of the sperm, never penetrate the oocyte.) Any mutation present in the maternal mitochondria will be passed to offspring (Figure 3-123E). Not all mutations cause disease, however. Even within a single individual, mitochondrial DNA is heterogenous, and often a defect in one or many mitochondria can be compensated for by others.

These modes of inheritance are summarized in Table 3-36.

Inheritance Properties

- **Incomplete penetrance** occurs when a person with a mutant genotype does not show signs of the **disease** (phenotype).
- **Variable expression** occurs when the severity and nature of the disease phenotype varies between individuals with the same mutant **genotype.**

TRISOMIES

Trisomies occur when three homologous chromosomes are present in a zygote.

Nondisjunction

Either the sperm or the egg may carry the extra chromosome, as shown in Figure 3-124.

Chromosomal Translocation

Trisomy can also occur when a piece of one chromosome attaches to another and "hitches a ride" during meiosis. As a result, two homologous chromosomes can be sorted to the same zygote, as shown in Figure 3-125.

Common Trisomies

All trisomies are characterized by mental retardation, abnormal facies, and often heart disease (Figure 3-126). Few fetal trisomies survive to birth (ie, most terminate in spontaneous abortion).

Trisomy 21 (Down syndrome) is the most common trisomy and the most common cause of mental retardation. Mothers may express **low α-ferroprotein and high** levels of **beta human chorionic gonadotropin (β-hCG)** during pregnancy and ultrasound may show **nuchal translucency.** Patients are characterized by:

- Epicanthal folds
- Simian crease

TABLE 3-36.   Modes of Inheritance

MODE	CHROMOSOME CARRIED ON	SEX AFFECTED	GENERATIONS AFFECTED	PARENT WHO TRANSMITS	TYPES OF DISEASE	HINTS WHEN LOOKING AT PEDIGREE TREE
Autosomal dominant	Non-X, non-Y chromosomes	Both equally	Multiple serial generations.	Parent who is also affected.	Often structural and not fatal at early age.	Most generations affected.
Autosomal recessive	Non-X, non-Y chromosomes	Both equally	Usually multiple offspring of one generation.	Both parents are carriers.	Most metabolic diseases and cystic fibrosis.	Often sporadically appears in one generation.
X-linked recessive	X chromosome	Males	Variable depending on presence of male offspring.	Mother.	Fragile X, muscular dystrophy, hemophilias, Lesch-Nyhan syndrome.	Mostly males.
X-linked dominant	X chromosome	Females > males	Multiple serial generations.	Both parents can give gene to a female, only mother gives to male offspring.	Hypophosphatemic rickets.	All female children of affected male are affected.
Mitochondrial	None (carried in mitochondrial DNA)	Both equally	Multiple serial generations.	Mother.	Leber's optic neuropathy, MELAS, many myopathies.	Only affected mothers can pass mutant alleles to offspring.

MELAS = mitochondrial encephalomyopathy with lactic acidosis and stroke-like episodes.

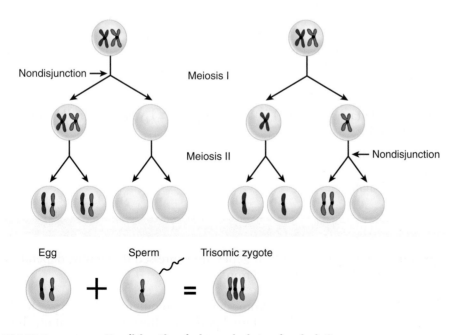

FIGURE 3-124.   Nondisjunction during meiosis I and meiosis II.

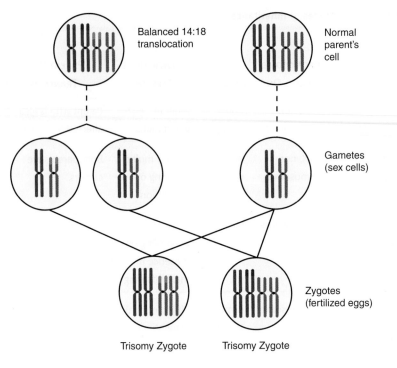

FIGURE 3-125. Robertsonian translocation resulting in Down syndrome.

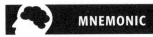

FLASH BACK

The normal allocation of chromosomes during gametogenesis is reviewed in Chapter 4 of this book. Briefly, each gamete is a haploid cell that contains one of two sister chromatids.

MNEMONIC

Drink at 21, **E**lection age is 18, **P**uberty at 13.
Down = Trisomy 21
Edward = Trisomy 18
Patau = Trisomy 13
Trisomy 8 is rare, but can also result in live births.
Trisomy 16 is a common cause of miscarriage.

- Atrial septal defect (ASD) or other congenital heart disease
- Acute lymphocytic leukemia (ALL)
- Duodenal atresia
- Celiac disease

Trisomy 18 (Edward syndrome) is often fatal by < 1 year of age. Patients are characterized by:

- Micrognathia
- Overlapping, clenched fingers
- Rocker-bottom feet
- Large occiput

Trisomy 13 (Patau syndrome) is often fatal by < 1 year of age. Patients are characterized by:

- Microphthalmia
- Polydactyly
- Cleft lip/palate

IMPRINT DISORDERS

Imprinting occurs when identical genes are expressed differently, depending on which parent they are inherited from.

Prader-Willi and Angelman syndromes create two different phenotypes based on whether the paternal or the maternal portion of the same segment on chromosome 15 is deleted in the fetus.

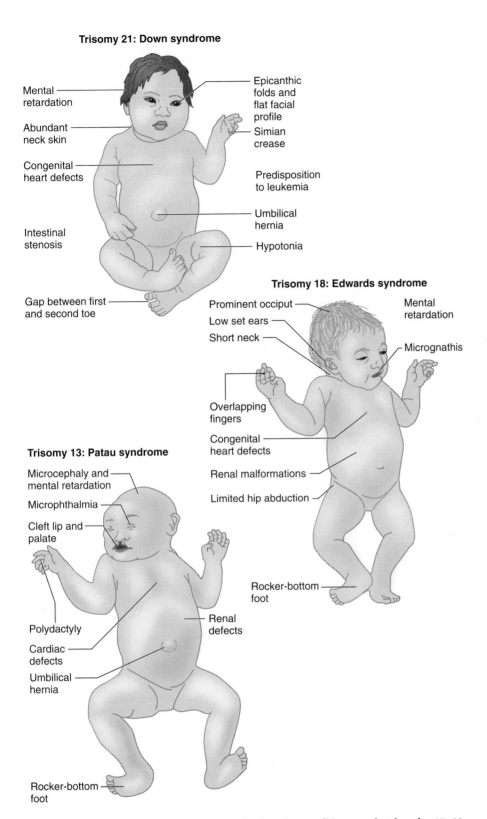

Trisomy 21: Down syndrome

Mental retardation

Abundant neck skin

Congenital heart defects

Intestinal stenosis

Gap between first and second toe

Epicanthic folds and flat facial profile

Simian crease

Predisposition to leukemia

Umbilical hernia

Hypotonia

Trisomy 18: Edwards syndrome

Prominent occiput

Low set ears

Short neck

Overlapping fingers

Congenital heart defects

Renal malformations

Limited hip abduction

Mental retardation

Micrognathis

Rocker-bottom foot

Trisomy 13: Patau syndrome

Microcephaly and mental retardation

Microphthalmia

Cleft lip and palate

Polydactyly

Cardiac defects

Umbilical hernia

Renal defects

Rocker-bottom foot

FIGURE 3-126. **Dysmorphic features and other abnormalities seen in trisomies 13, 18, and 21.**

Prader-Willi Syndrome

Occurs when a portion of the **paternal** chromosome 15 is deleted in the fetus:

- Neonatal hypotonia and failure to thrive
- Later childhood hyperphagia and obesity
- Mild mental retardation
- Aggressive/psychotic behavior
- Short stature, with small hands, feet, and gonads

Angelman Syndrome

Occurs when a portion of the **maternal** chromosome 15 is deleted in the fetus:

- Inappropriate laughter (also known as happy puppet syndrome)
- Jerky, flexed movements
- Microcephaly
- Minimal speech
- Severe mental retardation and seizures
- Sleep disturbance

Embryology

STAGES OF PRENATAL DEVELOPMENT

Human prenatal development is a complex process that allows a single cell to develop into an organism. The right cues must occur at the right time and in the right place to guide cellular proliferation, migration, differentiation and apoptosis. Development occurs in three main stages (Figure 4-1).

Germinal Stage (Weeks 0–2)

- Zygote formation
- Cell division
- Zygote attachment to the uterine wall

Embryonic Stage (Weeks 3–8)

- Organ formation
- Teratogen sensitivity

Fetal Stage (Week 9–Birth)

- Rapid fetal growth
- Sex organ formation
- Organ systems function

EMBRYOLOGY TERMS DECODER

Several key terms define the language of embryology and are instrumental to understanding the field (Table 4-1).

GAMETOGENESIS

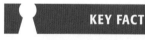

KEY FACT

Down syndrome (trisomy 21) is usually caused by a **nondisjunction** (failure of separation) during meiosis of the female gametes.

Meiosis

Prior to fertilization, the gametes that are going to fuse must undergo meiosis (Figure 4-2). During meiosis, the genetic information in diploid germ cells is ultimately halved ($2n \rightarrow n$). The genetic material is **initially doubled ($2n2\times$)** prior to the first meiotic division. Meiosis I separates homologous chromosomes producing **two haploid ($1n2\times$) daughter cells.** Each daughter cell then undergoes a second meiosis, in which sister chromatids are separated. This results in the production of **four haploid ($1n1\times$) daughter cells.** These haploid cells then fuse to produce a genetically unique offspring.

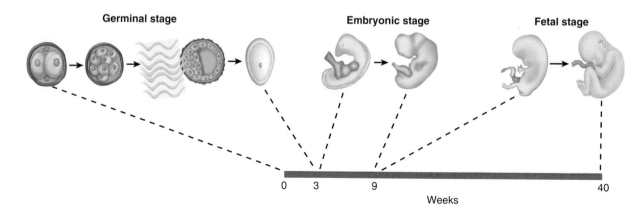

FIGURE 4-1. **Human prenatal development time line.** The germinal period (weeks 1 and 2) includes zygote formation and implantation. The embryonic period (weeks 3–8) includes organ formation. The fetal period (week 9 until birth) includes rapid growth and organ function.

TABLE 4-1.   **Embryology Vocabulary**

TERM	DEFINITION
Atresia	Blind pouch
Blast	Precursor cell
Caudal	Hind part, tail, posterior
Cephalic	Upper part, head
Coelom	Cavity
Cranial	Skull, head part, anterior
Dorsal	Back or top side
Ecto-	Outer
Endo-	Inner
Epi-	Above
Extraembryonic	Outside the embryonic body
Fistula	Abnormal connection
Gastrulation	Formation of the three germ layers
Hypo-	Below
Intraembryonic	Inside the embryonic body
Meso-	Middle
Mesenchyme	Any loosely organized tissue of fibroblast-like cells and extracellular matrix, regardless of the origin of the cells
Neurulation	Formation of the neural tube
Splanchnic	Belonging to the internal organs as opposed to its framework
Somatic	Belonging to the framework of the body rather than the internal organs
Ventral	Front, belly, or bottom side

Spermatogenesis

Just before **puberty,** the primordial sperm cells ($2n$) differentiate into **spermatogonia ($2n$)** (Figure 4-3) in the seminiferous tubules.

- **Type A spermatogonia:**
    - Stem cell population lining the basal compartment.
    - Produce progenitor type B spermatogonia.

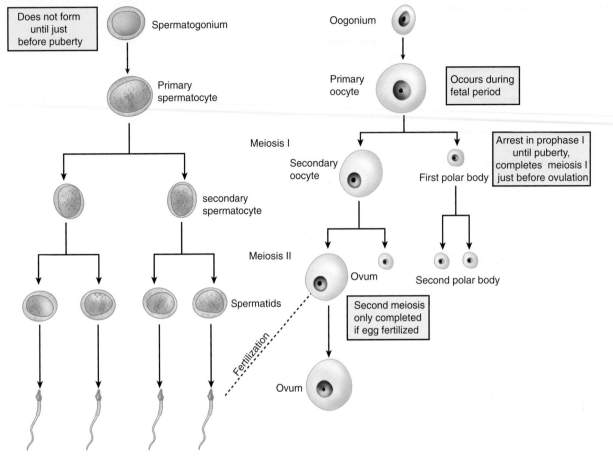

FIGURE 4-2. **Meiosis of male and female germ cells.** Gametogenesis begins with a doubling of the genetic information by mitosis. Subsequent meiosis results in halving of the DNA. This process takes place on a different timescale for male and female gametes.

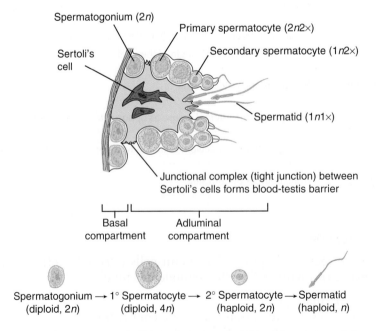

FIGURE 4-3. **Spermatogenesis.** Spermatogonia are produced from primordial germ cells just before puberty. Type A cells reside in the basal compartment and act as a stem cell population. As type B cells travel toward the testicular lumen, they continue to mature to the haploid spermatid state.

- **Type B spermatogonia:** Mature as they move toward the testicular lumen.
    - Mitosis → **primary spermatocytes ($2n2\times$).**
    - Meiosis after prolonged prophase → **secondary spermatocytes ($1n2\times$).**
    - Rapid second meiosis → **spermatids ($1n1\times$).**

The spermatids undergo several morphologic changes to form spermatozoa, including (Figure 4-4):

- **Cytoplasm reduction:** Discarded and phagocytosed by Sertoli cells.
- **Nuclear condensation.**
- **Flagellum formation:** Mitochondria pack tightly.
- **Acrosome formation:** Cap containing enzymes for penetration of the oocyte zona pellucida.

Components of a mature spermatozoon (Figure 4-4):

- **Head:** Nucleus covered by an acrosome and a cell membrane.
- **Neck:** Two centrioles + tightly packed mitochondria.
- **Tail:** A central pair of microtubules (**axoneme**) surrounded by nine doublets ($9 \times 2 + 2$).
    - Proximal: Axoneme + inner layer dense fibers + outer layer mitochondria.
    - Distal: Axoneme + dense fibers + outer fibrous sheath.
    - Terminal: Only axoneme.

Sertoli cells release spermatozoa into the lumen of the **seminiferous tubules,** which are connected to the rete testis. The **rete testis** is in turn connected to efferent ductules, which empty into the epididymis. In the **epididymis,** spermatozoa mature further and become motile.

Oogenesis

In contrast to spermatogenesis, primordial eggs differentiate into **oogonia ($2n$) during the fetal period** (Figure 4-5). By the end of the first trimester, after several mitotic divisions, the oogonia differentiate into **primary oocytes.** The primary oocytes replicate their DNA and **enter meiosis I ($2n2\times$),** but **arrest in prophase I until puberty.** After entry into meiosis I, further mitosis does not occur, and unlike in males, there is no stem cell system. Each primary oocyte becomes enveloped in a single layer of epithelial cells, which together form the **primordial follicle.** The follicle can develop through stages, but the primary oocyte remains dormant. After puberty, **a few primordial follicles begin to mature during each ovarian cycle,** but only one is ultimately released.

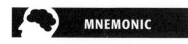
KEY FACT

Spermatogonia do not form until just before puberty and are then continually replenished by a resident stem cell.

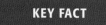
KEY FACT

The acrosome of the head is derived from the Golgi apparatus, the tail from a centriole, and the neck from mitochondria.

MNEMONIC

The neck, or **m**iddle part, of the sperm contains **m**itochondria.

KEY FACT

Oogonia form during fetal development (arresting in prophase I until puberty); there is no continual stem cell replenishment. The secondary oocyte, released into the fallopian tubes and fertilized by the sperm, is arrested in prophase II. The oocyte does not complete meiosis II until after fertilization.

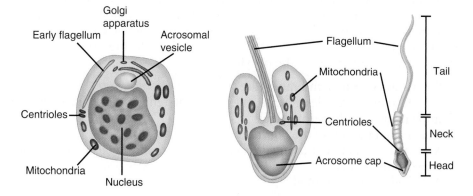

FIGURE 4-4.   Spermatid maturation. A fresh spermatid cell must undergo several morphologic changes on its way to becoming a mature sperm cell. These changes include cytoplasmic reduction, nuclear condensation, flagellum formation, and acrosome formation.

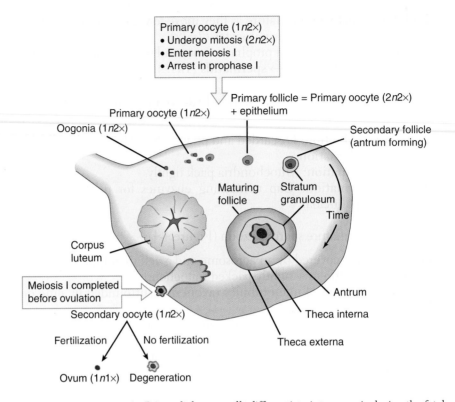

FIGURE 4-5. **Oogenesis.** Primordial germ cells differentiate into oogonia during the fetal stage. This maturation is arrested at the primary oocyte stage until puberty, although the surrounding follicle does continue to develop. Meiosis I is completed, creating a secondary oocyte just before ovulation. The secondary oocyte is arrested in prophase II when released.

>> **FLASH FORWARD**

Spermatogenesis and oogenesis are regulated by several crucial hormonal signals originating from both the endocrine and reproductive systems.

Prior to release, meiosis I is completed. Then a secondary oocyte ($1n2\times$) is released, which is arrested in prophase II. If the secondary oocyte is fertilized within 12–36 hours, it can escape degradation and complete meiosis II, forming the **ovum** ($1n1\times$).

EARLY LANDMARKS

Day 0: Fertilization

For the male and female gametes to fuse, they must first find their way to each other. Once introduced to the cervix, the **sperm traverses the hostile environment of the female genital tract to meet the secondary oocyte** in the fallopian tube at the infundibulum. During this journey, a maturation process called **capacitation** results in hyperactivity and activation of the sperm's acrosomal coat. When the sperm encounters the zona pellucida of the oocyte, the **acrosomal reaction** releases enzymes that degrade the zona pellucida. Once a single sperm reaches the oocyte:

- Sperm and oocyte membranes fuse.
- Oocyte cortex granules release enzymes that render the zona pellucida impenetrable (polyspermy block).
- The second meiosis of the oocyte is completed.
- Maternal and paternal pronuclei come together, and nuclear membranes between them dissolve.
- A diploid zygote is formed.

BLOCK TO POLYSPERMY

An oocyte is able to prevent multiple sperms from fertilizing it via both a fast and slow block to polyspermy.

- **Fast block to polysperm** occurs once one sperm has fused with the membrane of the oocyte, allowing Na^+ to enter the cell, depolarizing the oocyte and repelling other sperms.
- **Slow block to polysperm** is a cascade of events that occurs because Ca^{2+} has entered the cell, causing changes to the oocyte membrane, precluding other sperms from binding to receptors on the oocyte membrane.

Week 1: Cleavage and Implantation

CLEAVAGE

As the zygote travels through the fallopian tube, it rapidly divides. Cell division is occurring so quickly that each successive daughter cell is not accompanied by cell growth, therefore subdividing the larger zygote into smaller daughter cells (Figure 4-6).

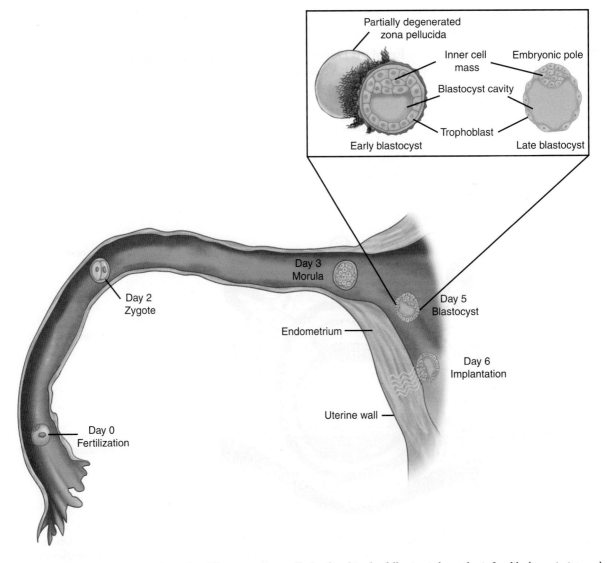

FIGURE 4-6. Fertilization to implantation. The oocyte is usually fertilized in the fallopian tube at the infundibulum. As it travels to the uterus, it goes through several maturational stages. While in the blastocyst stage, it "hatches" from the zona pellucida and implants in the uterine wall.

- **Morula:** 16- to 32-cell stages; resides at the cervical os.
- **Compaction:** Tight junction formation that leads to flattening and separation of the inner and outer blastomeres; a pole is formed.
- **Blastocoele:** Fluid pumped into the intercellular spaces of the morula.
- **Blastocyst:**
  - Free of the zona pellucida (hatching, "first birth").
  - Inner cell mass (**embryoblast,** embryonic stem cells).
  - Outer cell mass (**trophoblast**).

IMPLANTATION

The zygote attaches to and invades the endometrium, using the trophoblast cells over the embryoblast pole.

Week 2: "Week of Twos"

At this stage, the embryo has two germ layers (epiblast and hypoblast) surrounding two cavities (amniotic and yolk sac) (Figure 4-7).

TWO GERM LAYERS

The embryoblast organizes into two layers resembling a sandwich with only two slices of bread.

- **Epiblast:** Dorsal layer composed of high columnar cells.
- **Hypoblast:** Ventral layer composed of low cuboidal cells.

TWO CAVITIES

- **Amniotic cavity:** Dorsal to the epiblast, lined by proliferative edges of the epiblast.
- **Yolk sac:** Ventral to the hypoblast, lined by proliferative edges of the hypoblast.

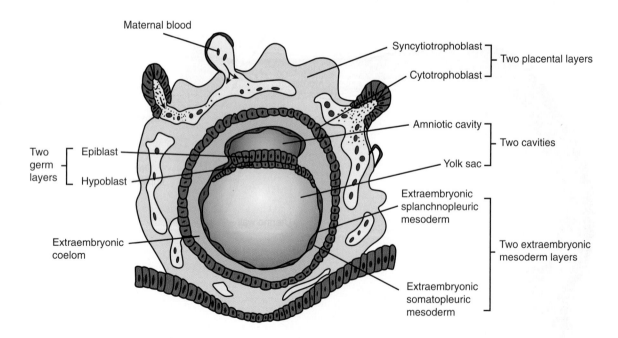

FIGURE 4-7. Second week of embryologic development. During the second week of embryologic development, there are two germ layers (epiblast and hypoblast), two cavities (amniotic cavity and yolk sac), two placental layers (syncytiotrophoblast and cytotrophoblast), and two extraembryonic mesoderm layers (splanchnopleuric and somatopleuric).

TWO PLACENTAL LAYERS

The trophoblast organizes into two layers:

- **Cytotrophoblast:** Inner proliferative layer that provides additional trophoblast cells.
- **Syncytiotrophoblast:** Thick outer layer without cell boundaries that invades the endometrium as the chorionic villi.

TWO EXTRAEMBRYONIC MESODERM LAYERS

Extraembryonic mesoderm, a **loose connective tissue layer,** forms between the cytotrophoblast and two cavities. During the second week, fluid-filled spaces appear, pushing aside the mesenchyme to **form a coelom,** or cavity (Figure 4-8). This **splits the mesoderm** into two layers that remain connected at the connecting stalk. The connecting stalk later contributes to the umbilical cord.

- **Splanchnopleuric:** Inner layer lining the yolk sac.
- **Somatopleuric:** Concentric layer lining the inner surface of the cytotrophoblast.

UTEROPLACENTAL CIRCULATION

The syncytiotrophoblast erodes the maternal vessels, forming **lacunae**—intervillous spaces—that allow for more efficient nutrient and gas exchange between the mother and embryo.

DECIDUAL REACTION

The cells of the decidua, the functional layer of the endometrium, enlarge. They accumulate lipid and glycogen to provide nourishment to the embryo until the placenta is vascularized.

Week 3: "Week of Threes"

THREE GERM LAYERS

During the process of **gastrulation,** the mesoderm fills in the middle of the bilaminar sandwich (Figures 4-8 and 4-9). Gastrulation begins with the forma-

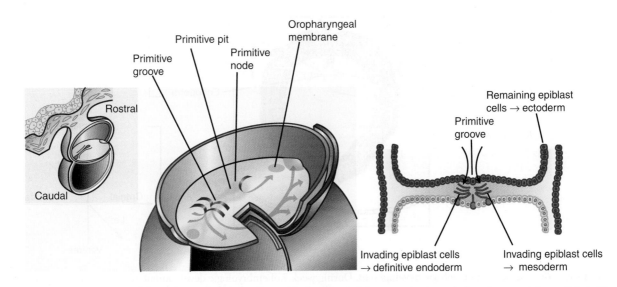

FIGURE 4-8.   Gastrulation. During gastrulation, epiblast cells detach, proliferate, and migrate below the remaining epiblast. The migrating cells displace the hypoblast, forming the endoderm, and fill in the space between the epiblast and hypoblast, forming the mesoderm. The remaining epiblast cells form the ectoderm.

tion of a groove and pit at the caudal end of the epiblast called the **primitive streak.** The pit and elevated cells around the cranial end constitute the **primitive node.** Cells proliferate from the streak and node, detach, and migrate beneath the remaining epiblast.

- **Ectoderm:** Remaining epiblast
- **Mesoderm:** New layer formed between old layers
- **Endoderm:** Original hypoblast displaced by the definitive endoderm

THREE CAVITIES

In addition to the yolk sac and amniotic cavity, the chorionic cavity is defined by complete separation of the mesoderm layers (Figure 4-9).

- **Chorionic:** Former extraembryonic coelom
- **Yolk sac**
- **Amniotic**

THREE PLACENTAL VILLI LAYERS

In addition to the two existing layers, the chorionic (extraembryonic) mesoderm invades the core (Figure 4-9).

- **Syncytiotrophoblast**
- **Cytotrophoblast**
- **Chorionic mesoderm**

THREE BODY AXES

- **Craniocaudal** (anteroposterior)
- **Dorsoventral**
- **Right-left**

NOTOCHORD AND NEURAL PLATE

The notochord is a **mesodermal derivative** that establishes the midline. It sends signals for **induction of the neural tube, somites, and other surrounding structures** (Figure 4-10).

> **KEY FACT**
>
> To visualize the process of notochord formation, picture a finger pressing into an inflated balloon while staying close to the surface.

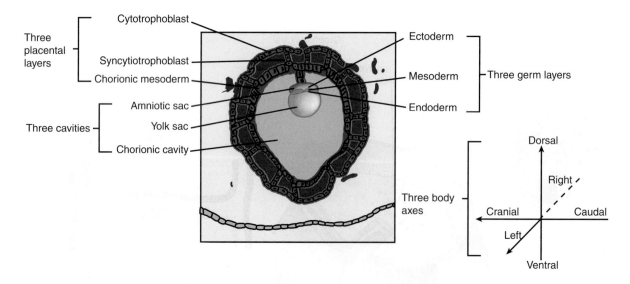

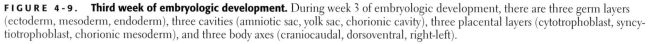

FIGURE 4-9. **Third week of embryologic development.** During week 3 of embryologic development, there are three germ layers (ectoderm, mesoderm, endoderm), three cavities (amniotic sac, yolk sac, chorionic cavity), three placental layers (cytotrophoblast, syncytiotrophoblast, chorionic mesoderm), and three body axes (craniocaudal, dorsoventral, right-left).

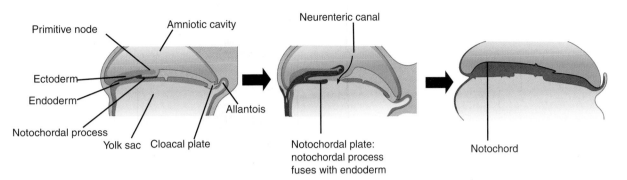

FIGURE 4-10. **Notochord development.** The notochord begins as an invagination of the mesoderm known as the notochordal process. This process then fuses with the endoderm, forming the notochordal plate. A portion of this plate degenerates, creating the neurenteric canal. Finally, a subset of the notochordal cells detaches from the endoderm, forming the definitive notochord.

- **Notochordal process:** Formed during gastrulation, when future notochord cells migrate through the primitive node.
- **Notochordal plate:** Formed when the chordal process fuses with underlying endoderm.
- **Neurenteric canal:** Formed when the floor of the chordal process and the fused endoderm degenerate, creating a temporary passage between the yolk sac and amniotic cavity.
- **Definitive notochord:** Formed when notochordal cells detach from the endoderm and reside in the middle of the mesoderm.
- **Neural plate:** Formed when the notochord induces a thickening of the ectoderm above it; this eventually forms the neural tube.

ALLANTOIS

The allantois, which is mostly vestigial in humans, begins as a diverticulum of the yolk sac at the posterior wall (Figure 4-10).

Weeks 3–8

During this time of rapid organ formation, the embryo is very fragile and susceptible to harmful teratogens.

ECTODERM

During week 3, the process of **neurulation** continues. The neural plate invaginates, forming the **neural groove** at the midline and **two neural folds** laterally (Figure 4-11). The plate rolls up like a tube fusing together at the midline. At the edges of these neural folds are the **neural crest cells. Neural tube** formation begins in the neck region, at the fourth somite, and proceeds in both cephalic and caudal directions, with the cephalic being completed first. The cephalic end dilates, forming the forebrain, midbrain, and hindbrain, and the rest of the neural tube forms the spinal cord.

As the neural folds elevate and join at the midline, cells at the neural crests differentiate, forming **neural crest cells** (Figure 4-11). When they reach their final destinations, they differentiate into numerous cell types, including spinal ganglia, melanocytes, and support cells of the nervous system. **Gut tube** formation is concurrently occurring ventrally, forming a **tube beneath a tube** held together by mesodermal glue.

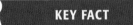

To visualize the process of neural tube formation, imagine a zipper starting in the middle and being pulled in both directions.

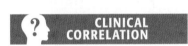

If the neural tube does not close completely, a variety of congenital **neural tube defects** can occur. A cranial defect results in **anencephaly,** and a defect along the spinal cord results in **spina bifida.**

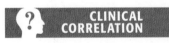

Neural crest cells migrate to become precursors of colonic ganglion cells. If this migration is incomplete, segments of the bowel cannot relax and a functional obstruction occurs. This disorder is known as **Hirschsprung disease.**

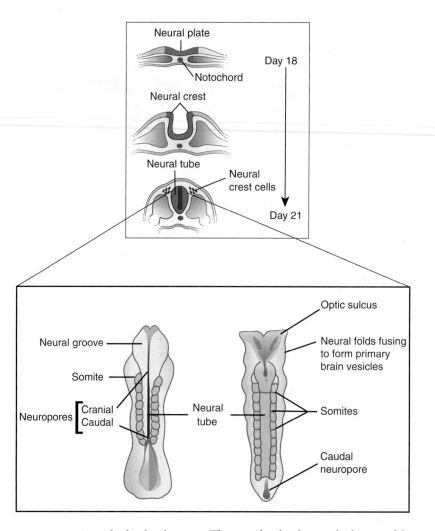

FIGURE 4-11. Neural tube development. The notochord induces a thickening of the ectoderm above it, known as the neural plate. This plate then rolls up to form the neural tube. The closing of the neural tube begins at the fourth somite and proceeds in both directions. A group of cells, the neural crest cells, migrate away from the tube and eventually form a variety of cell types, including spinal ganglia, melanocytes, and nervous system support cells.

MESODERM

While the neural and gut tubes are forming, the mesoderm proliferates and rearranges itself into **three distinct regions:** Paraxial, intermediate, and lateral.

The **paraxial mesoderm** forms paired, segmentally arranged columns on either side of the neural tube. These segments, called somites, divide into **sclerotomes, dermatomes,** and **myotomes** that give rise to bone/cartilage, dermis/subcutaneous, and skeletal muscles, respectively (Figures 4-11 and 4-12).

The **intermediate mesoderm** forms between the paraxial mesoderm and lateral mesoderm. Cranially, it arranges into segments of cell clusters that represent the future **nephrotomes** (Figure 4-12). In the lumbosacral region, an unsegmented mass of tissue known as the **nephrogenic cord** forms. These structures and their duct system contribute to the urogenital system.

The **lateral mesoderm** lies on the lateral edge of the embryo and is further divided by the intraembryonic coelom or cavity into **somatic or parietal** (wall), and **splanchnic or visceral** (organ). Vacuoles begin to form in the lat-

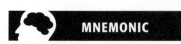

MNEMONIC

Mesoderm segment locations—

Paraxial mesoderm: Lies **next to (para)** the neural tube (axis).
Intermediate mesoderm: Lies **between (intermediate)** the other mesoderm segments.
Lateral mesoderm: Lies **lateral** to the other mesoderm segments.

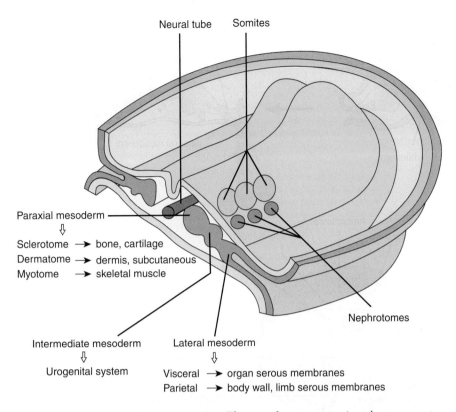

Neural tube   Somites

Paraxial mesoderm ⟶

Sclerotome ⟶ bone, cartilage
Dermatome ⟶ dermis, subcutaneous
Myotome ⟶ skeletal muscle

Nephrotomes

Intermediate mesoderm   Lateral mesoderm
⇩   ⇩
Urogenital system   Visceral ⟶ organ serous membranes
                           Parietal ⟶ body wall, limb serous membranes

FIGURE 4-12. Mesoderm segmentation. The mesoderm separates into three segments. Paraxial mesoderm lies alongside the neural tube and gives rise to sclerotomes, dermatomes, and myotomes. Intermediate mesoderm lies lateral to the paraxial mesoderm and forms the urogenital system. Lateral mesoderm lies lateral to the intermediate mesoderm and forms the serous membrane lining of organ systems, limbs, and the body wall.

eral mesoderm and ultimately fuse, creating a ∪-shaped cavity, the **intraembryonic coelom** (Figure 4-13). The outer parietal or somatic mesoderm layer form the serous membrane lining of the body wall, anterior abdominal wall, and limbs. The inner visceral or splanchnic mesoderm layer forms the serous membrane lining of the gut, pericardial, pleural, and peritoneal cavities and the smooth muscles and connective tissue components of the organs it lines.

ENDODERM

The endoderm forms the primitive **gut tube**—the future respiratory and digestive systems—via cephalocaudal and lateral folds of the embryonic disk. The folding is similar to pulling the strings on a cinched sac and leaves the embryonic disk in the traditional "fetal position." This folding is driven by rapid longitudinal growth of the central nervous system, creating caudal and cephalic bending known as the **head and tail folds.** The head fold brings the cardiogenic region cephalic to the brain. As the sac is cinched and folds in, part of the yolk sac is pinched off and is drawn into the embryo, becoming the **foregut** and **midgut,** and the allantois contributes to the **hindgut** (Figure 4-14).

Other Landmarks

WEEKS 3–4

- Body system appears in rudimentary form
- Heart beats
- Upper and lower limb buds form

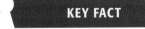

KEY FACT

Gut tube + neural tube = tube on top of a tube held together with mesodermal glue.

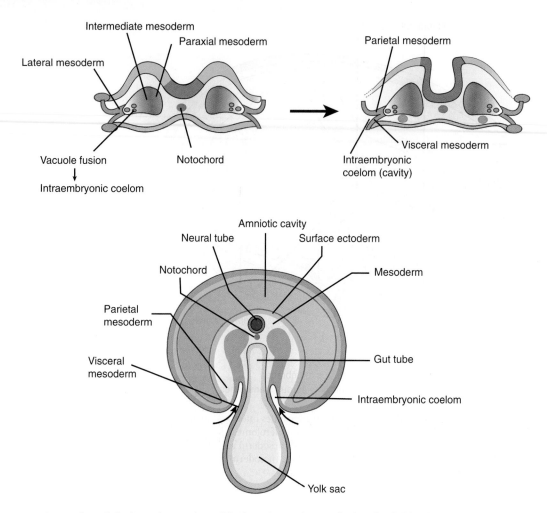

FIGURE 4-13. **Separation of the lateral mesoderm.** The lateral mesoderm is further divided by the formation of the intraembryonic coelom into parietal and visceral mesoderm. The outer parietal mesoderm forms the serous membrane lining of the body wall and limbs. The inner visceral mesoderm remains invested around the gut tube and forms the serous membrane lining of the gut and the pericardial, pleural, and peritoneal cavities.

WEEKS 4–5

- Muscle and cartilage formation begins
- Cardiac septa form and atrioventricular cushions fuse
- Craniofacial development begins

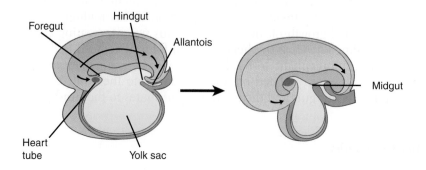

FIGURE 4-14. **Endodermal gastrulation.** The gut tube is formed by "cinching" the embryo with a combination of cephalocaudal and lateral folds. The yolk sac contributes to the formation of the foregut and midgut, and the allantois contributes to the hindgut.

WEEK 10

Genitalia have male or female characteristics.

FETAL MEMBRANES AND PLACENTA

The placenta supplies nutrients to and removes waste from the embryo via interaction with the maternal circulation.

Placenta

The **chorion** constitutes the **fetal contribution to the placenta** and includes the somatic extraembryonic mesoderm, cytotrophoblast, and syncytiotrophoblast. The **syncytiotrophoblast** invades and erodes maternal tissue and vessels, forming tissue lacunae, which fill with maternal blood. **Placental villi,** the exchange units, begin to form in stages.

- **Primary villi:** Syncytiotrophoblast covering + cytotrophoblast core.
- **Secondary villi:** Primary villi + invasion of the extraembryonic mesoderm at the core.
- **Tertiary villi:** Secondary villi + vessel formation in the extraembryonic mesoderm core.

On the maternal side, a **cytotrophoblastic shell** develops as the cytotrophoblast grows through the villi and connects with the cytotrophoblast of the adjacent villi (Figure 4-15). On the embryonic side, the extraembryonic mesoderm remains connected at its base, known as the **chorionic plate.** Extension of the villi from the chorionic plate to the cytotrophoblastic shell anchors the placenta to the uterus. The epithelial lining of the endometrium that participates in this anchoring is known as the **deciduas basalis.** As the heart develops, circulation is established in the placenta. The cytotrophoblast layer of the villi degenerates, thinning the wall and facilitating diffusion.

Similar to the polarization of the fetus, the placenta also becomes polarized, resulting in portions of the chorion and decidua becoming distinct (Figure 4-16).

- **Chorion frondosum:** Villi on the embryonic side grow and differentiate.
- **Chorion laeve:** Villi on the nonembryonic side degenerate, leaving this part of the chorion smooth.

> **CLINICAL CORRELATION**
>
> In **placenta previa,** the placenta implants in the lower part of the uterus, covering the cervix and effectively blocking entrance to the vagina. When this occurs, cesarean section is the preferred mode of delivery. In **placenta accreta,** the placenta is more deeply attached to the uterus, reaching the middle layer, or myometrium. This causes complications during birth in which bleeding becomes difficult to stop, and a hysterectomy may be required.

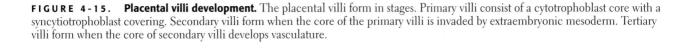

Endometrium (decidual plate)
Maternal vessels
Intervillous space
Syncytiotrophoblast
Cytotrophoblast
Extraembryonic mesoderm

Primary villi

Secondary villi
= primary villi + invasion extraembryonic mesoderm

Maternal side
Outer cytotraphoblast shell
Chorionic arteries and venis
Chorionic plate
Fetal side

Tertiary villi
= secondary villi + core vessel formation

FIGURE 4-15. Placental villi development. The placental villi form in stages. Primary villi consist of a cytotrophoblast core with a syncytiotrophoblast covering. Secondary villi form when the core of the primary villi is invaded by extraembryonic mesoderm. Tertiary villi form when the core of secondary villi develops vasculature.

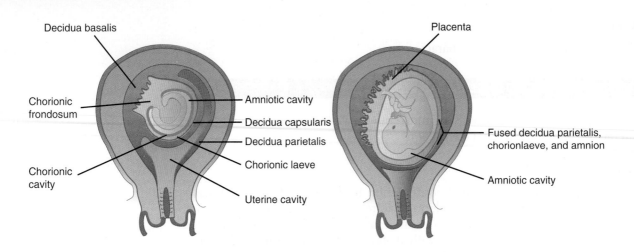

FIGURE 4-16. **Placenta polarization and cavity development.** As the embryo grows, the placenta becomes polarized, with different segments of the chorion and decidua developing different characteristics. These layers eventually degenerate and fuse, leaving one large amniotic cavity.

- **Decidua basalis:** Over the embryonic pole, the chorion frondosum adheres tightly, forming an anchoring decidual plate.
- **Decidua capsularis:** The decidual layer covering the embryonic side.
- **Decidua parietalis:** The decidua covering the remaining uterus.

As the fetus grows, the decidua capsularis contacts the decidua parietalis on the opposite uterine wall and degenerates. The underlying chorion laeve can then fuse directly with the decidua parietalis. As amniotic fluid fills the amniotic cavity, the amnion contacts the chorion laeve and also fuses, leaving one large amniotic cavity.

In the fourth month, the decidual plate begins to separate groups of villi into compartments called **cotyledons** by forming septa, or walls (Figure 4-17). The

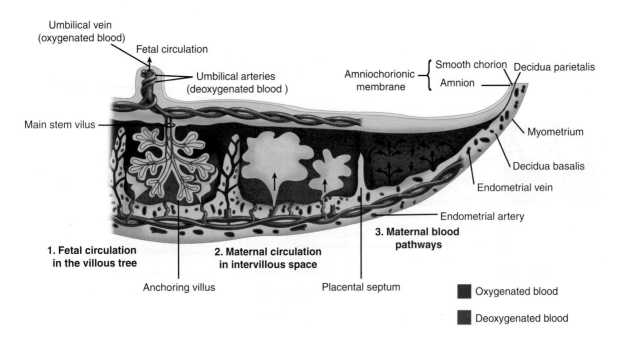

FIGURE 4-17. **Placental flow.** As the placenta matures, it separates the villi into communicating compartments. As oxygenated maternal blood enters these compartments, via spiral arteries, it has access to all of the compartments. The now deoxygenated maternal blood is returned to the circulation via endometrial veins. Deoxygenated fetal blood enters the placenta via two umbilical arteries, and oxygenated blood is returned via the umbilical vein.

septa grow toward but do not contact the chorionic plate, allowing maternal blood from the spiral arteries to flow between compartments. Maternal blood is subsequently drained by endometrial veins. Deoxygenated fetal blood is brought to the chorionic villi by two umbilical arteries, and oxygenated blood is returned by the umbilical vein. There is **no mixing of the maternal and fetal blood,** just an exchange of nutrients, gases, antibodies, and small molecules. The placenta is also responsible for producing hormones, such as progesterone, estrogen, and human chorionic gonadotropin.

Yolk Sac

The yolk sac functions as a **transfer agent for nutrients** from the trophoblast to the embryo (2–3 weeks), as a **source of primordial germ cells,** and as a **source of blood cells and vessels** that connect to the vitelline arteries and veins. The dorsal part of the yolk sac connects to the primitive gut and forms the epithelial linings and glands of the respiratory and digestive systems and the bladder, urethra, and lower vaginal canal in the female. The yolk sac is connected to the midgut via the **vitelline duct.** The body stalk with the vitelline duct and the umbilical vessels form the umbilical cord (Figure 4-18).

Allantois

The allantois is used in some animals for removal of nitrogenous waste. However, humans have a well-developed chorionic placenta that removes waste through the maternal circulation, thus the allantois is mostly vestigial. It does, however, **provide vessels for the establishment of the definitive placenta and forms the umbilical blood vessels.** Beginning as an outpouching from the yolk sac, it **forms the hindgut** (Figure 4-18). It also becomes incorporated into the umbilical cord and persists from the urinary bladder to the umbilicus as the **urachus.** After birth, the urachus becomes a fibrous cord known as the **median umbilical ligament.**

Amnion

The amnion is a **thin nonvascular membrane** derived from the epiblast. It **lines the fluid-filled amniotic cavity** that cushions the embryo. The fluid filling of the cavity is initially derived from the maternal blood, but is later derived from fetal urine. The fluid is rapidly turned over as the fetus swallows

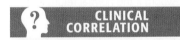

Mothers who lack the Rh antigen (Rh⁻) on the surface of their blood cells can develop an **Rh antibody** during pregnancy with a child who has the antigen (Rh⁺). Any subsequent Rh⁺ children are attacked by this maternal antibody, and **anemia, congestive heart failure,** and even **fetal death** may occur. Initial antibody development can be prevented with the delivery of **Rh immunoglobulin** to a mother immediately after birth.

CLINICAL CORRELATION

Meckel's diverticulum is a congenital outpouching in the small intestine and is a remnant of the **vitelline duct.** This uncommon malformation manifests in approximately 2% of the population, tends to be 2 inches long, and is found 2 feet from the ileocecal valve. When infected it can be mistaken for appendicitis.

CLINICAL CORRELATION

Amniotic fluid also contains cells that are sloughed from the fetus, placenta, and amniotic sac. This allows amniotic fluid sampling, or **amniocentesis,** to be used for karyotyping of the fetus. This procedure is usually performed after 15 weeks of gestation. Chorionic villus sampling can give similar results at an earlier gestational age (8 weeks) for higher risk mothers.

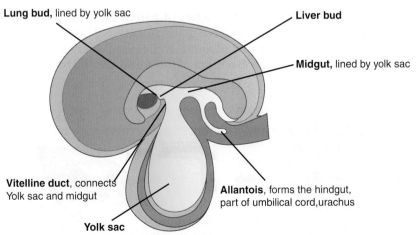

FIGURE 4-18. Yolk sac and allantois. The yolk sac connects to the primitive gut via the vitelline duct and forms the epithelial linings of the respiratory and digestive systems. The allantois contributes to the hindgut, part of the umbilical cord, and the urachus.

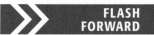

KEY FACT

A single umbilical artery is associated with congenital and chromosomal anomalies.

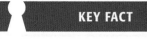

FLASH FORWARD

Physiologic intestinal herniation through the umbilical cord is a normal part of the development of the GI tract between five to ten weeks of gestation. It can present as **umbilical herniation** in the newborn if the normal return into the abdomen fails to occur.

KEY FACT

The **urachus** is part of the **allantoic duct** between the bladder and the umbilicus.

it and passes it via the placenta to the maternal blood for waste removal. In the fifth month, the fluid is swallowed and returned via the GI tract.

Umbilical Cord

The umbilical cord connects the embryonic circulation to the placenta. As the amniotic cavity is filled, the body stalk and yolk sac become incorporated into the umbilical cord. Initially, the umbilical cord is composed of:

- Vitelline vessels
- Umbilical vessels
- Allantois
- Chorionic cavity remnants
- Body stalk mesenchyme (Wharton's jelly)
- Intestinal loops (physiologic hernia)

Wharton's jelly is a gelatinous substance that contains no nerves and is a rich source for stem cells. As the umbilical cord develops, the vitelline vessels, allantois, yolk sac, and chorionic cavity remnants degrade and the intestinal loops are pulled back into the abdominal cavity. The cord ultimately consists of (Figure 4-19):

- Umbilical vessels: Two arteries (return deoxygenated blood) and one vein (supplies oxygenated blood to the growing fetus)
- Wharton's jelly
- Allantoic duct: Removes nitrogenous waste

EMBRYOLOGIC DERIVATIVES

Germ Layer Derivatives

As mentioned previously, the three embryonic germ layers form distinct subsets of adult tissue (Table 4-2).

Fetal-Postnatal Derivatives

Some embryonic structures persist in the adult, mostly as anatomic markers (Table 4-3).

Aortic Arch Derivatives

At the beginning of the fifth week, a **series of paired arteries and veins** supply the head, body, yolk sac, and developing placenta. The head and body are specifically supplied by a pair of aortic and carotid arteries that form on either side of the pharynx as an extension of the **aortic sac** (Figure 4-20, Table

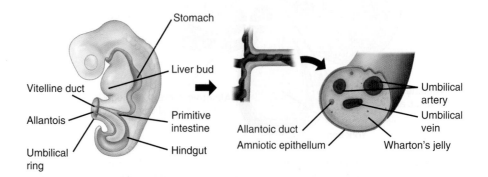

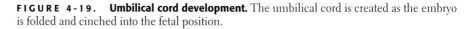

FIGURE 4-19. **Umbilical cord development.** The umbilical cord is created as the embryo is folded and cinched into the fetal position.

TABLE 4-2. Germ Layer Derivatives

GERM LAYER	DERIVATIVE
Ectoderm	
Surface ectoderm	▪ Adenohypophysis (anterior pituitary) ▪ Sensory epithelium: Nose, ear, eye ▪ Lens of eye ▪ Epidermis, hair, nails
Neuroectoderm	▪ Neurohypophysis (posterior pituitary) ▪ CNS neurons ▪ Oligodendrocytes ▪ Astrocytes ▪ Ependymal cells (glia) ▪ Pineal gland
Neural crest	▪ Autonomic nervous system ▪ Dorsal root ganglia ▪ Cranial nerves ▪ Melanocytes ▪ Chromaffin cells of adrenal medulla ▪ Enterochromaffin cells ▪ Pia and arachnoid ▪ Celiac ganglion, autonomic ganglia ▪ Schwann cells ▪ Odontoblasts ▪ Parafollicular (C) cells of thyroid ▪ Laryngeal cartilage ▪ Bones of face, jaw, and ossicles of ear
Mesoderm	
Paraxial	▪ Bones of skull ▪ Muscles ▪ Vertebrae ▪ Dura mater ▪ Connective tissue ▪ Bone
Intermediate	▪ Urogenital system ▪ Spleen
Lateral	Serous membranes around organs
Splanchnic/visceral	▪ Serous membranes and smooth muscles and connective tissue of viscera
Somatic/parietal	▪ Body wall ▪ Limbs
Endoderm	
	▪ Gut tube epithelium and glands ▪ Gut tube derivatives (lungs, liver, pancreas, thymus, parathyroid, thyroid follicular cells, gallbladder).

CNS = central nervous system.

TABLE 4-3. **Fetal-Postnatal Derivatives**

FETAL STRUCTURE	POSTNATAL DERIVATIVE
Umbilical vein	Ligamentum teres hepatic
Umbilical arteries	Medial umbilical ligament
Ductus arteriosus	Ligamentum arteriosum
Ductus venosus	Ligamentum venosum
Foramen ovale	Fossa ovalis
AllaNtois-urachus	MediaN umbilical ligament
Notochord	Nucleus pulposus of the intervertebral disk
Inferior epigastric artery, vein	Lateral umbilical ligament

MNEMONIC

Pharyngeal apparatus—

CAP covers outside from inside:

Clefts = ectoderm
Arches = mesoderm
Pouches = endoderm

4-4). The *aortic* arches appear in cranial to caudal order, and each travels through the center of a *pharyngeal* arch. During the fifth week, the vessels **fuse, sprout, and regress** to form the adult vascular system.

Pharyngeal (Branchial) Apparatus

Lower head and neck development begins with the appearance of the pharyngeal apparatus. This apparatus is composed of **clefts, arches,** and **pouches.**

The clefts are an external lining derived from ectoderm. The arches are a mesenchyme derived from mesoderm and neural crest cells. The pouches are an internal lining derived from endoderm (Figure 4-21).

Pharyngeal Arches

The mesenchymal core of the pharyngeal arches form the **bone and musculature of the face and neck** (Figure 4-22). The cranial nerves (CNs) present

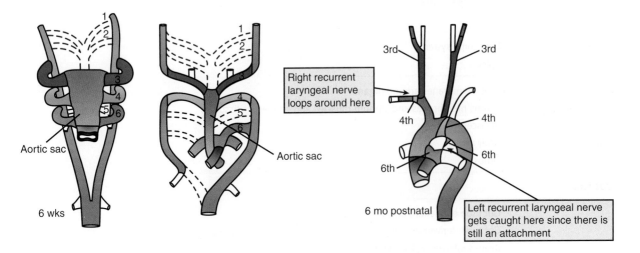

FIGURE 4-20. Aortic arch development. To develop the adult vascular system, the rudimentary paired arteries and veins fuse, sprout, and regress. This causes the right recurrent laryngeal nerve to get caught under the right subclavian artery, whereas the left recurrent laryngeal nerve is trapped under the ligamentum arteriosum.

TABLE 4-4. Aortic Arch Derivatives

ARCH	FATE	MNEMONIC
First	Part of **MAX**illary.	First arch is **MAX**imal.
Second	**S**tapedial artery, hyoid artery.	**S**econd = **s**tapedial.
Third	Common **C**arotid artery, proximal part of the internal carotid artery.	**C** is the third letter of the alphabet.
Fourth	Left = aortic arch; Right = proximal part of the right subclavian artery.	Fourth arch (four limbs) = systemic.
Fifth	(Fails to form).	
Sixth	Proximal part of pulmonary arteries; left only = ductus arteriosus.	Sixth arch = pulmonary and the pulmonary-to-systemic shunt (ductus arteriosus).

in the core of each arch innervate the structures that are derived from that arch (Table 4-5).

Pharyngeal Clefts and Pouches

The linings of the pharyngeal arches give rise to **epithelial linings, glandular structures,** and **cavities** (Figure 4-23, Table 4-6).

TONGUE DEVELOPMENT

The **anterior two thirds** of the tongue is derived from the **first pharyngeal arch** (Figure 4-24). Accordingly, its sensation is derived from V3 and its taste from cranial nerve (CN) VII. The **posterior one third** of the tongue is derived from the **third and fourth pharyngeal arches.** Accordingly, its sensation is derived from CN IX and the extreme posterior from CN X. All motor innervation for the tongue is derived from CN XII.

> **CLINICAL CORRELATION**
>
> **DiGeorge syndrome** is a congenital immunodeficiency resulting from aberrant development of the third and fourth pharyngeal pouches. The syndrome is marked by **T-cell deficiency** (thymic aplasia) and **hypocalcemia** (failure of parathyroid development).

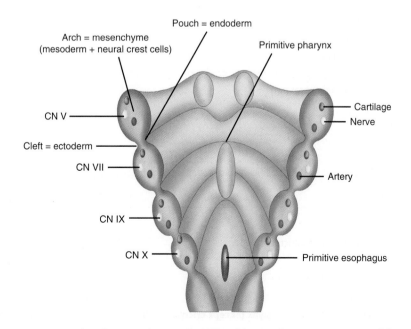

FIGURE 4-21. The pharyngeal apparatus. The pharyngeal apparatus consists of the outer pharyngeal clefts, the core pharyngeal arches, and the inner pharyngeal pouches.

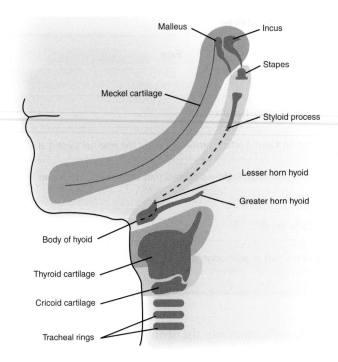

Malleus
Incus
Stapes
Meckel cartilage
Styloid process
Lesser horn hyoid
Greater horn hyoid
Body of hyoid
Thyroid cartilage
Cricoid cartilage
Tracheal rings

FIGURE 4-22. **The pharyngeal arch bone derivatives.** The pharyngeal arches contribute to the bone and musculature of the face.

TABLE 4-5. **Derivatives of the Pharyngeal Arches**

ARCH	CARTILAGE	MUSCLE	NERVE
1	Meckel • **M**andible • **M**alleus • Incus • Spheno **M**andibular ligament	• **M**uscles of **M**astication • Te**M**poralis • **M**asseter • Lateral pterygoid • **M**edial pterygoid • **M**ylohyoid • Anterior belly digastric • Tensor tympani • Tensor veli palatini	CN V$_3$
2	Reichert • **S**tapes • **S**tyloid process • Lesser horn of the hyoid • **S**tylohyoid ligament	• Muscles of facial expression • **S**tapedius • **S**tylohyoid • Posterior belly digastric	CN VII
3	Greater horn of the hyoid	Stylopharyngeus	CN IX
4–6	• Thyroid • Cricoid • Arytenoids • Corniculate • Cuneiform	From fourth arch • Most pharyngeal constrictors • Cricothyroid • Levator veli palatini From sixth arch • All intrinsic muscles of the larynx **(except cricothyroid)**	Fourth = CN X Sixth = CN X (recurrent laryngeal branch)

CN = cranial nerve.

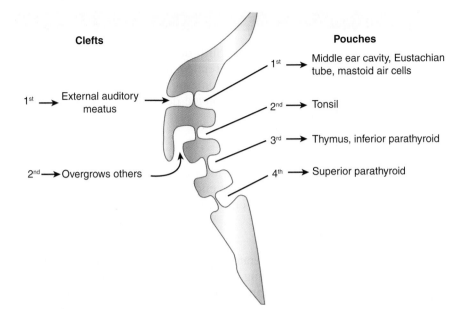

FIGURE 4-23. **The pharyngeal cleft and pouch derivatives.**

TABLE 4-6. **Pharyngeal Cleft and Pouch Derivatives**

ARCH	CLEFT DERIVATIVES	POUCH DERIVATIVES
1	External auditory meatus.	▪ Middle ear cavity. ▪ Eustachian tube. ▪ Mastoid air cells.
2		Epithelial lining of the palatine tonsil.
3	Temporary cervical sinuses obliterated by proliferation of the second arch mesenchyme.	▪ Dorsal wings → inferior parathyroids. ▪ Ventral wings → thymus.
4		Superior parathyroids.

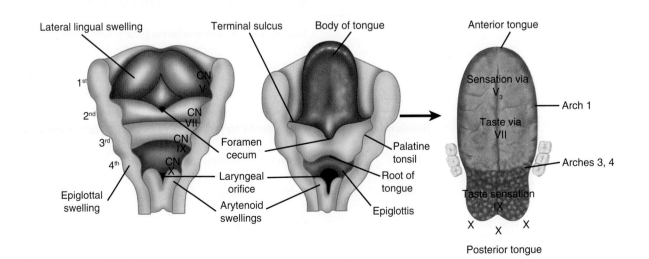

FIGURE 4-24. **Tongue development.** As the tongue develops from the pharyngeal arches, its taste and sensation are derived from the cranial nerves innervating the corresponding arches.

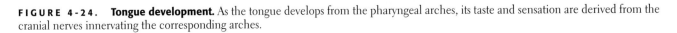

TERATOGENS

A teratogen is any agent that can cause birth defects following fetal exposure during a critical period of development. Teratogens include infectious agents, drugs, nutritional factors, chemicals, and ionizing radiation (Table 4-7). There are three different periods during embryologic development during which a fetus may be exposed to a teratogen:

"All or None" Period (Weeks 1–3)

In early embryogenesis, the fetus either dies due to cellular injury induced by the teratogen or survives unaffected if enough undifferentiated embryonic cells remain to replace the damaged or destroyed cells.

Embryonic Period (Weeks 3–8)

The fetus is most susceptible to teratogens because organ systems and body regions are being established during this period. Teratogen exposure during this period generally results in **organ malformation.** Each organ system develops at different times and at different rates; therefore, each organ system has different periods of susceptibility to various insults.

Fetal Period (Weeks 9–38)

The fetus has a decreased susceptibility to teratogens at this time because all organs have already been formed. Teratogen exposure during this period generally results in **organ malfunction** or growth disturbances.

Fetal infections can also cause congenital malformations.

KEY FACT

Weeks 3–8: Organs begin to form.

TABLE 4-7. Examples of Teratogens

TERATOGEN	EFFECTS ON FETUS
Alcohol	Birth defects and mental retardation (leading cause), fetal alcohol syndrome.
ACE inhibitors	Renal damage.
Cocaine	Abnormal fetal development and fetal addiction.
DES	Vaginal clear cell adenocarcinoma (occurs later in life).
Iodide	Congenital goiter or hypothyroidism.
13-*cis*-Retinoic acid	Extremely high risk of birth defects.
Thalidomide	Limb defects ("flipper" limbs), cardiovascular defects, ear defects.
Tobacco	Preterm labor, placental problems, ADHD.
Warfarin	Multiple anomalies.
X-rays	Multiple anomalies.

ACE = angiotensin-converting enzyme, ADHD = attention deficit/hyperactivity disorder; DES = diethylstilbestrol.

TWINNING

Dizygotic (Fraternal) Twins

Dizygotic twins are formed when **two different sperm** fertilize **two different secondary oocytes** (Figure 4-25). This produces two separate zygotes, which form two separate blastocysts. These unique blastocysts implant into the endometrium of the uterus independently and eventually form **two distinct placentas, chorions,** and **amniotic sacs.** The end result is two siblings that are genetically distinct, just like siblings born at two different times.

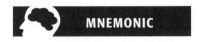

MNEMONIC

Dizygotic is **D**ifferent.

Monozygotic (Identical) Twins

Monozygotic twins are formed when **one sperm** fertilizes **one secondary oocyte.** This produces one zygote, which forms one blastocyst. Instead of the single blastocyst forming a single fetus, however, the inner cell mass splits into two, resulting in the formation of two genetically identical siblings. Monozygotic twins most commonly develop a **single placenta and chorion** and two separate amniotic sacs (65% of the time), but may also develop two separate placentas, chorions, or share an amniotic sac.

Conjoined (Siamese) Twins

Conjoined twins are considered monozygotic twins in whom the inner cell mass never fully separated. The two embryos are genetically identical and remain fused by a tissue bridge of variable proportions at birth.

In Vitro Fertilization (IVF)

IVF of oocytes and the subsequent transfer of cleaving embryos into the uterus is an assisted reproductive technology that includes several steps:

- Gonadotropins are given to the female to stimulate growth and maturity of the ovarian follicles.
- Maturing oocytes are monitored via ultrasound, and oocytes are collected from the ovary via needle aspiration.

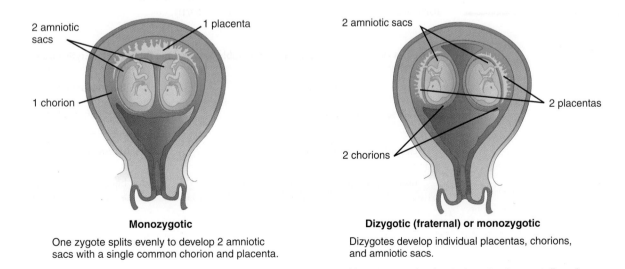

Monozygotic

One zygote splits evenly to develop 2 amniotic sacs with a single common chorion and placenta.

Dizygotic (fraternal) or monozygotic

Dizygotes develop individual placentas, chorions, and amniotic sacs.

Monozygotes develop 2 placentas (separate/fused), chorions. and amniotic sacs.

FIGURE 4-25.   Twinning.

- Sperm is collected via masturbation.
- In vitro culture of capacitated sperm and secondary oocytes is performed in a specialized medium to allow fertilization to occur.
- Once fertilization occurs, the zygote (an oocyte that has been fertilized) undergoes two to three rounds of cell division to become a 4- to 8-cell totipotent blastocyst.
- The cleaved embryo or blastocyst is then implanted into the uterus. (Typically, three or more blastocysts are implanted to increase the chances of success.)
- The remaining blastocysts are frozen for safekeeping for future use if needed or desired.

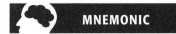

MNEMONIC

Young Liver Synthesizes The Blood:

Yolk sac (3–8 weeks)
Liver (6–30 weeks)
Spleen and **T**hymus (9–28 weeks)
Bone marrow (28 weeks onward)

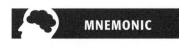

MNEMONIC

Fetal **F**ights (with the mother for O$_2$).

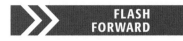

FLASH FORWARD

Thalassemia syndromes are disorders characterized by defects in either the α-globin (α-thalassemia) or β-globin (β-thalassemia) chain of hemoglobin.

FETAL ERYTHROPOIESIS

Erythropoiesis begins in the **third week of development,** when blood islands appear in the **mesoderm** around the wall of the yolk sac. Within the center of the blood islands are hemangioblasts, the pluripotent hematopoietic stem cells that will form all future blood cells. Although the first blood cells arise in the yolk sac, this site of blood formation is only temporary. By the fifth week, intraembryonic hematopoiesis begins to take place in different organs in a sequential manner:

1. Yolk sac (3–8 weeks)
2. Liver (6–30 weeks)
3. Spleen and thymus (9–28 weeks)
4. Bone marrow (28 weeks onward)

Hemoglobin

Three types of hemoglobin, corresponding to the organ involved in production, are synthesized during fetal erythropoiesis (Table 4-8). Fetal hemoglobin ($\alpha_2\gamma_2$) is the primary form during gestation because it has a higher affinity for O$_2$ than the adult form ($\alpha_2\beta_2$) and is therefore able to "steal" O$_2$ from maternal blood for fetal use. The switch between the fetal and adult forms occurs gradually, beginning at 30 weeks' gestation, and ultimately results in the fetal form being entirely replaced by the adult form.

TABLE 4-8. Timing of Various Hemoglobin Expressions During Fetal Erythropoiesis

PERIOD	HEMOGLOBIN TYPE
Yolk sac (3–8 weeks)	Embryonic hemoglobin = $\delta_2\varepsilon_2$
Liver period (6–30 weeks)	Fetal hemoglobin = $\alpha_2\gamma_2$
Bone marrow period (28 weeks onward)	Adult hemoglobin = $\alpha_2\beta_2$

Microbiology

Bacteriology

BACTERIAL STRUCTURES

Prokaryotic organisms exhibit several structural components (Figure 5-1).

Cytoplasmic Structures

Eukaryotes and prokaryotes differ in their cytoplasmic structures (Table 5-1). Bacteria carry the following intracellular components:

- **Bacterial chromosome:** Circular, double-stranded, and contained within the nucleoid.
- **Plasmids:** Smaller extrachromosomal DNA, often containing important genes, such as those that confer resistance to antibiotics.
- **Bacterial ribosome:** Consists of 30S and 50S subunits that form a 70S ribosome. Coupled in bacterial transcription and translation.

Bacterial Cell Walls

With the exception of **Mycoplasma,** which has **no cell walls,** the cell walls of bacteria are composed of layers of **peptidoglycan** that surround their cytoplasmic membranes (Figure 5-1). Important functions of the cell wall include:

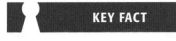

KEY FACT

Because bacterial ribosomes and RNA polymerases differ from those in humans, they are ideal targets for antibiotics.

KEY FACT

Mycoplasmas do not have cell walls and therefore cannot be seen with Gram stain.

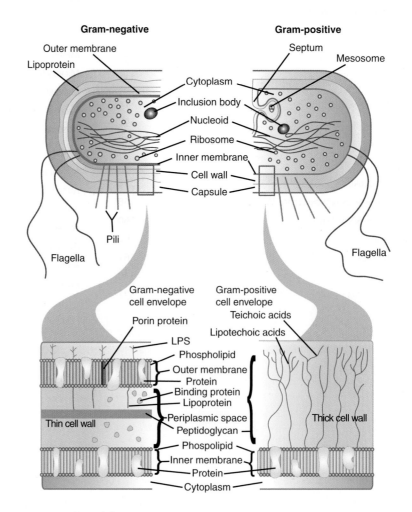

FIGURE 5-1. Bacterial structures.

TABLE 5-1. **Eukaryotic Versus Prokaryotic Cytoplasmic Structures**

CYTOPLASMIC STRUCTURES	EUKARYOTE	PROKARYOTE
Nucleus	Nuclear membrane present	Nuclear membrane absent
Chromosomes	Linear, diploid DNA	Circular, haploid DNA
Ribosome	80S (60S + 40S)	70S (50S + 30S)
Cell membrane	Contains sterols	No sterols[a]
Mitochondria	Present	Absent
Golgi bodies	Present	Absent
Endoplasmic reticulum	Present	Absent
Respiration	Via mitochondria	Via cell membrane

[a]Mycoplasmas are an exception, as they incorporate sterols.

- Resisting osmotic stress.
- Serving as a primer for its own synthesis, which is necessary for cell division.
- Defining the shape of the bacteria; **coccus, bacillus** (*Staphylococcus, Vibrio*), **spirillum** (spirochete).
- Providing some protection from innate immune responses in humans.

Peptidoglycan synthesis occurs in several steps:

- **Glucosamine** is converted into N-acetylmuramic acid (MurNAc) and activated by UTP (uridine triphosphate) to UDP (uridine diphosphate)-MurNAc.
- A UDP-MurNAc-pentapeptide precursor is assembled.
- The UDP-MurNAc pentapeptide is attached to bactoprenol in the cytoplasmic membrane.
- N-acetylglucosamine (GlcNAc) is added to make a disaccharide.
- The bactoprenol translocates the disaccharide: **Peptide precursor** to the outside of the cell.
- The GlcNac-MurNac disaccharide is attached to a peptidoglycan chain by a transglycosylase.
- The pyrophosphobactoprenol is converted back to a phosphobactoprenol and recycled.
- Peptide chains from adjacent glycan chains are cross-linked to each other by **transpeptidation.**

External Bacterial Structures

There are several external bacterial structures of interest (Figure 5-1):

- **Bacterial capsules** are usually composed of **glycocalyx,** with the exception of *Bacillus anthracis* (polypeptide capsule).
- Important virulence factor. Capsules help to resist opsonization and phagocytosis.

> **KEY FACT**
>
> **Encapsulated bacteria:**
> *Streptococcus pneumoniae,*
> *Klebsiella pneumoniae,*
> *Haemophilus influenzae, Neisseria*
> *meningitidis, Salmonella, Group B*
> *Strep*
>
> **S**ome
> **K**illers
> **H**ave
> **N**ice
> **S**hiny
> **B**odies

Fimbriae adhering to other bacteria = F (sex) pili; transfer bacterial chromosomes to each other.

Fimbriae adhering to the **host cell** (adhesion) = bacterial virulence factor.

For example, fimbriae account for the virulence of *Escherichia coli* (in urinary tract infections [UTIs]) and of *Neisseria* (in gonorrhea).

- **Biofilms** are bacterial communities that can protect bacteria from antibiotics and host immune defenses.
- **Flagella** are **coiled protein subunits (flagellin)** anchored in bacterial membranes. They provide bacterial motility and express **antigenic (H antigen)** and **strain determinants** useful for serotyping bacteria.
- **Fimbriae** are hair-like structures on the outside of bacteria, composed of repeating subunits of the protein **pilin.** Fimbriae often promote **adherence** to other bacteria or to host cells.

Bacterial cell walls differ between gram-positive and gram-negative bacteria (Figure 5-1 and Tables 5-2 and 5-3):

- **Gram-positive bacteria:** Thick cell wall, composed of many layers of **peptidoglycan.** The linkage between one layer of peptidoglycan and another (via the third and fourth amino acids of glucosamine pentapeptide) is further extended by a pentaglycine bridge, whereas gram-negative bacteria link their pentapeptide changes directly. Without peptidoglycan, the bacteria would lyse due to the differential in osmotic pressure across the cytoplasmic membrane. Gram-positive bacteria are also associated with **teichoic** and **lipoteichoic acids,** useful in distinguishing bacterial serotypes, promoting bacterial interactions with human cell receptors, and initiating host immune responses.
- **Gram-negative bacteria:** Consist of both a **peptidoglycan layer,** making up only 5–10% of the cell wall, and **an outer membrane.**

TABLE 5-2. **Gram-Positive and Gram-Negative Bacterial Membrane Structures**

GRAM-POSITIVE		**GRAM-NEGATIVE**	
STRUCTURE	**CHEMICAL CONSTITUENTS**	**STRUCTURE**	**CHEMICAL CONSTITUENTS**
Peptidoglycan	Chains of GlcNAc and MurNAc peptide bridges cross-linked by pentaglycine chains.	Peptidoglycan	Thinner version of that found in gram-positive bacteria with direct peptide bridging and no pentaglycine chains.
Teichoic acid	Glycerol phosphate or polyribitol phosphate cross-linked to peptidoglycan.	**Periplasmic space**	Enzymes involved in transport, degradation, and synthesis.
Lipoteichoic acid	Lipid-linked teichoic acid.	**Outer membrane**	Fatty acids and phospholipids.
Proteins	Porins, transport proteins.	Proteins	Porins, lipoprotein, transport proteins.
Plasma membrane	Phospholipids, proteins, and enzymes involved in generation of energy, membrane potential and transport.	Plasma membrane	Same as gram-positive bacteria.
Capsule	Disaccharides, trisaccharides, and polypeptides.	Capsule	Polysaccharides and polypeptides.
Pili	Pilin, adhesions.	Pili	Pilin, adhesions.
Flagellum	Flagellin, motor proteins.	Flagellum	Flagellin, motor proteins.
		Lipopolysaccharide (LPS)	Core polysaccharide, O antigen, lipid A.

TABLE 5-3. Summary of Gram-Positive and Gram-Negative Bacteria

Membrane Characteristic	Gram-Positive	Gram-Negative
Outer membrane	–	+
Cell wall	Thick	Thin
Lipopolysaccharide (endotoxin)	–	+
Exotoxin	Some	Some
Teichoic acid	Often present	–
Sporulation	Some strains	–
Capsule	Sometimes present	Sometimes present
Lysozyme	Sensitive	Resistant

- **Periplasmic space:** Area between the cytoplasmic membrane and the outer membrane. Contains **enzymes** necessary for metabolism and **virulence factors,** such as proteases, phosphatases, lipases, nucleases, collagenases, hyaluronidases, and β-lactamases.
- There is no teichoic or lipoteichoic acid in gram-negative bacteria.
- Gram-negative bacteria contain **lipopolysaccharide (LPS-endotoxin),** used for serotyping gram-negative bacteria. LPS is a potent activator of immune cells and stimulates release of major pyrogenic substances such as **interleukin-1 (IL-1), IL-6,** and **tumor necrosis factor (TNF),** the major cytokine responsible for shock.

> **KEY FACT**
>
> *Neisseria* contains a shorter version of LPS called lipo-oligosaccharide (LOS).

BACTERIAL GROWTH AND METABOLISM

Bacterial Growth and Death

The **minimum requirements** for bacterial growth are a source of carbon and nitrogen, an energy source, water, and various ions. When these conditions are met, bacteria must also obtain or synthesize the **amino acids, carbohydrates,** and **lipids** necessary for building proteins, structures, and membranes. A cascade of regulatory events then initiates **DNA synthesis,** which then runs to completion.

Bacterial growth occurs in **four phases** (Figure 5-2):

- **Lag phase:** Gathering of necessary growth requirements, no divisions occur during this phase.
- **Log phase** (or **exponential phase**): Growth and cell division begins. The doubling time varies among different strains and conditions.
- **Stationary phase:** Depicts the point at which bacteria run out of metabolites and toxic (metabolic) products start building up, ultimately causing cessation of bacterial growth. This is the phase where sporulation occurs.
- **Decline phase:** Death of bacterial cells after stationary phase.

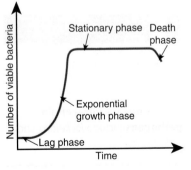

FIGURE 5-2. **Bacterial growth curve.** Depicted are lag phase, exponential growth phase, and stationary phase.

Bacterial growth is assessed in three ways: Viable cell counts, optical density, and metabolic products.

- **Viable cell counts** (colony-forming units—CFU/mL).
- **Optical density** (spectrophotometry).
- **Indirect measurement** of bacterial numbers by detection of metabolic by-products (CO_2).

Bacterial growth is **controlled** by subjecting bacterial populations to heat, antimicrobial chemicals, and antibiotics (see following discussion).

Key mechanisms of bacterial growth control include (Table 5-4):

- Alteration of membrane permeability.
- Denaturation of proteins.
- Interference with DNA replication—alkylating agents.
- Oxidation.

Bacterial Metabolism

Major **essential elements** necessary for bacterial metabolism include carbon, hydrogen, nitrogen, sulfur, phosphorus, potassium, magnesium, calcium, iron, sodium, chloride, and O_2.

Bacterial needs for O_2 can be divided into four groups:

- **Obligate (or strict) anaerobes:** Cannot grow in the presence of O_2.
- **Facultative anaerobes:** Can grow either in the presence or absence of O_2.
- **Obligate (or strict) aerobes:** Require molecular O_2.
- **Microaerophilic:** Require very low levels of O_2 for growth.

A **carbon source** is required by all bacteria. Genera can be differentiated based on the type of carbon they use (ie, **lactose, glucose,** and **galactose**).

Bacteria can produce energy via aerobic respiration, anaerobic respiration, or fermentation.

- **Aerobic respiration:** Completely converts glucose into CO_2 and H_2O and forms adenosine triphosphate (ATP) through **substrate level** and **oxidative phosphorylation.**
- **Anaerobic respiration:** ATP is also formed through substrate level phosphorylation; however, other high-energy molecules such as SO_4^{2-} and NO_3^- are used as the terminal electron acceptors rather than O_2. Anaerobic respiration produces slightly less ATP than aerobic respiration, but is more efficient than fermentation.
- **Fermentation:** In the absence of O_2 and following substrate level phosphorylation, certain bacteria are able to ferment pyruvic acid. The **end products** of this process are two- and three-carbon compounds. These organic molecules act in lieu of O_2 as **electron acceptors** to recycle the **reduced form of nicotinamide adenine dinucleotide (NADH) to nicotinamide adenine dinucleotide (NAD).**

The end products of fermentation can also be used to distinguish particular bacteria.

KEY FACT

Not all bacteria require O_2 for survival and replication.

MNEMONIC

Obligate aerobes: Nagging Pests Must Breathe—

Nocardia
Pseudomonas
Mycobacterium tuberculosis
Bacillus

Obligate anaerobes: Can't Breathe Air—

Clostridium
Bacteroides
Actinomyces

KEY FACT

Some bacteria are incapable of generating their own ATP and must dwell inside host cells that can. These **obligate intracellular pathogens** include *Rickettsia* and *Chlamydia.*

TABLE 5-4. **Methods of Controlling Bacterial Growth**

METHOD	ACTIVITY LEVEL, MECHANISM	SPECTRUM
Heat		
Steam autoclave 121°C for 15 min	Sterilizing, membrane-active, protein denaturant.	All bacterial growth phases, viruses, fungi. Spores can only be destroyed by autoclaving.
Boiling	Highly effective, membrane-active, protein denaturant.	Most growth phases, some spores, viruses, fungi.
Pasteurization	Intermediate, membrane-active, protein denaturant.	Vegetative cells.
Dry heat	High, membrane-active, protein denaturant.	All bacterial growth phases, viruses, fungi.
Chemical		
Ethylene oxide gas	Sterilizing, alkylating agent.	All bacterial growth phases, viruses, fungi.
Sodium hypochlorite (bleach)	High, oxidizing agent.	*Clostridium difficile.*
Alcohol	Intermediate, membrane-active, protein denaturant.	Vegetative cells, some viruses, fungi.
Hydrogen peroxide	High, membrane-active, oxidizing agent.	Vegetative cells, viruses, fungi.
Chlorine	High, oxidizing agent.	Vegetative cells, viruses, fungi.
Iodine compounds	Intermediate, iodination, oxidation.	Vegetative cells, viruses, fungi.
Phenolics, phenol, hexachlorophene, chlorhexidine	Intermediate, membrane-active.	Vegetative cells, some viruses, fungi.
Glutaraldehyde	High, alkylating agent.	Vegetative cells, viruses.
Formaldehyde	High, alkylating agent.	Bacteria, viruses, fungi.
Quaternary ammonium compounds	Low, membrane-active, cations.	Bacteria, viruses, fungi.
Radiation		
Ultraviolet	Sterilizing.	Bacteria, viruses, fungi.
Ionizing	Sterilizing.	Bacteria, viruses, fungi.
Physical		
Filtration	High, size exclusion.	Bacteria, fungi, some viruses.

Bacterial Genetics

The bacterial **genome** consists of the single **haploid chromosome** of the bacteria in addition to extrachromosomal genetic elements (**plasmids** and **bacteriophages**). These elements may be independent of the bacterial chromosome and, in most cases, can be transmitted from one cell to another.

Exchange of genetic material between bacterial cells can occur via three mechanisms:

- **Conjugation** (Figure 5-3): **One-way transfer of DNA** from a donor cell to a recipient cell through the sex (**F**) pilus. Conjugation typically occurs between members of the same species or related species. The transfer of DNA gives the recipient bacterium the ability to function as a viable donor itself.
    - The **donor bacterium** must carry the **F plasmid** (**F⁺, male**) and the other must not (**F⁻, female**). The F plasmid carries all the genes necessary for its own transfer.
    - Integration of the F plasmid into chromosomal DNA results in the **HFR** (high-frequency recombination) **state**. This allows the donor to transfer whole pieces of the chromosome into the recipient bacteria.
    - If the F plasmid sequence is excised from the host chromosome, it may take some genes from the chromosome with it. This plasmid is called the **F′** (F prime). Like F⁺, the prime plasmid can be transferred to an F⁻ recipient and transfer the host gene along with it. The conjugative R plasmid confers antibiotic resistance.
- **Transformation:** Bacteria take up **fragments of naked DNA** and **incorporate** them into their genomes if the recipient chromosome is sufficiently

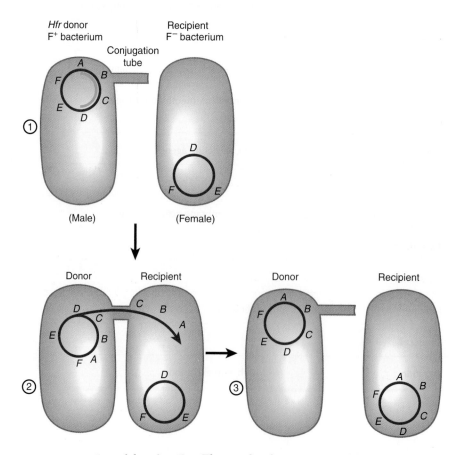

FIGURE 5-3.   Bacterial conjugation. The transfer of genetic material from a donor bacterium to a recipient bacterium through contact is conjugation.

homologous for **recombination** to occur. The new genetic material obtained by the recipient cannot be passed down to progeny. Certain species of bacteria such as *H influenzae*, *S pneumoniae*, *Bacillus* species, and *Neisseria* species are capable of taking up exogenous DNA.

■ **Transduction:** Genetic transfer mediated by bacterial viruses (**bacteriophages**). This is a very efficient way for bacteria to pass genetic information such as antibiotic resistance. There are two forms of transduction:

■ Generalized: A "packaging" event. **Lytic** phage infects bacterium, leading to cleavage of bacterial DNA and synthesis of viral proteins. Parts of bacterial chromosomal DNA may become packaged in viral capsid. Phage infects another bacterium, transferring these genes.

■ Specialized: An "excision" event. **Lysogenic** phage infects bacterium; viral DNA is incorporated into bacterial chromosome. When phage DNA is excised, flanking bacterial genes may be excised with it. DNA is packaged into phage viral capsid and can infect another bacterium.

Bacterial Defenses—Pathogenic Factors

Bacteria have multiple defensive **virulence factors** that protect themselves from the human immune system while also enabling them to enter the host and promote disease. A few of these factors include capsules (explained above), spores, toxins, proteases, hemolysins, coagulase, and catalase (Table 5-5).

SPORE

The spore is a dehydrated, multicelled structure that allows bacteria to survive when nutrients are limited. The spores are composed of:

■ Inner membrane
■ Two peptidoglycan layers
■ Outer protein coat

MNEMONIC

Genes for toxins that are acquired via specialized transduction (lysogenic phage)—

ABCDE

Shig**A**-like toxin
Botulinum toxin (certain strains)
Cholera toxin
Diphtheria toxin
Erythrogenic toxin of *Streptococcus pyogenes*

KEY FACT

Only certain **gram-positive rods** can form spores. Examples include *Clostridium* species and *B anthracis*.

TABLE 5-5. Defensive Virulence Factors

DEFENSE MECHANISMS	SPECIES OF BACTERIA
Spores	*Clostridium tetani*, *C botulinum*, or *C difficile*, *Bacillus anthracis*
IgA proteases	*S pneumoniae*, *Neisseria meningitidis*, *N gonorrhoeae*, *H influenza*
Cellular invasion	*Rickettsia* and *Chlamydia*, *Salmonella*, *Shigella*, *Brucella*, *Mycobacterium*, *Listeria*, *Francisella*, *Legionella*, *Yersinia*
Hemolysis	*Streptococcus pneumoniae*, *Streptococcus pyogenes*, *Streptococcus agalactiae*, *Staphylococcus aureus*, *Listeria monocytogenes*, *Enterococcus*
Catalase	*Staphylococcus*, *Micrococcus*, *Listeria*
Coagulase	*S aureus*
Toxins	*Streptococcus pyogenes*, *S aureus*, *Clostridium diphtheriae*, *Pseudomonas aeruginosa*, *Shigella dysenteriae*, *E coli*, *V cholerae*, *Bordetella pertussis*, *C difficile*, *Clostridium perfringens*, *Clostridium tetani*, *C botulinum*

The complete copy of the bacterium's chromosome, as well as the essential proteins and ribosomes necessary for germination, are confined within the spore. A spore can survive for decades, protecting bacterial DNA from heat, radiation, enzymes, and chemical agents (eg, most disinfectants).

PIGMENT PRODUCTION

Pigment is often useful in the identification of particular bacteria. Three important pigment-producing bacteria are *S aureus* (yellow), *P aeruginosa* (blue-green), and *Serratia marcescens* (red).

IgA PROTEASES

Streptococcus pneumoniae, N *meningitidis*, N *gonorrhoeae*, and H *influenzae* carry IgA proteases. These proteases cleave immunoglobulin A (IgA), which is found on mucosal surfaces and functions as a first line of defense against pathogens. Cleavage by the proteases prevents opsonization of these bacteria, thus allowing bacteria to enter unnoticed by the host's immune system.

CELLULAR INVASION

Some bacteria are able to live and replicate intracellularly to avoid the host's immune system. There are **obligate** and **facultative** intracellular bacteria.

HEMOLYSIS

Hemolysis is the breakdown of red blood cells in culture by hemolytic enzymes. Hemolysis is useful in categorizing types of streptococci. **Three types** of hemolysis are identified (Figure 5-4):

- α-**Hemolysis** results in greenish darkening of the blood agar. The green color change of the agar is caused by peroxide produced by the bacteria, not hemolysin, and therefore α-hemolysis is often referred to as **partial hemolysis** (*S pneumoniae*) (Figure 5-5).
- β-**Hemolysis** results in complete clearing of the blood agar (complete hemolysis by hemolysin) (*S pyogenes*) (Figure 5-5).
- γ-**Hemolysis** designates no hemolysis (there is no change to the blood agar) (*Enterococcus*).

KEY FACT

Obligate intracellular bacteria: *Rickettsia* and *Chlamydia*.
Facultative intracellular bacteria: *Salmonella, Shigella, Brucella, Mycobacterium, Listeria, Francisella, Legionella,* and *Yersinia*.

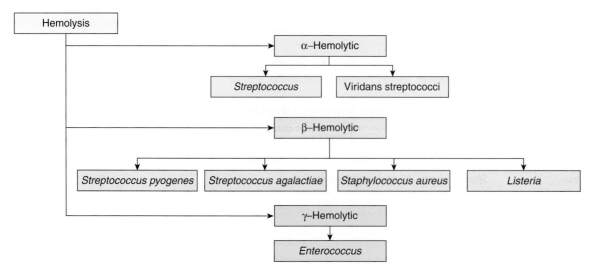

FIGURE 5-4. **Types of hemolysis.** Note that many other organisms besides enterococci are nonhemolytic, whereas enterococci can also be β, α, or γ.

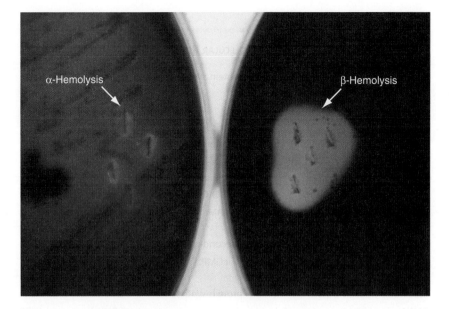

FIGURE 5-5. **Alpha hemolysis and beta hemolysis on blood agar.** (Image courtesy of CDC's Public Health Image Library; content provider Dr. Richard R. Facklam.)

CATALASES

Catalases are enzymes that catabolize hydrogen peroxide (H_2O_2) into water and O_2. The presence or absence of catalase can be used to categorize gram-positive cocci.

COAGULASE

This enzyme is used to **distinguish** *S aureus* (the most common species of staphylococci found in humans that produces the enzyme coagulase) from other forms of staphylococci (*S epidermidis*).

> **KEY FACT**
>
> In plasma, coagulase binds to serum factor and coverts fibrinogen to fibrin, forming a clot.

TOXINS

Three major types of toxins exist: endotoxin, exotoxin, and enterotoxin.

- **Endotoxin,** or lipopolysaccharide (**LPS**), is found in the outer cell membrane of gram-negative bacteria and can cause fever and shock.
- **Exotoxins** are **polypeptides** secreted by bacteria that cause harm to the host by altering cellular structure or function. Exotoxins are very potent and a very low dose may be lethal to the host.
- **Enterotoxins** are toxins that act on the gut.

Through the following **seven major mechanisms of action** (Table 5-6), toxins:

1. **Facilitate spread through tissues:** Enzymes break down the extracellular matrix or degrade cellular debris in necrotic tissue.
2. **Damage membranes:** Cytolysins, pore-forming toxins cause death of the host cell.
3. **Stimulate production of excessive amounts of cytokines:** Superantigens bind to a site distinct from the antigen-binding site on the T-cell receptor, stimulating excess synthesis of cytokines, such as IL-2 and interferon gamma (IFN-γ).

TABLE 5-6. Bacterial Toxicity in Brief

Microorganism	Toxin Type	Mechanism	Molecular Result	Clinical Result
Corynebacterium diphtheriae	Diphtheria toxin.	Inactivates EF-2 via ADP–ribosyltransferases.	Inhibits protein synthesis.	Upper respiratory tract infection. Sore throat. Low fever.
P aeruginosa	Exotoxin A.	Inactivates EF-2 via ADP–ribosyltransferases.	Inhibits protein synthesis.	Urinary tract infection.
E coli	Heat-labile (LT) enterotoxin (ETEC).	Activates adenylate cyclase via ADP ribosylation of *Gs*.	Activates second-messenger pathway ↑ cAMP.	Secretory diarrhea.
	Heat-stabile (ST) enterotoxin (ETEC).	Activates guanylate cyclase.	Activates second-messenger pathway ↑ cGMP.	Secretory diarrhea.
	Shiga toxins, (eg, EHEC strain O157:H7).	Inactivates ribosome via RNA N-glycosidase.	Inhibits protein synthesis.	Abdominal pain, fever. Bloody, mucoid, WBCs in stools. Reiter symptoms. Toxin binds to Gb3 receptor on glomerular epithelial cells. Swelling and fibrin deposits in glomerulus.
Shigella dysenteriae	Shiga toxin.	Inactivate ribosome via RNA N-glycosidase by binding 60S ribosome.	Inhibits protein synthesis.	
V cholerae	Cholera toxin.	Activates adenylate cyclase via ADP ribosylation of *Gs*.	Activates second-messenger pathway ↑ cAMP. Cl (–) out Na (+) in	Hypersecretory diarrhea with great loss of fluid and electrolytes.
	Heat-labile (LT) enterotoxin.			
B pertussis	Pertussis toxin.	Activates adenylate cyclase via ADP ribosylation of *Gi*.	Activates second-messenger pathway ↑ cAMP.	↑ Secretion in upper respiratory tract. Other tissue effects.
Clostridium tetani	Tetanus toxin.	Blocks release of glycine and GABA from inhibitory neurons.	Zinc-dependent proteases cleave VAMP.	Uncontrolled muscle spasms. Spastic paralysis.
C botulinum	Botulinum toxin (A, B, E).	Blocks release of acetylcholine at neuromuscular junctions.	Zinc-dependent proteases cleave VAMP.	Flaccid paralysis.
Bacillus anthracis	Anthrax toxin factor.	Calmodulin-dependent calcium activation.	Activates second-messenger pathway ↑ cAMP.	Edema, lethal.

GABA = γ-aminobutyric acid; VAMP = vessel-associated membrane protein.

4. **Inhibit protein synthesis:**
   - **Diphtheria toxin** and **P aeruginosa exotoxin A** are ADP ribosyltransferases, which ribosylate and inactivate eukaryotic elongation factor 2 (EF-2), resulting in the cessation of protein synthesis.
   - **Shiga toxins** of **Shigella dysenteriae** and **Escherichia coli** are highly specific RNA N-glycosidases that remove one particular residue from the 28S RNA, thereby inactivating the ribosomes and halting protein synthesis.

5. **Activate second-messenger pathways:** Exert hormone-like effects on the target cell, thus altering cell function without killing the cell.
   - **Heat-labile enterotoxins** *Vibrio cholerae* and *E coli* are ADP ribosyltransferases that activate cell membrane–associated adenylate cyclase, thus activating **stimulatory (Gs) proteins.**
   - **Pertussis toxin (A and B components)** is an ADP ribosyltransferase that activates cell membrane–associated adenylate cyclase by ADP ribosylating the **inhibitory (G_i) protein** of the cyclase complex. Pertussis toxin can increase intracellular cyclic adenosine monophosphate (cAMP) in many different target tissues, causing tissue-specific effects such as hypoglycemia (islet cell activation), ↑ histamine sensitivity, and inhibition of immune effector cells.
   - **Heat-stable enterotoxin I of E coli** activates cell membrane–associated guanylate cyclase. Increased intracellular cGMP in enterocytes causes secretory diarrhea.
   - **Anthrax edema factor** is an adenylate cyclase toxin similar to that of *B pertussis*. Toxins enter target cells, increase intracellular cAMP, and produce cAMP-dependent effects. Their enzymatic activity is activated by **calmodulin**-dependent **calcium activation** in target cells.

6. **Inhibit release of neurotransmitters:** Botulinum and tetanus toxins.
   - **Botulinum toxin** causes **flaccid paralysis** by inhibiting the release of **acetylcholine** (ACh) at myoneural junctions. The toxin targets the SNAP25 fusion protein, preventing neurotransmitter-filled vesicles from fusing to the membrane and releasing ACh.
   - **Tetanus toxin** inhibits the release of neurotransmitters (**glycine and GABA**) from **inhibitory** interneurons in the spinal cord, resulting in stimulation of muscular contraction and tetany (**spastic paralysis**).

7. **Modify the cytoskeleton** of the target cell by glucosylating RhoA (a small GTP-binding protein), causing disaggregation of actin filaments. This results in the formation of pseudomembranes in the colon (eg, *C difficile* **cytotoxin B**).

MICROBIOLOGIC STAINS

The microscopic examination and subsequent identification of microorganisms are greatly aided by the use of stains, which generate artificial contrast so the organism can be visualized. Bacteriologic specimens are always subjected to one or more **differential stains,** which aid in identification by permitting visualization of certain characteristic cellular substructures. Further biochemical tests are used to precisely identify the organism.

Staining Methods

Bacteria can be seen microscopically via:

- **Direct examination:** Performed by suspending bacteria in liquid (sometimes called a **wet mount**). This is useful for detecting motility, for distin-

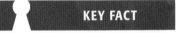

KEY FACT

Superantigens: Scarlet fever toxin of *Streptococcus pyogenes,* toxic shock syndrome toxin (TSST) of *S aureus,* and *Staphylococcus* enterotoxins.

KEY FACT

Toxins that inhibit protein synthesis: Diphtheria toxin, exotoxin A of *P aeruginosa,* Shiga toxins of *S dysenteriae,* and *E coli.*

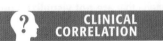

CLINICAL CORRELATION

Increased cAMP in enterocytes causes secretory diarrhea.

KEY FACT

Toxins that activate second-messenger systems: Edema factor of *B anthracis,* adenylate cyclase toxin and pertussis toxins of *B pertussis,* heat-stable enterotoxin and heat-labile toxin of *E coli,* heat-labile toxin of *V cholerae.*

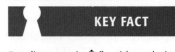
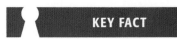
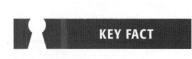
guishing larger organisms (eg, yeasts and parasites) from bacteria, and for visualizing *Treponema pallidum*, using darkfield microscopy.

- **Acid-fast stains** include **Ziehl-Neelsen, Kinyoun,** and **auramine-rhodamine.** They are used to stain the bacteria only if pretreated with acid-alkali solutions because the bacteria resist decolorization. Acid-fast staining is particularly useful in identifying **mycobacteria.** However, other acid-fast organisms include *Nocardia, Rhodococcus, Cryptosporidium, Isospora,* and *Cyclospora.*
- **Fluorescent stains** include acridine orange, auramine-rhodamine, calcofluor, and direct/indirect fluorescent antibody staining.
- The **acridine orange** stains DNA so that bacteria or fungi fluoresce a reddish orange at acidic pH.
- **Calcofluor staining** is used on fungi. **Fluorescent antibody staining** is based on the recognition of pathogens by staining with fluorescently labeled antibodies specific for the pathogens.

Gram Stain

Gram stain is the best-known and most widely used differential stain for bacteria (Table 5-7; depicting respective staining patterns of different bacterial species) because it permits identification of the bacteria based on the chemical and physical properties of their cell walls. This method is fast and reliable when rapid diagnosis is needed. It is usually performed on bodily fluids (eg, cerebrospinal fluid [CSF] for meningitis or synovial fluid for septic arthritis).

In a Gram stain preparation, gram-positive bacteria appear dark blue to **purple,** and gram-negative bacteria are **red.** The procedure includes:

- Application of a sample to a glass slide and fixation under a flame.
- Application of the primary stain—crystal violet (CV).
- Application of iodine to bind and "set" the dye.
- Washing away of unbound CV from gram-negative organisms during decolorization.
- Counterstaining of gram-negative organisms with the red dye safranin.

The mechanism of staining is based on the following properties or interactions:

- CV penetrates the cell wall and membrane of both gram-positive and gram-negative cells.
- **Iodine** interacts with CV and forms complexes of CV and iodine within the inner and outer layers of the bacterial cells.
- **Decolorizer** disintegrates the lipids of the cell membranes, thus gram-negative cells lose their outer membrane, exposing the peptidoglycan layer, whereas gram-positive cells dehydrate following treatment with ethanol.
- Decolorization washes out the CV–iodine complexes and outer membrane from gram-negative cells.
- CV–iodine complexes remain "trapped" within the gram-positive cells owing to the multilayered composition of their peptidoglycan.

TABLE 5-7.   Gram-Staining Patterns of Various Bacterial Species

STAIN	GRAM-POSITIVE	GRAM-NEGATIVE
Bacteria	*Staphylococcus, Streptococcus, Clostridium, Listeria, Bacillus, Corynebacterium*	*Neisseria, H influenzae, Pasteurella, Brucella, B pertussis, Klebsiella, E coli, Enterobacter, Citrobacter, Serratia, Shigella, Salmonella, Proteus, Pseudomonas*

- Following decolorization:
  - **Gram-positive** bacteria remain (stain) **purple.**
  - **Gram-negative** bacteria **lose** their **purple** color.

GRAM-POSITIVE CELL WALL

The cell wall of gram-positive organisms consists principally of **peptidoglycan**, which form multiple layers of a thick mesh outside the plasma membrane, and captures the Gram stain (Figure 5-6). **Teichoic acids** are exclusively found in gram-positive organisms and are covalently linked to the peptidoglycan molecules and can act as virulence factors. The laboratory algorithm for biochemically identifying gram-positive organisms is shown in Figure 5-7.

GRAM-NEGATIVE CELL WALL

Compared with the cell wall of gram-positive bacteria, a gram-negative cell wall has a much thinner layer of peptidoglycan immediately outside the plasma membrane. Crystal violet is easily washed out of this thin mesh by the decolorizer.

External to the peptidoglycan layer is the **outer membrane,** a porous structure unique to gram-negative bacteria that contains phospholipids, embedded proteins, and most significantly LPS, a phospholipid molecule largely responsible for the virulence of gram-negative organisms.

LPS is often referred to as **endotoxin** (as opposed to an *exotoxin*) because it is an integral part of the bacteria. The space between the plasma membrane and the outer membrane is referred to as the **periplasmic space,** which contains various membrane-associated proteins as well as the thin peptidoglycan layer.

Cell wall structures related to motility, including **pili** and **flagella,** are common to both gram-positive and gram-negative cell walls. The laboratory algorithm for biochemically identifying gram-negative organisms is shown in Figure 5-8.

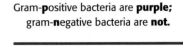

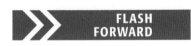

Gram-**p**ositive bacteria are **purple;** gram-**n**egative bacteria are **not.**

β-Lactam antibiotics target the enzymes—PBPs—responsible for cross-linking amino acids in peptidoglycan molecules. Eukaryotes (like us) possess neither peptidoglycan nor PBPs and thus are intrinsically "resistant" to these antibiotics.

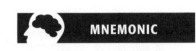

Gram-**n**egative bacteria are the only ones containing **en**dotoxin.

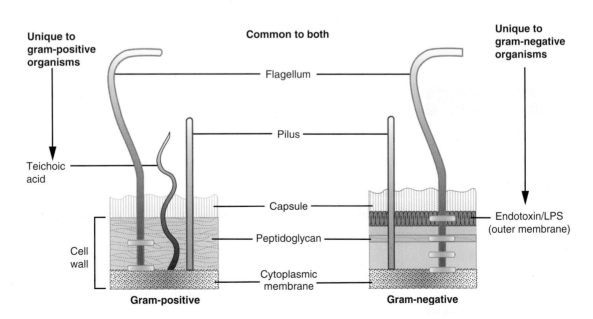

FIGURE 5-6. **Gram-positive and gram-negative cell wall structures.** The thick peptidoglycan mesh of the gram-positive cell wall effectively traps the crystal violet stain. LPS, lipopolysaccharide. (Modified with permission from Levinson W, Jawetz E. *Medical Microbiology and Immunology: Examination and Board Review,* 9th ed. New York: McGraw-Hill, 2006: 7.)

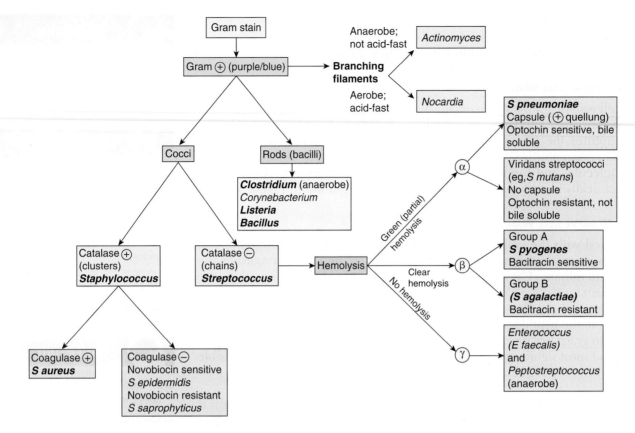

FIGURE 5-7. **Gram-positive laboratory algorithm.** Important pathogens are in bold type. Enterococcus is either α- or γ-hemolytic.

GRAM-INDETERMINATE ORGANISMS

Several medically important microorganisms are, for a variety of reasons, impossible to visualize on Gram stain preparation. Other techniques are necessary to visualize and identify these organisms in the laboratory.

MYCOBACTERIA

These intracellular organisms have a cell wall composed largely of mycolic acids, which are lipid-rich and prevent crystal violet from penetrating the cell wall. Mycobacteria can be visualized using an **acid-fast** (carbol fuchsin) stain.

MYCOPLASMA

Truly gram-indeterminate organisms, these microbes possess **no cell wall.** Conventional laboratory stains do not work, so culture and serologic cold agglutinin tests are used to make the diagnosis.

SPIROCHETES

The thin, corkscrew-shaped organisms in the genera *Treponema, Borrelia,* and *Leptospira* are too thin to be visualized via Gram stain. Hence, darkfield microscopy, indirect immunofluorescence, serologic assays, and specialized tests (eg, those for *T pallidum*) are used. Note that *Borrelia* microbes, larger than the other two, can generally be seen on peripheral blood smears—the preferred mechanism for the laboratory identification of relapsing fever. (Think: *Borrelia* = Big).

MNEMONIC

Gram-indeterminate organisms–

Some Errant Rascals May Microscopically Lack Color

Spirochetes
Ehrlichia
Rickettsia
Mycobacterium
Mycoplasma
Listeria
Chlamydia

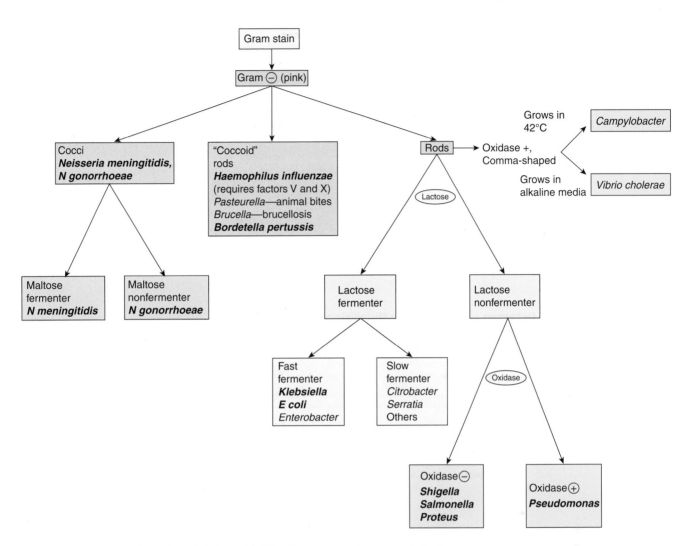

FIGURE 5-8. **Gram-negative laboratory algorithm.** Important pathogens are in bold type.

INTRACELLULAR MICROORGANISMS

Rickettsia spp. (*Coxiella*), *Ehrlichia* spp., and *Chlamydia* spp. are all small, obligate intracellular parasites that live in the cytosol of infected cells. They stain poorly with Gram stain, but share membrane characteristics with gram-negative organisms. Microscopy is generally not useful in the diagnosis of diseases caused by these organisms. *Listeria monocytogenes*, a gram-positive rod that is primarily intracellular, also does not take up crystal violet and is usually visualized on clinical specimens via a silver stain.

The limitations of Gram staining (due to differences in composition of various microorganisms) are bypassed by using other staining methods (Table 5-8).

Other Microbiologic Stains and Microscopic Techniques

For most common bacteria, Gram stain is sufficient to make an accurate diagnosis. However, in certain cases, such as the identification of nonstainable organisms, fungi, and parasites, other techniques must be used (Tables 5-9 and 5-10).

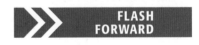
FLASH FORWARD

Don't forget the important nonmicrobiologic tissue–based stains: **Congo red** for **amyloid; Sudan black** for **fat droplets; periodic acid–Schiff** for **glycogen,** and **trichrome** for **tissue collagen.**

TABLE 5-8. Gram Stain Limitations

BACTERIA	PREFERRED STAINING METHOD
Treponema	Darkfield microscopy and fluorescent antibody staining.
Rickettsia	Immunofluorescent and immunoperoxidase staining.
Mycobacterium	Acid-fast.
Mycoplasma	Do not stain.
Legionella pneumophila	Silver stain.
Chlamydia	Immunofluorescent staining.

TABLE 5-9. Microscopy Techniques and Stains Used in Microbiology

	ORGANISMS	RATIONALE
Darkfield microscopy	Spirochetes.	Thin organisms are more easily identified by this technique.
KOH (potassium hydroxide) preparation	Fungi.	Bacteria are killed in this strong alkali solution, leaving fungi behind (which are stable in alkali solution).
India ink	*Cryptococcus* in CSF specimens.	Cryptococcal polysaccharide capsule scatters ink, rendering it bright against dark background. (However, latex agglutination test to detect polysaccharide capsular antigen is preferred for identification of *Cryptococcus.*)
Wright/Giemsa	*Borrelia recurrentis.* Blood parasites (*Plasmodium* spp., *Trypanosoma* spp. and *Babesia microti*). *Chlamydia* and *Rickettsia.*	A routine stain for peripheral blood.
Silver (methenamine silver)	Fungi. *Listeria monocytogenes.* *Pneumocystis jiroveci.*	Tissue stain for fungus; is also used to detect certain poorly Gram-staining organisms. Technically difficult.
Acid-fast (Ziehl-Neelsen or carbol-fuchsin)	*Mycobacterium.* *Nocardia.* Some protozoa.	High lipid content of cell wall prevents stain from being washed out by acid alcohol decolorizer.
Iron hematoxylin and trichrome	Protozoa.	
Fecal wet mount (ova and parasites)	Protozoa, helminth eggs.	

TABLE 5-10. Specialized Media for Microbial Growth

ORGANISM	MEDIUM
All bacteria	Blood agar
Gram-negatives, lactose fermenters	MacConkey agar
Gram-negatives, lactose fermenters	EMB (eosin-methylene blue) agar
H influenzae	Chocolate agar
Neisseria	Thayer-Martin (VCN) agar
B pertussis	Bordet-Gengou medium
Corynebacterium diphtheriae	Tellurite agar
Group D streptococci	Bile esculin agar

VCN = vancomycin, colistin, nystatin.

BACTERIAL CULTURE

Growing bacteria on agar plates can provide additional diagnostic information for the identification of clinically relevant microorganisms. Bacteria often have a characteristic colony appearance when growing on conventional media. For example, bacteria with polysaccharide capsules generally have "wet" or **mucoid**-appearing colonies. Some bacteria also produce visibly pigmented colonies on agar:

- *Pseudomonas aeruginosa* produces a fluorescing blue-green pigment.
- *Staphylococcus aureus* produces a **gold** pigment (think of **Au**reus, the abbreviation for gold on the periodic table).
- *Serratia marcescens* produces a red pigment. (Think: maraschino red cherries).

Generally, bacteria from clinical specimens are grown on an agar-based, permissive, nonselective medium, with an additional nutrient source (either hydrolyzed soy protein or sheep's blood). Isolated colonies from these agar plates can then be aseptically selected and used for further laboratory diagnosis via molecular, biochemical or serologic techniques, microscopy, or further culture.

- **Selective media** are supplemented with antibiotics or other substances that **prevent the growth** of certain contaminating bacteria.
- **Differential media** contain **indicators** that provide further biochemical information about the microorganisms.

MacConkey Agar

- Selective and differential medium.
- Inhibits the growth of gram-positive bacteria.

- Also differentiates whether a microorganism can use lactose as a nutrient source.
- Lactose utilizers form red colonies (vs. white colonies in lactose non-fermenters).
- Used to distinguish among different enteric bacteria.

Eosin-Methylene Blue (EMB) Agar

- Like MacConkey's, EMB agar inhibits gram-positive bacterial growth and allows assay of lactose as a sugar source.
- Lactose utilizers form dark-green, metallic-appearing colonies.

Chocolate Agar

- *Haemophilus* spp. are pathogens that are highly fastidious in their growth requirements and require enriched medium to survive in vitro.
- **X factor** (hemin) and **V factor** (nicotinamide adenine dinucleotide [NAD]) are required. *Haemophilus* can also be grown in media with *S aureus*, which lyses RBCs and provides *Haemophilus* with the factors it needs to grow.
- Present in sheep's blood agar, but gentle heating (or "chocolatizing") is required to remove V factor inhibitors.

Thayer-Martin (VCN) Agar

Like *Haemophilus*, *Neisseria* spp. are highly fastidious microbes and require X and V factors for growth in the laboratory. Thayer-Martin (VCN) agar is a selective medium made of **chocolate agar supplemented with vancomycin, colistin, and nystatin.** It is used for the isolation of *Neisseria gonorrhoeae* from mucosal surfaces. The three powerful antimicrobial agents strongly suppress growth of other commensal organisms present in vaginal, rectal, and pharyngeal specimens.

Bordet-Gengou Medium

Bordetella pertussis is a highly fastidious respiratory pathogen that is very difficult to grow under typical laboratory conditions. Specimen collection must be performed with a calcium alginate swab (because ordinary sterile cotton is toxic to the microbe), and freshly prepared special medium (charcoal and horse blood required for growth).

Tellurite Agars

Various selective and differential media (potassium tellurite agar, cysteine tellurite agar) are used to isolate *Corynebacterium diphtheriae* from the respiratory tracts of affected individuals. Positive colonies are characteristically black on these agar plates.

Bile Esculin Agar

This selective medium is used to differentiate group D streptococci (including *Enterococcus* spp.) from other streptococci, which are unable to grow in the presence of bile salts.

GRAM-POSITIVE COCCI

Microbes from the genera *Streptococcus* and *Staphylococcus* make up the bulk of medically relevant gram-positive cocci and are responsible for diseases affecting diverse organ systems. Streptococci and staphylococci can be easily differentiated based on microscopic morphology; staphylococci appear in clusters (often referred to as "bunches of grapes"), whereas streptococci are always seen in pairs (or **diplococci**) and chains (Figure 5-9). In addition, the **catalase** test easily discerns between the two genera; staphylococci are catalase-positive, and streptococci are catalase-negative.

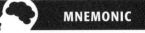

Streptococcus and *Enterococcus*

The catalase-negative, gram-positive cocci (*Streptococcus* and the closely related *Enterococcus*, from now on referred to together as streptococci for simplicity) are a diverse group of coccoid organisms. Many medically important streptococci were first classified serologically by their **Lancefield group antigen**, a polymorphic immunogen located on the C carbohydrate component of the cell wall. Today, only three medically important groups of streptococci are known by their Lancefield antigens. Streptococci can be differentiated from one another on the basis of hemolysis patterns on blood agar.

Streptococcus pyogenes (Lancefield Group A)

Characteristics

- **Pyogenic**, or pus-producing organism.
- Responsible for a diverse collection of diseases.
- By microscopy, classically a 1- to 2-μm spherical coccus found in chains (Figure 5-9).
- Easily discerned while growing on blood agar based on its wide zones of β-hemolysis.
- Like all streptococci, it is catalase-negative and sensitive to the antibiotic bacitracin.
- Colonizes the upper respiratory mucosa (especially the oropharynx). Asymptomatic carriage in healthy individuals is common.
- Spread by respiratory droplets, so crowded conditions (eg, day-care facilities) facilitate person-to-person transmission.

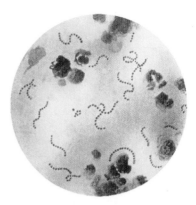

FIGURE 5-9. **Photomicrograph of *Streptococcus pyogenes* in long chains.** (Image courtesy of CDC's Public Health Image Library.)

Pathogenesis

Streptococcus pyogenes has a number of virulence factors that are important in causing a variety of diseases.

- **M protein** is a part of the cell wall that inhibits complement activation and thus prevents opsonization. Antibodies to M protein can cause rheumatic fever. Specific antibodies produced by the immune system are directed against the M protein.
- **Streptolysins S** and **O** are enzymes capable of causing hematopoietic cell death and are responsible for the characteristic β-hemolytic pattern in vivo.
- Streptolysin O is also a target for host cell antibodies and can be detected in blood as an antistreptolysin O (**ASO**) titer.
- **Pyrogenic exotoxins** are superantigens capable of causing the characteristic rash of scarlet fever as well as the multiple-organ system failure seen in streptococcal toxic shock syndrome.
- **Streptokinases** mediate the rapid spread of infection through infected tissues.

Clinical Symptoms

Clinical sequelae of *Streptococcus pyogenes* infection can be easily divided into diseases caused by toxic effects of the bacteria themselves (often termed

suppurative infections) and diseases caused by inappropriate activation of the host immune system.

- Local invasion or toxin released by the microbe:
  - Pharyngitis
  - Skin and soft tissue infection
  - Toxic shock syndrome (discussed under *S aureus* infections)
- Cross-reacting antibodies produced by an infected host:
  - Rheumatic fever
  - Poststreptococcal glomerulonephritis

STREPTOCOCCAL PHARYNGITIS

CLINICAL SYMPTOMS

Strep throat is a common cause of sore throat among children and young adults. It is characterized by pain on swallowing, high fever, regional lymphadenopathy, and, most notably, erythema and frank white exudate on the palatine tonsils. Distinguishing viral from streptococcal sore throat can be difficult, and throat culture or a "rapid Strep test" is usually required. A complication of streptococcal pharyngitis, caused by strains containing a lysogenized pyrogenic exotoxin, is **scarlet fever.** Following the sore throat, a sandpaper-like rash appears on the chest and spreads centrifugally (outward), sparing the palms, soles, and face. Complications from untreated pharyngitis include retropharyngeal and parapharyngeal abscesses, as well as immunologic complications (described later).

SKIN AND SOFT TISSUE INFECTIONS

CLINICAL SYMPTOMS

Several distinct syndromes are caused by *Streptococcus* infection of epidermal, dermal, or fascial components.

- **Impetigo** is a common childhood colonization of the upper epidermis characterized by perioral vesicular/blistered lesions that eventually develop a honey-colored crust (Figure 5-10). (Impetigo can also be caused by *S aureus.*)
- **Erysipelas** and **cellulitis** are both acute infections of the skin characterized by erythema, edema, warmth, and systemic symptoms; cellulitis also involves deeper subcutaneous/dermal tissues. Both can be caused by other organisms as well (mainly *S aureus* in immunocompetent individuals).
- **Necrotizing fasciitis** (or "flesh-eating bacteria") is a rapidly progressive infection of deep subcutaneous tissues. Symptoms include purple-blue **bullae** on the overlying skin following a cellulitis-like picture; overt gangrene, systemic symptoms, and multiorgan failure soon follow.

RHEUMATIC FEVER

PATHOGENESIS

Rheumatic fever is caused by cross-reaction of antibodies raised against the *Streptococcus* bacteria with antigens in the heart, causing an initial **pancarditis.** Further cardiac damage in the form of valvular disease may occur many years later.

CLINICAL SYMPTOMS

In addition to symptoms of valvular cardiac disease, joint, epidermal, and neurologic involvement is common.

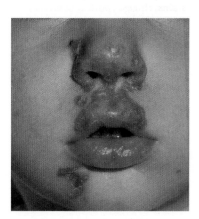

FIGURE 5-10. Impetigo.
(Reproduced with permission from Wolff K, Johnson RA, Suurmond D. *Fitzpatrick's Color Atlas & Synopsis of Clinical Dermatology,* 5th ed. New York: McGraw-Hill, 2005: 589.)

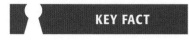

KEY FACT

Rheumatic fever follows untreated streptococcal pharyngitis, **not** strep skin or soft tissue infection!

TREATMENT

Rheumatic fever can recur after subsequent streptococcal infections, so patients are placed on lifelong prophylactic antibiotics.

POSTSTREPTOCOCCAL GLOMERULONEPHRITIS

PATHOGENESIS

Unlike rheumatic fever, renal sequelae of streptococcal infection can occur following either pharyngitis or skin or soft tissue infection. **Immune complexes** (antigen-antibody complexes) arising from streptococcal infection are deposited in the basement membrane of the glomerulus.

CLINICAL SYMPTOMS

The immune complex deposition causes typical glomerulonephritic symptoms of hematuria, hypertension, gross proteinuria, and tissue edema all secondary to glomerular inflammation. Prognosis is generally good in the pediatric population.

TREATMENT

In the case of poststreptococcal glomerulonephritis, treatment is generally supportive; immunosuppressive therapy to eliminate the immune complex deposition has been shown to have no effect on the disease course. *Streptococcus pyogenes* is highly sensitive to penicillin and other β-lactam agents, as well as macrolide antibiotics. Skin and soft tissue infections are usually treated with an antistaphylococcal penicillin (eg, oxacillin) to cover for *S aureus* as well. Prevention of rheumatic fever is effectively accomplished by the early diagnosis and treatment of streptococcal pharyngitis with antibiotics, thus preventing the synthesis of the responsible antistreptococcal antibodies.

STREPTOCOCCUS AGALACTIAE (LANCEFIELD GROUP B STREPTOCOCCUS)

Streptococcus agalactiae, a common cause of neonatal infection, is indistinguishable from *Streptococcus pyogenes* by microscopy and is also characterized by **β-hemolysis** on blood agar.

- Unlike *Streptococcus pyogenes*, *S agalactiae* is resistant to the antibiotic bacitracin.
- Approximately 10–30% of pregnant women are asymptomatically colonized with this organism. Transmission can occur transplacentally in utero or during delivery.

CLINICAL SYMPTOMS

Streptococcus agalactiae infections fall broadly into two classes. It is a relatively common cause of **UTI** in pregnant women, for whom the prognosis is excellent. Other group B streptococcal (GBS) infections of adults are uncommon and generally occur in immunocompromised individuals.

Given the high rate of asymptomatic carriage in pregnant females, it is no surprise that *Streptococcus agalactiae* is the most common cause of **neonatal septicemia** (sepsis) and meningitis. GBS can also cause **pneumonia in neonates.**

TREATMENT

Like *Streptococcus pyogenes*, GBS is also **penicillin-sensitive,** although higher concentrations are required for treatment. To prevent neonatal disease, cur-

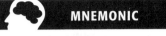

MNEMONIC

The **J♥NES** cr**ITERIA** are used to formally diagnose rheumatic fever.
Required criterion—documented evidence of recent group A streptococcal infection.

Major criteria:

Joint pains (migratory arthritis)
♥ (carditis)
Nodules (subcutaneous)
Erythema marginatum (spreading circular rash with red edges)
Sydenham chorea

Minor criteria:

Inflammatory cells (leukocytosis)
Temperature (fever)
ESR (erythrocyte sedimentation rate) or CRP (C-reactive protein) ↑
Rheumatic fever (history of rheumatic disease)
Increased PR interval
Arthralgias
Two major criteria, or one major and two minor criteria are required for diagnosis.

rent recommendations call for **screening** of pregnant women at 35–37 weeks' gestational age for GBS colonization via vaginal swab and culture. Women with positive cultures and those at high risk for intrapartum infection are given prophylactic penicillin G (or ampicillin) during delivery.

VIRIDANS STREPTOCOCCI

CHARACTERISTICS

The viridans group of *Streptococcus* consists of several **nongroupable** (ie, not classified according to the Lancefield classification) streptococci that produce α-hemolysis on blood agar. Important members of this group include:

- *Streptococcus mutans*, which is responsible for dental caries (cavities).
- *Streptococcus sanguis*, which causes subacute bacterial endocarditis (SBE).
- *Streptococcus intermedius* group, which can be found in abscesses.

The viridans group is resistant to **optochin,** which allows discrimination from *S pneumoniae*, which is optochin-sensitive.

CLINICAL SYMPTOMS

Several members of the viridans streptococci group are normal oropharyngeal flora; *S mutans* is well known to cause dental caries. Several other members of the group are associated with SBE, an indolent infection affecting previously damaged (ie, secondary to rheumatic fever or congenital bicuspid aortic valve) cardiac valves. Transient bacteremia is caused by dental procedures, and bacteria settle on the damaged valves. Associated symptoms include fevers, night sweats, fatigue, and new-onset murmurs. Resolution of this serious infection generally requires long-term use of parenteral antibiotics (typically ampicillin and an aminoglycoside).

ENTEROCOCCUS AND OTHER GROUP D STREPTOCOCCI

CHARACTERISTICS

The genus *Enterococcus*, members of which possess the group D Lancefield antigen, are distinguished from nonenterococcal group D streptococci by their growth under harsh conditions, namely 6.5% sodium chloride and 40% bile salts. Hemolysis patterns on blood agar vary. Two species of enterococci, *Enterococcus faecalis* and *Enterococcus faecium*, are clinically relevant.

- Responsible for disease in immunocompromised and up to 10% of all infections in hospitalized patients. Patients on extended courses of broad-spectrum antibiotics are also at risk.
- UTIs in catheterized patients, postsurgical peritonitis, and SBE are the most common clinical entities caused by these microorganisms.

Of note, *Streptococcus bovis* is an uncommon cause of endocarditis. It is associated with gastrointestinal malignancy for an unknown reason; all patients with documented *S bovis* infections should receive a complete work-up for GI malignancies.

TREATMENT

In the past, therapy for enterococcal infections, like many serious blood-borne gram-positive coccal infections, has been the synergistic combination of ampicillin and an aminoglycoside. In the 1990s, rising resistance to these agents has prompted the use of vancomycin to treat resistant strains. Unfortunately, resistance to vancomycin is rising (up to 20% of *E faecium* isolates), and novel antibiotic therapy has been required to treat these **vancomycin-resistant enterococci** (VRE) infections.

- **Linezolid** (Zyvox) and dalfopristin/quinupristin (**Synercid**) are two new antimicrobial agents with activity against VRE; unfortunately they are bacteriostatic and have significant side effects.
- Urinary sterilizers such as nitrofurantoin are another option for the treatment of VRE UTIs.

STREPTOCOCCUS PNEUMONIAE

CHARACTERISTICS

The nontypable *S pneumoniae*, commonly known as **pneumococcus**, is one of the most clinically important gram-positive cocci; it is the **most common cause of bacterial pneumonia in adults.** Microscopically, pneumococci are commonly seen as **"lancet-shaped"** organisms in pairs or **diplococci.** Most pathogenic strains are encapsulated with a polysaccharide capsule (which serves as a virulence factor), and thus colonies appear mucoid (jelly-like) on blood agar. Hemolysis patterns on blood agar vary, but usually α-hemolysis is seen.

Given the importance of this organism, it is fortunate that laboratory identification of the pneumococcus is facilitated by several individualized assays.

- The **Quellung** reaction can identify pneumococci in a clinically derived sample such as sputum; the polysaccharide capsule is microscopically visualized by the addition of anticapsular antibodies, which cause the capsule to swell.
- Colonies of *S pneumoniae* are differentiated from other α-hemolytic streptococci (eg, viridans streptococci) on agar plates by using optochin susceptibility and by adding bile to the culture medium.

PATHOGENESIS

Virulence of pneumococcus is in large part mediated by the presence of a polysaccharide capsule, which serves to inhibit the microorganisms' phagocytosis by first-line immune cells such as macrophages and neutrophils.

A pyogenic immune response is ensured because of the ability of pneumococcal teichoic acid and peptidoglycan to activate the alternative complement pathway, thereby recruiting vast numbers of neutrophils.

Transmission of *S pneumoniae* is respiratory, and prolonged; asymptomatic carriage is common. The capsule is highly immunogenic, and 84 serotypes have been identified in capsular antigens. Disease is caused by oropharyngeal infection with a noncolonizing serotype. The microorganism then spreads from the oropharynx via respiratory mucosa to the paranasal sinuses, the lower respiratory tract, or the meninges.

CLINICAL SYMPTOMS

- Pneumococcus is the most common cause of bacterial **pneumonia** in adults. A lobar pattern is seen on chest film, and high fevers with shaking chills are common. Frank blood and diplococci are found in an induced sputum sample.

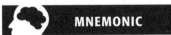

MNEMONIC

The **Quellung** reaction causes **swelling** of the polysaccharide capsule.

KEY FACT

Six key organisms with polysaccharide **capsules:** *S pneumoniae, K pneumoniae, H influenzae, N meningitidis, S typhi, S pyogenes.* The capsule serves as an antiphagocytic virulence factor. Patients without their spleens **(asplenia)** are at increased risk of becoming infected with one of these organisms.

- *Streptococcus pneumoniae* is also the number one cause of **meningitis** in adults.
- Pneumococcal **sinusitis** in adults and **otitis media** in children are commonly seen, owing to facilitated transmission on mucosal surfaces.
- Pneumococcus can also cause **sepsis**, often preceded by meningitis. Individuals with **asplenia** (including functional asplenia seen in sickle cell disease) are also at increased risk for pneumococcal bacteremia and sepsis.

TREATMENT

Penicillin was once the mainstay of treatment for pneumococcal infection. However, rapidly increasing resistance has forced the use of alternative therapies in certain areas with intermediate or high rates of resistance. **Ceftriaxone** or **vancomycin** (or both) are used in these cases.

A seven-valent conjugated pneumococcal vaccine is recommended for all infants younger than 2 years. Adults at high risk—including immunocompromised, asplenic, and elderly individuals as well as some transplant recipients—should receive a 23-valent polysaccharide vaccine to protect against pneumonia and invasive disease.

Staphylococcus

Staphylococci make up the other major medically relevant group of gram-positive cocci. Like streptococci, they are common colonizers of body surfaces and commonly cause skin and soft tissue substructure infections. Fortunately, they are easily differentiated from streptococci based on microscopy and the laboratory test for the **catalase** enzyme (using hydrogen peroxide as a substrate) (Table 5-11). Staphylococci always assume the form of purple clusters (often called a "bunch of grapes") when gram-stained.

Three common and medically relevant species of *Staphylococcus* include *S aureus*, *S epidermidis*, and *S saprophyticus*.

STAPHYLOCOCCUS AUREUS

CHARACTERISTICS

Because of its propensity for colonization and high degree of virulence, *S aureus* is a major cause of both community-acquired and nosocomial morbidity and mortality. Like other staphylococci, its microscopic appearance looks like purple clusters (Figure 5-11). Large β-hemolytic mucoid colonies that produce a **gold pigment** are seen when the organism is grown on blood agar.

Staphylococcus aureus is unique among the staphylococci in that it contains the enzyme **coagulase**. Other species of *Staphylococcus* do not have this enzyme and are thus often referred to in laboratory reports as "coagulase-negative *Staphylococcus*."

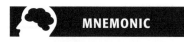

MNEMONIC

It takes a **Staph** of hard-working grape-squishers to produce wine from the **purple clusters** of grapes.

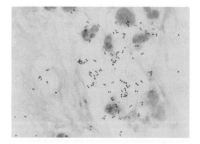

FIGURE 5-11. *Staphylococcus aureus.* Clusters of gram-positive cocci.

TABLE 5-11. *Staphylococcus* Compared With *Streptococcus*

	STAPHYLOCOCCUS	**STREPTOCOCCUS**
Microscopy	Clusters.	Pairs and chains
Catalase test	Positive.	Negative
Penicillin-sensitive	Rarely (except *S saprophyticus*).	Commonly

Staphylococcus aureus is a part of the normal flora of human skin, and transient colonization of moist skin folds and the nasopharyngeal cavity is common. It also survives for long periods of time on dry surfaces. Transmission is either via shedding of microbes or contaminated **fomites,** inanimate objects that serve as vectors for microbial transmission. The rate of hospital-acquired multidrug-resistant *S aureus* infections is almost certainly due to transmission via fomites such as bed linens and the nares of hospital staff.

PATHOGENICITY

Like *Streptococcus pyogenes, Staphylococcus aureus* features a number of different virulence factors that can be divided into several groups. Not all strains carry all virulence factors.

Immune modulators:

- **Protein A:** Specifically binds the F_c component of immunoglobulin, preventing immune-mediated destruction via **opsonization.**
- **Coagulase:** An enzyme that builds an insoluble fibrin capsule that surrounds the microorganism, thus preventing immune cell access.
- **Hemolysins** (also known as cytotoxins) α, β, γ, and δ—directly toxic to hematopoietic cells.
- **Leukocidin:** A toxin specific for white blood cells.
- **Catalase:** Prevents toxic action of neutrophil-derived hydrogen peroxide.
- **Penicillinase:** A secreted form of β-lactamase, can inactivate penicillin and derivatives.

Factors permitting penetration through tissues:

- **Hyaluronidase:** Hydrolyzes hyaluronic acid present in connective tissue.
- **Fibrinolysin** (also known as **staphylokinase**)—dissolves fibrin clots.
- **Lipases** allow for the survival and spread of *S aureus* in fat-containing areas of the body, especially sebaceous glands.

Secreted toxins:

- **Exfoliatin:** Result in the exfoliation of the middle skin layer, causing staphylococcal scalded skin syndrome.
- **Enterotoxins** (heat-stable): Cause vomiting and diarrhea.
- **Toxic shock syndrome toxin (TSST-1): A superantigen** that cross-links the major histocompatability complex (MHC) class II molecules on antigen-presenting cells, causing a massive nonspecific T-cell response, leading to toxic shock syndrome.

CLINICAL SYMPTOMS

Staphylococcus aureus is capable of invading almost any organ. Signs and symptoms obviously differ but, because of the myriad virulence factors symptoms, they can be severe in any organ system. Both toxin-mediated (sterile) and invasive diseases are common (Table 5-12).

STAPHYLOCOCCAL SCALDED SKIN SYNDROME (SSSS)

A relatively common disease of infants that presents with perioral exfoliation of the middle layer of the epidermis followed by the diffuse formation of blisters containing sterile fluid (Figure 5-12). Unless there is bacterial superinfection, the disease resolves within approximately one week without further sequelae; morbidity and mortality rates are low.

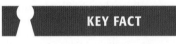

FLASH FORWARD

The development of multidrug (or methicillin)-resistant *S aureus* (MRSA) has complicated the treatment of *S aureus* infections. Stronger drugs such as vancomycin are now needed to treat such infections.

KEY FACT

Superantigens are substances that can cause a massive, **nonspecific** overstimulation of the immune system by chemically cross-linking the MHC class II molecules on antigen-presenting cells.

TABLE 5-12. **Spectrum of Staphylococcal Disease**

Exotoxin-Mediated	Invasive
Staphylococcal scalded skin syndrome (SSSS)	Skin and soft-tissue infections
Food poisoning	Endocarditis
Toxic shock syndrome	Pneumonia and empyema
	Osteomyelitis
	Septic arthritis

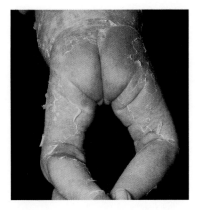

FIGURE 5-12. **Staphylococcal scalded skin syndrome.** The exfoliative dermatitis is widespread but not severe. (Reproduced with permission from Wolff K, Johnson RA, Suurmond D. *Fitzpatrick's Color Atlas & Synopsis of Clinical Dermatology*, 5th ed, New York: McGraw-Hill, 2005: 623.)

GASTROENTERITIS

CHARACTERISTICS

Caused by *S aureus*, gastroenteritis is common and notable for its rapid onset (within 4–6 hours of ingestion of the tainted foodstuffs).

PATHOGENESIS

Unusually rapid onset owing to the ingestion of **preformed heat-stable enterotoxin** (not the bacterium itself) found in food.

CLINICAL SYMPTOMS

Illness is often characterized by a rapid, abrupt onset of copious vomiting and nonbloody diarrhea. The illness generally runs a short (< 24 hours) and uncomplicated course. Common culprit food items are room-temperature "salads" made with mayonnaise, such as **potato and tuna salad,** processed meats, custard, and nondairy creamer. The source is usually a human food preparer with a skin infection or asymptomatic nasal carriage.

TREATMENT

Supportive only; antibiotics do not significantly shorten the course of the diarrhea.

TOXIC SHOCK SYNDROME

CHARACTERISTICS

Occurs primarily in menstruating women using superabsorbent tampons left in place for long periods of time, but can also occur in wounds with draining fluid collections.

PATHOGENESIS

Staphylococcus aureus microbes multiply in the nutrient-rich menstrual or wound fluid and secrete TSST-1, which causes a systemic inflammatory response due to the nonspecific activation of T cells.

CLINICAL SYMPTOMS

Abrupt onset of fever and hypotension, and multiple organ dysfunction are seen; a **desquamating rash of the palms and soles** is typical as well.

TREATMENT

Antibiotics have limited effectiveness, and supportive care is the rule.

SKIN AND SOFT TISSUE INFECTIONS

CHARACTERISTICS

Like group A *Streptococcus*, *S aureus* can also cause various **skin and soft tissue infections,** such as cellulitis and impetigo. The following skin substructure infections are more commonly caused by *S aureus*:

- **Folliculitis** is an infection of the base of the hair follicle. Patients present with a small, raised, erythematous bump. This infection can occur anywhere on the skin, but is most common in areas with abundant hair.
- A **furuncle** is a conglomeration of several adjacent inflamed follicles. It presents as a large, painful nodule that requires drainage.
- **Carbuncles** are coalesced furuncles that often extend into the dermis. They can cause systemic symptoms such as fever as well as staphylococcal bacteremia.
- **Staphylococcal wound infections** are common and are generally seen in a "dirty wound" containing foreign matter.

TREATMENT

Appropriate antibiotic therapy can be administered either systemically or locally via topical creams or ointments.

INFECTIVE ENDOCARDITIS (IE)

CHARACTERISTICS

IE of undamaged (native) valves is commonly caused by *S aureus* migrating from infected surgical wounds or contaminated IV catheters. It is a serious disease with high (> 50%) mortality, especially when untreated.

CLINICAL SYMPTOMS

Unlike SBE, IE is characterized by a **rapid onset** of high fever with rigors, myalgias, and possibly a loud murmur. Large infective vegetations are seen on the affected valves (Figure 5-13) and can embolize to the pulmonary or cerebral parenchyma.

PNEUMONIA

CHARACTERISTICS

Staphylococcal **pneumonia** is rare in the community but a relatively more common cause of nosocomial pneumonia, especially in the elderly following infection with influenza.

CLINICAL SYMPTOMS

Characterized by the rapid onset of fever and chills and a nonspecific radiographic pattern. **Cavitations** in the lung tissue are seen on gross dissection. Infected parapneumonic effusions (known as **empyema**) are common as well. Certain strains can cause an even more severe variant known as **necrotizing** pneumonia, characterized by massive hemoptysis and septic shock.

OSTEOMYELITIS

CHARACTERISTICS

A deep-seated infection of the bone most often seen in preadolescent boys.

> **KEY FACT**
>
> Most cases of IE occur on **left-sided** valves and have a poor prognosis due to brain emboli; IV drug users get **right-sided** IE, which has a much better prognosis.

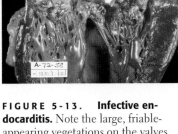

FIGURE 5-13. Infective endocarditis. Note the large, friable-appearing vegetations on the valves. (Image courtesy of CDC's Public Health Image Library; content provider Dr. Edwin P. Ewing, Jr.)

PATHOGENESIS

Seeded hematogenously from distant sites (usually cutaneous staphylococcal infections) or from contiguous, overlying skin infections (eg, diabetic foot ulcers).

CLINICAL SYMPTOMS

Localized pain and fever are presenting symptoms, and further hematogenous spread is common. Bone scans are used to screen for distant disease.

TREATMENT

Several weeks to months of appropriate antibiotic therapy usually results in a complete cure.

SEPTIC ARTHRITIS

CHARACTERISTICS

Staphylococcus aureus is the most common organism implicated in **septic arthritis** seen in pediatric and elderly age groups (*N gonorrhoeae* is the most common cause among sexually active individuals).

PATHOGENESIS

Disease can be caused by local introduction of the organism by synovial puncture via needle or via hematogenous spread from distant foci of infection.

CLINICAL SYMPTOMS

Classic symptoms include an erythematous, swollen joint with decreased range of motion; the key laboratory finding from **arthrocentesis** (joint aspiration) is an elevated neutrophil count.

TREATMENT

Drainage and prompt antibiotics generally produce an effective cure, especially in children.

Since most S *aureus* isolates carry a penicillinase enzyme, first- and second-generation penicillins are not used for antibiotic therapy.

Methicillin-sensitive *Staphylococcus aureus* (MSSA) make up approximately 70% of S *aureus* strains and are appropriately treated with semisynthetic penicillins such as nafcillin, oxacillin, and dicloxacillin, which are not broken down by penicillinase. First-generation cephalosporins are also highly efficacious. Note that methicillin is no longer used clinically because of concerns about nephrotoxicity.

Unfortunately, multidrug-resistant strains of S *aureus* have developed in the past half-century. These strains, termed **methicillin-resistant *Staphylococcus aureus*,** or **MRSA,** contain an altered PBP, rendering them resistant to the semisynthetic penicillins. Previously, these strains were found only in settings where broad-spectrum antibiotics were commonly used. However, community-acquired MRSA is seen increasingly, especially as skin and skin substructure infections. **Vancomycin** is the cornerstone of MRSA therapy. However, clindamycin, tetracycline, and trimethoprim-sulfamethoxazole (TMP-SMX) may be effective for mild infection.

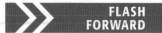

FLASH FORWARD

Osteomyelitis is an important infection, especially in adolescents and immunocompromised individuals. *Staphylococcus aureus* is the **most common causative organism,** but *Salmonella* osteomyelitis is common in patients with sickle cell disease.

Coagulase-Negative *Staphylococcus*

Characteristics

Staphylococcus epidermidis and *S saprophyticus* are commonly isolated *Staphylococcus* species, but are much less clinically significant than *S aureus*. Both appear as gram-positive cocci in small clusters and are catalase-positive, but do not contain the coagulase enzyme. Of note, *S epidermidis* is sensitive to the antibiotic **novobiocin,** whereas *S saprophyticus* is resistant.

Clinical Symptoms

Staphylococcus epidermidis is a constituent of normal bacterial skin flora. In healthy, individuals, this species is not a major cause of disease. However, it can cause major infections of **mechanical prostheses** (eg, prosthetic joints, mechanical heart valves) as well as **indwelling catheters** (vascular) because of the organism's unique polysaccharide capsule. These diseases are usually characterized by an indolent course with systemic symptoms developing slowly, if at all.

Staphylococcus saprophyticus is the second most common cause of community-acquired UTIs in sexually active women (*E coli* being the most common). Symptoms are typical and include dysuria, pyuria, and bacteruria.

Treatment

Over 50% of *S epidermidis* isolates are methicillin-resistant and thus require vancomycin or alternative treatment. *Staphylococcus saprophyticus* responds to typical empiric treatment for urinary tract infections with TMP-SMX, fluoroquinolones, and others.

> **KEY FACT**
>
> *Staphylococcus epidermidis* is one of the most frequently isolated organisms from blood cultures in hospitals. This is usually due to contamination of the venipuncture needle rather than true *S epidermidis* bacteremia.

GRAM-POSITIVE RODS

Gram-positive rods fall into two general categories: The spore-forming—or **sporulating**—rods, and the non–spore-forming rods. The anaerobic *Clostridium* spp. and the aerobic *Bacillus* spp. form **endospores** under conditions of metabolic stress, and these spores are seen under phase (wet-mount) microscopy, enabling easy differentiation. *Listeria monocytogenes*, *C diphtheriae*, and the actinomycetes (*Actinomyces* spp. and *Nocardia* spp.) make up the heterogeneous group of nonsporulating gram-positive rods.

Sporulating Gram-Positive Rods

The medically important gram-positive rods in this category are universally soil microbes. The endospore that they produce is actually thought to be an evolutionary adaptation to the dehydration these organisms can experience in exposed environments. Pathogenically, these microorganisms cause disease by secreting powerful exotoxins. Invasive disease is not characteristic and, since the toxins are usually preformed, antibiotics are of limited efficacy in treatment of disease.

Clostridium Botulinum

Characteristics

Clostridium botulinum is a gram-positive, sporulating rod that is anaerobic, thus growing only in specially designed anaerobic environments. It produces a highly virulent exotoxin that leads to **flaccid muscular paralysis.**

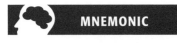
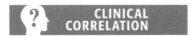
PATHOGENESIS

The botulism exotoxin is a **heat-labile A-B neurotoxin** that inhibits the release of acetylcholine (ACh) at neuromuscular junctions, leading to flaccid paralysis. There are seven serotypes, A–G; however, the serotypes that most commonly cause disease are **A, B,** and **E.** People never develop natural immunity to botulism toxin because of its extreme toxicity; even amounts too small to initiate an immune response can be fatal if untreated. Botulism toxin is a potential biologic weapon and is listed as a CDC category A **bioterrorism agent.**

CLINICAL SYMPTOMS

There are three clinical presentations of botulism toxicity.

- **Food-borne botulism** is the only form that results from ingestion of pre-formed toxins.
  - Patients complain of blurred or double vision, difficulty speaking or swallowing, droopy eyes or muscle weakness, and GI symptoms. The paralytic effects progress in a descending fashion.
  - This disease often occurs 1–2 days after eating homemade canned or preserved foods. Improperly processed food offers the anaerobic environment that spores need to germinate and synthesize botulism toxin.
  - Once ingested, the exotoxin is absorbed through the gut and travels in the blood to nerve synapses.
  - Patients need to be treated immediately because the toxin may compromise respiratory muscles. Treatment includes antitoxin and respiratory support.
- **Infant botulism** results when babies ingest spores found in household dust or (the classic scenario) **honey.**
  - The spores germinate in the gut and produce the exotoxin, which is absorbed into the blood.
  - Symptoms include constipation, limp body, loss of head control, dysphagia, weak feeding, and weak crying. This disease is sometimes referred to as **floppy baby syndrome** because of the severe loss of muscle tone and control.
  - Treatment includes respiratory support and human-derived polyvalent antitoxin (serotypes A, B, and E). A human-derived antitoxin rather than the equine-derived antitoxin is given to prevent any risk of type III hypersensitivity reaction.
  - Prognosis is good, even without the use of humanized antitoxin.
- **Wound botulism** occurs from traumatic implantation and germination of spores at the wound site.
  - Botulism toxin is produced in vivo and disseminated throughout the body. Symptoms are the same as those for food-borne botulism, without GI symptoms.
  - Patients are treated with respiratory support, equine-derived polyvalent antitoxin, and antibiotics to eradicate the bacteria.

TREATMENT

Antitoxin is the cornerstone of treatment for all varieties of botulism. Antitoxin is a fraction of serum (usually equine) obtained from an animal that has been inoculated with the antigen in question. This serum contains polyclonal antibodies that can neutralize the botulism toxin. Antibiotics and supportive care are also important in selected situations.

CLOSTRIDIUM TETANI

CHARACTERISTICS

Like other *Clostridium* species, this anaerobic gram-positive rod produces spores that are generally found in the soil. These spores are inoculated into puncture wounds, which provide an ideal environment for germination.

PATHOGENESIS

The bacteria produce **tetanus toxin,** also known as tetanospasmin, a neuro-toxin that binds peripheral nerve terminals and travels intra-axonally from the site of entry to the CNS. Like botulism toxin, tetanus toxin does not induce an immune response because of its sheer potency. It binds ganglioside receptors at the presynaptic inhibitory nerve ending, selectively cleaves synaptobre-vin, a protein component of the synaptic vesicle, and **prevents the release of the inhibitory neurotransmitters** (GABA and glycine). Without inhibitory signals, excitatory neurons are unopposed, causing sustained muscle contraction or **tetany.**

CLINICAL SYMPTOMS

Patients with tetanus present with severe, unopposed muscle contractions. Often, this is most evident in the muscles of the jaw, producing the characteristic **risus sardonicus** (strange grin), or lockjaw (Figure 5-14).

TREATMENT

The major modality for control and prevention of tetanus is the **tetanus toxoid** vaccine. This is a formalin-inactivated toxin that is first injected as part of the **DTaP** vaccine (diphtheria-tetanus-acellular pertussis). Since immunity is fleeting, booster shots are given every 10 years.

Treatment of active tetanus infection is accomplished with antibiotics (usually metronidazole), antitetanus immune globulin, an immediate tetanus booster, extensive debridement, and muscle relaxants. Rapid response is critical to prevent death secondary to respiratory complications.

CLOSTRIDIUM PERFRINGENS

CHARACTERISTICS

This anaerobic, spore-forming soil bacterium is well known for causing **gas gangrene,** a debilitating and often fatal infection of muscle tissue.

PATHOGENESIS

Traumatic implantation of the spores into muscle tissue (ie, by a puncture wound) causes germination and the release of the α **toxin,** a lecithinase that can necrotize tissue and destroy blood and vascular cells. Other toxins are released as well, some of which are capable of catalyzing a **fermentation reaction,** causing the release of intraparenchymal **gas.**

CLINICAL SYMPTOMS

The most serious infection caused by *C perfringens* is the aforementioned gas gangrene, also known as **clostridial myonecrosis.** This infection is characterized by **tissue crepitus** (the palpable and audible presence of subcuticular air or gas) and rapid, widespread necrosis of muscular tissue with rapidly ensuing death. Other soft tissue infections with significantly less severe presentations, and gastroenteritis (watery diarrhea), are also possible sequelae.

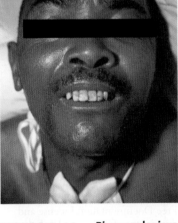

FIGURE 5-14. **Risus sardonicus of tetanus.** (Image courtesy of CDC's Public Health Image Library; content provider Dr. Thomas F. Sellers.)

TREATMENT

Treatment of gas gangrene involves debridement, high-dose penicillin, and hyperbaric O_2 (to provide a toxic atmosphere for the anaerobic clostridia). Mortality is unfortunately still high in the most severe infections.

CLOSTRIDIUM DIFFICILE

CHARACTERISTICS

Clostridium difficile is another anaerobic, spore-forming organism that causes **antibiotic-associated colitis** (the severe variant is known as **pseudomembranous colitis**), which is common among hospitalized patients, especially those on broad-spectrum antibiotics.

PATHOGENESIS

Clostridium difficile is a normal component of the intestinal flora of some people (and is easily spread to others via its hardy spores). Because of its relative antibiotic resistance, it has the tendency to proliferate in the colon during treatment with broad-spectrum antibiotics, thus outcompeting the susceptible normal enteric flora. At this point, the organism produces **enterotoxin** and **cytotoxin**, which cause the characteristic secretory diarrhea.

CLINICAL SYMPTOMS

Clinically, patients present with an acute episode of watery diarrhea and abdominal cramping. In severe cases, a **pseudomembrane** composed of sloughed inflammatory cells, fibrin, and mucus is seen overlying intact colonic mucosa (Figure 5-15).

TREATMENT

Appropriate treatment is discontinuation of broad-spectrum antibiotics and treatment with **oral metronidazole** (preferred) or **oral vancomycin.**

BACILLUS ANTHRACIS

CHARACTERISTICS

This spore-forming facultative anaerobe is the causative agent of **anthrax.** The microbe has received much press in recent years because of its potential as a bioweapon. It is a relatively large, sporulating, nonmotile gram-positive rod that primarily infects herbivores or lives in the soil as a resilient spore. Transmission to humans is usually via traumatic implantation or inhalation of spores from infected animals or, more recently, via inhalation of intentionally placed spores.

PATHOGENESIS

Three virulence factors are largely responsible for most of the clinical manifestations of *B anthracis.* The organism possesses a unique, immunogenic **capsule** composed of a polypeptide that prevents phagocytosis. **Protective antigen** allows entry of other toxins into cells, and **edema factor** activates adenylate cyclase, causing osmotic cell swelling. The ominous-sounding **lethal factor** is a cytotoxic protein that causes inflammation, macrophage activation, and cell death.

CLINICAL SYMPTOMS

There are three categories of clinical anthrax, which correspond completely with the route of contact with the pathogen or its spores.

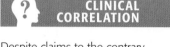

CLINICAL CORRELATION

Despite claims to the contrary, *C difficile* colitis cannot be diagnosed based on the smell of the offending stool alone. One or both toxins must be isolated from stool specimens.

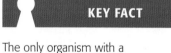

FIGURE 5-15. Pseudomembranous colitis. Note the confluent pseudomembrane covering the colon. (Image courtesy of Wikipedia; permission granted per the GNU Free Documentation License and the Creative Commons Attribution ShareAlike 3.0 license.)

KEY FACT

The only organism with a polypeptide capsule is *B anthracis.* All other known capsules are composed of polysaccharides.

■ **Cutaneous anthrax** occurs when humans have direct epidermal contact with *B anthracis* spores. A characteristic papule progresses to vesiculation/ulceration and subsequently to black eschar and central necrosis, all at the original site of inoculation (Figure 5-16). The lesion itself is painless, but painful regional lymphadenopathy and systemic disease can develop. The mortality rate is approximately 10%.

■ **Pulmonary (inhalational) anthrax** occurs when spores are inhaled, either from animals (**woolsorter's disease**) or from **weaponized** preparations. Nonspecific symptoms such as fever, headache, cough, malaise, and chest pain are the usual initial manifestations. Untreated, this disease leads to **massively enlarged mediastinal lymph nodes,** pulmonary hemorrhage, meningeal symptoms, and often (50%) death.

■ **Gastrointestinal anthrax** is caused by ingestion of live spores; it is highly lethal but rare.

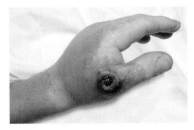

FIGURE 5-16. Cutaneous anthrax on the thumb of a child. (Reproduced with permission from Wolff K, Johnson RA, Suurmond D. *Fitzpatrick's Color Atlas & Synopsis of Clinical Dermatology*, 5th ed. New York: McGraw-Hill, 2005: 631.)

TREATMENT

Immediate antibiotic treatment as soon as the diagnosis is suspected is the key to preventing fatality. Ciprofloxacin is the agent of choice, although several alternatives are available. Prevention is focused on **animal vaccination;** a human vaccine is available but has major side effects and is routinely given only to at-risk populations.

BACILLUS CEREUS

CHARACTERISTICS

Bacillus cereus is another motile, spore-forming gram-negative rod, but its virulence is much lower than that of *B anthracis*.

PATHOGENESIS

The spores are ubiquitously found in nature and are typically ingested in food sources. **Reheated fried rice** is a common source, since microwaving typically does not kill the spores.

CLINICAL SYMPTOMS

Two forms of GI disease are possible: An **emetic** form manifesting as rapid-onset vomiting and diarrhea, and a **diarrheal** form characterized by a watery, secretory diarrhea.

TREATMENT

Both forms typically resolve without sequelae, and antibiotic treatment is not indicated.

Nonsporulating Gram-Positive Rods

LISTERIA MONOCYTOGENES

Listeria is an uncommon human pathogen responsible for important diseases affecting neonates. It is a short gram-positive rod that exhibits **tumbling motility** at room temperature and is easily grown on agar, **even at cold temperatures.** Like many opportunistic pathogens, it is ubiquitous in nature and can be found in animals, soil, and even as asymptomatic colonizers of the human GI tract. When a source is identified, it is often a refrigerated, contaminated food product such as soft cheese, cabbage, or milk.

PATHOGENESIS

Infection is often precipitated by ingestion and subsequent transmucosal uptake by cells of the GI tract. *Listeria monocytogenes* is also a facultative intracellular organism, enabling it to evade clearance by phagocytosis.

CLINICAL SYMPTOMS

Neonatal listeriosis can take on two forms. **Early-onset disease** (also known as **granulomatosis infantiseptica**) occurs as a result of transplacental transmission and is characterized by late miscarriage or birth complicated by sepsis, multiorgan abscesses, and disseminated granulomas. The mortality rate is extremely high. **Late-onset disease** typically is transmitted during childbirth and manifests as meningitis or meningoencephalitis occurring 2–3 weeks later. Therefore, pregnant women should avoid eating soft cheeses.

Adult listeriosis (in pregnant, elderly, or immunocompromised individuals) can present as bacteremia, sepsis, or meningitis. Signs and symptoms are not unique to this organism, so other causes need to be ruled out. Mortality is rare.

TREATMENT

Listeria monocytogenes is intrinsically resistant to cephalosporins, and the mainstays of treatment are IV penicillin or ampicillin, often combined with gentamicin for synergy.

CORYNEBACTERIUM DIPHTHERIAE

This important comma-shaped bacteria is the causative agent of the once-prevalent childhood pharyngitis **diphtheria.** They are small, pleomorphic irregular-staining gram-positive rods that are observed to contain **metachromatic** (red or blue) **granules** when stained with methylene blue (Figure 5-17). They can grow on most media, but **tellurite-containing medium** is often used to selectively isolate the organism from pharyngeal swab specimens.

Because of an extensive childhood vaccination campaign, *C diphtheriae* has become rare in the developed world, but cases are still relatively common in impoverished urban areas in the Third World. Transmission is via respiratory droplets from unvaccinated individuals or asymptomatic vaccinated carriers.

PATHOGENESIS

The virulence of *C diphtheriae* is almost entirely due to the **diphtheria toxin,** an exotoxin that is encoded on a lysogenic bacteriophage virus called **β-phage.** Not all bacteria express the toxin, since expression relies on infection with the bacteriophage. The toxin itself is a classic A-B toxin; component B allows entry of the A subunit into the cells. The A subunit in this case is an ADP-ribosyltransferase enzyme that **inactivates elongation factor EF-2** via ADP-ribosylation, thereby inhibiting protein synthesis.

CLINICAL SYMPTOMS

Diphtheria generally manifests as an **exudative pharyngitis** causing dysphagia (pain on swallowing), fever, and malaise following an incubation period of less than 1 week. As the disease progresses, a thick **pseudomembrane** (made up of fibrin, dead cells, bacteria, and leukocytes) forms on the posterior oropharynx and tonsils. This membrane is gray and tightly adherent and **cannot be scraped off** without causing bleeding of the underlying tissue. After another

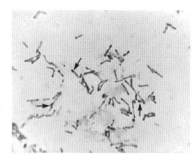

FIGURE 5-17. *Corynebacterium diphtheriae.* This specimen was stained with methylene blue; metachromatic granules are designated with arrows. (Reproduced with permission from Brooks GF, Butel JS, Morse SA. *Jawetz, Melnick, & Adelberg's Medical Microbiology*, 23rd ed. New York: McGraw-Hill, 2004: 214.)

week, this membrane spontaneously dislodges, although complications can arise from airway compromise from the membrane. Other features of the disease include cervical lymphadenopathy and edema, resulting in the characteristic **bull-neck** appearance. Cardiac and lower respiratory complications are rare but potentially fatal.

Diagnosis of diphtheria is usually clinical, but clinical specimens are generally tested for pathogenicity using the **Elek test,** an in vitro assay that tests for the production of exotoxin.

TREATMENT

The cornerstone of treatment of active diphtheria is the early administration of **diphtheria antitoxin** to neutralize extant exotoxin, and appropriate antibiotic therapy (penicillin or erythromycin).

PREVENTION

Prevention has been largely successful in the United States, owing to routine childhood immunization with nontoxic **diphtheria toxoid** as part of the DTaP vaccine series.

ACTINOMYCETES

The actinomycetes are a group of gram-positive rods that typically live in soil and have unique, fungus-like microscopic morphology with branching and hyphal forms. There are a staggering number of these organisms, many of which cause rare opportunistic or pulmonary infections. Two actinomycetes are particularly important and are discussed here.

NOCARDIA SPECIES

CHARACTERISTICS

Nocardia is a strictly aerobic actinomycete that is distinguished from many others because it is partially **acid-fast** on carbol-fuchsin stain (unlike *Actinomyces*).

CLINICAL SYMPTOMS

This organism causes indolent bronchopulmonary infections, especially in individuals with **decreased T-cell immunity.** Cavitary pulmonary lesions as well as hematogenous spread to the skin and CNS are common. Primary cutaneous lesions such as cellulitis, subcutaneous abscesses, and **mycetomas** can develop as well. Mycetomas are chronic, destructive cutaneous lesions caused by actinomycetes that generally feature sinus tracts communicating with the epidermal surface, painless edema, and subcutaneous abscesses.

TREATMENT

Treatment is with sulfonamides or TMP-SMX.

ACTINOMYCES ISRAELII

CHARACTERISTICS

Unlike its partner *Nocardia*, *Actinomyces israelii* is an anaerobic actinomycete that is not acid-fast. It is a constituent of the normal mouth flora of some humans.

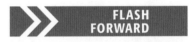

FLASH FORWARD

The causative agent of **Whipple disease, *Tropheryma whipplei,*** is also an actinomycete.

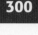
CLINICAL SYMPTOMS

Typically causes slowly developing oral and facial abscesses with an underlying yellow color due to the presence of so-called **sulfur granules**. These granules are actually massive collections of *Actinomyces* organisms. Sinus tract drainage of these abscesses to the skin surface is common. Other potential sites for actinomycosis are the brain, chest cavity, and abdominopelvic region. Mycetomas are also possible.

TREATMENT

Via surgical incision and drainage coupled with penicillin or ampicillin.

GRAM-NEGATIVE COCCI

Neisseria

The only two medically important gram-negative cocci are N *meningitidis* or **meningococcus,** which causes meningitis and sepsis; and N *gonorrhoeae* or **gonococcus,** which causes gonorrhea, disseminated gonococcal disease, and ophthalmia neonatorum. All *Neisseria* are small aerobic gram-negative cocci typically seen on microscopy as coffee-bean-like **diplococci** or in clumps (Figure 5-18). Both are oxidase-positive (in contrast to the oxidase-negative Enterobacteriaceae). *Neisseria meningitidis* can be differentiated from N *gonorrhoeae* by two distinguishing features:

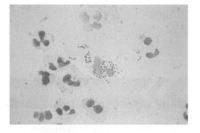

FIGURE 5-18. *Neisseria gonorrhoeae* **as seen on preparation from urethral discharge.** Microorganisms are arranged in side-by-side pairs and small clumps. (Image courtesy of Wikipedia; permission granted per the GNU Free Documentation License and the Creative Commons Attribution ShareAlike 3.0 Unported license.)

- A polysaccharide capsule that inhibits phagocytosis.
- Metabolizes both glucose and maltose (*Neisseria gonorrhoeae* only metabolizes glucose).
- *Eikenella* and *Kingella* are uncommon opportunistic pathogens and rarely are implicated in SBE.

PATHOGENESIS

Except for the aforementioned meningococcal capsule, N *meningitidis* and N *gonorrhoeae* share the same virulence factors:

- **Pili** mediate mucosal surface attachment. The pili of N *gonorrhoeae* undergo rapid antigenic variation, so there is a corresponding **lack of long-term immunity** to gonococcal infection.
- **Por** proteins form outer membrane pores that allow passage of nutrients and waste materials and, in some cases, prevent complement-dependent killing of the bacteria.
- **Opa** proteins are involved in surface adhesion.
- **LOS** (lipooligosaccharide) is a variant of gram-negative endotoxin (LPS) that does not possess the O-polysaccharide moiety present in LPS but still possesses endotoxin-like cytotoxic capabilities.
- **IgA proteases** cleave the immunoglobulin IgA into its inactive constituents thus foiling mucosal adaptive immunity.
- **Siderophores** allow collection of iron from human iron-binding proteins (transferrin).

NEISSERIA MENINGITIDIS

CHARACTERISTICS

Meningococcus is the organism responsible for most cases of bacterial meningitis in adolescents and certain at-risk populations (military trainees, dormitory residents). In addition, it can cause debilitating sepsis known as **meningococ-**

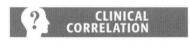

cemia. The microorganism is transmitted by respiratory droplets and can be a normal constituent of the oropharyngeal flora.

Pathogenesis

As stated, this important pathogen possesses an antiphagocytic polysaccharide capsule, which is the basis of its subclassification into several serogroups. Serogroups A, B, C, Y, and W-135 are responsible for most infections. This capsule is immunogenic and is used to synthesize the meningococcal vaccine.

Clinical Symptoms

Once resident in the nasopharynx, N meningitidis can cause local symptoms, such as painful swallowing and fever. More important, it can easily spread to other subepithelial locations and cause significant disease.

Meningococcemia is a life-threatening meningococcal sepsis that results in severe multiorgan disease characterized pathologically by small-vessel thrombosis and overwhelming consumptive coagulopathy. As a result, a characteristic **petechial,** or **purpuric, rash** is often seen on the trunk and lower extremities (Figure 5-19). Fulminant meningococcemia can result in septic shock and bilateral **hemorrhagic destruction of the adrenal glands;** this symptom complex is known as **Waterhouse-Friderichsen syndrome.**

Meningococcal meningitis is a sequela of meningococcal invasion of the meninges of the CNS. Typical symptoms include an abrupt onset of fever, chills, stiff neck, headache, and vomiting. Meningeal signs are often present as well. Mortality rate is approximately 10% in appropriately treated patients, and complications such as long-term neurologic damage are rare.

Meningococcus is an uncommon cause of pneumonia and is usually observed with signs and symptoms of pharyngitis.

Treatment

Neisseria meningitidis is almost universally sensitive to penicillin, which, owing to the severity of the disease, is usually given parenterally in cases of severe meningococcal infection. **Rifampin** can be used for chemoprophylaxis of close contacts of affected individuals. Currently, the American Academy of Pediatrics recommends vaccinating all adolescents at age 11–12 with the meningococcal conjugate vaccine, which covers four of the five most common disease-causing serogroups (capsule polysaccharide from serogroup B is not sufficiently immunogenic to synthesize a vaccine).

Neisseria gonorrhoeae

Characteristics

Like N meningitidis, N gonorrhoeae is an aerobic gram-negative coccus that is responsible for serious infections in humans. It possesses the same virulence factors as N meningitidis except that it lacks a polysaccharide capsule. It is responsible for the sexually transmitted infection **gonorrhea** as well as a disseminated variant. Passage through an infected vaginal canal during parturition can result in purulent gonococcal infection of the eye, termed **ophthalmia neonatorum.** Transmission is otherwise via unprotected sexual contact.

Attempts to isolate gonococcus from clinical samples (eg, urethral swabs) are usually performed on **Thayer-Martin (VCN) medium,** which is supplemented with antibiotics to prevent overgrowth of normal genital flora.

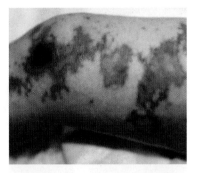

FIGURE 5-19. Purpura fulminans due to acute meningococcemia. (Reproduced with permission from Wolff K, Johnson RA, Suurmond D. *Fitzpatrick's Color Atlas & Synopsis of Clinical Dermatology,* 5th ed. New York: McGraw-Hill, 2005: 643.)

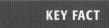

KEY FACT

Meningeal signs include **nuchal rigidity** and **Kernig** and **Brudzinski signs.** All are signs of **meningeal irritation** (though have fairly low sensitivity) and their presence should prompt a meningitis work-up.

Kernig sign is positive when the leg is fully bent at the hip and knee, and extension of the knee is painful. Brudzinski sign is elicited while the patient is lying supine and is positive when lifting of the patient's head causes the patient's legs to involuntarily lift as well.

KEY FACT

Gonorrhea is the second most common sexually transmitted infection in the United States, following only *Chlamydia trachomatis.*

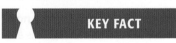

KEY FACT

Pelvic inflammatory disease is usually polymicrobial; however, gonococcus or *C trachomatis* (or both) are commonly involved.

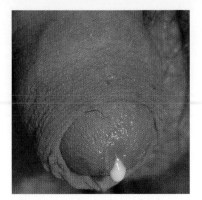

FIGURE 5-20. Urethral discharge secondary to gonorrhea. Frank purulent discharge is a common feature, especially in infected males. (Reproduced with permission from Wolff K, Johnson RA, Suurmond D. *Fitzpatrick's Color Atlas & Synopsis of Clinical Dermatology,* 5th ed. New York: McGraw-Hill, 2005: 907.)

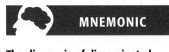

MNEMONIC

The diagnosis of disseminated gonococcal infection is an ART:

Arthralgia
Rash
Tenosynovitis

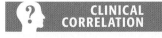

CLINICAL CORRELATION

Empiric antibiotic therapy for genital gonorrhea should always include coverage for coinfection with **C trachomatis.** For this reason, **azithromycin** or **doxycycline** is usually added to standard single-dose intramuscular **ceftriaxone** for gonorrhea.

KEY FACT

Haemophilus influenzae does **not cause influenza,** although it is an important cause of postinfluenza pneumonia.

CLINICAL SYMPTOMS

- Uncomplicated genital gonorrhea is generally found as acute, purulent **urethritis** in males (Figure 5-20) and either as acute **cervicitis** or an asymptomatic finding in females. Most infected men present with acute onset of dysuria and discharge. Infected women may experience abdominal pain, vaginal discharge, and dysuria; however, the infection is often asymptomatic in women.
- **Gonococcal pharyngitis** is an uncommon cause of sore throat, inevitably caused by orogenital contact.
- A significant complication of untreated disease in females is ascending genital tract infection, termed **pelvic inflammatory disease (PID),** in which the infection spreads to the uterus, salpinges, and ovaries. Symptoms are protean and include abdominal pain, cervical motion tenderness, dysuria, fever, nausea, and vomiting. Serious sequelae of PID include **tubo-ovarian abscess, infertility,** and increased probability of **ectopic pregnancy.**
- **Disseminated gonococcal infection** via hematogenous spread is also possible following local gonococcal infection. This is often manifested as acute, painful, asymmetrical migratory polyarthralgia, frequently seen in a clinical triad with **tenosynovitis** (inflammation of the tendon capsule, often on the dorsum of the hand) and a painless, nonpruritic **rash.** Acute suppurative **septic arthritis** with swollen, painful knees, wrists, and ankles is also seen in disseminated infection.
- **Gonococcal ophthalmia neonatorum** manifests as an acute purulent conjunctivitis several days after birth. All newborns in the United States routinely receive intraocular antibiotics as prophylaxis against ocular gonococcal and chlamydial infections.

TREATMENT

Resistance rates to penicillin and tetracycline are high, and resistance to the previous first-line therapy of fluoroquinolones is on the rise. Therefore, first-line therapy is usually a **third-generation cephalosporin,** such as intramuscular ceftriaxone. Prior infections do not confer immunity, so efforts at disease prevention are currently focused on barrier methods of contraception.

GRAM-NEGATIVE RODS

Because of the plethora of medically important gram-negative rods, many medical students find that keeping them straight is a difficult proposition. In this book, the microorganisms are grouped according to the major site of disease to allow for easier learning by categorization (Table 5-13).

Gram-Negative Rods Causing Respiratory and Mucosal Infections

These organisms all appear as small, gram-negative "coccoid" rods when viewed under the microscope and are sometimes described as "coccobacillary" for this reason. The zoonotic bacteria *Brucella* spp. and *Pasteurella multocida* can also fall into this group, although for convenience they are described in the Zoonotic Bacteria section.

HAEMOPHILUS INFLUENZAE

CHARACTERISTICS

Certainly the most clinically important member of the above-defined respiratory group is *H influenzae.* Formerly a major cause of severe childhood respiratory disease, the highly virulent *H influenzae* serotype b (Hib) has now

TABLE 5-13.   Gram-Negative Rods

Respiratory/Mucosal Pathogens	Enteric Pathogens	Zoonotic Pathogens
H influenzae	Enterobacteriaceae family	Yersinia pestis
Haemophilus ducreyi	Vibrio spp.	Francisella tularensis
Gardnerella vaginalis	P aeruginosa	Brucella spp.
B pertussis	Bacteroides fragilis	Pasteurella multocida
Legionella pneumophila	Campylobacter	Bartonella henselae

been largely relegated to the annals of pediatric history owing to remarkable success in vaccination.

- *H influenzae* culture requires the addition of factors V and X, which are found in hydrolyzed blood ("chocolate") agar.
- They appear as small, gram-negative, nonmotile coccobacillary organisms.
- Both encapsulated and nonencapsulated (nontypable) strains exist.
- Encapsulated strains have been characterized as **serotypes a through f.**
- In the prevaccination era, **serotype b** (also known as **Hib**) was responsible for over 95% of invasive pediatric disease.
- Most *H influenzae* disease is now caused by serotypes c, f, and nontypable strains (which can only cause local disease).

Nontypable *H influenzae* contribute to normal bacterial flora of the nasopharyngeal mucosa from an early age, and endogenous infection from these sites is responsible for most localized disease (otitis media, sinusitis, pneumonia). Transmission is by respiratory droplets.

Children younger than 3 years old are uniquely susceptible to infection with encapsulated serotypes of *H influenzae* because specific adaptive immune response to polysaccharide antigens is deficient in young children. Infants younger than 6 months have relative protection due to maternal antibodies passed transplacentally and via breast milk. Immunocompromised, nonvaccinated, and asplenic patients are also at risk.

Pathogenesis

Like all gram-negative organisms, *H influenzae* possesses endotoxin, which is responsible for many of its deleterious effects. Other virulence factors include pili and nonpilus adhesins, which mediate attachment, and the antiphagocytic polysaccharide capsule if present.

Clinical Symptoms

Haemophilus influenzae is responsible for a number of respiratory diseases with varying degrees of severity.

- **Epiglottitis** is perhaps the most memorable of the clinical entities caused by *H influenzae*. It is uncommon now because it is **caused only by Hib.** Affected children are 2–4 years old and present sitting bolt upright with copious drooling, stridor, sore throat, fever, and dyspnea. Rapid airway obstruction leading to death can occur, and **laryngoscopy in the operating room** is required for definitive diagnosis.

MNEMONIC

HaEMOPhIuS influenzae **causes:**

Epiglottitis
Meningitis
Otitis media
Pneumonia
eye –"**I**"–infections (conjunctivitis)
Sinusitis

■ **Meningitis** also only results from infection with serotype b. Formerly, it was the major causative organism of meningitis in infants 6 months to 3 years old. Since children at this age do not commonly present with the typical meningitic symptom of stiff neck, the diagnosis is suspected based on nonspecific signs such as fever, poor feeding, vomiting, and irritability. Mortality is low, but residual neurologic deficits are common.

■ Upper and lower respiratory tract disease (**otitis media** in children, and **pneumonia, conjunctivitis,** and **sinusitis** in anyone) are common manifestations of endogenous *H influenzae* infection caused by colonization with nontypable strains. The organism is among the top two causative agents of otitis media and sinusitis (*S pneumoniae* is the other); pneumonia usually occurs only in previously damaged lungs (smokers and patients recovering from influenza viral pneumonia, for example).

TREATMENT

Minor respiratory tract infections generally respond to treatment with ampicillin or amoxicillin, although resistance rates are increasing (currently approximately 30%). Other options are azithromycin or a "respiratory" cephalosporin. Meningitis requires prompt therapy with CNS-penetrant third-generation cephalosporins (ceftriaxone or cefotaxime).

Chemoprophylaxis of susceptible close contacts is required and rifampin is the drug of choice. More important, immunization of all children with the univalent conjugate vaccine against the *H influenzae* serotype b polysaccharide capsule is recommended—three doses are generally given before 6 months of age.

HAEMOPHILUS DUCREYI

CHARACTERISTICS

The causative organism of **chancroid,** a sexually transmitted infection.

CLINICAL SYMPTOMS

Patients have a tender perineal nodule that eventually ulcerates (Figure 5-21) and is associated with inguinal lymphadenopathy. The differential diagnosis of this condition is important (Table 5-14).

TREATMENT

Treatment is with erythromycin. The major complication is increased rate of transmission of other sexually transmitted diseases through the open sore.

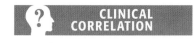

CLINICAL CORRELATION

A **chancroid** is **painful** and should not be confused with the **chancre** of **syphilis,** which is **painless.**

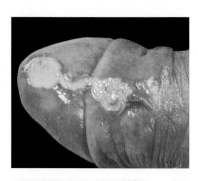

FIGURE 5-21. **An enlarging chancroid with gray exudate.** (Reproduced with permission from Wolff K, Goldsmith LA, Katz SI, et al. *Fitzpatrick's Dermatology in General Medicine,* 7th ed. New York: McGraw-Hill, 2008: Figure 202-2.)

TABLE 5-14. **Differential Diagnosis of Genital Ulceration**

	CHANCROID (*H DUCREYI*)	CHANCRE (SYPHILIS)	GENITAL HERPES (HSV-2)	LYMPHOGRANULOMA VENEREUM (*CHLAMYDIA* L1-3)
Number of ulcers	Single.	Single, rolled edges.	Multiple, vesicular.	Single.
Ulcer painful?	Pain**ful.**	Pain**less.**	Pain**ful.**	Pain**less.**
Regional lymphadenopathy	Unilateral, painful, suppurative.	Bilateral, painless, nonsuppurative.	None, but systemic symptoms present.	Pain**ful,** suppurative; appear after ulcer disappears.

GARDNERELLA VAGINALIS

CHARACTERISTICS

Gardnerella vaginalis is a coccobacillary gram-negative organism that has been isolated from the vaginal mucosa of both asymptomatic females and those with **bacterial vaginosis (BV).**

CLINICAL SYMPTOMS

BV is a polymicrobial colonization of the vagina with *G vaginalis* in addition to a number of anaerobic bacteria. Clinically, it is characterized by intense pruritus, dysuria, and a characteristic **fishy odor** of the copious, frothy secretions when treated with KOH prep. **Clue cells,** which are vaginal epithelial cells covered with coccobacillary bacteria, are seen on wet mount of the discharge (Figure 5-22).

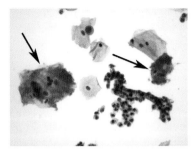

FIGURE 5-22. **Clue cells of bacterial vaginosis.** The image shows the organisms coating squamous cells forming a purple, velvety coat. (Image courtesy of USMLERx.com.)

TREATMENT

Treatment is with metronidazole to cover both *G vaginalis* and anaerobes.

BORDETELLA PERTUSSIS

CHARACTERISTICS

Like *H influenzae* serotype b, *B pertussis* is a former major cause of pediatric respiratory morbidity and mortality that has been largely controlled by an effective vaccination program. It is responsible for **whooping cough.**

- *Bordetella pertussis* is an extremely small, coccobacillary, gram-negative rod.
- It is highly sensitive to drying, so care must be taken when collecting and transporting patient samples.
- The microbe has fastidious nutritional requirements, so specialized media (Bordet-Gengou or Regan-Lowe agars) are required for growth.
- Only 50% of all clinically diagnosed patients have positive cultures.

Bordetella pertussis is highly infective via the nasopharyngeal/respiratory route and infects only humans. Although it is traditionally considered a pediatric disease, whooping cough is now seen in older individuals as well, a phenomenon thought to be secondary to decreased protective effects of childhood vaccination.

PATHOGENESIS

Bordetella pertussis has a number of virulence factors that contribute to its toxicity. **Filamentous hemagglutinin** and **pertactin** are proteins that mediate specific adhesion to ciliated respiratory epithelial cells. **Tracheal cytotoxin** destroys respiratory epithelium directly and may be responsible for the characteristic violent cough. **Pertussis toxin** is a two-part (A-B) exotoxin in which the B component binds the respiratory epithelial cell, allowing entry of the A component. The A component then constitutively inactivates the inhibitory G protein $G\alpha_i$, causing increased cAMP levels and therefore increased respiratory secretions. The **adenylate cyclase toxin** also increases cAMP levels to the same effect.

CLINICAL SYMPTOMS

Pertussis, or whooping cough, is characterized by four stages with relatively distinct clinical features.

- The asymptomatic **incubation** period is 7–10 days.
- The **catarrhal stage** lasts about 10 days. This stage is characterized by typical upper respiratory infection symptoms such as sneezing, low fever, and rhinorrhea. Despite its nonspecific symptoms, this stage harbors the period of maximum infectivity.
- The **paroxysmal stage** then lasts for 2 weeks to 1 month and is characterized by the "whoops" of whooping cough. Patients have periodic paroxysms consisting of repetitive nonproductive coughing followed by an inspiratory "whoop"; this then continues to cycle and is often terminated only by posttussive emesis or exhaustion. Hypoxemia and cyanosis are also seen.
- Finally, the **convalescent stage** lasts for approximately 1 month and is characterized by the gradual reduction in intensity and frequency of paroxysms.

TREATMENT

Macrolide antibiotic therapy is effective only when given during the incubation or catarrhal stages of the disease. Other treatment is generally supportive in nature and is focused on maintenance of a patent airway. Household contacts of patients with pertussis undergo chemoprophylaxis with 14 days of erythromycin.

The acellular pertussis vaccine—which has replaced the complication-prone whole-cell pertussis vaccine—is a key component of the diphtheria-tetanusacellular pertussis combination vaccine (DTaP) recommended for all infants. Five total doses are given. TdaP (tetanus-acellular pertussis) was recently approved as a booster vaccine to reimmunize adolescent and adult individuals who have probable waning immunity from their childhood DTaP series.

LEGIONELLA PNEUMOPHILA

CHARACTERISTICS

Legionella pneumophila, the causative organism of **Legionnaires' disease**, was discovered in 1976 after an outbreak of severe lower respiratory disease at a convention in Philadelphia. During the work-up of this epidemic, this novel organism was discovered to preferentially inhabit natural and artificial bodies of water. Transmission is usually via the inhalation of infectious aerosols. In the case of the Legionnaires' convention, the microbe was found in the air-conditioning system.

Legionella pneumophila is a highly motile, pleomorphic, gram-negative rod that is poorly visualized on Gram staining; therefore, silver or fluorescent antibody staining is generally used. Culture is possible on **buffered charcoal yeast extract agar** supplemented with **cysteine and iron**, but diagnosis is usually made using urine serology.

PATHOGENESIS

The *Legionella* organism is a facultative intracellular microbe, meaning that it multiplies inside the phagosomes of alveolar macrophages following phagocytosis, specifically inhibiting lysosome fusion so that it is not destroyed.

CLINICAL SYMPTOMS

The mild form of legionellosis is an influenza-like illness called **Pontiac fever.** It is characterized by epidemic outbreaks with a high attack rate, as well as

MNEMONIC

Imagine a French **legionnaire** sitting around campfire **(charcoal)** with **iron** dagger—he is no sissy **(cysteine).**

a clinical syndrome of fever, chills, and myalgias with resolution in about 1 week without treatment. Legionnaires' disease itself is a severe community-acquired pneumonia that generally affects elderly persons with underlying lung disease. Clinically presentation includes a nonproductive cough, high fevers, and headache, with a rapid deterioration often leading to death if antibiotic therapy is not promptly started.

TREATMENT

The mainstay of treatment is erythromycin; fluoroquinolones are also highly effective; penicillins are not effective because of the presence of β-lactamase. Following diagnosis, an effort to discover and eradicate the source of infection should be undertaken.

Enteric Gram-Negative Rods

Enteric microbes constitute the normal flora of the GI tract or infect the lumen of the lower alimentary canal. **Pathogenic** enteric microbes can produce syndromes along **two** clinical spectra: diarrheal disease and systemic disease.

Four taxonomic families of enteric organisms are important in medicine:

1. **Enterobacteriaceae:** A large family consisting of organisms such as *Shigella dysenteriae*, *Escherichia coli*, *Salmonella enterica*, and *Klebsiella pneumoniae*. Other notable members of the family include *Yersinia enterocolitica*, *Proteus mirabilis*, *Enterobacter cloacae*, and *Serratia marcescens*.
2. **Vibrionaceae:** Notable organisms are *Vibrio cholerae*, *Campylobacter jejuni*, and *Helicobacter pylori*.
3. **Pseudomonadaceae:** *Pseudomonas aeruginosa*, commonly seen in hospitalized patients.
4. **Bacteroidaceae:** *Bacteroides fragilis*, an anaerobe that can cause gastrointestinal infections.

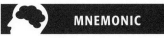

MNEMONIC

COFFEe

Capsulated
O antigen
Flagellar antigen
Ferment glucose
Enterobacteriaceae

ENTEROBACTERIACEAE

CHARACTERISTICS

- **All** are oxidase-negative, facultative anaerobes.
- The **lactose fermentation test** (often accomplished on the selective and differential eosin-methylene blue (EMB) or MacConkey agar) and the ability to **produce hydrogen sulfide (H₂S) gas** are two biochemical tests that help characterize and differentiate members of the Enterobacteriaceae family.
- Nonlactose fermentation and production of H₂S are signs of pathogens associated with severe illness, such as *Shigella*, *Salmonella*, and *Yersinia*.
- If motile, flagella are usually peritrichous (ie, numerous flagella projecting in many directions).
- *Shigella* and *Klebsiella* are nonmotile. *Yersinia* is nonmotile at 37°C but motile at 22°C.

PATHOGENESIS

All Enterobacteriaceae have **O, K,** and **H** antigens, which differ between genera and species and are used to serologically classify clinical isolates. The heat-stable **O antigen** is the outermost polysaccharide layer of the lipopolysaccharide (LPS) (endotoxin) component of the cell wall. The heat-labile **K antigen** refers to the polysaccharide capsule if present, and the heat-labile **H antigen** is a flagellar protein that may be present.

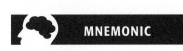

MNEMONIC

OKH antigens—

Outside Kapsule Hello

Outside
Kapsule
H is a flagellum waving **"hello"**

SHIGELLA SPECIES

CHARACTERISTICS

- **Nonmotile,** gram-negative rod-shaped organisms that do **not ferment lactose** but are able to produce H_2S **gas.**
- The four species that make up the genus *Shigella* are **highly virulent** enteric bacteria responsible for many cases of GI disease, especially in pediatric populations and in areas with potentially substandard hygiene (eg, day-care centers)
- Humans are the only host of *Shigella*; unlike many other Enterobacteriaceae, there is **no animal reservoir.** Transmission is from person to person via the fecal-oral route, and as few as 10 organisms may cause symptomatic infection!

PATHOGENESIS

Shigella species cause **invasive** gastroenteritis by specifically attaching to and invading immune cells located in Peyer patches. Much of *Shigella's* virulence can be ascribed to the presence of the highly virulent exotoxin called **Shiga toxin.** The Shiga toxin is a typical A-B toxin in which the B subunit binds to enterocytes, allowing the A unit to penetrate the cells and cause cell death.

CLINICAL SYMPTOMS

The invasive diarrhea caused by *Shigella* species is called **shigellosis** and is characterized by **bloody stools** with pus, fever, and abdominal pain occurring 1–3 days after ingestion of the organism. Initially, diarrhea is often watery. *Shigella dysenteriae* specifically produces the Shiga toxin and can cause a more severe form of the disease termed **bacterial dysentery;** this species is also occasionally associated with the **hemolytic-uremic syndrome.**

TREATMENT

Empiric antibiotic therapy with a fluoroquinolone or trimethoprim-sulfamethoxazole (TMP-SMX) can shorten the course of disease. Other treatments are supportive in nature.

SALMONELLA SPECIES

CHARACTERISTICS

- *Salmonella* species are **motile,** gram-negative rods that, like *Shigella,* produce H_2S **gas,** and do **not ferment lactose.**
- Unlike infection with *Shigella, Salmonella* is normally acquired by eating **contaminated** food products such as contaminated **chicken, egg, or dairy** products.
- Several species exist due to antigenic variation, but the most important distinction is between *Salmonella typhi* (the causative agent of typhoid fever) and the other species.
  - *Salmonella typhi* is the only *Salmonella* that does **not** produce H_2S. Also, *Salmonella typhi* is able to cause the systemic disease called **typhoid fever** because it expresses on its polysaccharide capsule—the rather unusual virulence factor known as the **Vi antigen.**
  - Unlike other *Salmonella* subspecies, *Salmonella typhi* is propagated by a **human host** (fecal-oral route), often from asymptomatic carriers that harbor the organism in their gallbladders.

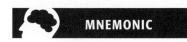

MNEMONIC

The four **F**'s of *Shigella* transmission: **F**ood, **F**ingers, **F**lies, and **F**eces.

PATHOGENESIS

Like *Shigella*, the main route of *Salmonella* invasion is via the M cells of the Peyer patches of the intestine, which may result in hematogenous spread. *Salmonella typhi* can **reside in macrophage vesicles,** allowing it to be carried to extraintestinal sites to cause typhoid fever.

CLINICAL SYMPTOMS

Four different clinical symptoms can result from *Salmonella* infection: gastroenteritis, bacteremia/sepsis, typhoid fever, and an asymptomatic carrier state.

- *Salmonella* **gastroenteritis** is the most common form of salmonellosis. It manifests as an invasive diarrhea characterized by nausea, frequent stools ranging from watery to slightly bloody with mucus, and abdominal pain. Antibiotic therapy does not shorten the course of the disease.
- *Salmonella* **sepsis** is uncommon and has a higher incidence in immunocompromised, pediatric, or elderly patients. Asplenic individuals have difficulty clearing the organism due to its polysaccharide capsule, so hematogenous spread to various end organs (bone, joints, heart) is possible in these individuals.
- **Typhoid fever** (also known as enteric fever) results from *Salmonella typhi* invasion of enterocytes and subsequent intracellular residence in circulating macrophages. It is characterized by the onset of fever, headache, and abdominal pain, **mimicking appendicitis,** approximately 1–3 weeks after exposure. Clinical signs include splenomegaly and occasionally a transient rash (termed **rose spots**) on the abdomen of the patient (Figure 5-23).
- **Asymptomatic carriers** of *Salmonella typhi* constitutively excrete the organism in stool due to colonization of the gallbladder but are completely asymptomatic. This represents the source and reservoir of salmonellosis.

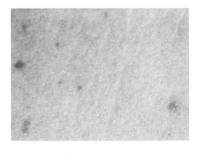

FIGURE 5-23. Rose spots of typhoid fever. These pathognomonic spots appear transiently on light-skinned individuals. (Reproduced with permission from Kasper DL, Braunwald E, Fauci AS, et al. *Harrison's Principles of Internal Medicine,* 16th ed. New York: McGraw-Hill, 2005: 899.)

TREATMENT

Ciprofloxacin or ceftriaxone, among other agents, are appropriate treatments for disseminated disease or typhoid fever. Treatment of asymptomatic carriers is strongly suggested as a public health measure and may require surgical excision of the gallbladder. A vaccine for *Salmonella typhi* is available but is only routinely given to individuals traveling to endemic areas.

ESCHERICHIA COLI

Escherichia coli is the most important of the enteric bacteria. It is associated with many diseases affecting different organ systems.

- *Escherichia coli* is a **motile,** gram-negative, medium-sized rod.
- It is a **lactose fermenter,** thus appearing purple on MacConkey agar.
- *Escherichia coli* does **not** produce H$_2$S gas.
- It is the most common gram-negative rod in the digestive tract.

CLINICAL SYMPTOMS

Diseases caused by *E coli* are numerous and varied. The spectrum ranges from relatively trivial infections such as bacterial cystitis and traveler's diarrhea to neonatal meningitis and gram-negative sepsis.

- *Escherichia coli* **infectious diarrhea** is a major cause of infant mortality worldwide, usually due to dehydration. Several variants of diarrheal illness caused by *E coli* have been characterized in humans. They differ from each other based on affected populations, clinical presentation, pathogenic factors, and severity (Table 5-15).

- The **hemolytic-uremic syndrome (HUS)** is one of the most feared complications of enterohemorrhagic *E coli* (EHEC) infection in children. Approximately 5–10% of infected children younger than 10 years develop the clinical **triad of renal failure, hemolytic anemia,** and **thrombocytopenia,** in addition to bloody diarrhea.
- *Escherichia coli* is by far the **number one** cause of urinary tract infections. Strains of *E coli* possess **pili**-bound adhesion factors, allowing them to attach to the urethral wall and ascend the urinary tract, causing **bacterial cystitis.** This is characterized by dysuria and increased urinary frequency. A common complication of cystitis is **pyelonephritis** or ascending infection of the kidney parenchyma; this complication is commonly associated with **fever, flank pain,** and **vomiting.**
- *Escherichia coli* is the second most common cause of **neonatal meningitis.**
- Gram-negative sepsis is usually nosocomially acquired and caused by *E coli.* It primarily affects debilitated, hospitalized patients, especially following instrumentation or intra-abdominal surgery. Septic shock is the most common cause of death in this group, presumably caused by the endotoxin component of the cell wall.

TABLE 5-15. Diarrhea Caused by *Escherichia coli*

Variant	Epidemiology	Presentation	Pathogenesis	Severity
ETEC—traveler's diarrhea. Found in contaminated water.	Affects infants in developing countries, travelers.	Copious, watery, nonbloody diarrhea up to 20 L/day, abdominal cramping.	Cholera-like heat-labile toxin **LT-I** and heat-stable toxin **STa** stimulate secretion of Cl$^-$ and HCO$_3^-$ ions into intestinal lumen; water follows osmotic load.	Can be fatal in infants if not rehydrated.
EPEC.	Affects infants in developing countries.	Watery diarrhea.	Microcolony formation on the surface of intestinal epithelium with subsequent loss of microvilli → decreased absorption.	Mild to moderate disease.
EIEC.	Rare in developed countries, uncommon worldwide.	Bloody diarrhea with pus, fever, and abdominal pain.	Shares virulence factors with *Shigella* (not Shiga toxin) and can invade enterocytes directly, causing an inflammatory reaction and colitis.	Usually mild; can progress to dysentery.
EHEC, including strain O157:H7. Found in ground beef.	Most common strains causing disease in developed world; **O157:H7** most common in United States.	Hemorrhagic colitis—abdominal pain, bloody diarrhea, no fever; can cause HUS.	**Expresses Shiga-like toxin,** inhibiting protein synthesis and causing enterocyte death.	Usually resolves without treatment; HUS can be fatal.

EHEC = enterohemorrhagic *E coli*; EIEC = enteroinvasive *E coli*; EPEC = enteropathogenic *E coli*; ETEC = enterotoxigenic *E coli*; HUS = hemolytic-uremic syndrome.

TREATMENT

Antibiotics are often **not** indicated in diarrheal infections. Antibiotic choice is dictated by susceptibility testing in the case of disseminated or serious disease. UTIs are usually treated empirically with TMP-SMX, and fluoroquinolones.

KLEBSIELLA PNEUMONIAE

CHARACTERISTICS

Klebsiella is an **encapsulated, lactose-fermenting** member of the Enterobacteriaceae family that causes community-acquired pneumonia.

CLINICAL SYMPTOMS

Alcoholics and others with conditions causing **aspiration** of oral secretions are particularly at risk for this condition, which is characterized by bloody, **currant-jelly** sputum. The pneumonia is **lobar**, severe, often **necrotizing**, and **cavitating**. It can also cause gram-negative sepsis.

PROTEUS MIRABILIS

CHARACTERISTICS

This organism is characterized by its extreme **motility** and its ability to chemically split urea into two molecules of ammonia via its **urease** enzyme.

CLINICAL SYMPTOMS

Proteus mirabilis is a common cause of **urinary tract infections**; in these cases, urinalysis confirms the bacterial diagnosis owing to the **alkaline pH of the urine**.

YERSINIA ENTEROCOLITICA

CHARACTERISTICS

This bacterium is a zoonotic pathogen, infecting mostly farm animals and pets. It is transmitted by ingestion of contaminated water or milk.

CLINICAL SYMPTOMS

Yersinia enterocolitica causes an **invasive gastroenteritis** associated with fever, abdominal pain, and diarrhea (sometimes bloody). It can also spread to the **mesenteric lymph nodes** and produce symptoms of abdominal pain that **closely mimic acute appendicitis**.

CITROBACTER, ENTEROBACTER, MORGANELLA, SERRATIA, EDWARDSIELLA, AND PROVIDENCIA

CHARACTERISTICS

Certain other Enterobacteriaceae **rarely infect immunocompetent patients** and are included here for completeness. *Enterobacter* infections are known for **broad antibiotic resistance**. *S marcescens* infections are usually nosocomially acquired. *S marcescens* culture produces characteristic **bright-red** colonies on agar.

VIBRIONACEAE

CHARACTERISTICS

- Important members of the family are *V cholerae, C jejuni,* and *H pylori.*
- *Vibrio* species are **curved, motile, oxidase-positive** gram-negative rods with a **single polar flagellum**.

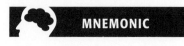

- Three medically relevant members of the *Vibrio* genus exist. The well-known *V cholerae* produces the profuse watery diarrhea of cholera. *Vibrio parahaemolyticus* and *V vulnificus* are both acquired by eating **contaminated shellfish** and cause self-limiting gastroenteritis and wound infections, respectively.

VIBRIO CHOLERAE

CHARACTERISTICS

Vibrio cholerae is a major cause of infant mortality worldwide due to the effects of its **exotoxin**. It is a comma-shaped gram-negative rod that has no specific culture requirements (Figure 5-24). Many serogroups are found in nature; the **O1 and O139 serogroups** are specifically associated with epidemic full-blown cholera.

Vibrio cholerae is generally found in developing or impoverished countries in standing or brackish water contaminated by human feces. The organism can easily multiply and contaminate drinking water, causing epidemics and pandemics. The **"El Tor"** biotype of serogroup O1 was responsible for the most recent worldwide pandemic in the latter half of the previous century. Person-to-person transmission is rare, and inhabitants of endemic areas are often immune.

PATHOGENESIS

The **cholera toxin**, also known as choleragen, is an A-B exotoxin that is secreted upon binding of the cholera bacteria to enterocytes. Once the A subunit gains entry into the cell, it causes constitutive activation of the G protein, $G_{\alpha s}$, which results in the **buildup of cAMP** in a manner similar to the action of pertussis toxin. Because of this cAMP accumulation, sodium and chloride ions are actively extruded into the colon lumen and reabsorption is inhibited.

CLINICAL SYMPTOMS

Affected individuals are rapidly afflicted with **"rice-water stools"** named for their appearance. Massive fluid diarrhea due to osmotic pull of secreted sodium chloride occurs, with **isotonic** fluid losses potentially up to 20 L/day. Electrolyte imbalances (hypokalemia, metabolic acidosis) and hypovolemic shock can occur and lead to death if affected persons are untreated.

TREATMENT

The cornerstone of therapy for cholera is fluid replacement; the use of inexpensive **oral rehydration therapy** in developing countries has saved countless lives. Antibiotic therapy with doxycycline or TMP-SMX in children can shorten the course of the disease.

CAMPYLOBACTER JEJUNI

CHARACTERISTICS

- Similar to *V cholerae*, *Campylobacter jejuni* is a small, curved (comma-shaped), motile gram-negative rod with a polar flagellum.
- Culture conditions require special nutrients contained in **Campy agar** as well as a **microaerophilic** atmosphere (3–15% O_2) and a temperature of 42°C for growth.
- Acquisition of the organism is from contaminated food and water; **undercooked chicken,** and **unpasteurized milk** are common sources.

FIGURE 5-24. *Vibrio cholerae* **in broth culture.** These organisms appear black because this is a phase-contrast micrograph; on Gram stain they would appear red. (Reproduced with permission from Brooks GF, Butel JS, Morse SA. *Jawetz, Melnick, & Adelberg's Medical Microbiology,* 23rd ed. New York: McGraw-Hill, 2004: 271.)

- Although usually not stressed in microbiology textbooks, *Campylobacter* is the single **most common cause of invasive diarrhea.** Over two million incident cases of *C jejuni* infection occur in the United States each year.

PATHOGENESIS

As indicated by its species name, *C jejuni* causes an invasive diarrhea with tissue invasion largely in the **distal small bowel.** Pathologic specimens show ulceration, crypt abscesses, and acute inflammation.

CLINICAL SYMPTOMS

Like other invasive infectious diarrheas, *C jejuni* enteritis is characterized by **bloody diarrhea,** fever, malaise, and abdominal pain. The disease is self-limited. Complications are rare and include sepsis and spontaneous abortion.

TREATMENT

Routine regional enteritis of *C jejuni* infection usually responds to fluid replacement and does not require antibiotic therapy. More serious infections require erythromycin, tetracycline, or fluoroquinolones.

HELICOBACTER PYLORI

CHARACTERISTICS

Helicobacter pylori is an important cause of gastroduodenal pathology.

- It is a corkscrew-shaped, highly motile, gram-negative rod that grows best under microaerophilic conditions.
- Although it shares many characteristics with *C jejuni, H pylori* does **not** grow at 42°C.
- It is found in biopsy specimens of **duodenal ulcers** and **chronic gastritis,** but without evidence of tissue invasion.
- It possesses a **urease** enzyme capable of splitting urea into alkaline ammonia, which allows it to survive in the highly acidic gastric microenvironment.
- Diagnosis is usually made by:
  - Examination of endoscopic biopsies
  - Testing for serum antibodies against *H pylori*
  - Performing the highly specific **urease breath test**
  - Applying immunoassay detection of *H pylori* antigen in stool
- **Triple therapy** (either bismuth-metronidazole-tetracycline/amoxicillin or metronidazole-omeprazole-clarithromycin) eradicates the organism and prevents recurrence of ulcer and gastritis.

PSEUDOMONACEAE

CHARACTERISTICS

Pseudomonas aeruginosa and related organisms constitute a group of microbes that are **opportunistic pathogens** of humans; that is, they mainly infect immunocompromised patients. These **strictly aerobic,** gram-negative rods **do not ferment lactose** and are differentiated from the nonfermentative Enterobacteriaceae (*Shigella, Salmonella,* and others) by the fact that they are **oxidase-positive.** *Pseudomonas aeruginosa* is by far the most common and important of these organisms; the others that make up this group are listed only for completeness: *Burkholderia* spp., *Stenotrophomonas maltophilia,* and *Acinetobacter* spp.

PSEUDOMONAS AERUGINOSA

CHARACTERISTICS

Pseudomonas is an oxidase-positive, gram-negative rod that can be easily identified in a microbiology lab because of its characteristic odor and color. Cultures of this organism (as well as infected surface wounds) have a **bluish green tint** due to the production of the **water-soluble** pigments **pyocyanin** and **fluorescein**. In addition, the bacteria produce a sweet (some people liken it to **grapes**) odor.

The epidemiology of *Pseudomonas* is relatively uncomplicated. It is naturally a **soil** contaminant and is commonly found in **moist** environments, especially within hospitals such as in respiratory ventilators. The organism is **resistant** to many antibiotics and disinfectants, and is primarily transmitted from contaminated surfaces.

PATHOGENESIS

This organism features a number of virulence factors that are key to its unique patterns of toxicity. It does not possess significant invasive ability in healthy hosts, but easily infects hospitalized, immunocompromised patients.

- **Exotoxin A** serves as an inhibitor to elongation factor 2 (EF-2), effectively disrupting protein synthesis in mammalian cells.
- **Endotoxin** (LPS) is a major player in pseudomonal sepsis.
- Some strains have an antiphagocytic polysaccharide **capsule.**
- The organism has connective tissue hydrolases, including **elastases** and an **alkaline protease,** allowing facile spread through infected tissues.
- Through different mechanisms, *Pseudomonas* is **resistant to multiple antibiotics,** and therapy must be carefully chosen.

CLINICAL SYMPTOMS

Pseudomonas has a predilection for causing certain diseases in immunocompromised individuals (Table 5-16).

TREATMENT

Pseudomonas can acquire **resistance** to many commonly used antibiotics, including aminoglycosides, penicillins, and fluoroquinolones. Appropriate therapy is **multiagent** for synergy and generally consists of a parenteral aminoglycoside coupled with an antipseudomonal penicillin such as piperacillin/tazobactam (Zosyn) or ticarcillin/sulbactam (Timentin). Ciprofloxacin and the third-/fourth-generation cephalosporins as well as the carbapenem agents are also usually active against *Pseudomonas*.

The cornerstones of prevention of pseudomonal infection are **sterilization of medical equipment** and prevention of overgrowth of resistant organisms via **appropriate use of broad-spectrum antibiotics,** since elimination of the pathogen from all contaminated surfaces is usually not feasible.

BACTEROIDIACEAE

Although the anaerobic Bacteroidiaceae family has several medically relevant members, the most important is *Bacteroides fragilis*, commonly implicated in visceral abscesses. Other members of the family include organisms causing periodontal disease and aspiration pneumonia such as *Bacteroides* spp., *Fusobacterium* spp., and *Porphyromonas* spp. In general, **anaerobic infections tend to be polymicrobial,** with a number of different organisms responsible for pathology.

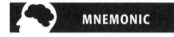

MNEMONIC

PSEUDO*monas* **causes:**

Pneumonia
Sepsis/**S**kin infections
Endocarditis/**E**xternal otitis
Urinary tract infection/corneal **U**lcers
Diabetic infections
Osteomyelitis

TABLE 5-16. Diseases Caused by *Pseudomonas aeruginosa*

DISEASE	SUSCEPTIBLE POPULATION(S)	CLINICAL SYNDROME
Pneumonia	Cystic fibrosis (CF).	Almost all CF patients are **colonized** with *Pseudomonas,* and exacerbations of the underlying disease are often associated with a necrotizing, destructive pseudomonal pneumonia. In CF patients, *Pseudomonas* forms **mucoid biofilms** that inhibit phagocytosis and decrease antibiotic penetration, thus establishing pseudomonal colonization of the CF patient's lungs.
	Prior therapy with broad-spectrum antibiotics, or respiratory instrumentation.	Diffuse, bilateral necrotizing pneumonia with high mortality rate.
Urinary tract infections	Urinary instrumentation, broad-spectrum antibiotics.	Typical UTI symptoms of dysuria, pyuria, and urgency.
Osteomyelitis	Diabetics.	*Pseudomonas* is often the causative agent of infected **diabetic** foot ulcers.
	Children after puncture trauma.	Through-and-through **puncture** into the foot can lead to the introduction of *Pseudomonas* from the moist shoe environment into the wound.
Malignant otitis externa (OE)	Diabetics.	Typical OE is characterized by **pain on ear traction** and sometimes discharge; malignant OE is a severe and potentially fatal complication characterized by spread into the mastoid, with resultant destruction of bone and cranial nerves.
Wound infections	Burn patients.	The moist environment of the burn surface is an ideal breeding ground for *Pseudomonas.* One of the most feared complications of topical burns, is that it can lead to gram-negative sepsis.
Hot tub folliculitis	Anyone.	Inflammation of hair follicles with characteristic rash after immersion in warm, contaminated water.
Sepsis	Neutropenia, diabetics, extensive burns, leukemia.	Extremely high mortality rate for gram-negative sepsis.
Endocarditis	Intravenous drug abusers.	Infects right-sided heart valves.
Corneal ulcers	Contact lens wearers.	Usually occurs after incidental trauma to the eye; can rapidly progress if untreated.

UTI = urinary tract infection.

Culturing obligate anaerobic bacteria presents a special problem; specific culture media as well as an O_2-free atmosphere are required. Treatment of these infections must include clindamycin, metronidazole, or other antibiotics with activity against anaerobes.

BACTEROIDES FRAGILIS

CHARACTERISTICS

This **obligate anaerobe** is a gram-negative organism that lives within the alimentary and female reproductive tracts. When an **interruption** occurs in the wall of these areas (eg, due to surgery, septic abortion, pelvic inflammatory disease, intestinal rupture), these organisms seed the intraperitoneal cavity, forming **abscesses.**

CLINICAL SYMPTOMS

Fever and localized pain are the presenting symptoms of *B fragilis* abscesses, and systemic hematogenous spread can result.

Zoonotic Gram-Negative Bacteria

Zoonotic infections are, by definition, acquired from reservoirs principally existing in animals: humans are usually accidental hosts. Wild or domesticated animals are the principal sources of infection of the following organisms. Transmission usually occurs by direct contact with the animal in question.

YERSINIA PESTIS

CHARACTERISTICS

Yersinia pestis is the causative organism of the **plague,** the "Black Death" that decimated the population of Europe during the 1300s. As a gram-negative, lactose-fermenting rod, it is related to the enteric pathogen *Y enterocolitica* but produces a markedly different clinical syndrome. It is a facultatively intracellular organism and is disseminated throughout the body by macrophages following phagocytosis.

The natural reservoirs of *Y pestis* are **rats** in the urban setting and other **wild rodents** in more rural areas. Transmission is accomplished either by the bite of an infected rodent or by a secondary vector such as fleas. Currently, very few cases are reported in the United States, with most cases restricted to the American Southwest.

PATHOGENESIS

Yersinia pestis possesses an antiphagocytic **protein** capsule (called **F1**) as well as the **V** and **W** antigens, of unknown function. These antigens allow the organisms to reside in the phagosomes of macrophages without destroying them. Very few organisms are required for infection to occur.

CLINICAL SYMPTOMS

Two syndromes are associated with *Y pestis* infection: **bubonic plague** and **pneumonic plague.**

- **Bubonic plague** occurs after direct contact with an infected rodent or flea and is characterized by the presence of **buboes**—erythematous, painful, and swollen inguinal or axillary lymph nodes that become indurated about 1 week after exposure (Figure 5-25). High fever and cutaneous hemorrhage follow, and bacteremia and multiorgan involvement are inevitable without treatment. The mortality rate is approximately 75% if untreated.
- **Pneumonic plague** has an incubation period of only 3 days and represents an instance when the microorganism is aerosolized, causing the exhalations of affected humans to be infectious. Constitutional and respiratory symptoms predominate, and the mortality rate is even higher (90% if untreated) than that for bubonic plague.

TREATMENT

Appropriate treatment for plague involves the administration of a parenteral aminoglycoside: streptomycin or gentamicin. Rodent control and vaccination of at-risk populations can help control the spread of this disease.

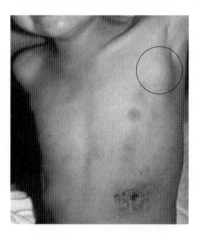

FIGURE 5-25. Bubonic plague. Note the bubo in the left axilla (*circle*). The ulcer is an unusual manifestation at the initial site of infection. (Reproduced with permission from Kasper DL, Braunwald E, Fauci AS, et al. *Harrison's Principles of Internal Medicine,* 16th ed. New York: McGraw-Hill, 2005: 923.)

FRANCISELLA TULARENSIS

CHARACTERISTICS

Francisella tularensis is another rare zoonotic bacterium, which is the causative agent of **tularemia.** It is an extremely small gram-negative coccobacillus that, like *Y pestis,* is a facultative intracellular bacterium that spreads from the point of entry into the body via macrophage phagosomes. It is fastidious to culture and requires either "chocolate" or buffered charcoal yeast extract agar and an extended incubation period for growth in the lab.

The animal reservoirs for *F tularensis* are wild rodents, especially **rabbits, voles,** and the like. Humans are usually infected either by contact with a domestic animal that has killed an infected rodent or by a tick bite. In the United States, tularemia is seen mostly in the Central Plains states, although most states have reported cases. The species is **highly virulent;** only a few organisms are required to produce infection.

PATHOGENESIS

Francisella tularensis has an antiphagocytic polysaccharide capsule, which protects against opsonization. It is resistant to intracellular killing in the phagosomes of macrophages.

CLINICAL SYMPTOMS

Tularemia can manifest as a variety of different syndromes.

- The **ulceroglandular** variant is the most common form. Lesions resemble bubo formation at the site of initial infection except that the skin surface ulcerates as well; the bacteria can spread from there to the blood.
- **Pneumonic** tularemia results from contact with aerosolized bacteria and can lead to a bilateral pneumonia.
- **Oculoglandular** tularemia affects the eye and cervical lymph nodes.
- **Typhoidal** tularemia has GI and systemic symptoms.

TREATMENT

Streptomycin and gentamicin are standard therapies for tularemia. Tick prophylaxis (light-colored clothing, insect repellents, and long sleeves) and avoidance of known reservoirs of infection serve to decrease the incidence of disease in endemic areas.

BRUCELLA

CHARACTERISTICS

Brucella species (*B melitensis, B abortus, B suis,* and *B canis*) are facultatively intracellular, small, nonmotile, encapsulated gram-negative organisms that infect mammals such as **cows, goats,** and **pigs.** Spread to humans is usually through contact with infected meat, aborted placentas, or unpasteurized milk products. Brucellosis is rare in the United States owing to cattle immunization and milk pasteurization.

CLINICAL SYMPTOMS

Brucellosis generally manifests with nonspecific symptoms; one common finding is an intermittent fever (**undulant fever**), which rises during the day and resolves at night. Progressive involvement of the GI, respiratory tracts or skeleton is possible.

TREATMENT

A combination of doxycycline and rifampin are used to eradicate the organism.

PASTEURELLA MULTOCIDA

CHARACTERISTICS

Pasteurella is a nonmotile, encapsulated gram-negative organism distantly related to *Haemophilus*, which asymptomatically colonizes the mouths of dogs and especially **cats.**

CLINICAL SYMPTOMS

Common cause of localized wound infection, cellulitis, and lymphadenopathy following a bite or scratch from an infected cat or dog.

TREATMENT

Doxycycline or penicillin as well as appropriate wound care.

BARTONELLA

CHARACTERISTICS

Bartonella species are **aerobic** gram-negative rods that are poorly characterized to date. They are found in a number of animal reservoirs, often with insects as intermediate vectors. The most clinically important member of the genus is *B henselae*, the causative agent of **cat-scratch fever.** However, worth mentioning is *B quintana*, which causes **trench fever,** a 5-day illness frequently seen during World War I, characterized by fever and bone pain. *Bartonella quintana* has no known animal reservoir; transmission occurs via the bite of the human body louse.

CLINICAL SYMPTOMS

Cat-scratch fever is a **chronic lymphadenitis** occurring mainly in children after being scratched by an infected cat (hence the name, cat-scratch fever). Lymph nodes near the site of infection become enlarged and painful, and chronic, low-grade fevers may develop.

TREATMENT

The infection is worrisome to parents but self-limited and does not respond to antibiotic therapy.

GRAM-INDETERMINATE BACTERIA

Several other groups of medically important bacteria do not have a definitive Gram stain because of the makeup (or utter lack) of their cell walls or their obligate localization within the phagosomes of eukaryotic cells. These bacteria include *Mycobacteria, Mycoplasma, Chlamydia,* and *Rickettsia*.

MYCOBACTERIUM

Mycobacteria are small, nonmotile, **aerobic** rods with a complex cell wall that differs from both gram-positive and gram-negative organisms. The cell walls of mycobacteria possess complex lipids called **mycocides—mycolic acid** residues on the most external surface—and various additional membrane proteins and cross-linkages of the peptidoglycan layer. This cell wall structure causes mycobacteria to stain positive with **acid-fast stains (Ziehl-Neelsen stain),** as described previously. It also acts as a virulence factor, resulting in resis-

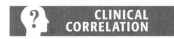

CLINICAL CORRELATION

Because of the risk of *Pasteurella* (and other) infections, animal (and human) bite wounds are generally **not** closed with sutures.

tance to common antimicrobial agents, such as β-lactam and cephalosporin antibiotics.

Many pathogenic mycobacteria are either **very slow-growing** or unable to be grown in bacterial cultures. The three most important members of the genus are *M tuberculosis*, the causative agent of **tuberculosis**, *M leprae*, which causes **Hansen disease** (formerly known as leprosy) and *M avium–intracellulare* (MAC or MAI), an opportunistic pathogen that causes disseminated infection in immunodeficient persons.

MYCOBACTERIUM TUBERCULOSIS

CHARACTERISTICS

Mycobacterium tuberculosis infection (TB) is a major, life-threatening chronic condition affecting individuals in both impoverished and developed countries.

- *Mycobacterium tuberculosis* is a small, acid-fast, obligate aerobe that resides inside macrophages and can establish lifelong infection.
- It is found worldwide—primarily in Southeast Asia, Africa, and Eastern Europe—and is spread by infectious aerosols from person-to-person (without animal reservoirs).
- One-third of the world's population carries some form of infection, but because of efficacious treatment regimens and strict reporting of cases, disease burden in the United States has been steadily decreasing.
- Risk factors for TB (in the United States) include:
  - Incarceration
  - Immunodeficiency—especially active, untreated HIV infection
  - Homelessness
  - Travel to endemic areas
  - Exposure to individuals with known active TB
  - Drug and alcohol abuse
  - Employment in a health care setting

PATHOGENESIS

Primary *M tuberculosis* infection usually begins when infectious particles are inhaled and phagocytosed by alveolar macrophages. The microbe evades intravesicular killing by lysosomes by **inhibition of lysosomal fusion;** however, a chronic inflammatory response is produced. This inflammatory response damages tissue parenchyma, especially the lungs, resulting in the soft, deliquescent **caseous granulomas** composed of multiple infected macrophages and debris. Eventual control of the infection is achieved with **cell-mediated** (T_H1-based) immunity, but viable *M tuberculosis* bacteria continue to exist within the granulomas and can **reactivate** when host immune function is depressed. **Virulent** strains can form microscopic "serpentine **cords**" (hence the term *cord factor* to describe virulence) in which the bacilli are arranged in parallel chains.

CLINICAL SYMPTOMS

The first exposure to the pathogen, termed **primary tuberculosis,** usually results in an asymptomatic lung infection. Primary infection is generally established in **central (perihilar) lung fields** (Figure 5-26). The characteristic finding on chest radiograph is a **Ghon complex,** which consists of **enlarged perihilar lymph nodes adjacent to a calcified granuloma.** Symptomatic infection can occur in the elderly, pediatric, or immunosuppressed populations.

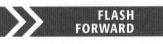

KEY FACT

Acid-fast bacteria: *Mycobacterium* spp. and *Nocardia* spp.

FLASH FORWARD

TB is the prototypical example of a T_H1-based infection. HIV patients with decreased CD4+ T-cell counts are especially susceptible to this infection.

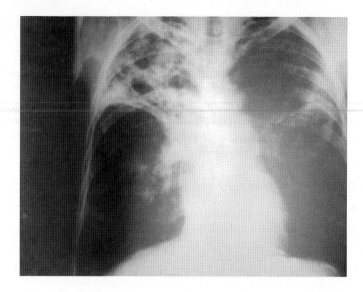

FIGURE 5-26. **An anteroposterior X-ray of a patient diagnosed with advanced bilateral pulmonary tuberculosis.** This anteroposterior X-ray of the chest reveals the presence of bilateral pulmonary infiltrate, and "caving formation" present in the right apical region. The diagnosis is far-advanced tuberculosis. (Image courtesy of CDC's Public Health Image Library.)

- **Latent tuberculosis** is an asymptomatic state in which the bacterium lies dormant inside caseous granulomas.
- **Reactivation (secondary) tuberculosis** occurs when the host undergoes a transient decrease in immune function, allowing escape of the organism from the granuloma and seeding of end organs. Most commonly, the **apices of the lungs** are affected because of the microbe's predilection for areas of high O_2 concentration (Figure 5-26).
- Symptoms in this case are highly suggestive and include **fever, night sweats, weight loss,** and **hemoptysis.**
- Without treatment, the bacteria and resultant inflammatory response slowly erode the lung parenchyma.
- TB can also reactivate in a number of **extrapulmonary organs:** The CNS (causing lymphocytic meningitis), vertebra (causing compression fractures and referred to as **Pott disease**), kidneys, lymphoreticular system, and GI tract.
- **Miliary tuberculosis** occurs when tubercular bacteremia causes distal seeding. This is seen mainly in immunosuppressed populations and has a high mortality rate. The radiographic and pathologic presentations of this disease are remarkable.

Diagnosis of active TB is usually clinical and radiographic, but the **purified protein derivative (PPD)** skin test provides a measure of whether individuals can mount a cell-mediated response to *M tuberculosis*. Purified protein particles from killed bacteria are injected intradermally; a few days later, the area of induration (hard, raised bump; not the area of redness) is measured. Positive tests correlate with active, latent, or resolved infection; unfortunately, false-positive results are common (due to cross-reactivity in recipients of the bacillus Calmette-Guérin [BCG] vaccine) and false-negative (due to anergy in immunosuppressed patients).

TREATMENT

The mainstay of treatment for active TB is **prolonged multidrug therapy** to prevent the onset of resistance.

■ Generally, a four-drug regimen consisting of isoniazid (INH), ethambutol, pyrazinamide, and rifampin for 2 months followed by INH/rifampin for 4–6 more months is used, although alternative combinations are required if resistance or drug intolerance develops.

■ Chemoprophylaxis for exposure to active TB or a positive PPD test without symptoms is generally 9 months of INH; again, alternative regimens are possible depending on resistance patterns. The BCG vaccine is given in some endemic countries to prevent primary infection. It prevents major sequelae of TB (disseminated or miliary) without actually preventing spread.

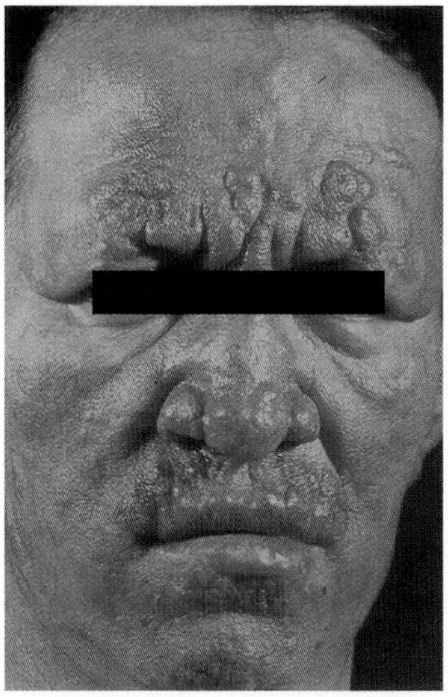

MYCOBACTERIUM LEPRAE

CHARACTERISTICS

Mycobacterium leprae is an acid-fast, aerobic rod that causes the disfiguring disease known as **leprosy,** or **Hansen disease.** Humans and armadillos are the only known hosts. The disease is spread through contact with infected lesions. Better control of Hansen disease has caused a 90% reduction in its incidence since 1985. *Mycobacterium leprae* **cannot** be grown in artificial culture.

PATHOGENESIS

Mycobacterium leprae has a predilection for **cool** surfaces, and therefore most of its pathogenic features occur in superficial tissues such as the **skin** and the **peripheral nerves.**

CLINICAL SYMPTOMS

Two clinical forms of leprosy are known: Tuberculoid leprosy and lepromatous leprosy (Figure 5-27). They develop based on differential responses of the immune system to the bacteria (Table 5-17).

TREATMENT

Therapy for the tuberculoid variant involves the antibiotics **dapsone** and **rifampin** for 6 months. Longer therapy of 12 months and the addition of clofazimine are required for the lepromatous variant.

FIGURE 5-27. Lepromatous leprosy. Thickened and nodular facial skin produces the characteristic leonine facies and saddle-nose deformity. (Reproduced with permission from Kasper DL, Braunwald E, Fauci AS, et al. *Harrison's Principles of Internal Medicine,* 16th ed. New York: McGraw-Hill, 2005: 968.)

TABLE 5-17. Pathogenesis and Clinical Features of Lepromatous and Tuberculoid Leprosy

FEATURE	LEPROMATOUS LEPROSY	TUBERCULOID LEPROSY
Immunopathogenesis	Failed cell-mediated (T_H1) immunity; primarily ineffective humoral response.	Successful cell-mediated immunity; lesions contained.
Skin lesions	Many nodular growths with tissue compromise; stocking-and-glove peripheral neuropathy but no anesthesia around lesions; skin thickening.	Few, hypopigmented macules; complete sensory loss in/around lesions; presence of granulomas and vigorous chronic inflammatory response.
Organism presence in skin lesions	Always, innumerable.	Few to none.
Infectivity of skin lesions	Highly.	Minimal.
Prognosis	Poor; can lead to death, if untreated.	Can be self-limiting.

ATYPICAL MYCOBACTERIA

CHARACTERISTICS

The atypical mycobacteria such as *M avium-intracellulare*, *M kansasii*, *M scrofulaceum*, and so on, tend to cause disease in specific populations. They are ubiquitous in the environment, are not readily transmitted from person to person, and are often opportunistic infections. Atypical bacteria are grouped according to speed of growth in media as well as pigmentation.

Mycobacterium avium-intracellulare (MAI) (also known as *M avium* complex, or **MAC**) is a ubiquitous atypical mycobacterium present in **soil and water.**

CLINICAL SYMPTOMS

Rarely, *M avium-intracellulare* can cause pulmonary infections or lymphadenitis in immunocompetent individuals. Pulmonary infections are typically **nodular** and **bronchiectatic.** More importantly, MAC is a major cause of chronic disseminated disease in **patients with active AIDS.** This infection generally afflicts patients who have CD4+ T-cell counts below $10/mm^3$. The disease manifests as an overwhelming, disseminated infection in virtually all tissues. Patients present with cough, diarrhea, osteomyelitis, anemia, and wasting.

TREATMENT

Multidrug resistance is common. Susceptible AIDS patients are routinely treated **prophylactically** for MAI with **macrolide** antibiotics (usually azithromycin).

Other atypical mycobacteria include:

- *Mycobacterium kansasii*, which is a **rare** cause of a syndrome clinically **identical** to pulmonary tuberculosis.
- *Mycobacterium scrofulaceum* is the causal agent of the pediatric disease **scrofula,** a chronic cervical lymphadenitis.
- *Mycobacterium marinum* inhabits standing water and can cause ulceration and granulomas at sites of open wounds.

MYCOPLASMA

Mycoplasma are the smallest free-living bacteria in nature. They are so small that they were originally thought to be viruses. They are unique in that they **do not possess cell walls,** therefore drugs that inhibit cell wall synthesis (penicillins, cephalosporins and vancomycin) are ineffective against mycoplasma. Mycoplasma also have a plasma membrane reinforced with **cholesterol,** a sterol usually found in eukaryotic cells. Mycoplasma can be grown (very slowly) on artificial media in the lab but have complex nutritional requirements. They assume a **fried-egg** appearance after a few weeks of culture. The most important of the species is *M pneumoniae*, which causes atypical pneumonia. *Ureaplasma urealyticum* can cause nongonococcal urethritis (like *C trachomatis*).

MYCOPLASMA PNEUMONIAE

CHARACTERISTICS

This bacterium is actually smaller than some large viruses in nature. Its plasma membrane possesses the **P1 protein,** which is capable of binding specifically to respiratory epithelial cells. *M pneumoniae* plasma membrane is antigenic. Unfortunately, human anti-*Mycoplasma* cell membrane antibodies **cross-react** with erythrocyte antigens and agglutinate RBCs but **only at low** temperatures (4°C but not 37°C). Thus, the **cold agglutinin test** is a simple (but nonspecific) test for an anti-*Mycoplasma* immune response that can be performed at the bedside.

CLINICAL SYMPTOMS

Mycoplasma pneumoniae is a common cause of **atypical pneumonia** in young adults and manifests as gradual-onset, persistent low fever with a hacking, nonproductive cough and associated pharyngitis and malaise. Chest radiograph usually reveals patchy bilateral infiltrates that appear much worse than the clinical picture.

TREATMENT

Tetracyclines, macrolides, or fourth-generation fluoroquinolones.

CHLAMYDIAE AND RICKETTSIAE

Chlamydiae and rickettsiae are tiny organisms (between the size of viruses and bacteria). They are **obligate intracellular,** meaning that they are unable to live outside eukaryotic cells because they do not produce their own ATP. They have **both** DNA and RNA. They stain gram-negative and possess a modified gram-negative cell wall, but the organisms are so small that they are invisible under conventional microscopy.

Chlamydia spp. cause a variety of **respiratory and mucosal diseases** because of its **tropism to ciliated columnar epithelial cells,** whereas *Rickettsia* spp. (and the closely related pathogens *Coxiella* and *Ehrlichia*) tend to cause **fever and rash syndromes** owing to a **predilection for endothelium.** Diseases caused by these organisms are also commonly treated with tetracyclines, macrolides, or (rarely) chloramphenicol.

CHLAMYDIA SPECIES

Chlamydia spp. are distinguished from all other bacteria because of their **unique replicative cycle.** The infectious particle associated with *Chlamydia* infection is the **elementary body (EB),** which is structurally similar to a spore in that much of its exterior peptidoglycan is cross-linked, protecting it from the elements. This peptidoglycan does **not** possess **muramic acid** and is not susceptible to disruption by penicillin antibiotics.

Once the EB form is taken up by the host cell, the cross-linkages are lost, and it transforms into a **reticulate body** (RB, also known as an **initial body**). In this form, the microbe is metabolically active and amplifies its DNA, RNA, and protein production, **using host ATP.** These RBs are visible under microscopy as **cytoplasmic inclusions.** Intracellular EBs are produced when the number of RBs is sufficient to sustain production; these are extruded from the host cell and the cycle begins again.

The three medically important members of the *Chlamydia* genus are *C trachomatis*, which causes optic, genital tract, and neonatal pulmonary infections, and *C pneumoniae* and *C psittaci*, both of which cause atypical pneumonia.

The EB of *C trachomatis* is capable of infecting only certain types of cells—generally columnar or transitional epithelium, depending on the **serovar** or **serologic variant** of the organism. Different serovars have different epidemiologic and disease patterns (Table 5-18).

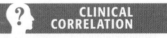

KEY FACT

Atypical "walking" pneumonia can be caused by *Legionella*, *Mycoplasma*, or *Chlamydia*.

CLINICAL CORRELATION

Cases of mucopurulent urethritis and cervicitis are usually treated with ceftriaxone and doxycycline because of the high rate of gonococcal and chlamydial coinfection!

TABLE 5-18. Disease Patterns of *Chlamydia* Infections

Symptoms	Susceptible Populations	Transmission Pattern	Clinical Symptoms	Serovar
Trachoma	Impoverished children in endemic areas (Middle East, India).	Hand-to-eye, eye-seeking flies, and contaminated clothing.	Follicular conjunctivitis, repeated infections leading to scarring and blindness.	A, B, C
Inclusion conjunctivitis	Neonates.	Passage through infected birth canal.	Purulent conjunctivitis occurring about 1 week after birth.	D–K
Infantile pneumonia	Neonates.	Passage through infected birth canal.	Rhinitis and cough without fever, occurs about 2–3 weeks after birth.	D–K
Urethritis	Sexually active individuals.	Sexual transmission.	Asymptomatic, or dysuria with mucoid urethral discharge; can be a polymicrobial infection with *N gonorrhoeae*.	D–K
Cervicitis	Sexually active females.	Sexual transmission.	Mostly asymptomatic, may progress to pelvic inflammatory disease (PID), may have purulent cervical discharge.	D–K
Pelvic inflammatory disease (PID)	Females with untreated cervicitis.	Ascending infection.	Vaginal bleeding or discharge, suprapubic pain, cervical motion tenderness, fever, nausea, vomiting; can lead to infertility or ectopic pregnancies.	D–K
Lymphogranuloma venereum	Sexually active individuals.	Sexual transmission.	Painless inguinal papule progressing to painful unilateral lymphadenopathy.	L1–L3
Psittacosis	Individuals with close contact with birds.	Aerosolized dust and feathers from birds.	Atypical pneumonia (fever, headache, dry nonproductive cough) 1–3 weeks after exposure.	*C psittaci*
Chlamydial pneumonia	Common.	Person-to-person via aerosolized droplets.	Atypical pneumonia.	*C pneumoniae*

RICKETTSIA SPECIES AND RELATED ORGANISMS

Like *Chlamydia* spp., *Rickettsia* spp. and the closely related organisms *Coxiella burnetii*, *Orientia tsutsugamushi*, and *Ehrlichia chaffeensis* are tiny obligate intracellular organisms with structures similar to gram-negative rods. As with *Chlamydia* infections, treatment is almost always with doxycycline, or with chloramphenicol in children. However, these organisms differ from *Chlamydia* spp. in several ways:

- Unlike *Chlamydia* infections, which affect only humans, these organisms generally have **arthropod vectors (tick, mite, and louse)** (except for *Coxiella*).
- Reproduction is by **binary fission**.

TABLE 5-19.   **Rickettsial Diseases**

Organism/Disease	Affected Locations	Vector/Reservoir	Clinical Symptoms	Rash
R rickettsii: Rocky Mountain spotted fever.	Southeastern and south central United States.	"Hard" *Dermacentor* ticks.	High fever, chills, headache, and myalgias.	Macular, centripetal spread (extremities to trunk) and palms/soles.
R akari: Rickettsialpox.	Rare in United States.	Mites that live on field mice.	Fever, chills, headache; mild.	Vesicular, generalized.
R prowazekii: Epidemic typhus.	Latin America, Africa in areas of poor hygiene.	*Pediculus* body louse.	Fever, chills, myalgias, headache, arthralgias, mental status changes.	Petechial or macular, centrifugal spread (trunk to extremities).
R typhi: Endemic typhus.	Warm areas.	Fleas that live on rodents.	Gradual onset of fever, chills, myalgias, nausea.	Maculopapular, restricted to chest/abdomen.
O tsutsugamushi: Scrub typhus.	Asia, Pacific islands.	Larvae (chiggers) of mites.	High fever, headache, myalgias.	Maculopapular, centrifugal spread.
C burnetii: Q fever.	Worldwide.	Endospore inhalation.	Headache, high fever, chills, myalgias, atypical pneumonia.	None.
E chaffeensis: Ehrlichiosis.	Southern United States, Asia.	*Amblyomma* ticks.	Headache, fever, chills, myalgias; GI symptoms; leukopenia.	Macular, centripetal spread.

- Intracellular localization is within the **cytoplasm** and **nucleus.**
- Disease symptoms usually consist of headache, fever, and rash, resulting from the **vasculitis** secondary to the replication of the rickettsiae inside endothelial cells (Table 5-19).

Spirochetes

Spirochetes are spiral-shaped bacteria with an **internal flagellum:**

- Technically gram-negative (ie, contain endotoxin), but not well visualized with light microscopy. Can be visualized with **darkfield** or fluorescent microscopy.
- Three clinically important genera: *Borrelia, Treponema,* and *Leptospira* (Table 5-20).
- Treated with tetracyclines or β-lactams.

TREPONEMA

The *Treponema* genus consists of **venereal** treponema (*T pallidum,* subspecies *pallidum* (**simply referred to as *Treponema pallidum***) as well as **nonvenereal** treponema that cause various infections such as **yaws, pinta,** and **bejel.**

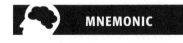

MNEMONIC

BLT
***B**orrelia*
***L**eptospira*
***T**reponema*

TABLE 5-20. Summary of Spirochete Diseases

Pathogen	General	Transmission	Diagnosis	Infection	Treatment
Treponema pallidum (syphilis)	Microaerophilic, extracellular.	Skin-skin contact Transplacental (**TO**RCH).	Serology: VDRL, then FTA-Abs.	*Primary:* Painless chancre. *Secondary:* Condylomata lata, palm and sole rash. *Tertiary:* Aortitis, gummas, Argyl-Robertson pupil, tabes dorsalis.	Penicillin G.
Borrelia burgdorferi (Lyme disease)	Most common vector-borne disease. Microaerophilic, intracellular.	Deer tick (*Ixodes scapularis*).	Clinical, serology.	*Stage 1:* Erythema, chronicum migrans, flulike symptoms. *Stage 2:* Bell palsy, AV block. *Stage 3:* Chronic arthritis, encephalopathy.	Doxycycline.
Borrelia recurrentis	Antigenic variation.	*Pediculus humanus corporis* (human body louse).	Blood samples during fever.	Sudden onset of fever, etc. Spontaneous resolution and relapse.	Tetracycline, penicillin.
Leptospira interrogans	Aerobic.	Animal urine.	Microscopy.	*Initial:* Flulike symptoms, photophobia. *Later:* Liver damage with jaundice, renal failure.	Penicillin G; doxycycline for prophylaxis.

AV = atrioventricular; FTA-Abs = fluorescent treponemal antibody absorption; TORCH = Toxoplasmosis; Other infections (syphilis, parvovirus B19, hepatitis B virus, HIV, varicella-zoster virus), Rubella, Cytomegalovirus, Herpes simplex virus); VDRL = Venereal Disease Research Laboratory.

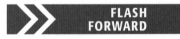
FLASH FORWARD

Symptoms of **congenital** syphilis:
- May result in stillbirth.
- Early: rhinitis and mucocutaneous lesions.
- Late (more than 2 years): deafness and recurrent arthropathies.
- Affects organ systems: Skin, mucous membranes, lymph nodes, aorta, and CNS.

Treponema pallidum (Syphilis)

Characteristics

- Gram-negative.
- Microaerophilic.
- Extracellular.
- Typically spiral-shaped, with an internal flagellum between outer membrane and cell wall.
- Diagnosed using **darkfield** microscope (**cannot** be grown in culture).
- Transmitted through **sexual contact, contact with open chancre,** or **transplacentally.**
- Humans are the only host.

Pathogenesis

- Outer membrane carries endotoxin-like lipids.
- Spirochetes penetrate mucous membranes, leading to bacteremia and seeding of organs throughout the body.

Clinical Symptoms

There are **three** clinical stages of syphilis (Table 5-21):

- **Primary syphilis** (following a 3–6 week incubation period).
  - A single **painless**, indurated ulcer with smooth margins (**chancre**) at **site of inoculation,** that heals within 3–6 weeks (Figure 5-28).

TABLE 5-21.   Summary of Syphilis

GENERAL	TRANSMISSION	DIAGNOSIS	INFECTION	TREATMENT
Microaerophilic, extracellular	Skin-skin contact, transplacental (**TO**RCH).	Serology: VDRL, then FTA-Abs.	*Primary:* Painless chancre. *Secondary:* Condylomata lata, rash on palms and soles. *Latent:* Usually asymptomatic. *Tertiary:* Aortitis, ascending aortic aneurysm, gummas, Argyll-Robertson pupil, tabes dorsalis, neurosyphilis.	Penicillin G

FTA-Abs = fluorescent treponemal antibody absorption; TORCH = Toxoplasmosis, Other infections (syphilis, parvovirus B19, hepatitis B, virus, HIV, varicella-zoster virus), Rubella, Cytomegalovirus, Herpes simplex virus); VDRL = Venereal Disease Research Laboratory.

- Early spread to regional lymph nodes and early bacteremia.
- Self-limited primary stage, but **highly contagious.**
- **Secondary syphilis** (1–3 months later; rarely coexists with primary syphilis):
  - Manifests with flulike symptoms and a maculopapular rash on **palms, soles,** and mucous membranes.
  - May include condylomata lata (**highly infectious** wartlike lesions on perianal skin).
  - May cause infection in any organ or part of body (eg, hepatitis, arthritis, meningitis, etc).
  - Relapsing and remitting course, with cyclic symptoms and episodes of latency.
- **Tertiary syphilis** (decades later):
  - **Aortitis**—aortic insufficiency, ascending aortic aneurysm.
  - Neurosyphilis—**tabes dorsalis** (posterior column disease); **Argyll Robertson pupil** (accommodates but does not react to light), psychosis, and meningitis.
  - **Gummas**—soft granulomas of bone, skin, viscera (Figure 5-29).

DIAGNOSIS

Based on clinical presentation, microscopy, and especially **serology:**

- *Treponema pallidum* enzyme-linked immunosorbent assay (ELISA, TP IgG).

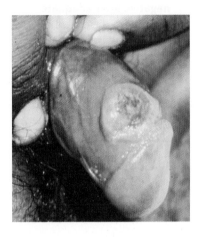

FIGURE 5-28.   Chancre of primary syphilis. (Reproduced with permission from Kasper DL, Braunwald E, Fauci AS, et al. *Harrison's Principles on Internal Medicine,* 16th ed. New York: McGraw-Hill, 2005: 978.)

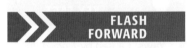

FLASH FORWARD

Tabes dorsalis occurs late and is characterized by demyelination of the posterior columns and dorsal roots. Corresponding symptoms include:

- Ataxia and wide-based gait (particularly in the dark or with eyes closed).
- Paresthesias and anesthesias (loss of proprioception and vibration sense).
- "Shooting" pains in lower extremities, loss of deep tendon reflexes and joint damage (Charcot joints)

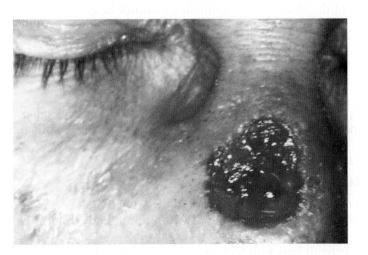

FIGURE 5-29.   Gumma of nose due to a long-standing tertiary syphilitic *Treponema pallidum* infection. (Image courtesy of CDC's Public Health Image Library; content provider J. Pledger.)

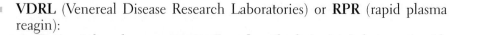

- **VDRL** (Venereal Disease Research Laboratories) or **RPR** (rapid plasma reagin):
  - Testing is based on a **nontreponemal** antibody (reagin) that reacts with cow heart cardiolipin-lecithin *in vitro*.
  - **Screening** tests: **High sensitivity,** low specificity.
  - Turn positive 1 week after infection.
  - False-positive in systemic lupus erythematosus, Epstein-Barr virus infection, leprosy, hepatitis B infection, and many others.
- **FTA-Abs:**
  - Tests for **antitreponemal** antibody.
  - **Confirmatory** test—used to follow up positive VDRL/RPR.
  - Highly sensitive and **highly specific.**
  - Expensive.

TREATMENT

- Benzathine penicillin G is used for primary and secondary syphilis as well as for prophylaxis to contacts. Aqueous penicillin G is used to treat neurosyphilis (due to poor CNS penetration of benzathine penicillin).
- Complication of treatment due to lysis of treponeme = Jarisch-Herxheimer reaction (fevers, chills, myalgias).
- No vaccine.
- Reinfection can occur as immunity to previous syphilis infection is incomplete.

PROGNOSIS

Dependent on stage of infection and affected organs. Early syphilis and neurosyphilis tend to resolve well; however, aortitis may result in permanent structural defects.

NONVENEREAL TREPONEMAL INFECTIONS

- Nonvenereal treponemal infections (yaws, pinta and bejel) generally occur in **hot, humid areas** such as sub-Saharan Africa, the Middle East, Southeast Asia, Central and South America, and sometimes Mexico.
- **All** cause **cutaneous** disease sometimes with internal organ involvement.
- Unlike syphilis, nonvenereal treponemal infections are **not** transmitted sexually and do **not** cause congenital disease. These infections are transmitted by direct person-to-person contact.
- Like syphilis, the causative spirochetes **cannot** be grown in culture. Importantly, nonvenereal treponemal infections yield **positive** VDRL/RPR and FTA-Abs test results.
- **All** treponemal infections are treated with penicillin G.

BORRELIA

Generally, microbes of the *Borrelia* genus are more loosely coiled than treponemes and are **arthropod-borne** (not sexually or transplacentally transmitted).

BORRELIA BURGDORFERI (LYME DISEASE)

CHARACTERISTICS

- **Most common tick-borne** disease in the United States.
- Can sometimes live intracellularly. As a result, body fluid samples may be polymerase chain reaction (PCR)-negative.
- Some patients have coinfection with *Ehrlichia* or *Babesia.*
- Transmission via bite of ***Ixodes scapularis*** (deer or black-legged tick).
- Successful transmission requires more than 24 hours of feeding.
- Reservoirs include the **white-tailed deer** and the **white-footed mice.**

PATHOGENESIS

- **Antigenic variation.**
- Invades skin and spreads hematogenously; leads to immune complex deposition.
- Can access immunoprivileged sites such as CNS, tendons, and synoviae.

CLINICAL SYMPTOMS

There are **three** clinical stages of Lyme disease:

1. **Primary (early):** Erythema chronicum migrans (spreading, red target lesion, Figure 5-30) and constitutional symptoms—fever, chills, fatigue, headache, myalgias or arthralgias.
2. **Secondary,** disseminated phase (days to weeks after infection):
    - Bell's palsy (CN VII), aseptic meningitis, peripheral neuropathy.
    - Atrioventricular (AV) block, carditis.
    - Multiple erythema chronicum migrans (secondary lesions).
    - Migratory myalgias, transient arthritis.
    - Other: Fever, stiff neck, headache, limb numbness or pain, malaise, fatigue.
3. **Tertiary,** late (months to years after infection):
    - Chronic polyarthritis.
    - Neurologic impairment, fatigue.
    - Acrodermatitis chronicum atrophicans (skin atrophy).

DIAGNOSIS

Often clinical, based on history of tick bite with characteristic erythema chronicum migrans. Serology may also be tested, although many false-negatives result, owing to antigenic variation and intracellular location. **Skin biopsy** can also be performed and is a positive result if motile spirochetes are visible under darkfield microscopy. Other diagnostic tests include **PCR** and **culture** (modified Kelly medium).

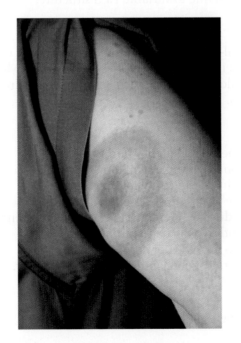

FIGURE 5-30. **Pathognomonic erythematous rash (*erythema chronicum migrans*) in the pattern of a "bull's-eye" of stage 1 Lyme disease.** (Image courtesy of CDC's Public Health Image Library; content provider James Gathany.)

TREATMENT

Doxycycline (oral) for primary-stage Lyme disease and **ceftriaxone (IV)** for later-stage disease.

BORRELIA RECURRENTIS (RELAPSING FEVER)

PATHOGENESIS

Antigenic variation allows new variants to evade the immune system and proliferate in the bloodstream, which then stimulates a subsequent immune response.

CLINICAL SYMPTOMS

- Inoculation: Transmitted by **human body louse.**
- Infection: Sudden onset of shaking chills, fever, myalgias, headache, delirium, cough, lethargy, hepatosplenomegaly.
- Spontaneous resolution and recurrence (less severe) due to antigenic variation and recurrent septicemia.
- Can be diagnosed from blood sample when febrile; darkfield microscopy shows spirochete (Giemsa stain).
- Serology for serum antibodies against *Borrelia.*

TREATMENT

Penicillin or tetracycline. Treatment may cause Jarisch-Herxheimer reaction via lysis of bacteria and release of antigens.

LEPTOSPIRA INTERROGANS (LEPTOSPIROSIS, ICTEROHEMORRHAGIC FEVER)

CHARACTERISTICS

- Aerobic.
- **Two** periplasmic flagella.
- Fine spirochete with hooked ends (Figure 5-31).
- Antigenic variation due to **variable LPS** structure.

PATHOGENESIS

Transmission is fecal-oral through **animal urine** (variety of wild and domesticated animals, especially rodents, dogs, fish, and birds). Most common modes of transmission: puddle stomping, recreation in contaminated water, working in sewers (rat urine).

CLINICAL SYMPTOMS

- Disease syndrome is called leptospirosis.
- Leptospiremic phase: Flulike symptoms, photophobia.
- Immune phase: Increasing antileptospira IgM.
- Mild → anicteric leptospirosis: Aseptic meningitis.
- Severe → **Weil disease:** Hemorrhagic vasculitis leading to kidney damage (renal failure) and hepatic damage (jaundice).
- Mortality is high in cases of severe infection (Weil disease). Otherwise, prognosis is generally good, and most patients recover.

DIAGNOSIS

Microscopy (spirochetes in blood, CSF, urine), serology.

TREATMENT

- Penicillin G
- Doxycycline prophylaxis

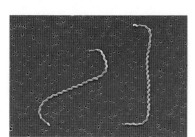

FIGURE 5-31. Scanning electron micrograph of *Leptospira interrogans.* (Image courtesy of CDC's Public Health Image Library; content provider Rob Weyant.)

Mycology

FUNGI

General Characteristics

- **Nonmotile** organisms that form hyphae or spores.
- Cause an array of diseases including skin, lung, opportunistic, and systemic infection.
- Grow on **Sabouraud** agar which is selective for fungi due to its low pH, which inhibits growth of most bacteria.
- Cell **membrane** contains **ergosterol** and cell **wall** is composed of **chitin.**
- Fungi can cause **systemic** infections as well as **localized** infections (ie, **superficial, cutaneous,** or **subcutaneous**). Some fungi are **opportunistic** pathogens that cause disease in immunocompromised hosts.

Life Forms

Fungi exist in **two** forms: yeast and molds. Many fungi can be found in either life form, depending on the **temperature** at which they are growing (Figure 5-32 and Table 5-22).

Systemic Fungal Infections

- **Inhaled** particles primarily cause pulmonary infections but can disseminate system-wide through the bloodstream, producing systemic symptoms involving several organs.
- Pathogens include *Histoplasma, Coccidioides, Blastomyces,* and *Paracoccidioides,* all of which:
  - Are dimorphic fungi (existing in two forms) and can be treated with **fluconazole.**
  - Can be diagnosed with sputum cytology, sputum cultures on blood agar, special media, and peripheral blood cultures (*Histoplasma* in particular).
  - Can induce **granuloma formation** that may calcify over time.
- Systemic fungal infections are **not** transmittable from person to person.

COCCIDIOIDES IMMITIS

CHARACTERISTICS (FIGURE 5-33)

- Found in the **southwestern United States,** known as "desert rheumatic fever" or "valley fever."
- At 25°C (room temperature), grows as cylindrical arthroconidia.
- At 37°C (body temperature), grows as spherules in endospore (spores with spherules).

PATHOGENESIS

- Reservoir: **Soil.**
- Transmission: Airborne. Inhaled arthroconidia become endospores in body.

CLINICAL SYMPTOMS

- Erythema nodosum
- Pneumonitis
- CNS involvement

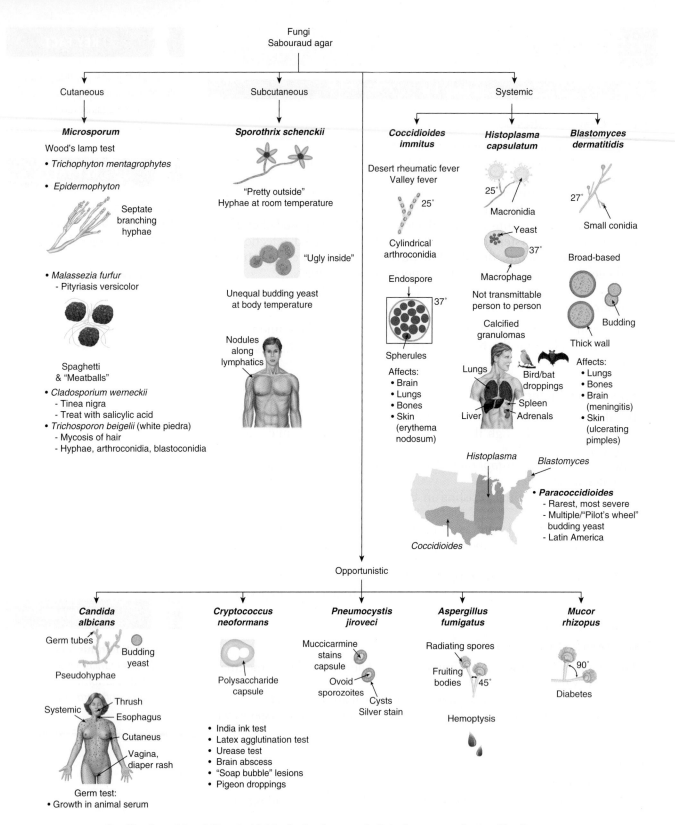

FIGURE 5-32. **Classification of fungi.** Fungi with histologies shown and clinical symptoms depicted by diagrams.

TABLE 5-22.   Life Forms of Fungi

	YEAST	MOLDS
Cellularity	Unicellular.	Multicellular.
Form	Budding cells.	Hyphae (long filamentous tubular cells).
Other forms	**Pseudohyphae** (long chains of cells formed by incomplete budding).	**Septate** hyphae—membranes separate cells. **Aseptate** hyphae—no membranes between cells, multinucleated cells.

- Arthritis
- AIDS patients: Meningitis, mucocutaneous lesions
- Pregnancy: Disseminated in third trimester

DIAGNOSIS

- Dimorphic yeast (no hyphae).
- Thick-walled spores.
- Granulomas.
- Biopsy specimen shows **endospores inside spherules,** all inside giant cells.

TREATMENT

- **Cell-mediated immunity** is required.
- Itraconazole for mild infections.
- Amphotericin B for severe infections without CNS involvement.
- Fluconazole for CNS involvement (good CNS penetration).

PROGNOSIS

Fair, but may be fatal for elderly.

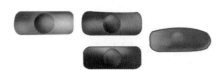

Tissue form:
arthraconidia

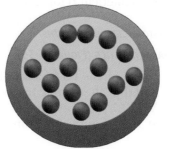

Spore form:
endospores, spherules

FIGURE 5-33.   *Coccidioides* forms.

HISTOPLASMA CAPSULATUM

CHARACTERISTICS (FIGURE 5-34)

- Found in **Mississippi River Valley** transmitted by inhalation of **bird** and **bat droppings.**
- At 25°C, grows as hyphae with macronidia and micronidia.
- At 37°C, found as yeast inside macrophages in the body.

PATHOGENESIS

- Reservoir: **Soil, bird,** and **bat droppings** contain spores.
- Transmission: Spores are inhaled from dust.
- Macrophages phagocytose spores and carry them systemically.
- Budding yeast form **inside** macrophages, causing local infections throughout the body.

CLINICAL SYMPTOMS

- Asymptomatic in immunocompetent patient.
- Systemic infection in immunocompromised patient.
- Calcified granulomas in tissues involved.
- Pneumonitis that appears similar to miliary TB.
- Infection may involve liver, spleen, and adrenals in immunocompromised patients.

DIAGNOSIS

- Dimorphic yeast.
- Thick-walled spores.
- Granulomas.
- Small budding cells within macrophages on biopsy.
- Calcified lung lesions; may become **cavitary** in chronic progressive form.

TREATMENT

- Cell-mediated immunity required.
- Itraconazole for moderate infection.
- Amphotericin B for severe infection

BLASTOMYCES DERMATITIDIS

CHARACTERISTICS (FIGURE 5-35)

- Found on the **East Coast of the United States and Mexico.**
- **Rarest** of all systemic mycoses.
- At 27°C, found as hyphae with small conidia.
- At 37°C, found as budding yeast with broad base in tissue.

> **KEY FACT**
>
> *Histoplasma capsulatum* is named because it is found in histiocytes (macrophages). However, despite the name, it is *not* encapsulated.

> **MNEMONIC**
>
> **BBB**
>
> **B**lastomyces are found as **B**udding yeast with **B**road **B**ase.

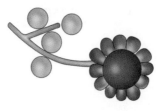
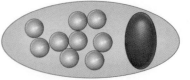

Tissue form   Intracellular form in a reticuloendotheial cell

FIGURE 5-34. *Histoplasma* **forms**.

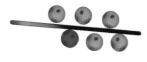 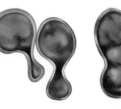

Endemic form   Budding yeast forms in tissue

FIGURE 5-35. ***Blastomyces* forms.**

PATHOGENESIS

- Reservoir: **Soil** and **rotten wood** contain spores.
- Transmission: Inhaled spores.
- Spores form yeast in the body, causing local infections.
- Yeast spread systemically over time and cause granulomas throughout the body (lungs, bones, and skin).

CLINICAL SYMPTOMS

- Ulcerating pimples, verrucous.
- Pneumonitis, night sweats, weight loss.
- Meningitis.
- Arthritis.
- Does **not** reactivate.

DIAGNOSIS

- Dimorphic yeast
- Thick-walled spores
- Lung lesions do **not** calcify
- Granulomas

TREATMENT

- Cell-mediated immunity required.
- Itraconazole for moderate infection or meningeal involvement.
- Amphotericin B for severe infection without meningeal involvement.

PROGNOSIS

Poor, **most severe** of systemic mycoses.

PARACOCCIDIOIDES

CHARACTERISTICS (FIGURE 5-36)

- Found in **Latin America.**
- Appears as multiple budding yeast often described as **"spokes of a wheel,"** or **"pilot's wheel."**
- Affected population: 90% **male.**

PATHOGENESIS

- Reservoir: Spores found in **soil.**
- Transmission: Inhalation of spores.

CLINICAL SYMPTOMS

Symptoms are similar to those of *Coccidioides.*

> **KEY FACT**
>
> Remember **Blastomyces dermatitidis** is the only systemic fungus that causes ulcerating pimples.

> **KEY FACT**
>
> Systemic infection with **Blastomyces dermatitidis** often occurs in the absence of lung disease.

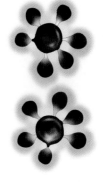

FIGURE 5-36. ***Paracoccidioides*—"pilot's wheel."**

DIAGNOSIS

Dimorphic yeast.

TREATMENT

- Bactrim
- Amphotericin B
- Itraconazole

PROGNOSIS

Good.

Opportunistic Fungal Infections

Opportunistic fungi include *Candida, Cryptococcus, Pneumocystis, Aspergillus,* and *Mucor.* These fungi cause symptoms almost exclusively in immunocompromised hosts. However, candidal disease can occur after prolonged **antibiotic** use or contamination of **indwelling catheters** in immunocompetent hosts.

CANDIDA ALBICANS

CHARACTERISTICS (FIGURE 5-37)

- **Natural flora** of skin.
- Appear as budding yeast with **pseudohyphae** in tissue biopsy.
- Common cause of yeast infection and skin infection (in the immunocompromised host).

PATHOGENESIS

- Reservoir: GI flora and normal skin flora in moist areas like underneath breasts or in skin folds.
- Growth: Forms **"germ tubes"** (Figure 5-38) at 37°C and pseudohyphae when invading tissue. Grows rapidly if not controlled.
- **Antibiotic use,** immunocompromise, and cancer increase risk of infection.

CLINICAL SYMPTOMS

- In immunocompetent hosts:
  - Oral **thrush**
  - **Vulvovaginitis** ("yeast infection")
  - **Diaper rash**

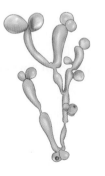
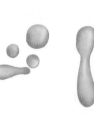
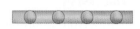

Pseudohyphage

Budding yeast

True hyphae

FIGURE 5-37. *Candida* **forms.**

- In immunocompromised hosts:
  - **Esophagitis**
  - Skin infection
  - Disseminated systemic infection and septicemia
- Endocarditis in **IV drug users.**

DIAGNOSIS

- **Silver** stain.
- **KOH** stain for pseudohyphae, budding yeast.
- **Germ tube test**—grow in animal serum.

TREATMENT

- Nystatin/fluconazole for cutaneous infection.
- Amphotericin B for systemic infection.

PROGNOSIS

Good.

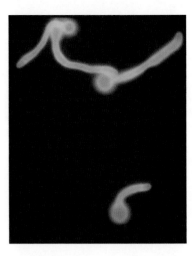

FIGURE 5-38. *Candida: "germ tube"* **morphology.** (Image courtesy of CDC's Public Health Image Library; content provider Dr. Brian Harrington.)

CRYPTOCOCCUS NEOFORMANS

CHARACTERISTICS

- Appears as budding yeast in **India ink stain.**
- Has **thick polysaccharide capsule.**
- Mostly affects patients with AIDS patients or lupus.

PATHOGENESIS

- Reservoir: Bird (especially **pigeon**) droppings.
- Transmission: Inhaled yeast from droppings results in lung infection.
- Spreads hematogenously to CNS, causing meningitis, abscess formation, and increased intracranial pressure.
- Can grow within Virchow-Robinson space (space between vessel wall and surrounding connective tissue).
- Affects people with poor T-cell-mediated immunity.

CLINICAL SYMPTOMS

- Pneumonia
- Fungemia
- Meningitis

DIAGNOSIS

- **Latex agglutination test** for capsular antigen in blood.
- "Soap bubble lesions."
- Budding yeast on **India ink stain.**

TREATMENT

- Amphotericin B plus flucytosine for meningitis.
- Fluconazole for lifetime suppression in AIDS patients.

PROGNOSIS

Poor.

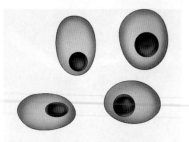

FIGURE 5-39. *Pneumocystis jiroveci* in tissue with silver stain.

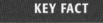

KEY FACT

Pneumocystis jiroveci pneumonia is still called **PCP** (**P**neumocystis **c**arinii **p**neumonia) in the medical community. In AIDS patients, PCP **prophylaxis** is initiated when the CD4 count is < **200.**

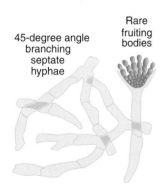

FIGURE 5-40. *Aspergillus.*

PNEUMOCYSTIS JIROVECI (FORMERLY KNOWN AS PNEUMOCYSTIS CARINII)

CHARACTERISTICS (FIGURE 5-39)

- Appears as dark **ovoid sporozoites within cysts** on **silver stain.**
- Frequently affects AIDS patients.
- May also affect premature infants.

PATHOGENESIS

- Transmission: Cyst is inhaled by most people in childhood, leading to an asymptomatic or mild pneumonia, then to a latent infection in the lungs.
- In immunocompromised hosts: Reactivation, uncontrolled growth, and an inflammatory response can lead to pneumonia.

CLINICAL SYMPTOMS

- Pneumonitis.
- Classically may cause **pneumothorax.**

DIAGNOSIS

Silver stain showing cysts containing **dark oval bodies.**

TREATMENT

- Bactrim or pentamidine.
- Bactrim, aerosolized pentamidine, or dapsone for **prophylaxis.**

PROGNOSIS

Fair.

ASPERGILLUS FUMIGATUS

CHARACTERISTICS (FIGURE 5-40)

- Found in wheat stacks.
- **Septate** hyphae **branching at a 45-degree angle.**
- Fruiting bodies at ends of hyphae.
- Affects **neutropenic** patients.

PATHOGENESIS

- Reservoir: Mold grows on **decaying vegetation.**
- Transmission: Spores are inhaled.
- May stimulate IgE response, leading to bronchospasm and **allergic** bronchopulmonary aspergillosis.
- May deposit in existing lung cavity to form aspergillus ball (aspergilloma, or fungus ball).
- May invade lung tissue and enter bloodstream in the immunocompromised host. Can occlude blood vessels leading to pulmonary **infarction.**

CLINICAL SYMPTOMS

- Various lung diseases, including fungus ball, acute and chronic pneumonitis, and disseminated systemic disease.
- Pneumonitis often with **hemoptysis.**

DIAGNOSIS

- Tissue biopsy reveals branching hyphae (45-degree angle).
- Sputum culture shows radiating chains of spores.
- **X-ray** may detect aspergilloma.
- Overall, diagnosis is difficult.

TREATMENT

- Allergic bronchopulmonary aspergillosis: Corticosteroids, no antifungals needed.
- Aspergilloma: Surgery.
- Invasive aspergillosis: Amphotericin B.

PROGNOSIS

Depends on type of disease. For disseminated disease, prognosis is poor.

RHIZOPUS MUCOR

CHARACTERISTICS (FIGURE 5-41)

- **Aseptate** hyphae branch at **90-degree angle.**
- Afflicts patients with diabetic **ketoacidosis** or **leukemia.**

PATHOGENESIS

- Reservoir: Spores in the environment.
- Transmission: Spores inhaled.
- In immunocompromised hosts: Colonizes tissue and invades blood vessels, leading to necrosis (similar to aspergillosis).

CLINICAL SYMPTOMS

- Invasive **rhinocerebral** infection, a medical and surgical emergency.
- Pneumonitis similar to *Aspergillus.*

DIAGNOSIS

- Tissue biopsy shows branching hyphae (branching at 90-degree angle) without septae.
- Shows a broad ribbon-like growth pattern.

TREATMENT

- Control of diabetes
- Surgery for rhinocerebral infections
- Amphotericin

PROGNOSIS

Fair.

Cutaneous Fungal Infections

MICROSPORUM

CHARACTERISTICS

- Includes multiple types of fungi that infect the skin.
- *Trichophyton* and *Epidermophyton* affect the nails specifically.
- Septate branching hyphae with arthroconidia and cross-walls.

PATHOGENESIS

- Reservoir: **Soil, animals, humans.**
- Transmission: Spread by contact with infected individuals or animals.
- Colonize **keratinized** epithelium (dead, horny layer) in warm, moist areas.
- Infection spreads centrifugally with curvy worm-like borders ("ringworm").

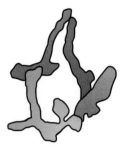

FIGURE 5-41. *Rhizopus mucor.* Irregular broad (empty-looking) aseptate hyphae, wide-angle branching.

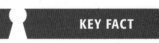

KEY FACT

Aspergillus fumigatus and *Rhizopus mucor* appear very similar, but *Aspergillus* branches at 45 degrees and *Rhizopus* branches at 90 degrees. Also, *Aspergillus* has septate hyphae, but *Rhizopus* hyphae are aseptate.

- Fungal antigens are released from the hyphae and may induce **delayed-type hypersensitivity** reaction (dermatophytoses: Inflammation, itching, scaly skin, pustules).
- Fungal antigens may diffuse systemically and cause dermaphytid reactions: Hypersensitivity responses (vesicles) at distant sites such as fingers.

CLINICAL SYMPTOMS

- Ringworm (tinea corporis): Ring lesion on the skin that appears to spread centrifugally.
- Athlete's foot (tinea pedis).
- Jock itch (tinea cruris).
- Onychomycoses (tinea unguium): Nail infection, discoloration of nails.
- Body infection (tinea corporis).

DIAGNOSIS

- Scrapings of infected skin are placed in KOH preparation, which destroys nonfungal cells and allows visualization of fungal hyphae.
- Wood's lamp (**UV** light) detects *Microsporum*.

TREATMENT

- Topical antifungal creams for skin infections (imidazole).
- Oral antifungals for hair follicle and nail infections.

PROGNOSIS

Good, but relapse is common.

MALASSEZIA FURFUR

CHARACTERISTICS

Natural flora of skin.

PATHOGENESIS

- Reservoir: Animals, humans, soil.
- Transmission: Contact.

CLINICAL SYMPTOMS

Pityriasis (tinea) versicolor: **Pale** spots on the skin, often on the back, chest, and neck.

DIAGNOSIS

- KOH prep.
- Spherical yeast.
- "Spaghetti and meatballs" appearance (Figure 5-42).

PROGNOSIS

Good.

TREATMENT

Topical antifungals: Imidazole.

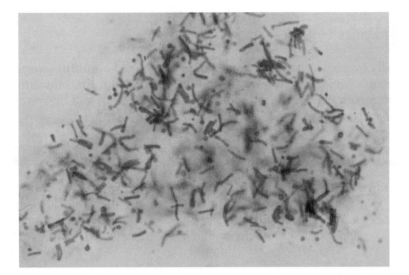

FIGURE 5-42. *Malassezia furfur,* "spaghetti and meatballs" appearance, shown on **Gram stain.** (Image courtesy of CDC's Public Health Image Library; content provider Dr. Lucille K. Georg.)

Subcutaneous Fungal Infections

SPOROTHRIX SCHENCKII

CHARACTERISTICS (FIGURE 5-43)

- Found in soil.
- "Gardener's nodule": Often transmitted via prick of finger on **rose thorns**.
- At 25°C, appears as branching hyphae with macronidia-shaped-like flowers.
- At 37°C, appears as unequally budding yeast.

PATHOGENESIS

- Subcutaneous infections affect skin and surrounding lymphatics.
- Reservoir: Spores in soil.
- Transmission: Spores enter skin through cuts and puncture wounds such as puncture of rose thorn.

CLINICAL SYMPTOMS

Subcutaneous nodules form along lymphatics usually in the upper extremity that was infected via break in the skin. Primary nodule becomes necrotic and ulcerates. Secondary nodules form along lymphatic tracts draining primary infection.

DIAGNOSIS

- Culture at different temperatures reveals branched hyphae at 25°C and single cells (**cigar-shaped** budding yeast) at 37°C.
- Produces **black** pigment.
- Rosette conidia.
- Neutrophilic **microabscesses** in skin.

TREATMENT

- Oral potassium iodide (mechanism unclear).
- Antifungals for extracutaneous involvement: Amphotericin B, itraconazole.

PROGNOSIS

Good.

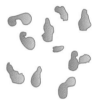

FIGURE 5-43. *Sporothrix schenckii.* Yeast forms, unequal budding.

Parasitology

Medically important parasites comprise **two** groups: **helminths** (worms) and **protozoans.** Notable helminths are the tapeworms and the pinworm. Relevant protozoa include *Plasmodium* (the malaria parasite) and organisms such as *Entamoeba* and *Giardia*.

HELMINTHS

Helminths are multicellular parasites (worms) often associated with **eosinophilia.** Two general types of helminths include the flatworms (Platyhelminthes) and roundworms (nematodes). The flatworms may be segmented (ie, cestodes, or tapeworms) or nonsegmented (ie, trematodes, or flukes) (Figure 5-44).

Cestodes (Tapeworms)

Cestodes are **segmented** flatworms, and **all** are transmitted by **ingestion.** In general, infected persons are treated with albendazole, praziquantel, or niclosamide (Table 5-23).

TAENIA SAGINATA (BEEF TAPEWORM)

CHARACTERISTICS

Composed of scolex ("head") and proglottids (segmented "tail"). *Taenia saginata* can grow to several meters long.

PATHOGENESIS

Adheres to mucosa via **scolex** and absorbs nutrients from host.

CLINICAL SYMPTOMS

- Ingestion of larvae in undercooked beef leads to infection that may be asymptomatic or may present with abdominal discomfort or malnutrition (or both).
- Diagnosis is by detection of proglottids or eggs in **stool.**

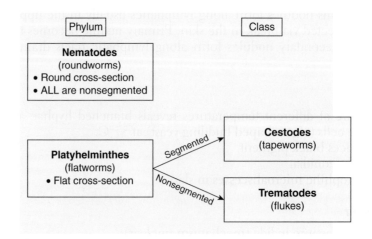

FIGURE 5-44. Helminth classification scheme.

TABLE 5-23.   Summary of Cestodes

Mode of Transmission	Type of Infection	Worm	Symptoms	Buzzwords/ Associations	Lab Findings
Ingestion of larvae	GI	*T saginata* (**beef** tapeworm)	None, abdominal discomfort, malnutrition.	Undercooked beef, proglottids.	Eggs in stool.
	GI	*T solium* (**pork** tapeworm)	None, abdominal discomfort, malnutrition.	Undercooked pork, proglottids.	Eggs in stool.
Ingestion of eggs	Tissue	*T solium* (pork tapeworm)	Cysticercosis, seizures, blindness.	Worm can be seen in vitreous humor!	Tissue calcifications on X-ray.
	GI	*Diphyllobothrium latum* (broad**fish** tapeworm)	None, B$_{12}$ deficiency, macrocytic anemia.	Undercooked or pickled fish.	Eggs in stool.
	GI	*Echinococcus granulosus* (**dog** tapeworm)	Right upper quadrant pain, hepatomegaly, anaphylaxis.	Liver cysts, hydatid cyst disease, sheep, dogs.	Cysts on X-ray or CT.

TREATMENT

Niclosamide or praziquantel.

TAENIA SOLIUM (PORK TAPEWORM)

CHARACTERISTICS

Body plan similar to that of *Taenia saginata*. Ingestion of the *T solium* egg versus larva causes different diseases (Figure 5-45).

PATHOGENESIS

Ingesting the larval form through contaminated pork leads to infestation of intestines. The egg form is ingested through fecal contamination, and hatches in the intestines. The larvae then penetrate the intestinal wall to enter the bloodstream and cause systemic infection.

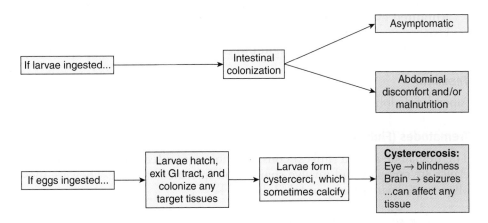

FIGURE 5-45.   Mechanisms of *Taenia solium* infection.

Clinical Symptoms

Diagnosis rests on **calcified cysticerci** on radiograph and serology.

Treatment

- GI infection: Niclosamide or praziquantel.
- Cysticercosis: Albendazole with prednisone.

Diphyllobothrium latum (Fish Tapeworm)

Characteristics

Can grow to several meters long.

Pathogenesis

Ingestion of infected undercooked or pickled freshwater fish results in intestinal colonization. May absorb nutrients and **outcompete host for vitamin B_{12}.**

Clinical Symptoms

Diagnosis is based on finding eggs in **stool.** Infection is often asymptomatic, but can also cause B_{12} **deficiency** with a megaloblastic, macrocytic anemia.

Treatment

Praziquantel.

Echinococcus granulosus (Dog Tapeworm)

Characteristics

Smaller than other tapeworms.

Pathogenesis

Ingestion of eggs from canine fecal contamination allows larvae to hatch in the GI tract. They can then penetrate the intestinal wall and migrate to target tissues, where they form **hydatid cysts.**

Clinical Symptoms

- **Diagnosis** is based on plain film or CT visualization of cysts in tissue. Clinical manifestations of infection include **hydatid cyst disease,** which can affect the liver, lungs, and brain, resulting in organ **dysfunction.**
- **Ruptured cysts** can release high levels of antigen and may cause **anaphylaxis.**
- **Liver cysts** can present with **right upper quadrant pain** and **hepatomegaly.**

Treatment

Albendazole followed by careful cyst aspiration.

Trematodes (Flukes)

The trematode genera (flukes) consist of **nonsegmented** flatworms. Their life cycles are complex and involve **snails** as an intermediate host. They are most often treated with **praziquantel** (Table 5-24).

Clonorchis sinensis (Chinese Liver Flukes)

Characteristics

Endemic in Southeast Asia.

KEY FACT

Modes of transmission:
- Undercooked seafood: *Clonorchis sinensis, Paragonimus westermani, Diphyllobothrium latum*
- Undercooked beef: *Taenia saginata*
- Undercooked pork: *Taenia solium, Trichinella spiralis*
- Human feces: *Ascaris lumbricoides, Enterobius vermicularis, Trichuris trichiura*
- Dog feces: *Toxocara, Echinococcus*
- Drinking water: *Dracunculus*

TABLE 5-24. **Summary of Trematodes**

Mode of Transmission	Type of Infection	Worm	Symptoms	Buzzwords/ Associations	Lab Findings
Ingestion of encysted larvae	GI	*Clonorchis sinensis* (Chinese liver fluke).	Biliary tree infection.	Undercooked fish, **cholangiocarcinoma.**	Eggs in stool.
Ingestion of eggs	Lung	*Paragonimus westermani.*	Hemoptysis, cough, fever.	Shellfish (crab meat).	Eggs in stool and sputum.
Larval penetration of skin	Tissue	*Schistosoma mansoni* and *Schistosoma japonicum.*	Pruritus at entry sites, constitutional symptoms (Katayama fever).	**Portal hypertension,** intestinal polyps, snails.	Eggs in stool.
	Tissue	*Schistosoma haematobium.*	Pruritus at entry sites, constitutional symptoms (Katayama fever), **hematuria.**	**Squamous cell carcinoma of bladder,** snails.	Eggs in stool and urine.

PATHOGENESIS

Encysted larvae are ingested in **raw or undercooked freshwater fish.** The larvae migrate through the GI tract and mature in the **biliary tree.**

CLINICAL SYMPTOMS

Diagnosis is by eggs in stool. Manifestations range from asymptomatic to vague right upper quadrant pain, cholangitis, and/or biliary obstruction. Associated with **cholangiocarcinoma.**

TREATMENT

All flukes are treated with praziquantel.

PARAGONIMUS WESTERMANI (LUNG FLUKE)

CHARACTERISTICS

Endemic in Asia, Africa, and South America.

PATHOGENESIS

Ingestion of eggs from infected **shellfish.**

CLINICAL SYMPTOMS

Diagnosis is via eggs in sputum and stool. Clinical manifestations of infection include **hemoptysis,** cough, and fever.

TREATMENT

All flukes are treated with praziquantel.

SCHISTOSOMES (BLOOD FLUKES)

CHARACTERISTICS

- Male folds its body ventrally to hold female in **permanent copulation.**
- Eggs are highly **immunogenic,** resulting in chronic inflammation and erosion of tissues.

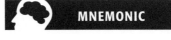

MNEMONIC

PPPP

Paragonimus causes hemo**P**tysis, eggs in s**P**utum, and **P**ulmonary disease.

- Transmission: Larvae released into freshwater penetrate through the skin, then enter the bloodstream to reach target tissues.
- Clinical manifestations of infection: Patient may be asymptomatic or may present with constitutional symptoms (Katayama fever) or early dermatitis with pruritus at the entry site (or both). Late manifestations are due to chronic inflammation of target tissue.
- **Three species: *Schistosoma japonicum, S haematobium,* and *S mansoni.***
- Clinical manifestations: *Schistosoma japonicum* and *S mansoni* can mature in the **portal circulation,** resulting in periportal fibrosis and portal hypertension. They can also affect the mesenteric circulation, resulting in intestinal polyps.
- *Schistosoma haematobium:*
  - Clinical manifestations: *S haematobium* can mature in the blood vessels supplying the **bladder,** resulting in **hematuria,** dysuria, frequency, and urgency. Long-term infection is associated with **squamous cell carcinoma of the bladder,** presumably as a result of chronic inflammation. (Note that most primary bladder cancers are transitional cell carcinoma.)
  - Diagnosis: Eggs found in stool (all *Schistosoma*) and eggs in urine (*S haematobium*)

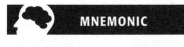

MNEMONIC

*Schistosoma **hemat**obium* causes **hemat**uria.

TREATMENT

All flukes are treated with praziquantel.

Nematodes (Roundworms)

Nematodes are **nonsegmented** worms with a **circular** cross-section and complete digestive system. Table 5-25 contains a summary of nematodes.

ASCARIS LUMBRICOIDES

CHARACTERISTICS

Ascaris is a large nematode that can grow up to 13 inches long. It is the **most common helminthic infection in the world** and is especially prevalent in tropical areas with poor sanitation.

PATHOGENESIS

Transmission is **fecal-oral** via ingestion of eggs from contaminated soil. Eggs hatch in the digestive tract, and larvae then penetrate the intestinal wall and enter the vasculature.

CLINICAL SYMPTOMS

Ascariasis may be **asymptomatic** but may result in **pneumonia.** Larvae can also mature into adult worms in the intestines. As a result, *Ascari* infection may cause **malnutrition,** bowel obstruction, or biliary obstruction. Diagnosis is made by eggs in the stool and **eosinophilia.**

TREATMENT

Pyrantel pamoate, mebendazole, albendazole.

ENTEROBIUS VERMICULARIS (PINWORMS)

CHARACTERISTICS

Pinworms are small nematodes, about 1 cm long. Pinworm infection is the **most common helminthic infection in the United States.**

PATHOGENESIS

Transmission is **fecal-oral** via ingestion of eggs from contaminated surfaces or household dust. Eggs hatch in the digestive tract, where the larvae then mature and mate. Adult females migrate out through the anus and **lay eggs in perianal skin.**

TABLE 5-25.   Summary of Nematodes

MODE OF TRANSMISSION	TYPE OF INFECTION	WORM	SYMPTOMS	BUZZWORDS	LABORATORY DIAGNOSIS
Ingestion of eggs	GI	*Ascaris lumbricoides.*	None, pneumonia, malnutrition.	Bowel obstruction, bile obstruction.	Eggs in stool.
	GI	*Enterobius vermicularis* (pinworm).	Anal pruritus.		Scotch tape test.
	GI	*Trichuris trichiura* (whipworm).	None, diarrhea without pruritus.		
Ingestion of larvae	Tissue	*Trichinella spiralis* (pork roundworm).	Diarrhea, myalgias, periorbital edema.	Pork, wild game.	
	Tissue	*Dracunculus medinensis* (Guinea worm).	Painful subcutaneous nodules.	Copepods.	Roll out on a stick, surgery.
Ingestion of eggs	GI	*Toxocara canis* (dog ascaris).	Hepatosplenomegaly, blindness.	Visceral larva migrans.	
Larvae penetrate skin (usually feet)	GI	*Strongyloides stercoralis* (threadworm).	None, pneumonitis, gastroenteritis.		Larvae in stool, string test.
	GI	*Necator americanus* (New World hookworm).	Pneumonitis, gastroenteritis, microcytic anemia.		Eggs in stool.
	GI	*Ancylostoma duodenale* (Old World hookworm).	Pneumonitis, gastroenteritis, microcytic anemia.		Eggs in stool.
	GI	Cat or dog hookworm.	Itching along worm's path.	Cutaneous larva migrans.	
Arthropod bite					
Blackfly	Systemic	*Onchocerca volvulus.*	River blindness, skin nodules, rash, hyperpigmentation.		
Mosquito	Systemic	*Wuchereria bancrofti.*	Elephantiasis, edema, fever, scaly skin.	Enter bloodstream at night.	
Deer fly	Systemic	*Loa loa* (eye worm).	Blindness, swelling in skin.		

CLINICAL SYMPTOMS

Pinworms most often affect **children,** and the eggs cause **intense perianal itching.** Diagnosis is made using the **Scotch tape test,** in which a piece of tape is pressed against the perianal skin and then examined for eggs.

TREATMENT

Pyrantel pamoate, mebendazole, albendazole.

TRICHURIS TRICHIURA (WHIPWORM)

CHARACTERISTICS

Adult worms are typically 3–5 cm long, with a whiplike shape (narrow anterior, wide posterior).

PATHOGENESIS

Similar to pinworms, whipworm transmission is fecal-oral via ingestion of eggs. Eggs hatch in the digestive tract, where the larvae then mature and mate. Adult whipworms attach to the **superficial mucosa.**

CLINICAL SYMPTOMS

Usually **asymptomatic,** but heavier worm burdens may result in malnutrition, abdominal pain, **bloody diarrhea,** tenesmus, and/or **rectal prolapse.** No anal pruritus. Diagnosis of whipworm is made by eggs in the stool.

TREATMENT

Mebendazole, albendazole.

TRICHINELLA SPIRALIS (PORK ROUNDWORM)

CHARACTERISTICS

Most common cause of parasitic **myocarditis.**

PATHOGENESIS

Transmission occurs by ingestion of encysted larvae in **undercooked pork** or wild game. Larvae mature and mate in the human digestive tract and may subsequently penetrate the intestinal wall to enter the bloodstream. From the blood, larvae often migrate to skeletal **muscle.**

CLINICAL SYMPTOMS

Trichinellosis is characterized by different stages of symptoms that correlate to the worm's life cycle. Early symptoms occur while the larvae are still within the digestive tract and include **nausea, vomiting, diarrhea,** and other constitutional symptoms. Migrating larvae that have entered the bloodstream and reached peripheral tissues may then cause both a local and a systemic response. Symptoms may include high **fever, eosinophilia, periorbital edema,** conjunctival and splinter hemorrhages, and urticarial rash. Once the larvae have migrated to skeletal muscle, **myalgias** may occur. Over time, these larvae may become surrounded by calcified fibrous tissue, thus forming **calcified cysts.** Higher inocula may lead to larval infiltrations of the heart and brain, leading to myocarditis and encephalitis, respectively. Diagnosis is confirmed by **muscle biopsy** or positive anti-*Trichinella* **serology** (or both). Note that there are **no eggs in the stool** because *Trichinella* eggs hatch in the intestinal submucosa.

TREATMENT

Mebendazole, albendazole, and thiabendazole are effective for the intestinal stages of infection. Although there is no effective treatment for muscle cysts, **glucocorticoids** may be beneficial in cases of severe myositis or myocarditis.

DRACUNCULUS MEDINENSIS (GUINEA WORM)

CHARACTERISTICS

Larvae live in tiny aquatic crustaceans (called **copepods**).

PATHOGENESIS

Copepods are ingested in drinking water. *Dracunculus* larvae are then free to mature and mate in the human host.

CLINICAL SYMPTOMS

Adult worms migrate to the **skin** to release their eggs back into the environment. They form painful subcutaneous nodules and can reach lengths up to 3 feet.

TREATMENT

Nodules can be removed surgically or by slowly pulling out the worm by rolling it on a stick. If the worm were to break during this process, **anaphylaxis** may result.

TOXOCARA CANIS (DOG ASCARIS)

CHARACTERISTICS

Toxocara canis is similar to *A lumbricoides*, but can complete its life cycle only in dogs. Humans are a dead-end host.

PATHOGENESIS

Transmission is fecal-oral via ingestion of eggs soil contaminated with dog feces. Eggs hatch in the digestive tract, and larvae penetrate the intestinal wall and enter the vasculature.

CLINICAL SYMPTOMS

Larvae can migrate to many different organs. Therefore this disease is known as **visceral** larva migrans. Common manifestations include **hepatosplenomegaly** and **blindness**. Diagnosis is made by **eosinophilia** and anti-*Toxocara* **serology**.

TREATMENT

Infection is usually self-limited, but glucocorticoids may be helpful in severe cases.

STRONGYLOIDES STERCORALIS (THREADWORM)

PATHOGENICITY

Larvae in contaminated soil are able to directly penetrate the skin, usually through the feet.

CLINICAL SYMPTOMS

Strongyloidiasis can be **asymptomatic**. However, **local itching** may occur at the site of entry, and larvae are transported through the vasculature to the lungs, where they may result in **pneumonia.** From the lungs, they can migrate up the trachea and into the pharynx where they are subsequently swallowed. Larvae can then mature and mate in the digestive tract. Females lay their eggs in the intestinal wall, which may cause abdominal pain and **diarrhea.** Once the eggs hatch, larvae may exit with feces or may penetrate the abdominal wall and reenter the bloodstream. In the latter case, larvae can then travel to the lungs and repeat the life cycle (**autoinfection**). Diagnosis is made by eosinophilia and **larvae in the stool.** Serology is highly sensitive and specific and has replaced the "**string test,**" in which a patient swallows a long string that reaches the duodenum, after which larvae can then be pulled out via the string.

TREATMENT

Ivermectin, thiabendazole.

NECATOR AMERICANUS AND ANCYLOSTOMA DUODENALE (NEW WORLD AND OLD WORLD HOOKWORM)

CHARACTERISTICS

Both species of hookworms have characteristic "hooks" in their mouth that allow them to attach to the intestinal mucosa.

PATHOGENICITY

Similar to *Strongyloides*, larvae in contaminated soil are able to directly penetrate the skin, usually through the feet.

CLINICAL SYMPTOMS

Similar to *Strongyloides*, **local itching** may occur at the site of entry. Larvae are then transported through the vasculature to the lungs, where they may result in **pneumonia.** From the lungs, they can migrate up the trachea and into the pharynx, where they are subsequently swallowed. Larvae can then mature into adults in the GI tract. The adult form attaches to the intestinal mucosa using characteristic hooks. It can then feed off of the host's blood. Adults can also mate in the intestines and release eggs into the stool.

- Initial symptoms may include abdominal pain and **diarrhea.**
- Over time, the host may develop a **hypochromic microcytic anemia.**
- Diagnosis is made by eggs in the stool, along with **eosinophilia.**

TREATMENT

Mebendazole, pyrantel pamoate. Treat anemia with iron and folic acid.

CAT OR DOG HOOKWORM

CHARACTERISTICS

Lacks the necessary collagenase to be able to penetrate through the epidermal basement membrane in humans. The infection is especially prevalent in warm, humid climates and usually affects children.

PATHOGENESIS

Larvae reside in soil contaminated with dog or cat feces. Similar to human hookworms, they are able to directly penetrate the skin, usually through the feet.

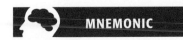

MNEMONIC

STrongyloides is the only helminth whose larvae are **ST**rong enough to get into the **ST**ool.

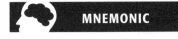

MNEMONIC

Remember that both hookworms can cause **iron deficiency anemia:**
Dracula sucks blood from your **Nec**(ator).
Ancylostoma forms an **an**astomosis with your gut.

CLINICAL SYMPTOMS

Because the larvae cannot penetrate human skin, they are only able to migrate along the dermal-epidermal junction. Their path is marked by a serpiginous erythematous rash that is intensely pruritic. This is known as **cutaneous larva migrans** (Figure 5-46).

TREATMENT

Infection is usually self-limited, and larvae usually die within several weeks.

ONCHOCERCA VOLVULUS (RIVER BLINDNESS)

CHARACTERISTICS

Arthropod-borne, endemic near rivers.

PATHOGENESIS

Larvae migrate through skin and mature into adults. Adults can mate and release microfilariae into subcutaneous tissues. To complete their life cycle, microfilariae are ingested via a second fly bite and then mature into larvae.

CLINICAL SYMPTOMS

- A bite from the **black fly** releases larvae into the **skin.**
- Fibrosis can occur around adults, resulting in **subcutaneous nodules.**
- Migrating microfilariae result in an inflammatory response consisting of a thick, hyperpigmented, pruritic **rash.**
- If microfilariae reach the eye, local inflammation can also cause blindness (**river blindness**).
- Diagnosis can be made with a skin biopsy of a subcutaneous nodule.

TREATMENT

Ivermectin is effective against microfilariae only. Subcutaneous nodules (ie, adults) must be surgically removed.

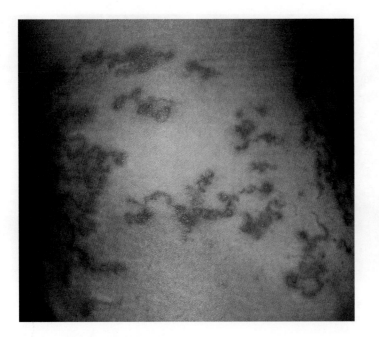

FIGURE 5-46. **Cutaneous larva migrans.** (Image courtesy of Wikipedia; permission granted per the GNU Free Documentation License and the Creative Commons Attribution ShareAlike 3.0 license.)

Loa Loa (Eye Worm)

Characteristics

Arthropod-borne, similar to *Onchocerca*. Found in Africa.

Pathogenesis

A bite from the **Chrysops** fly releases larvae into the skin.

Clinical Symptoms

Infection is most often asymptomatic, but can lead to episodic swelling (Calabar swellings). Adult worms can sometimes be seen **migrating through the subconjunctiva.**

Treatment

Diethylcarbamazine.

Wuchereria Bancrofti (Elephantiasis)

Characteristics

Arthropod-borne, endemic in tropical areas.

Pathogenesis

A **mosquito** bite releases microfilariae into the **blood.**

Clinical Symptoms

Microfilariae reach the lymphatic system and mature into adults. Fibrosis around adults results in obstruction, leading to edema and scaly skin (**elephantiasis**), which usually involves the **genitalia** and **lower extremities** (Figure 5-47). Other signs and symptoms of infection may include fever, chills, lymphadenopathy, and eosinophilia. Diagnosis can be made by detecting microfilariae in the blood at **night.**

> **MNEMONIC**
>
> *Arthropod-borne nematodes—*
>
> **OWL**
> **O**nchocerca
> **W**uchereria
> **L**oa loa

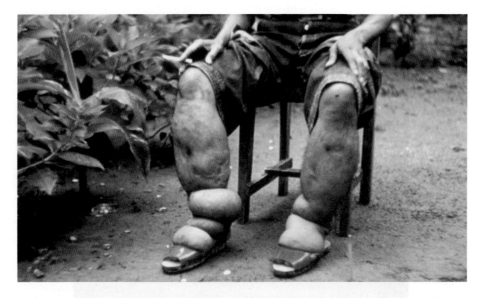

FIGURE 5-47. **Elephantiasis of the lower extremity.** (Image courtesy of CDC's Public Health Image Library.)

TREATMENT

Diethylcarbamazine treats the parasite; however, doxycycline treats an obligate intracellular parasite and has a high cure rate alone.

PROTOZOA

Protozoa are **unicellular,** eukaryotic parasites. They can be classified into two groups based on sites of pathogenesis:

1. Intestinal and mucocutaneous protozoa: *Entamoeba, Giardia, Cryptosporidium, Isospora, Balantidium,* and *Trichomonas.*
2. Blood and tissue protozoa: *Plasmodium, Babesia, Toxoplasma, Leishmania,* and *Trypanosoma.*

Intestinal and Mucocutaneous Protozoa

ENTAMOEBA HISTOLYTICA

- Infection may be **asymptomatic** or may cause amoebic **dysentery** (tenesmic diarrhea with blood and mucus) and visceral **abscess** especially in the liver (Figure 5-48).
- Fecal-oral transmission.
- Exists in **two** forms: trophozoite and cyst.
- Trophozoite contains **ingested** RBCs, whereas the cyst form has characteristic **four** nuclei.
- Treatment: Metronidazole.

GIARDIA LAMBLIA

- Causes noninvasive gastrointestinal disease characterized by abdominal cramps, flatulence, and **foul smelling, "explosive" stools** with **steatorrhea.**
- Often seen in **campers** or **hikers** who drank from streams contaminated with infected animal feces.
- Transmission between humans can be **fecal-oral** or **oral-anal** (homosexuals).
- Organism has characteristic "facelike" appearance.
- Treatment: Metronidazole.

> **KEY FACT**
>
> Helminths are **multicellular** parasites, but protozoa are **unicellular** parasites.

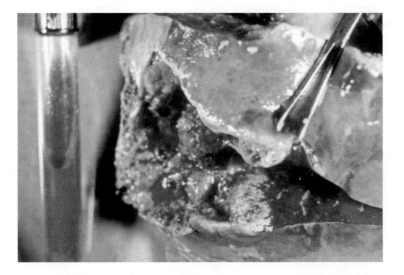

FIGURE 5-48. **Amebic abscess of the liver.** Tube of "chocolate pus" from abscess. (Image courtesy of CDC's Public Health Image Library; content provider Dr. Mae Melvin, Dr. E. West.)

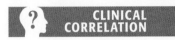
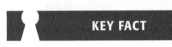
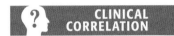
CRYPTOSPORIDIUM PARVUM

- Causes **self-limiting** watery diarrhea in **immunocompetent** persons but can result in massive, **chronic** watery diarrhea in **immunocompromised** patients such as AIDS patients.
- Fecal sample reveals **acid-fast** oocysts (Figure 5-49).
- Treatment: Supportive.

TRICHOMONAS VAGINALIS

- **Sexually transmitted** urogenital infection.
- Infection (**vaginitis** in females) characterized by **greenish, foul-smelling,** watery and **itchy** discharge. Infected cervix has punctate hemorrhages ("strawberry cervix").
- Infected males are usually **asymptomatic** but may present with **urethritis** or **prostatitis.**
- **Wet mount** reveals motile organism with four anterior flagella.
- Treatment: Metronidazole.

Blood and Tissue Protozoa

PLASMODIUM SPECIES

- Causes **malaria,** a mosquito-borne infection that affects 200–400 million people worldwide and kills about 1 million people annually.
- Five species: *Plasmodium falciparum, Plasmodium vivax, Plasmodium ovale, Plasmodium malariae,* and the newly recognized *Plasmodium knowlesi.*
- Vector: female *Anopheles* **mosquito.**
- Complex life cycle involving mosquito, human liver, and human erythrocytes.
- Malaria is characterized by **cyclical fever** with **hemolytic anemia** (parasites infect and rupture RBCs), **myalgias,** and sometimes **gastroenteritis and splenomegaly.**
- Giemsa-stained blood smear reveals **banana-shaped** gametocytes (*Plasmodium falciparum* only), and **"ring" forms** within RBCs (Figure 5-50).
- Sickle cell gene has **protective** effect against malaria.
- **Treatment:** Quinines (chloroquine, primaquine, mefloquine), artemisinin, sulfadoxine-pyrimethamine.
- **Drug-resistance** to antimalarial medications is common.

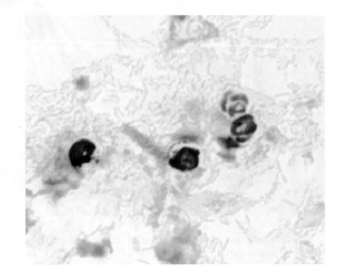

FIGURE 5-49. **Photomicrograph shows acid fast *Cryptosporidium* spp. oocysts (bright red coloration).** (Image courtesy of CDC's Public Health Image Library.)

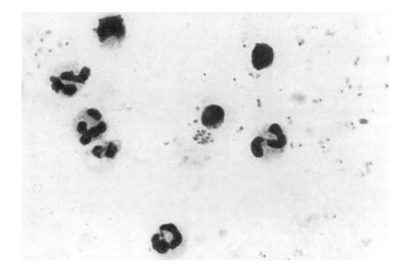

FIGURE 5-50. **Plasmodium.** Giemsa-stained photomicrograph of numerous ring-staged *Plasmodium falciparum* trophozoites, and a centrally-located mature schizont. (Image courtesy of CDC's Public Health Image Library; content provider Dr. Mae Melvin.)

TOXOPLASMA GONDII

- Causes toxoplasmosis, which resembles mononucleosis in immunocompetent persons but can be severe (especially in AIDS patients), resulting in encephalitis with multifocal CNS lesions.
- Routes of infection: **Ingestion** of undercooked, **cyst-contaminated meat,** exposure to **oocysts** in **cat feces,** and **transplacental** transmission.
- Congenital disease (TORCH) is characterized by hydrocephalus, cerebral calcifications, and chorioretinitis.
- Diagnosis: by serology (IgM antibodies to toxoplasmosis antigen). Brain CT scan shows **ring-enhancing lesions.**
- Treatment: Pyrimethamine.

TRYPANOSOMA SPECIES

- Includes *Trypanosoma brucei* and *Trypanosoma cruzi.*
- *Trypanosoma brucei* (*rhodesiense* and *gambiense*) transmitted by **tsetse fly,** causes **African sleeping sickness.**
- *Trypanosoma cruzi,* transmitted by the **reduviid (kissing) bug,** causes **Chagas disease.**
- **Chronic** manifestations of Chagas disease include **dilated cardiomyopathy, megaesophagus, megacolon,** and meningoencephalitis.
- **Treatment:** For sleeping sickness: suramin and pentamidine (blood infection) and melarsoprol (CNS infection). For Chagas disease: benznidazole and nifurtimox (if acute). Symptomatic therapy for chronic Chagas disease.

LEISHMANIA SPECIES

- Four species: *Leishmania donovani, Leishmania tropica, Leishmania mexicana,* and *Leishmania braziliensis.*
- Disease depends on species: *Leishmania donovani* causes visceral leishmaniasis, or "kala azar," resulting in fever, anemia, leukopenia and hepatosplenomegaly. The other *Leishmania* species cause cutaneous or mucocutaneous disease
- Transmission: **Sand fly.**
- Treatment: Stibogluconate. Amphotericin in severe cases.

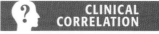

CLINICAL CORRELATION

Due to the risk of transplacental transmission, pregnant women are advised to **avoid cat-litter boxes and undercooked meat.**

CLINICAL CORRELATION

Chagas disease: Think **GIANT** organs!

Irreversible **dilated** cardiomyopathy leads to arrhythmias and heat failure.

Megaesophagus leads to achalasia (swallowing difficulties).

Megacolon leads to malnutrition and weight loss.

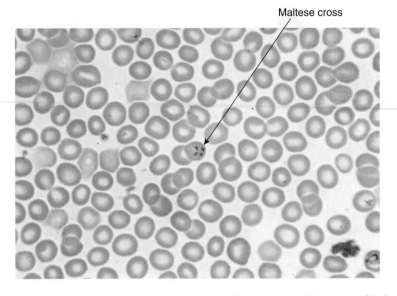

Maltese cross

FIGURE 5-51. **Babesia.** Blood smear showing "maltese cross" configuration of *Babesia* trophozoites. (Image courtesy of CDC's Public Health Image Library; content provider Dr. Mae Melvin.)

Other Notable Protozoa

BABESIA

- **Tick-borne** parasite that causes **malaria-like** illness in northeastern United States.
- Although *Babesia* infects RBCs and causes hemolytic anemia, it does **not** infect the liver like *Plasmodium*.
- Blood smear reveals RBCs containing trophozoites in a **"maltese cross"** configuration (Figure 5-51).
- **Treatment:** Clindamycin and quinine.

NAEGLERIA FOWLERI

- An amoeba that causes **highly fatal, rapid-onset meningoencephalitis.**
- Humans are infected while **swimming** in contaminated **fresh waters.**
- **Treatment:** Amphotericin B or supportive care (advanced cases).

Virology

BASIC STRUCTURE

Virus Particles: Virions

Viruses are obligate intracellular pathogens and can only replicate inside an appropriate host cell. Because they lack their own machinery for self-replication and are not technically living cells, viral infectious particles are instead dubbed "virions." They are composed of a genome encased in a protein coat (**capsid**). Depending on the life cycle of the virus, the capsid may or may not be surrounded by a lipoprotein envelope (Figure 5-52).

Viral genome + Capsid ± Virus-Encoded Enzymes = Nucleocapsid = Nonenveloped Virus

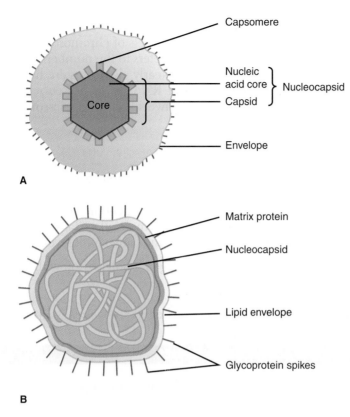

FIGURE 5-52.   **Schematic diagram of the components of the complete virus particle (the virion).** (A) Enveloped virus with icosahedral symmetry. (B) Virus with helical symmetry. (Modified with permission from Brooks GF, Carroll KC, Butel JS, et al. *Jawetz, Melnick, & Adelberg's Medical Microbiology*, 24th ed. New York: McGraw-Hill, 2007.)

Nucleocapsid + Host Membrane with Virus-Encoded Glycoproteins =
Enveloped Virus

Viral Genome

The viral genome is composed of a nucleic acid sequence made up of either DNA or RNA (but not both). There is great variation in genomic structure:

- Double-stranded (**ds**) or single-stranded (**ss**)
- Segmented or nonsegmented
- Linear, circular, or partial circular

A virus with a **single-stranded genome** can either be:

- **Positive-stranded (positive sense) RNA:** Genome exhibits mRNA-like characteristics; thus it can be directly translated by the host cell.
- **Negative-stranded (negative sense) RNA:** The virus must first make a complementary copy of its genome before it can undergo translation. Negative-stranded viruses must carry their own enzymes, such as **RNA-dependent RNA polymerases** to transcribe the complement strand after infecting a host cell. Most (+) strand RNA viruses also encode RNA-dependent RNA polymerase.
- **Ambisense:** Genome contains both positive-stranded and negative-stranded nucleic acid. This arrangement requires two rounds of transcription to be carried out.

KEY FACT

Most **DNA** viruses = **ds**
Many **RNA** viruses = **ss**

Viral Ploidy

Traditionally, ploidy refers to the number of sets of chromosomes in a biological cell. When referring to viruses, ploidy refers to the number of copies of the viral genome contained in each virion. Nearly all viruses are haploid, meaning they have one copy of their DNA or RNA genome. Retroviruses are the exception—they are diploid, possessing two identical copies of their ssRNA genome.

Capsid

The capsid forms an outer shell that holds and protects the viral genome and virus-encoded enzymes. It is composed of structural proteins called **capsomeres** that are uniquely determined by the viral genome and serve as antigenic stimuli for antibody production; that is, the molecular "tags" by the immune system identifies viruses as foreign. The capsid can exhibit several **shapes:**

- **Icosahedral** (symmetrically sided polygon—polyhedron with 20 symmetrical triangular faces)
  - **Helical**
  - **Complex** (including a mix of polyhedral and helical shapes)

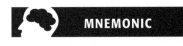

ENVELOPED VERSUS NONENVELOPED VIRUSES

General characteristics of viral species that are human pathogens are depicted in Figure 5-53.

Enveloped Viruses

Enveloped viruses are surrounded by a lipoprotein membrane acquired when the virus is nonlytically released from the host cell. **Virus-encoded glycoproteins present in the lipid membrane** are essential for attachment to the host cell and initiation of infection. The glycoproteins also serve as viral antigens and stimulate antibody production.

- **Most DNA** viruses acquire their envelopes from the host's nuclear plasma membrane as the virus exits the nucleus.
- **Exceptions** are **poxviruses,** because they replicate and acquire their envelope (through "Golgi wrapping") in the cytoplasm.

In addition to their primary function, viral glycoproteins also serve as **viral attachment proteins (VAPs)** that bind to host cell structures. Some examples are:

- Influenza **hemagglutinin (HA):** Binds to exposed sialic acid to mediate viral entry.
- Influenza **neuraminidase (NA):** Facilitates release of virion from host cell.
- **Fusion proteins (F):** Facilitates fusion of virion and the host cell.

Enveloped viruses are more "fragile" and thus require additional packing to protect them against the harsh acidic environment of the GI tract; conversely, nonenveloped viruses can "roam free." However, the lipid envelope carries its own set of susceptibilities, including lipid-dissolving organic solvents such as phenol, detergents, dehydration, and extremes of pH or temperature. Because of these weaknesses, enveloped viruses are limited to the following **modes of transmission:**

- **Direct contact** with bodily fluids: Respiratory droplets, blood, mucus, saliva, and semen.
- Injections or organ transplants.

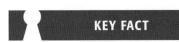

KEY FACT

Viral envelopes mediate attachment to the host cell and initiation of infection and also serve as antigenic stimuli for antibody production.

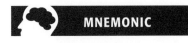

MNEMONIC

Pox (**Pox**viridae) in a box: **C**omplex, divides in **c**ytoplasm

KEY FACT

Many nonenveloped viruses are able to survive the harsh, acidic environment of the stomach and the detergent-like bile found in the intestines. So if you know a virus typically causes GI-related complaints (rotavirus, adenovirus), you know it's nonenveloped!

MNEMONIC

Naked DNA viruses—

A woman needs to be naked for a PAP smear.

Parvovirus
Adenovirus
Papovavirus (**P**apilloma/**P**olyoma)

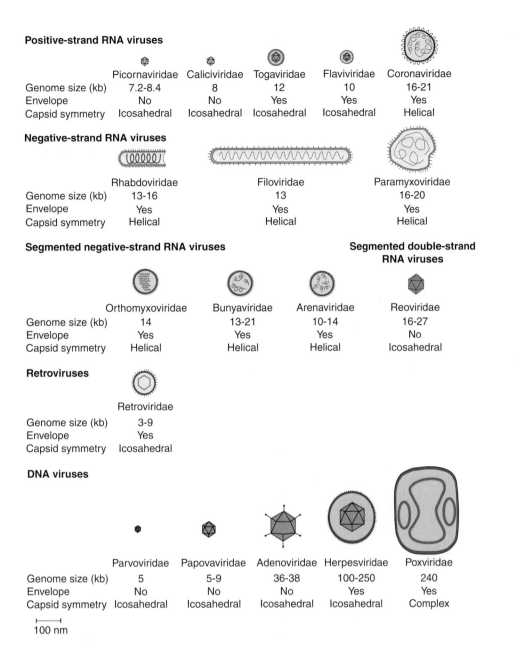

Positive-strand RNA viruses

	Picornaviridae	Caliciviridae	Togaviridae	Flaviviridae	Coronaviridae
Genome size (kb)	7.2-8.4	8	12	10	16-21
Envelope	No	No	Yes	Yes	Yes
Capsid symmetry	Icosahedral	Icosahedral	Icosahedral	Icosahedral	Helical

Negative-strand RNA viruses

	Rhabdoviridae	Filoviridae	Paramyxoviridae
Genome size (kb)	13-16	13	16-20
Envelope	Yes	Yes	Yes
Capsid symmetry	Helical	Helical	Helical

Segmented negative-strand RNA viruses   **Segmented double-strand RNA viruses**

	Orthomyxoviridae	Bunyaviridae	Arenaviridae	Reoviridae
Genome size (kb)	14	13-21	10-14	16-27
Envelope	Yes	Yes	Yes	No
Capsid symmetry	Helical	Helical	Helical	Icosahedral

Retroviruses

	Retroviridae
Genome size (kb)	3-9
Envelope	Yes
Capsid symmetry	Icosahedral

DNA viruses

	Parvoviridae	Papovaviridae	Adenoviridae	Herpesviridae	Poxviridae
Genome size (kb)	5	5-9	36-38	100-250	240
Envelope	No	No	No	Yes	Yes
Capsid symmetry	Icosahedral	Icosahedral	Icosahedral	Icosahedral	Complex

├─────┤
100 nm

FIGURE 5-53. **Schematic diagrams of the major virus families including species that infect humans.** The viruses are grouped by genome type and are drawn approximately to scale. (Modified with permission from Kasper DL, Braunwald E, Fauci, et al. *Harrison's Principles of Internal Medicine*, 16th ed. New York: McGraw-Hill, 2005: 1021.)

Nonenveloped Viruses

Nonenveloped viruses have no envelopes and are usually more stable than enveloped viruses because they are better equipped to withstand injury from the damaging agents mentioned earlier. Enteric viruses such as reoviruses and picornaviruses are transmitted via the **fecal-oral** route. Other viruses are transmitted via respiratory droplets and contact with fomites.

There are four families of **nonenveloped DNA** viruses:

- Parvoviridae
- Adenoviridae
- Papovaviridae (now classified into separate Papilloma and Polyoma families)

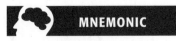

MNEMONIC

Nonenveloped RNA viruses—

A virus needs to be nonenveloped for **A PCR** reaction

Astrovirus
Picornavirus
Calicivirus
Reovirus

For DNA viruses–

Think HHAPPPPy

Herpesviridae
Hepadnaviridae
Adenoviridae
Papillomaviridae
Polyomaviridae
Parvoviridae
Poxviridae

Single-stranded DNA genome–

Like a one-**PAR** hole in golf.
PARvoviridae.

There are four families of **naked RNA** viruses:

- Astroviridae
- Reoviridae
- Picornaviridae
- Caliciviridae

DNA VERSUS RNA VIRUSES

DNA Viruses

There are **six families** of viruses **with DNA genomes** (Figure 5-54). These viruses share the following common characteristics:

1. **Double-stranded genome** with the exception of:
   - Parvoviridae (B19)—**single-stranded** DNA genome.
   - Hepadnavirus—**incomplete double-stranded** genome.
2. **Linear** viral genomes with the exception of: Papovaviruses (papilloma/polyoma) and hepadnavirus—**circular.**
3. **Icosahedral capsid** with the exception of: Poxviruses, which have a complex **capsid.**
4. **Replication** in the nucleus with the exception of: Poxviruses, which carry their own DNA-dependent RNA polymerase and can replicate in the cytoplasm.

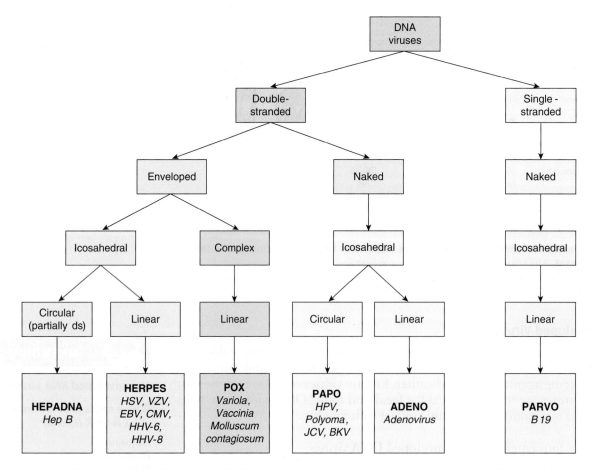

FIGURE 5-54. Flowchart of DNA viruses. Each family is categorized by the type of viral genome and capsid shape. Important examples of each viral family are highlighted.

RNA Viruses

There are **14 major** families of medically important **RNA viruses** (Figure 5-55), which are generally categorized into **three** major groupings: Positive-sense (positive-strand), negative-sense (negative-strand), and ambisense RNA viruses. The terms *sense* and *strand* are used interchangeably.

- Genomes of **positive-sense RNA** viruses act as mRNA and can be directly translated once the virus invades the host cell.
- **Negative-sense RNA** viruses carry their own **RNA-dependent RNA polymerase** and make a positive-sense copy once the virus infects the host cell. The copy is then used as both a genomic template and as mRNA for protein synthesis.
- The genomes of **ambisense RNA** viruses have portions that are both positive- and negative-sense.
- **Segmented viral genomes** are seen mostly in human RNA viruses. After replication, these viral genomes are cleaved into two or more smaller, physically separate segments of nucleic acid. When the virion attaches to and infects another cell, these segments reassemble noncovalently, and join to form a complete genome.

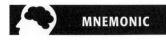

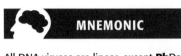

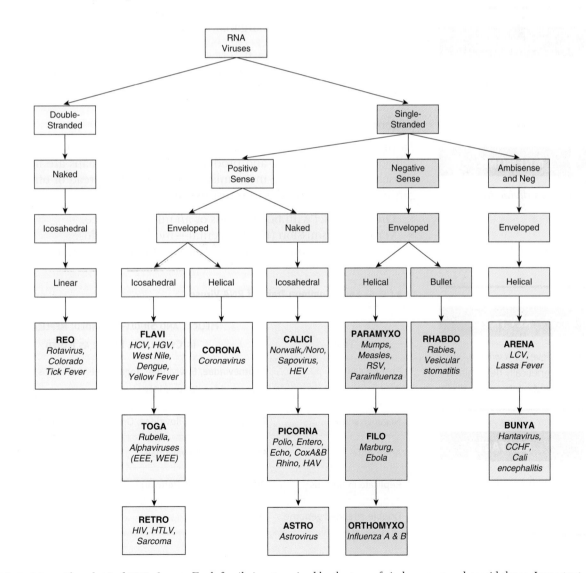

FIGURE 5-55. Flowchart of RNA viruses. Each family is categorized by the type of viral genome and capsid shape. Important examples of each viral family are highlighted.

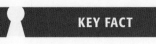

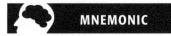

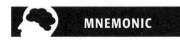

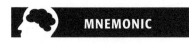

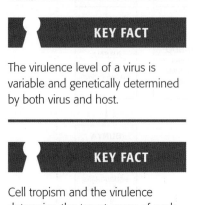

Because of the great number and diversity of the RNA viruses, they have fewer shared characteristics than the DNA viruses. However, they do share a few **common traits** (Table 5-26):

- Single-stranded genome—except for reoviruses, which have a double-stranded RNA genome.
- Replicate in the cytoplasm—except for orthomyxoviruses and retroviruses, both of which replicate at least partially in the nucleus.

PATHOGENESIS

General Considerations

Several key properties influence viral **pathogenesis** (the interaction of viral and host factors that lead to production of disease):

- **Virulence:** Ability of the virus to cause disease by avoiding or otherwise overcoming the host's defense mechanisms.
- **Cellular tropism:** The specificity of a virus for a given host cell or host tissue, determined by surface receptors and intracellular content within the host cell. Infection by a certain virus tends to affect a specific organ or group of organs (**target organs**), causing classic symptoms for that particular virus.
- **Host range:** Range of cells (or species) that can become a host to a virus or bacteriophage; dictated by the presence or absence of specific receptors that enable active viral infection.

Infection

To produce a disease, viruses must enter the host, interact with susceptible cells or tissues, replicate, and produce cell injury. Humans are infected with viruses by the same basic mechanisms that allow the spread of other microorganisms. Common **modes of transmission** include:

- Direct contact with bodily fluids or an infected source.
- Vertical transmission (transplacental—mother to child).
- Direct inoculation through injections or trauma; organ transplant.

TABLE 5-26. **Common Traits of RNA Viruses**

TRAIT	HELICAL AND SINGLE-STRANDED; REPLICATE IN CYTOPLASM, EXCEPT AS NOTED
Positive sense	Picornaviridae, Flaviviridae, Togaviridae, Calicivirus, Coronaviridae, Retroviridae
Negative sense	Paramyxoviridae, Filoviridae, Orthomyxoviridae, Rhabdoviridae
Ambisense	Arenaviridae, Bunyaviridae
Replicate in nucleus	Orthomyxoviridae, Retroviridae
Double-stranded genome	Reoviridae

- **Vectors,** such as insects and small rodents. Humans can become infected through bites of vector species or inhalation of viral particles from the vector's hair, fur, or bodily fluids.
    - **Arthropod-borne viruses—arboviruses:** Mainly belong to four families of viruses—Flaviviridae, Togaviridae, Bunyaviridae, and Reoviridae. The most common arthropod vectors are mosquitoes and ticks. Classic examples of arboviruses include Dengue or "break-bone" fever and yellow fever (both flaviviruses).
    - **Rodent-borne viruses—roboviruses:** Belong to the Arenaviridae and Bunyaviridae families. These viruses are generally transmitted by rats and mice. Perhaps the most well known examples are lymphocytic choriomeningitis virus (LCMV) and Lassa fever, both arenaviruses.
- **Reinfection:** Secondary infection that occurs after recovery from a previous infection and is caused by the same agent.
- **Coinfection:** Concurrent infection of a host (single cell/tissue) by two or more viruses.
- **Superinfection:** Process by which a host previously infected by one virus acquires coinfection with another virus at a later point in time. Superinfection can also be caused by other microorganisms owing to the host's compromised immune system or the microorganisms' resistance to previous antibiotics.

Replication

As obligate intracellular parasites, viruses must infect host cells in order to replicate. This process involves several sequential steps:

- **Attachment to host cell:** Binding of viruses to host cells is mediated through the interaction of viral surface proteins with specific and nonspecific host cell surfaces.
- **Penetration and entry:**
    - Most nonenveloped viruses enter host cells through **receptor-mediated endocytosis.**
    - **Viropexis:** Upon attachment to the host cell surface, hydrophobic (lipophilic) structures of certain naked viruses' capsid proteins are exposed, thus enabling them to directly penetrate the host cell.
    - **Enveloped viruses** enter host cells by **fusing** with the cell membrane, thus allowing the nucleocapsid or the viral genome to be delivered directly into the cytoplasm.
    - The fusion activity can be mediated by **VAPs,** fusion proteins, or other glycoproteins found in the viral membrane.
    - Optimal fusion pH is specific to each type of virus.
    - If the optimal pH is neutral, the enveloped virus can fuse with the outer cell membrane.
    - If the optimal pH is acidic, the virus must first be internalized by endocytosis and fuse with the endosomal membrane in low pH.
- **Uncoating of the virion:** Once a virus is internalized, the nucleocapsid must be brought to the site of replication and removed. Uncoating of a virion results in the loss of infectivity.

REPLICATION OF DNA VIRUSES

DNA viruses (except for poxviruses; Figure 5-54) enter the nucleus and utilize the host cell's DNA-dependent RNA polymerase to transcribe its mRNA from

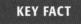

CLINICAL CORRELATION

ARBOvirus = **AR**thropod-**BO**rne virus, including some members of **F**lavivirus, **T**ogavirus, and **B**unyavirus, ie, **F**ever **T**ransmitted by **B**ites.

KEY FACT

Enveloped viruses mediate host cell attachment through their glycoproteins (**VAPs**—viral attachment proteins).
Nonenveloped viruses use **capsid surface proteins** to attach to host cells (receptor-mediated endocytosis).

KEY FACT

Early transcripts encode proteins important for viral replication, gene transcription, and takeover of the host cell.
Late transcripts commonly encode structural proteins, which serve to build new virions later released to infect other cells.

KEY FACT

Adenoviruses use the host cell's enzymes.
Herpesviruses carry their own.

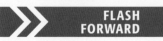

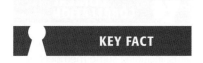

FLASH FORWARD

Hepatitis B virus needs a reverse transcriptase to replicate; therefore, infection can be treated with reverse transcriptase inhibitors used to inhibit retroviruses such as in HIV.

KEY FACT

Poxviruses have their own DNA-dependent RNA polymerase and are capable of replicating in the cytoplasm.

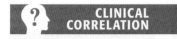

FLASH BACK

Inhibitors of DNA polymerase: Acyclovir, vidarabine, foscarnet, ganciclovir.
Neuraminidase inhibitors zanamivir and oseltamivir specifically inhibit release of progeny virus.

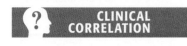

CLINICAL CORRELATION

Nonenveloped viruses cannot cause persistent productive infections, because productive (nonlatent) infection with these viruses characteristically results in cell lysis and death.

CLINICAL CORRELATION

Hepatitis B virus can establish persistent productive infections; that is, infected cells produce virus by slowly spreading in a noncytolytic fashion, remaining morphologically intact over time.

the negative-strand template. There is a specific **temporal pattern of transcription:** immediate early, delayed early, and late mRNA transcripts.

Key steps in DNA virus replication:

- mRNA transcripts undergo modification: Addition of poly A tail and methylated cap takes place in the host cell's **nucleus.**
- Transcripts then are transported to the **cytoplasm** and translated on cytoplasmic polysomes.
- Newly synthesized proteins are then transported **back** to the nucleus, where the capsid is assembled and the viral genome and enzymes are packaged before the virus is released.

Genomic replication is performed by a **DNA-dependent DNA polymerase. Hepatitis B virus** is a **unique DNA virus** because the genome is partially double-stranded with single-stranded regions scattered throughout. Before it can be delivered to the nucleus and replicate, this virus must first generate a fully double-stranded genome. Hepatitis B virus carries a **RNA-dependent DNA polymerase** with reverse transcriptase properties that uses an RNA template to synthesize the DNA.

REPLICATION OF RNA VIRUSES

Both replication and transcription of RNA viruses (except for orthomyxoviruses and retroviruses) occur **in the cytoplasm** (Figure 5-56). This is possible because RNA viruses encode for their own **RNA-dependent DNA polymerases (replicases** and **transcriptases).**

Negative-sense RNA viruses carry these enzymes in their capsids. The genomes of positive-sense RNA viruses can serve as mRNA. Once inside the host cell, the genome can be directly translated to synthesize proteins (Table 5-27).

RELEASE OF NEWLY SYNTHESIZED VIRUS

The process of releasing newly synthesized viruses differs between nonenveloped and enveloped viruses:

- **Naked viruses** kill the host cell through cytolysis in order to be released; thus, they are unable to establish persistent productive infections because infected cells are lysed in the process.
- **Enveloped viruses** are released from infected host cells through a process referred to as **"budding"**; thus, the infected host cell survives and budding can lead to **cell senescence.** Budding involves synthesis of virally encoded glycoproteins within the host cell, which are temporarily anchored in the host cell's membrane. As the virus is released through the process of exocytosis, it is surrounded by the region of the cell membrane studded with glycoproteins, thus creating the viral envelope.

Once viruses are surrounded by the lipoprotein membrane and are released from the host cell, they are considered infective.

Patterns of Infections

Patterns of infection can be divided as follows (Figure 5-57):

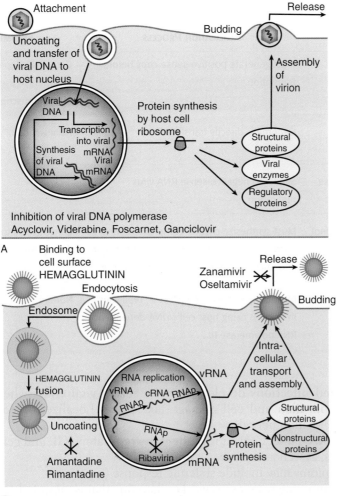

FIGURE 5-56. **Replicative cycles of DNA and RNA viruses.** The replicative cycles of herpesvirus (A) and influenza A virus (B) are examples of DNA-encoded and RNA-encoded viruses, respectively. Sites of action of antiviral agents also are shown. An X on top of an arrow indicates a block to virus growth. The neuraminidase inhibitors zanamivir and oseltamivir specifically inhibit release of progeny virus. Small capitals indicate virus proteins. mRNA, messenger RNA; vRNA, viral RNA; RNAp, RNA polymerase; cRNA, complementary RNA. (Modified with permission from Brunton LL, Parker KL, Buxton ILO, Blumenthal DK. *Goodman & Gilman's The Pharmacological Basis of Therapeutics*, 11th ed. New York: McGraw-Hill, 2006.)

SUBCLINICAL INFECTIONS

Subclinical infections are either asymptomatic or cause a less severe, nonspecific illness that may not be recognized or identified as the result of a specific virus.

- The virus inoculum is small, or only a few host cells are infected.
- The virus may reach its target tissue but replication is curtailed.

ACUTE INFECTIONS

- Acute infections develop apparent clinical symptomatology within a short period of time after the incubation period of the virus. Infections can be **localized** or **disseminated**. In addition, acute infections can be **rapidly cleared** or they can develop into either **persistent** or **latent** infection.

TABLE 5-27. **Specifics of Genomic Replication of the RNA Viruses**

VIRUS	GENOME	REPLICATION PROCESS	ENZYMES
Negative-sense RNA viruses	Complementary to mRNA.	Must generate positive-sense copy before translation.	Carry RNA-dependent RNA polymerase used to make mRNA transcript.
Positive-sense RNA viruses	Acts as mRNA transcript.	Genome is directly translated.	None.
Ambisense RNA viruses	Some portions are positive-sense and others are negative-sense.	Similar to negative-sense RNA virus replication.	
Retroviruses	Positive-sense genome, but cannot be used as mRNA transcript.	Must synthesize circular complementary DNA (cDNA) copy in cytoplasm, which is brought into nucleus and integrated into host DNA.	Carry reverse transcriptases that synthesize cDNA.
Delta virus	Single-stranded RNA genome.	Most unique replication process; replicates in nucleus using host cell's DNA-dependent RNA polymerase II.	None.

- **Localized infections** develop near the site of viral entry, where the primary replication and cell damage take place. Localized infections have short incubation periods.
  - Localized infections mostly affect the respiratory, GI, and genitourinary tracts, as well as the eye.
  - Symptoms may include systemic response (eg, fever).
  - The immune response is weaker than one that is mounted against a disseminated infection.

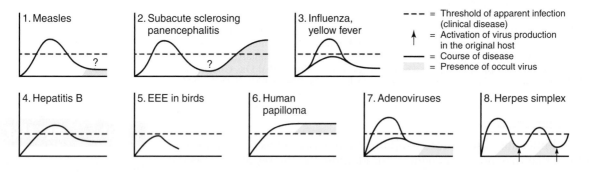

FIGURE 5-57.   Types of virus-host interactions: Apparent (clinical disease), inapparent (subclinical), chronic, latent, occult, and slow infections. (1) Measles runs an acute, almost always clinically apparent course resulting in long-lasting immunity. (2) Measles may also be associated with persistence of latent infection in subacute sclerosing panencephalitis. (3) Yellow fever and influenza follow a pattern similar to that of measles, except that infection may be more often subclinical than clinical. (4) In hepatitis B, recovery from clinical disease may be associated with chronic infection in which fully active virus persists in the blood. (5) Some infections are, in a particular species, always subclinical, such as eastern equine encephalomyelitis (EEE) in some species of birds that then act as reservoirs of the virus. (6) For human papillomavirus, the course of infection is chronic; when cervical cancer develops, the virus present is occult (not replicating). (7) Infection of humans with certain adenoviruses may be clinical or subclinical. There may be a long latent infection during which virus is present in small quantity; virus may also persist after the illness. (8) The periodic reactivation of latent herpes simplex virus, which may recur throughout life in humans, often follows an initial acute episode of stomatitis in childhood. (Modified with permission from Brooks GF, Carroll KC, Butel JS, et al. *Jawetz, Melnick, & Adelberg's Medical Microbiology*, 24th ed. New York: McGraw-Hill, 2007: 400.)

- **Disseminated infections** tend to have longer incubation periods (weeks rather than days) and generally cause **viremia.**
  - Disseminated infections affect multiple organ systems.
  - Symptoms are systemic, reflecting affected organ(s).
  - The immune response is usually greater than in localized infections; however, it typically takes longer to eradicate the virus and clear the infection in these cases.
  - **Congenital malformations** result from acute maternal infections that result in viremia. The virus can cross the placental barrier (**vertical transmission**) and easily infect the fetus because of its immature immune system.
- **Persistent infections** refer to continued presence of the infectious virus over an extended period of time (months, years, or possibly a lifetime).
  - **Carriers** live with a persistent viral infection (hepatitis B virus) and may or may not have clinical manifestations.
  - Other viruses (eg, **herpesvirus**) are able to establish persistent infections in patients in a noninfectious form (no symptoms, viral antigen or viral cytopathology are detected) and periodically reactivate into an infectious form (full-blown symptomatology/disease).

VIRAL GENETICS

Viral variations and alterations that lead to new strains can result from a number of different processes:

- Changes directly affecting the genome: **Genetic drift,** and genetic reassortment resulting in **genetic shift.**
- Strictly phenotypic changes that do not modify viral genomes: **Complementation, phenotypic mixing,** and **phenotypic masking.**

Many of these processes occur when a single cell is infected by multiple strains of a virus or by multiple viruses.

Genetic Reassortment

When two strains of a segmented virus infect the same cell, respective segments can intermingle in the cytoplasm during replication.

- As viral particles undergo assembly, the segmented genomes from the respective strains can trade segments during replication, thus creating a new (progeny) strain with a genome containing sequences from both (parental) strains.
  - Recombination can also occur between genes within the same segment. In general, the recombination frequency between genetic loci increases as the distance between the loci increases.
  - Changes in the **genome** resulting from genetic reassortment are referred to as **genetic shift.**
  - Genetic shift alters the antigenic properties (gene expression profiles) of the affected viruses; hence the term **antigenic shift** (Figure 5-58). This creates phenotypic variation; for example, novel surface proteins may allow viruses to infect previously resistant hosts or gain increased virulence or allow immune escape (antigenic).
- Generated changes in the genome are drastic, yet positively selected, thus providing a source for major viral outbreaks and epidemics or pandemics.

MNEMONIC

Congenital infections—

TORCH

Toxoplasmosis
Other infections*
Rubella
Cytomegalovirus
Herpes simplex virus
*Other infections include syphilis, parvovirus B19, hepatitis B, virus, HIV, and varicella-zoster virus.

KEY FACT

Persistent infection = recurring disease with cycles of symptomatic outbreaks and silent periods.

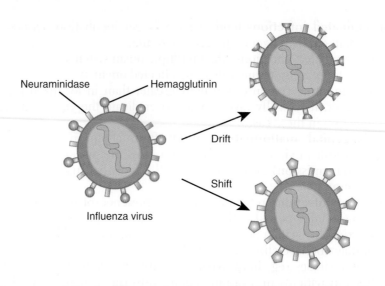

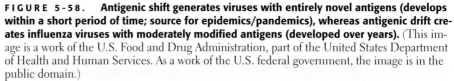

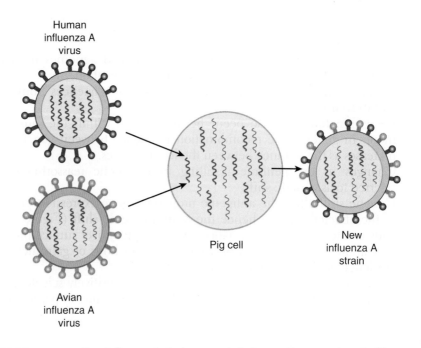

FIGURE 5-58. **Antigenic shift generates viruses with entirely novel antigens (develops within a short period of time; source for epidemics/pandemics), whereas antigenic drift creates influenza viruses with moderately modified antigens (developed over years).** (This image is a work of the U.S. Food and Drug Administration, part of the United States Department of Health and Human Services. As a work of the U.S. federal government, the image is in the public domain.)

▪ A prototypic example of a virus with ability to produce great genetic diversity via genetic reassortment is **influenza A** virus. This ability is secondary to its wide host range (Figure 5-59). Influenza B and C viruses do not exhibit antigenic shift because few related viruses exist in animals.

Genetic (Antigenic) Drift

Genetic drift comprises the spontaneous mutations in viral genomes that create slight antigenic changes, which may or may not alter the virulence of the virus (Figure 5-58).

FIGURE 5-59. **New influenza A strain generated via genetic reassortment of human and avian strains of the virus.**

It is **most notable in RNA viruses,** especially in **HIV** and **orthomyxoviruses,** because their replication processes are error-prone.

Complementation

A defective mutant strain of a virus may be missing a gene encoding an enzyme or factor necessary for replication. Complementation refers to the **rescue** of such a mutant via **coreplication** with **another mutant** or cell line that expresses the missing protein.

- The newly established (**rescued**) genome, though still defective, is able to replicate and form progeny.
- The progeny derived from the original (**mutant**) genome still lack the same gene and are not able to replicate unless they, too, are rescued.

Phenotypic Mixing

When two related, yet **antigenically distinct** viruses infect a **single host cell,** their proteins can mingle. Capsid proteins can merge during the assembly process, resulting in a capsid composed of a mixture of structural and surface proteins from both strains. The **genomes** remain **unchanged,** but the **capsids** are **hybrids** of the two strains, which may then alter the host range or develop resistance to antibody neutralization (Figure 5-60).

Phenotypic Masking (Transcapsidation)

Similar to phenotypic mixing, phenotypic masking occurs when a **single** host cell is infected with **two related viral strains.**

- The genome of one strain is packaged in the capsid of the other.
- **Unlike** phenotypic mixing, the capsid is completely composed of proteins encoded by one strain.
- Phenotypic masking can occur with two completely different types of viruses and can result in what is called **"pseudotypes."**

Viral Vectors

With the use of recombinant DNA technology, viruses can be manipulated to serve as vectors, which deliver foreign genes into human cells. Viral vectors can be used to transfer DNA for gene therapy, as vaccines, and as killers that target specific tumor cells.

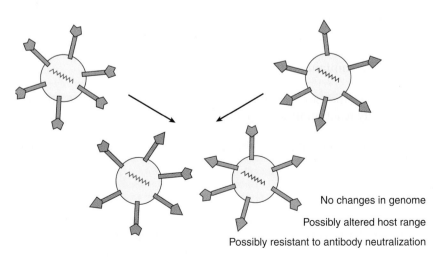

No changes in genome

Possibly altered host range

Possibly resistant to antibody neutralization

FIGURE 5-60. Phenotypic mixing.

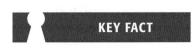
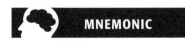

Defective viruses are usually used as vectors because they cannot replicate, but they can infect and deliver genetic material into a targeted cell.

VACCINES

Active immunization with virus vaccines exposes patients to a virus or its antigenic proteins, thus inducing an immune response that may protect from subsequent infection (protection immunity).

Live Virus Vaccines

Live vaccines incorporate **attenuated** viral strains that are relatively non-virulent. These viral vaccines are effective against enveloped viruses, which require cell-mediated immune response to clear the infection.

- The **immune response** to a live virus vaccine mimics natural infection by generating T_H1 and T_H2 responses, thus stimulating both humoral and cell-mediated antibody immunity.
- **Routes of administration** can be parenteral, oral, or by inhalation to mimic the natural route of infection.
- **Immunity** derived from a live virus vaccine is long-lasting; thus, "boosters" are generally not needed. Notable exceptions include measles and chickenpox.

Immunization with a live virus vaccine carries a greater risk than vaccination using an inactivated virus. Live virus vaccines carry the **potential to revert** to a virulent form of the virus and may actually cause disease. Measles, mumps, and rubella (MMR) is the **only** live-attenuated vaccine that can be given to HIV-positive patients, although there is currently a move to allow them to receive others.

Inactivated Vaccines

Contain either killed (inactivated) virus or viral subunits. Once inactivated vaccine is injected into the patient, the body mounts a response to the immunogenic surface antigens found on the viral capsid or envelope.

- The **immune response:**
  - Predominantly a T_H2 (antibody) response, generating immunoglobulin G (IgG) that neutralizes and opsonizes the inactive virus.
  - Local secretory immunoglobulin A (IgA) response is not sufficient.
  - There is not a strong cell-mediated response.
- **Routes of application:** Generally parenteral.
- **Immunity:** Not as long lasting as with live vaccines; **boosters** are usually required to maintain immunity.

Killed virus vaccines are generally very safe. However, they can stimulate a hypersensitivity reaction in some people.

Advantages and disadvantages of the respective types of vaccines are depicted in Table 5-28.

Recombinant Vaccines

Recombinant vaccines utilized bacteria or yeast to generate a large amount of a single protein, which is then purified and injected into the patient. Two recombinant vaccines widely used in the clinical setting are:

TABLE 5-28. Comparison of Advantages and Disadvantages of Live and Killed/Inactivated Vaccines

	LIVE	KILLED/INACTIVATED
Immunity duration	Long-lasting	Short-term
Doses	Single	Multiple (boosters)
Antibody response	IgG, IgA	IgG
Cell-mediated response	Good	Poor
Side effects	Mild symptoms	Soreness around injection site
Temperature-sensitive	Yes	No
Reversion to virulence	Possible	Never

- Hepatitis B (HBV) vaccine (containing the viral envelope protein known as recombinant hepatitis B surface antigen [HBsAg]).
- Human papillomavirus (HPV) vaccine (against types 16 and 18, associated with cervical cancer, and types 6 and 11, associated with genital warts).

DIAGNOSTIC TESTS

Although the history and clinical signs and symptoms are often used to diagnose many viral illnesses, collected specimens can be used in the laboratory to confirm or to diagnose atypical or unusual cases. Most commonly used tests are described below.

- **Cytology** is a rapid detection method. Direct microscopic examination of collected specimens or monolayer cell culture samples are used to detect viruses.
- **Cytopathic effects (CPE):** Viruses can also be characterized and identified by the type of cells they infect, the rate of viral growth, and specific patterns of cellular changes caused by infection.
  - **Syncytia** (multinucleated giant cells) form when individual infected cells fuse together. They are often observed with **HSV, paramyxoviruses,** and **VZV.**
  - **Inclusion bodies** can also be seen in the cytoplasm or nucleus of infected cells.
- **Detection of viral genetic material:** Northern and Southern blot analyses, restriction endonuclease fragment lengths, **genetic probes** and polymerase chain reaction (**PCR**) can all be used to detect viral genetic material.
- **Detection of viral proteins:** Immunohistochemistry is used to detect and quantify viruses or their antigens in clinical specimens or culture samples. **Immunofluorescence,** enzyme-linked immunosorbent assays (**ELISA**), radioimmunoassay (**RIA**), and latex agglutination (**LA**) tests are commonly used methods.
- **Serologic tests:** Virus-specific antibodies may be detected, identified, and quantified in blood or serum samples.
  - **Seroconversion** indicates current infection and is determined by observing at least a fourfold increase in the antibody titer between

KEY FACT

Inactivated vaccines:
Influenza
Adenovirus

KEY FACT

Owl's eye inclusion body = **CMV.**
Negri bodies = **rabies**-infected brain tissue.
Cowdry type A inclusion = individual cells or syncytia of tissues infected with **HSV** or **VZV.**

serum collected during the acute and convalescent phases of an infection.

- Virus-specific **IgM**—usually present during the first 2–3 weeks of a **primary infection.**
- High titers of **IgG** are usually detected a few weeks after infection; they may be detected earlier in a **reinfection.**
- In patients who experience frequent recurrence of disease, antibody titers tend to remain high.

DNA VIRUSES

All viruses have a protein capsid. The capsid of all known DNA viruses is either icosahedral or complex. In addition to their capsid, some DNA viruses also have an outer phospholipid envelope; those that do not are known as nonenveloped viruses. DNA viral genomes are either single-stranded or double-stranded and can be linear or circular (Table 5-29).

Parvovirus B19

CHARACTERISTICS

This is the **smallest** clinically important virus, with a size of 20–25 nm. It is also one of the **five** most common pediatric viral exanthems (diseases that cause a **rash**).

PATHOGENESIS

Transmitted via aerosolized droplets that inoculate the nasal cavity; infects erythroid progenitor cells.

CLINICAL SYMPTOMS

Immune complex deposition results in a lacy red rash (also called erythema infectiosum, fifth disease, or slapped-cheek fever) and arthralgias. Patients with thalassemia or sickle cell anemia may develop a **transient aplastic crisis.** Immunocompromised individuals may develop a **severe chronic anemia.** Infants may develop **hydrops fetalis** and severe anemia. Diagnosis can be confirmed with serology and complete blood count.

TREATMENT

Supportive care with blood transfusions as needed. Immunocompromised patients may require intravenous immunoglobulins.

Papovaviruses (Now Classified Separately as Papillomavirus and Polyomavirus Families)

PAPILLOMAVIRUSES—HUMAN PAPILLOMAVIRUS (HPV)

CHARACTERISTICS

Infects squamous epithelial cells.

PATHOGENESIS

Transmitted by close contact.

TABLE 5-29. Summary of DNA Viruses

Family	Structure	Disease	Route of Transmission	Important Facts
Hepadnaviridae				
Hepatitis B (HBV)	Partially dsDNA, ssDNA gap, enveloped, icosahedral, circular.	Infectious hepatitis.	Blood, blood products, sexual activity, shared needles.	Cause of primary hepatocellular carcinoma, cirrhosis, hepatitis.
Herpesviridae				
Herpes simplex virus (HSV)	dsDNA, enveloped, icosahedral, linear.	Cold sores (usually HSV-1), genital herpes (usually HSV-2), encephalitis (often with characteristic necrosis of the temporal lobes).	Mucous membranes, breaks in skin, sex.	Most common diagnosed cause of acute sporadic encephalitis in the United States.
Varicella-zoster virus (VZV)	dsDNA, enveloped, icosahedral, linear.	Chickenpox, shingles, pneumonia.	Airborne, close contact.	Remains latent in sensory nerve ganglia throughout the body after infection.
Epstein-Barr virus (EBV)	dsDNA, enveloped, icosahedral, linear.	Fever, pharyngitis, lymphadenopathy (heterophile-positive mononucleosis), encephalitis.	Airborne, close contact, mucous membranes.	Associated with malignancies, (eg, Burkitt lymphoma, nasopharyngeal carcinoma, oral hairy-cell leukoplakia).
Cytomegalovirus (CMV)	dsDNA, enveloped, icosahedral, linear.	Fever, pharyngitis, lymphadenopathy (heterophile-negative mononucleosis), infection in immunocompromised individuals (particularly transplant recipients), congenital abnormalities (TORCH).	Close contact (perinatal, venereal), transfusion, transplacental organ transplantation.	One of the TORCH viruses; causes teratogenic symptoms in fetus.
Human herpes-virus 6 (HHV-6)	dsDNA, enveloped, icosahedral, linear.	Fever, rash, adenopathy (cause of roseola or sixth disease), chemical hepatitis.	Saliva.	90% of all humans infected by age 3, usually benign course.
Human herpes-virus 8 (HHV-8)	dsDNA, enveloped, icosahedral, linear.	Primary infection asymptomatic; causes Kaposi sarcoma in AIDS patients.	Sexual and body fluids.	Causes purpuric, raised skin lesions.
Poxviridae				
Variola	dsDNA, enveloped complex, linear.	Smallpox.	Respiratory droplets or close contact.	Lesions develop at the same pace and so are all at the same stage of development.
Vaccinia	dsDNA, enveloped complex, linear.	Cowpox "milkmaid's blisters."	Contact.	Used to make smallpox vaccine.
Molluscum contagiosum	dsDNA, enveloped complex, linear.	Small, spontaneously regressing, umbilicated, flesh-colored skin lesions.	Contact.	Common among wrestlers, HIV+.

(continues)

TABLE 5-29. **Summary of DNA Viruses** *(continued)*

FAMILY	STRUCTURE	DISEASE	ROUTE OF TRANSMISSION	IMPORTANT FACTS
Papillomaviridae				
Human papillomavirus (HPV)	Naked, dsDNA icosahedral, circular.	Cervical or vaginal intraepithelial neoplasia (CIN/VIN), cervical carcinoma and anogenital cancers (types 16 and 18); genital warts/condylomata (types 6 and 11).	Sex, contact.	Highly restricted in tissue tropism and replicates only in epithelial cells. Many serotypes.
Polyomaviridae				
Polyomavirus	Naked, dsDNA icosahedral, circular.	Causes no disease in humans.	Sex, contact.	Causes no human malignancy.
JC virus	Naked, dsDNA icosahedral, circular.	Progressive multifocal leukoencephalopathy (PML).	Sex, contact.	Fatal disorder of CNS that can occur in immunodeficient patients.
BK virus	Naked, dsDNA icosahedral, circular.	Hemorrhagic cystitis, ureteral stenosis, and urinary tract infections.	Sex, contact.	Oncogenic in animal models, not in man.
Adenoviridae				
Adenovirus	dsDNA, naked, icosahedral, linear.	Pharyngitis/pneumonia, conjunctivitis, gastroenteritis.	Fecal-oral, aerosol, close contact.	51 known serotypes of human adenoviruses.
Parvoviridae				
Parvovirus B19	ssDNA, linear, naked, icosahedral.	Erythema infectiosum (fifth disease), aplastic anemia, hydrops fetalis.	Respiratory droplets, oral secretions, parenterally.	The only parvovirus known to cause human disease.

CLINICAL SYMPTOMS

Varies depending on the strain.

- HPV 6 and 11 cause benign warts, including anogenital and laryngeal warts.
- **HPV serotypes 16, 18, 31, 33, and 45 are associated with cervical cancer** (Figure 5-61).
- These strains produce two proteins that inactivate known tumor suppressor genes: E6 inhibits *p53*, E7 inhibits *Rb*.
- Diagnosis can be made by PCR, Papanicolaou (Pap) smear, and/or biopsy.

TREATMENT

Most warts regress spontaneously after 1 or 2 years. Warts can also be ablated or surgically removed. With respect to cervical abnormalities, low-grade

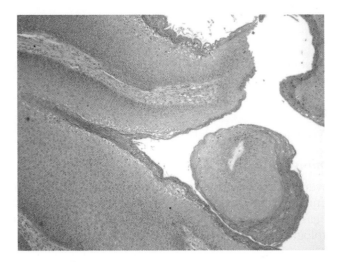

FIGURE 5-61.   Condyloma due to human papillomavirus (HPV). Large warty projections of thickened epidermis with scale; note that infected cells have prominent haloes and are visible in the most superficial layers. (Reproduced with permission from USMLERx.com.)

squamous intraepithelial lesions often regress and are monitored by regular Pap smears; higher-grade lesions are evaluated with a biopsy. Cervical cancer is managed according to stage (surgery or radiation, or both).

PREVENTION

Vaccination, barrier contraception.

POLYOMAVIRUSES: **BK** AND **JC** VIRUSES

CHARACTERISTICS

Both BK and JC viruses are common in the general population; most people are asymptomatic carriers by the age of 18.

PATHOGENICITY

Only cause clinical disease in immunocompromised individuals (eg, those with AIDS, chemotherapy, immunosuppressants).

CLINICAL SYMPTOMS

Reactivation of latent **JC virus** in immunocompromised individuals results in progressive multifocal leukoencephalopathy (**PML**). PML is a demyelinating, rapidly progressive, fatal disease that affects oligodendrocytes (ie, CNS) and is characterized by deficits in speech, coordination, and memory. Diagnosis is largely clinical, but can be confirmed by imaging and PCR of the CSF. PML has also been linked to use of the monoclonal antibody Tysabri in multiple sclerosis, currently a "black box" warning. **BK virus** causes kidney disease and can be found in patients with solid organ (kidney) and bone marrow transplants.

TREATMENT

Only treatment available is improving immune function or treating the underlying HIV/AIDS.

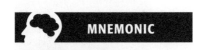

MNEMONIC

JC virus affects the **C**erebrum.
BK virus affects the **K**idneys.

Adenoviruses

CHARACTERISTICS

One of the **most common causes of the common cold;** also causes nonpurulent **conjunctivitis, pneumonia, gastroenteritis.**

PATHOGENESIS

Transmitted via aerosolized droplets, contact, or fecal-oral route.

CLINICAL SYMPTOMS

There are over 40 serotypes, each of which has different manifestations, including rhinitis, pharyngitis, atypical pneumonia, conjunctivitis, hematuria, dysuria, and gastroenteritis with nonbloody diarrhea. Diagnosis can be confirmed by serology or viral cultures.

TREATMENT

None.

Herpesvirus Family

GENERAL CHARACTERISTICS

Herpesviruses are unique in that they are assembled in the nucleus and are the only viruses whose envelope is derived from the **nuclear** membrane. Because they are assembled in the nucleus, infected cells can often be identified histologically by the presence of **intranuclear inclusion bodies.** Infections may also become **latent.**

HERPES SIMPLEX VIRUS 1 (HSV-1)

CHARACTERISTICS

Common; prevalence ranges from 65–90% worldwide. HSV-1 is also the **most common cause of sporadic encephalitis** in the United States.

PATHOGENESIS

Transmitted by respiratory secretions or saliva. The virus invades mucous membranes and can cause a local infection. HSV may also invade nearby sensory nerve endings; it is then transported back to the cell body and becomes latent.

CLINICAL SYMPTOMS

Most infections are **asymptomatic.** Initial symptoms may include vesicular ulcerating lesions of the mouth (**gingivostomatitis**) or eye (**keratoconjunctivitis**). HSV can also infect the hand, causing a vesicular lesion called **herpetic whitlow** (Figure 5-62). HSV-1 may become latent in the **trigeminal** ganglia and can be reactivated under conditions of stress. Reactivation can result in recurring gingivostomatitis, keratoconjunctivitis, or **herpes labialis** (cold sores or fever blisters, Figure 5-63). Recurrent keratoconjunctivitis may lead to blindness. In some cases, the virus can be transported into the brain (via cranial nerves), where it characteristically infects the temporal lobe. Symptoms of **temporal lobe encephalitis** include fever, headache, neck stiffness, and **olfactory hallucinations.** Permanent neurologic damage or death may ensue. Diagnosis of HSV encephalitis can be made by **PCR** of the CSF. Diagnosis of cutaneous lesions can be made by direct fluorescent antibody test (DFA), demonstration of multinucleate giant cells on a **Tzanck** smear of an opened

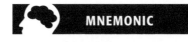

MNEMONIC

Get herpes in a **CHEV**rolet: **C**MV, **H**SV, **E**BV, **V**ZV.

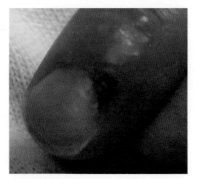

FIGURE 5-62. Herpetic whitlow. Painful, grouped, confluent vesicles on an erythematous edematous base on the finger. (Image courtesy of Dr. James Heilman.)

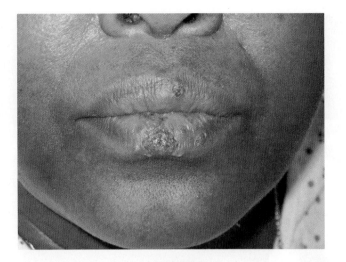

FIGURE 5-63. **Herpes labialis due to HSV-1 infection.** Connective tissue erosion of the lip with scalloped border and vesicles on an erythematous base. (Reproduced with permission from USMLERx.com.)

skin vesicle, or by the presence of intranuclear Cowdry A inclusion bodies on skin **biopsy.**

TREATMENT

Acyclovir to decrease the duration of active infection or prevent recurrence (not curative). Valacyclovir and famciclovir are also used and have increased bioavailability, allowing less frequent dosing. All three function by inhibiting viral DNA replication.

HERPES SIMPLEX VIRUS 2 (HSV-2)

CHARACTERISTICS

Less widespread than HSV-1, but still a common infection; approximately one in six adults between the ages of 14 and 49 are seropositive. HSV is one of the **TORCH** infections!

PATHOGENESIS

Transmitted by sexual contact or perinatally. Like HSV-1, HSV-2 invades mucous membranes and can cause a local infection (Figure 5-64). It may also invade nearby sensory nerve endings, where it is then transported back to the cell body and can become latent.

CLINICAL SYMPTOMS

Most infections are **asymptomatic.** Initial symptoms may include vesicular ulcerating lesions of the genitals and perianal area. Like HSV-1, HSV-2 can also cause **herpetic whitlow** (Figure 5-62). HSV-2 may become latent in the **lumbosacral** ganglia and can be reactivated under conditions of stress, resulting in recurring genital lesions. **Neonatal HSV** can occur via transplacental transmission (TORCH) or during delivery. Infection may be local (mouth, eyes, skin), may affect multiple organs and cause congenital defects, or result in spontaneous abortion. HSV-2 can also cause **neonatal encephalitis.** Diagnosis of cutaneous lesions can be made by DFA, by demonstration of multinucleate giant cells on a **Tzanck** smear, or by visualization of intranuclear inclusion bodies on skin **biopsy.**

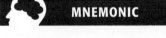

KEY FACT

HSV-1 above the waist; HSV-2 below (however, the reverse may be true in up to one-third of cases)

MNEMONIC

Tzanck goodness if you don't have herpes!

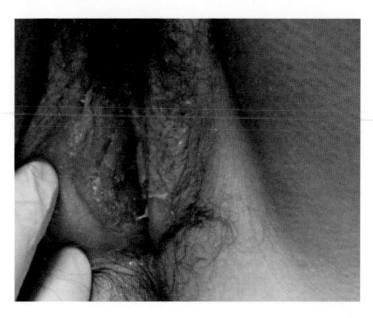

FIGURE 5-64.   Multiple genital lesions due to HSV-2 infection. (Reproduced with permission from USMLERx.com.)

TREATMENT

Acyclovir to decrease the duration of active infection or prevent recurrence (not curative). **Cesarean section** is indicated for mothers with active lesions in the birth canal or prodromal symptoms (fever, pruritus, paresthesias).

VARICELLA-ZOSTER VIRUS (VZV, CHICKENPOX, ZOSTER, SHINGLES)

CHARACTERISTICS

Highly contagious. More commonly occurs in the winter and early spring, with the highest prevalence rate in children aged 4–10 years (uncommon in preschoolers).

PATHOGENESIS

Transmitted by respiratory secretions or contact with active lesions. Like HSV, VZV also causes local infection and can invade sensory nerve endings, where it is then transported back to the cell body and can become latent.

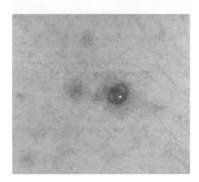

FIGURE 5-65.   Varicella-zoster virus (VZV) lesions. VZV lesions are characterized by multiple papules and vesicles on an erythematous base. (Image courtesy of Wikipedia; permission granted per the GNU Free Documentation License and the Creative Commons Attribution ShareAlike 3.0 license.)

CLINICAL SYMPTOMS

- In **children,** VZV typically causes a mild, flulike illness with characteristic skin lesions (**varicella** or **chickenpox**).
- Often described as "**dew drops on a rose petal**," these lesions appear initially as discrete papules on a macular erythematous base (Figure 5-65). The papules then vesiculate, become pustules, and eventually rupture and release additional virus particles before crusting over. However, children can remain infectious through respiratory contact for up to 10 days after crusting occurs.
- Lesions tend to spread distally from the trunk and are characteristically **asynchronous** (ie, multiple lesions observed at different stages of evolution).
- Infection is usually self-limited and resolves after a few weeks. In **adults,** primary infection can be much more severe and lead to **pneumonia** and **encephalitis.**
- **Reactivation** of latent VZV (**herpes zoster** or **shingles**) can also occur under conditions of stress.

- Zoster is often characterized by extremely **painful** vesicular lesions in a **unilateral dermatomal** distribution (due to reactivation of latent VZV in a single sensory nerve). In **immunocompromised** patients, both primary and reactivated VZV infections are much more severe.
- Diagnosis of cutaneous lesions can be made by DFA, demonstration of multinucleate giant cells on a **Tzanck** smear, or by the presence of intranuclear inclusion bodies on skin **biopsy.**

TREATMENT

Usually supportive. In severe cases, acyclovir can be given. In immunocompromised patients, anti-VZV Ig (VZIG) can be given intravenously. **Reye syndrome** has often been associated with the use of aspirin to treat chickenpox in children. There are two **VZV vaccines**—one for children to prevent chickenpox and one for adults to prevent shingles. Long-term efficacy has not been proven with regard to decreasing zoster incidence, but its use in the pediatric population is widely accepted.

EPSTEIN-BARR VIRUS (EBV, INFECTIOUS MONONUCLEOSIS)

CHARACTERISTICS

Symptomatic infections typically affect teenagers and young adults.

PATHOGENESIS

Transmitted by saliva and respiratory secretions. EBV binds to CD21 on B cells. This selective transformation causes B cells to proliferate abnormally. The host's response to these infected B cells results in the clinical presentation.

CLINICAL SYMPTOMS

EBV can cause **infectious mononucleosis (kissing disease)**, which presents with **flulike** symptoms, profound **fatigue**, painful **pharyngitis, lymphadenopathy** (characteristically occurring in the posterior cervical nodes), and **hepatosplenomegaly.** Peak incidence is at 15–20 years of age, consistent with the term *kissing disease* to describe disease transmission through the saliva. Patients are at risk for splenic rupture and should avoid contact sports. Infection is usually self-limited. In immunocompromised patients, sustained B-cell proliferation may result in mutations that predispose to future neoplasms (**Burkitt lymphoma** and **nasopharyngeal cancers**).

DIAGNOSIS

- Presence of **atypical T lymphocytes** in the blood (these are the cytotoxic T cells responding to the infection, not the proliferating B cells).
- **Monospot test** detects **heterophile antibodies** in the blood.
- Heterophile antibodies are produced during an active EBV infection and are able to agglutinate sheep RBCs.

TREATMENT
Supportive.

CYTOMEGALOVIRUS (CMV)

CHARACTERISTICS

Common. Also can cause neonatal infection (one of the **TOR<u>C</u>H** infections).

PATHOGENESIS

Transmitted by close contact, body fluids, organ **transplantation,** and through the placenta. Infects many cell types.

CLINICAL SYMPTOMS

Most infections are **asymptomatic** and become **latent.**

- Primary infections in **adults** can be similar to infectious mononucleosis, but do not result in the production of heterophile antibodies (**heterophile-** or **Monospot-negative mononucleosis**).
- In **newborns,** primary infection results in **cytomegalic inclusion disease.** Symptoms include microcephaly, hepatosplenomegaly, and CNS deficits.
- In **immunocompromised** patients, latent CMV can reactivate and cause severe infections such as retinitis, pneumonia, and esophagitis.
- Diagnosis can be made with a tissue biopsy, based on the visualization of large cells with characteristic purple intranuclear inclusion bodies surrounded by a halo (**owl's eye inclusion bodies,** Figure 5-66).

TREATMENT

Ganciclovir (not acyclovir) and foscarnet (in the rare case of a ganciclovir-resistant virus).

HUMAN HERPESVIRUSES 6 AND 7 (HHV-6, HHV-7, ROSEOLA)

CHARACTERISTICS

Affects infants or bone marrow transplant recipients (encephalitis). Route of transmission currently unknown.

PATHOGENESIS

Infects B and T cells.

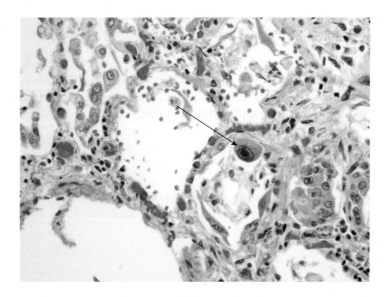

FIGURE 5-66. Cytomegalovirus infection. A CMV-infected cell with prominent "owl's eye" inclusion (*arrow*) is seen lining an alveolar space in an immunosuppressed patient with pneumonia. (Reproduced with permission from USMLERx.com.)

CLINICAL SYMPTOMS

Roseola (Figure 5-67) is characterized by a high fever for several days that can cause seizures, followed by the sudden appearance of a diffuse macular rash on the trunk.

TREATMENT

Foscarnet for HHV-6 encephalitis. Roseola goes away on its own and is treated supportively.

HUMAN HERPESVIRUS 8 (HHV-8, KSHV OR KAPOSI'S SARCOMA–ASSOCIATED HERPESVIRUS)

CHARACTERISTICS

Affects patients with **HIV**, especially men. Transmitted via sexual contact.

PATHOGENESIS

HHV-8 interacts with HIV to produce angioproliferative lesions.

CLINICAL SYMPTOMS

Kaposi's sarcoma (KS) lesions can affect any organ, but are often seen as raised violaceous skin nodules containing extravasated RBCs.

TREATMENT

Antiretroviral drugs can be effective by treating underlying HIV disease.

HEPADNAVIRUS (HEPATITIS B VIRUS, HBV)

CHARACTERISTICS

HBV has a complicated life cycle. After infecting host cells, the partial dsDNA genome is completed by viral DNA polymerase, thus becoming a

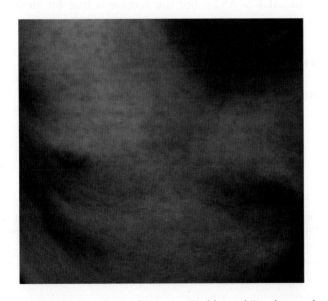

FIGURE 5-67.   Roseola. Exanthem subitum (ie, "sudden rash"), otherwise known as sixth disease, or roseola, is caused by human herpesvirus 6 (HHV-6) infection and characterized by high fever and truncal pink macules that appear 1 day after defervescence, as seen here. (Image courtesy of Emiliano Burzagli.)

KEY FACT

HBV: **Partially** dsDNA, **circular,** enveloped, icosahedral

fully double-stranded genome. Viral genes are then transcribed into mRNA. Viral mRNA is used both to make viral proteins **and** to regenerate the partially dsDNA viral genome through the action of a **viral reverse transcriptase.** Replicated genomic DNA and viral proteins are then repackaged into virion particles.

PATHOGENESIS

Transmitted through blood (**transfusions**), sexual contact, and transplacentally (one of the **TORCH** infections). Initial viremia leads to hepatocyte infection. A number of markers are used to track clinical course:

- **Hepatitis B surface antigen (HBsAg)** indicates either acute disease or a chronic carrier state.
- **Anti-HBsAg antibodies** (IgM or IgG) indicate immunity to HBV, which can occur either through immunization or recovery from prior infection.
- **Hepatitis B core antigen (HBcAg)** and **anti-HBcAg antibodies.** Anti-HBcAg antibodies are positive during the equivalence zone or **window period** when HBsAg and anti-HBsAg are roughly equal in quantity, complex with each other, and thereby evade serologic detection. Thus, a positive HBcAb is often a helpful indicator of infection when the serologic profile is otherwise normal-appearing. One can also ascertain whether disease is recent (IgM HBcAb) or chronic (IgG).
- **Hepatitis B infectivity "e" antigen (HBeAg)** is an important indicator of active viral replication and, thus, transmissibility.

Conversely, the presence of **anti-HBeAg antibodies** indicates low transmissibility: **HBV PCR** is also used to measure viral load and monitor response.

Thus, depending on the serologic pattern observed, one can reliably interpret a patient's infectious status (Table 5-30). Laboratory tests are also helpful in differentiating viral from other causes of hepatitis. As a rule of thumb, alanine aminotransferase (ALT) is greater than aspartate aminotransferase (AST) in viral hepatitis (ALT > AST), but the reverse is true for alcoholic hepatitis (AST > ALT).

TABLE 5-30.   Serologic Patterns and Interpretation of HBV Infection

HBsAg	Anti-HBs	Anti-HBc	HBeAg	Anti-HBe	Interpretation
+	–	IgM	+	–	Acute hepatitis B.
+	–	IgGa	+	–	Chronic hepatitis B with active viral replication.
+	–	IgG	–	+	Chronic hepatitis B with low viral replication.
+	+	IgG	+ or –	+ or –	Chronic hepatitis B with heterotypic anti-HBs (about 10% of cases).
–	–	IgM	+ or –	–	Acute hepatitis B (window period).
–	+	IgG	–	+ or –	Recovery from hepatitis B (immunity).
–	+	–	–	–	Vaccination (immunity).
–	–	IgG	–	–	False-positive; less commonly infection in remote past.

aLow levels of IgM anti-HBc may also be detected. (Reprinted with permission from McPhee SJ, Papadakis MA, Tierney LM. *Current Medical Diagnosis & Treatment 2008,* 47th ed. New York: McGraw-Hill, 2008: 571.)

CLINICAL SYMPTOMS

Infection may be acute or chronic, depending on the host response. Infected hepatocytes can be killed by cytotoxic T cells; therefore, a robust immune response may result in a severe but acute course that ultimately clears the infection. A weaker immune response results in a milder course, but the infection may not be cleared. Liver function tests are elevated in both cases. Acute infection is characterized by **jaundice** and **fever** (Figure 5-68). Chronic infection may result in an asymptomatic **carrier** state. However, if a chronic inflammatory response is present, the host may develop **cirrhosis** or **hepatocellular carcinoma** (or both).

TREATMENT

Interferon alpha (INF-α), adefovir, tenofovir, lamivudine. There is also a recombinant HBV **vaccine** that contains HBsAg. Passive immunization with anti-HBsAg Ig is used in some cases (needlesticks, and immediately after delivery of infants from infected mothers).

Poxvirus Family

Poxviruses are the **largest human viruses.** They are also the only viruses that **make their own envelope** and the only DNA viruses that replicate in the **cytoplasm.** Infected cells often have characteristic **cytoplasmic inclusion bodies** (in contrast to nuclear inclusion bodies in herpesvirus infections).

SMALLPOX (VARIOLA)

PATHOGENESIS

Transmitted as aerosolized droplets.

CLINICAL SYMPTOMS

Smallpox (variola) is characterized by constitutional symptoms and a disseminated rash that is initially maculopapular, then forms vesicles, and later pustules (Figure 5-69). The rash begins on the face and extremities and spreads

> **KEY FACT**
>
> Poxviruses: dsDNA, linear, enveloped
> - Large, complex viruses with a brick shape
> - Includes smallpox (variola) and molluscum contagiosum

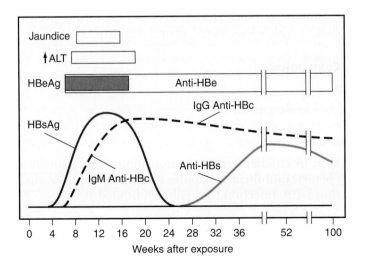

FIGURE 5-68. **Typical clinical and laboratory features of acute hepatitis B virus (HBV) infection.** ALT, alanine aminotransferase; HBc, hepatitis B core; HBeAg, hepatitis B infectivity "e" antigen; HBsAg, hepatitis B surface antigen; Ig, immunoglobulin. (Modified with permission from Kasper DL, Braunwald E, Fauci AS, et al. *Harrison's Principles on Internal Medicine,* 16th ed. New York: McGraw-Hill, 2005: 1825.)

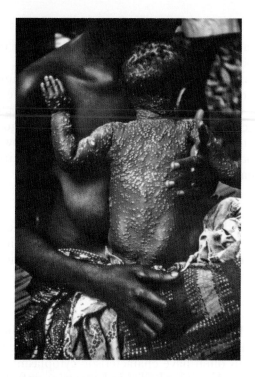

FIGURE 5-69. **Multiple pustules of smallpox can be seen on the back of this child.**
Note that all lesions are at the same stage of development. (Image courtesy of CDC's Public Health Image Library; content provider Dr. Lyle Conrad.)

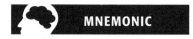

MNEMONIC

For the positive-sense RNA viruses, remember to **Cal/Pico** and **Flo To Come Right Away:**

Caliciviridae
Picornaviridae
Flaviviridae
Togaviridae
Coronavirus
Retro **A**stroviridae

to the trunk (centripetal). Systemic illness results in a 10–30% mortality rate during the second week of symptoms.

TREATMENT

Supportive. The smallpox vaccine successfully eradicated smallpox infections in 1977. The vaccine contained an attenuated virus similar to smallpox (**vaccinia**) that served as the antigen. While there are only two known repositories of the virus worldwide (United States and Russia), there is concern that smallpox could be utilized as a bioterrorism agent in the future given that populations are no longer widely vaccinated against the virus.

MOLLUSCUM CONTAGIOSUM

PATHOGENESIS

Transmitted by close contact.

CLINICAL SYMPTOMS

Most often seen in children and immunocompromised patients and is characterized by benign **umbilicated** papules on the skin that are small and flesh-colored (Figure 5-70). Infection is usually self-limited.

TREATMENT

None.

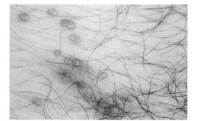

FIGURE 5-70. **Multiple umbilicated lesions, characteristic of molluscum contagiosum infection.** (Reproduced with permission from Kasper DL, Braunwald E, Fauci AS, et al. *Harrison's Principles on Internal Medicine*, 16th ed. New York: McGraw-Hill, 2005: 1053.)

POSITIVE (SINGLE)-STRANDED RNA VIRUSES–SS (+) RNA

GENERAL CHARACTERISTICS

All positive, single-stranded RNA viruses have an icosahedral capsid with the exception of coronavirus, which has a helical capsid. RNA can either be enveloped or naked (exits host cells through budding or lysis, respectively; Table 5-31). Another helpful generalization that can be made is that **all positive single-stranded RNA viruses replicate in the cytoplasm** with the exception of HIV, which replicates in the nucleus (carries its own RNA-dependent DNA polymerase—reverse transcriptase—RT).

TABLE 5-31. Positive-Stranded RNA Viruses

FAMILY	STRUCTURE	DISEASE	ROUTE OF TRANSMISSION	IMPORTANT FACTS
Caliciviridae				
Hepatitis E (HEV)	Naked, icosahedral, nonsegmented, linear	Enteric hepatitis.	Fecal-oral.	Self-limiting disease (except in pregnant women, for whom there is a high mortality rate).
Norwalk and Norovirus (Norwalk agent)	Naked, icosahedral, nonsegmented, linear	Epidemic adult gastroenteritis.	Fecal-oral.	Vomiting more frequent than diarrhea.
Sapovirus	Naked, icosahedral, nonsegmented, linear	Epidemic outbreaks of gastroenteritis.	Fecal-oral.	Associated with pediatric gastroenteritis.
Picornaviridae				
Polioviruses	Naked, icosahedral, nonsegmented, linear	Abortive poliomyelitis, paralytic poliomyelitis (1%), aseptic meningitis.	Fecal-oral.	Immunization: Natural infection confers lifelong immunity.
Echoviruses	Naked, icosahedral, nonsegmented, linear	Can cause mild or febrile illnesses, rashes, and aseptic meningitis.	Infection by viral invasion of nasopharyngeal mucosa.	High incidence during summer-fall.
Enteroviruses	Naked, icosahedral, nonsegmented, linear	Common cause of mild or febrile illness, aseptic meningitis. Enterovirus 70 can cause conjunctivitis.	Fecal-oral.	High incidence during summer-fall.
Rhinoviruses	Naked, icosahedral, nonsegmented, linear	Number 1 cause of common cold; > 100 serologic types.	Often spread by self-inoculation nose/throat.	Clinical diagnosis from symptoms.
Hepatitis A (HAV)	Naked, icosahedral, nonsegmented, linear	Acute viral hepatitis. Not a chronic disease; no carriers.	Fecal-oral.	Anti-HAV IgG: Indicates person had a previous infection.

(continues)

TABLE 5-31. Positive-Stranded RNA Viruses *(continued)*

FAMILY	STRUCTURE	DISEASE	ROUTE OF TRANSMISSION	IMPORTANT FACTS
Picornaviridae *(continued)*				
Coxsackieviruses	Naked, icosahedral, nonsegmented, linear	Group A viruses can cause herpangina, hand-foot-mouth disease, aseptic meningitis, and pharyngitis. Group B viruses can cause myocarditis and pleurodynia.	Infection by viral invasion of nasopharyngeal mucosa.	High incidence during summer-fall.
Flaviviridae				
Hepatitis C (HCV)	Enveloped, icosahedral	Acute, usually subclinical hepatitis; ~80% chronic.	Primarily parenteral (common cause of post-transfusion hepatitis and hepatitis among IV drug abusers); sexual.	Associated with hepatocellular carcinoma; cirrhosis.
Saint Louis encephalitis	Enveloped, icosahedral		*Culex* mosquito.	Most common encephalitis in elderly in the United States.
West Nile virus	Enveloped, icosahedral	Fever, nausea, vomiting, and rash.	*Culex* mosquito.	Peaks in summer.
Japanese encephalitis virus	Enveloped, icosahedral	Mild febrile illness, acute meningoencephalitis.	*Culex* mosquito.	Reservoirs in pigs and birds.
Yellow fever virus	Enveloped, icosahedral	Chills, fever, black vomit, headaches.	*Aedes* mosquito.	With liver involvement, patients have jaundice with Councilman bodies (acidophilic inclusions).
Dengue virus	Enveloped, icosahedral	Mild fever, headache, bone aches, hemorrhagic shock syndrome (Southeast Asian variant).	*Aedes* mosquito.	Biggest arbovirus problem.
Togaviridae				
Rubella (German measles, 3-day measles)	Enveloped, icosahedral, linear	Maculopapular rash, fever, conjunctivitis, sore throat.	Respiratory droplets.	Congenital rubella syndrome prevented if mother is vaccinated.
Western/Eastern/Venezuelan equine **encephalitis** virus	Enveloped, icosahedral, linear	Flulike illness, encephalitis.	Mosquito vector.	

TABLE 5-31. **Positive-Stranded RNA Viruses** *(continued)*

FAMILY	STRUCTURE	DISEASE	ROUTE OF TRANSMISSION	IMPORTANT FACTS
Coronaviridae				
Coronaviruses	Enveloped, helical, nonsegmented	Second leading cause of common cold. Implicated in infant gastroenteritis.	Aerosols and respiratory droplets.	The only positive sense ssRNA virus with a helical capsid.
Astroviridae				
Astroviruses	Naked, icosahedral, linear	Endemic gastroenteritis in neonates and young kids.	Fecal-oral.	Outbreaks similar to rotavirus; peaks in winter in temperate climates and during rainy season in tropics.
Retroviridae				
Human immunodeficiency virus (HIV)	Enveloped, icosahedral, linear; *diploid* ss(+) RNA RNA-dependent DNA polymerase	Primary infection: mononucleosis-like syndrome. As disease progresses, virus infects and kills more CD4+ T cells; without these cells both humoral and cell-mediated arms of the immune system are weakened (CDC criteria).	Vertical, perinatal via breast milk, sex, blood transfusions, and needles.	Common opportunistic infections. At risk for thrush when CD4+ T cells < 400. At risk for *Pneumocystis jiroveci* pneumonia when CD4+ T cells < 200. At < 100, risk of cytomegalovirus, *Mycobacterium avium* complex, and toxoplasmosis.
Human T-cell lymphotrophic virus type I (HTLV-I)	Enveloped, icosahedral, linear	Causes adult T-cell leukemia and tropical spastic paraparesis (TSP).	Vertical, perinatal via breast milk, sex, blood transfusions, and needles.	TSP/HTLV-1–associated myelopathy: Demyelination of the spinal cord pyramidal tract. Rapid onset.

Hepatitis E (Enteric Hepatitis)

CHARACTERISTICS

Unique 30-nm hepatitis virus. It does not appear to cause chronic infection and is serologically distinct from hepatitis A virus (HAV).

PATHOGENESIS

Like HAV, transmitted via the fecal-oral route and can cause water-borne outbreaks (water contamination with fecal material).

PicoRNAvirus = pico (small) RNA virus.

PERCH on a "peak" (pico)

Poliovirus
Echovirus
Rhinovirus
Coxsackievirus
HAV

CLINICAL SYMPTOMS

It resembles HAV in its incubation, course, and severity; typically causes mild hepatitis in healthy individuals. It is self-limited but can cause **fulminant hepatitis in pregnant women.**

TREATMENT

Supportive; no benefit from administering INF-α. **Vaccine is in development.**

Polioviruses

Abortive poliomyelitis, paralytic poliomyelitis, postpolio syndrome.

CHARACTERISTICS

Very small picornavirus (20–30 nm), which usually causes a subclinical syndrome. It is important, however, because it can also cause paralysis, which is completely preventable.

PATHOGENESIS

The portal of entry is the mouth, and viral replication occurs in the gut. Active virus is excreted in the feces for several weeks.

CLINICAL SYMPTOMS

- Most common outcome is **abortive poliomyelitis,** which is a mild febrile syndrome.
- **Paralytic poliomyelitis** occurs in 1% of all cases. Paralysis results from viral damage to **anterior horn motor neurons.**
- Many years after resolution, some patients can develop **postpolio syndrome,** which causes further muscle atrophy.
- Also causes **aseptic meningitis.** (Other picornaviruses, notably echoviruses and coxsackieviruses, commonly cause this condition.)
- Diagnosis can be confirmed by serology, virus isolation or RT-PCR (reverse transcriptase-polymerase chain reaction), and DNA hybridization.

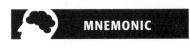

KEY FACT

Young children receive four doses of Salk (IPV) vaccine. Sabin (OPV) is no longer available in the United States.

TREATMENT

Supportive care.

- Prevention: Two types of vaccines are available: Killed (**Salk; IPV**) and live attenuated (**Sabin; OPV**) vaccinations.
- The IPV is given to immunocompromised patients.
- OPV contains three serotypes of poliovirus. This vaccine has also been known to cause **vaccine-associated paralytic poliomyelitis (VAPP)** as a result of reversion to wild-type virus.

Hepatitis A (HAV)

Enteric, short incubation acute viral hepatitis.

CHARACTERISTICS

Positive sense, single-stranded 27-nm RNA virus associated with poor sanitation. Common childhood infection in developing countries.

PATHOGENESIS

Similar to HEV, acquired by the **fecal-oral route.**

- Incubation is between 2 and 6 weeks, with shedding of virus occurring during late incubation period and the prodrome.

MNEMONIC

The Vowels Hit Your Bowels: Hepatitis A and E → Fecal-Oral Route

- The virus is shed in stool and thus can be contracted through exposure to contaminated water, food, and shellfish.
- The highest prevalence is in densely populated areas and developing countries.

CLINICAL SYMPTOMS

Often asymptomatic and anicteric; experienced as flulike illness. Often manifests with jaundice and GI disturbances (watery diarrhea is most common). Fulminant hepatitis or carrier states are rare. The infection is usually self-limited and is **not** associated with chronic hepatitis or hepatocellular carcinoma. Diagnosis can be confirmed with ELISA tests for HAV antigen and antibody.

TREATMENT

- Supportive care. Prevention involves hand washing.
- **Vaccine:** HAV vaccine is given to all patients with chronic liver disease (especially hepatitis C), travelers to high-risk countries, those with high-risk behavior, and those from high-risk communities. Anti-HAV antibody is 90% effective if given within 2 weeks of exposure.

Coxsackieviruses

Herpangina, hand-foot-and-mouth disease, aseptic meningitis.

CHARACTERISTICS

This small, 20- to 30-nm, virus is the most common cause of aseptic meningitis (far more than all bacterial forms), followed by echovirus and mumps virus. It is highly contagious and manifests with rash.

PATHOGENESIS

Fecal-oral transmission.

CLINICAL SYMPTOMS

- **Group A** coxsackievirus is responsible for **herpangina** (Figure 5-71) and hand-foot-and-mouth disease.
- **Group B** coxsackievirus is responsible for cardiomyopathy (acute myocarditis and pericarditis), aseptic meningitis, and pleurodynia.

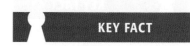

KEY FACT

Anti-HAV IgM indicates recent infection
Anti-HAV IgG = remote infection

KEY FACT

Coxsackievirus: ssRNA, linear, naked, icosahedral.

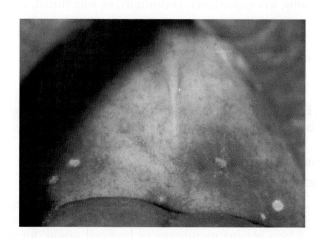

FIGURE 5-71. **Infectious enanthem: Herpangina.** Multiple, small vesicles and erosions with erythematous halos on the soft palate. (Reproduced with permission from Wolff K, Johnson RA, Suurmond D. *Fitzpatrick's Color Atlas & Synopsis of Clinical Dermatology,* 5th ed. New York: McGraw-Hill, 2005: 784.)

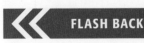
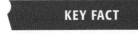

Most hepatitis C viral infections develop into chronic hepatitis.

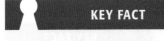

Retroviruses, including HIV, are the **only** diploid virus of clinical relevance to humans.

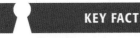

Structural genes:
- *Gag*—group-specific antigen; encodes p24; p6, p7, and p9; p17.
- *Pol*—encodes RT; integrase; protease.
- *Env*—encodes gp120; gp41.

Regulatory genes:
- *Tat*—encodes transactivator proteins.
- *Rev*—encodes regulatory virion proteins.
- *Nef*—encodes negative factor.

KEY FACT

Major **risk factors** for contracting HIV:
- Unprotected sexual intercourse.
- Sharing contaminated needles.
- Birth from an infected mother.
- In underdeveloped countries, blood products and transfusions still pose major risk factors.

TREATMENT

Supportive care.

Hepatitis C (HCV, Infectious Hepatitis)

CHARACTERISTICS

The HCV genome is a 10-kB positive-sense RNA genome, with a 42-nm capsid. It is a major cause of non-A, non-B (NANB) hepatitis worldwide.

PATHOGENICITY

Mainly acquired through IV drug use or blood products. It can also be transmitted perinatally or sexually.

CLINICAL SYMPTOMS

Presentation is similar to that of hepatitis B, but less severe. Persistent infections may progress to chronic active hepatitis, cirrhosis, and hepatocellular carcinoma. Enzyme-linked immunosorbent assay (ELISA) detects the antibodies to HCV, which indicate acute or chronic infection. RT-PCR and DNA assays are also used to determine the viral load.

TREATMENT

Supportive care and INF-α (or pegylated-α) + ribavirin.

Rubella (German Measles)

CHARACTERISTICS

This togavirus can persist in humans for years with no detectable signs or symptoms. Rubella virus readily crosses the placenta and is highly teratogenic, causing deafness, blindness, and/or heart or brain defects in fetuses of mothers infected in the first trimester.

PATHOGENESIS

Spreads primarily through aerosolized particles. The mucosa of the upper respiratory tract is the portal of viral entry and initial site of virus replication.

CLINICAL SYMPTOMS

Clinically apparent rubella is characterized by a truncal maculopapular rash, lymphadenopathy, low-grade fever, conjunctivitis, sore throat, and arthralgias.

TREATMENT

Supportive care.

PREVENTION

Live vaccine is available and confers long-term immunity to rubella. However, **the vaccine is not given to pregnant women.**

Human Immunodeficiency Virus (HIV)

CHARACTERISTICS

The genome consists of two identical subunits of (ss) RNA (**diploid linear**), surrounded by a conical truncated capsid (Figure 5-72). These components are surrounded by a plasma membrane of host-cell origin, formed when the capsid buds from the host cell.

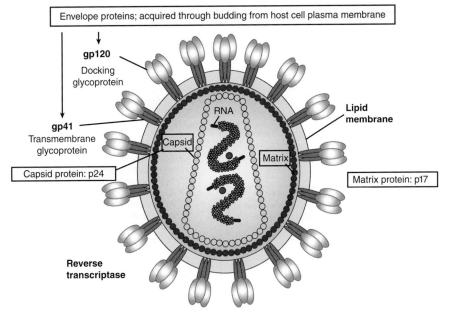

Envelope proteins; acquired through budding from host cell plasma membrane

gp120
Docking glycoprotein

gp41
Transmembrane glycoprotein

Capsid protein: p24

RNA

Capsid

Matrix

Lipid membrane

Matrix protein: p17

Reverse transcriptase

FIGURE 5-72. **Diagram of the HIV virus.**

- (ss) RNA: Tightly bound to the nucleocapsid proteins and enzymes, such as reverse transcriptase (**RT**), **integrase**, and **protease**.
- The main **matrix protein (p17)** surrounds the capsid (**p24–capsid protein**) and maintains the integrity of the virion particle.
- The **envelope** includes glycoproteins **gp120** and **gp41**.

The HIV genome is very complex and includes several major genes coding for **structural proteins** (expressed in all retroviruses), and several **regulatory genes,** unique to HIV.

PATHOGENESIS

Transmission of HIV may occur secondary to sexual contact (semen, vaginal secretions), blood transfusions, IV drug use, and contact with other infected bodily fluids (plasma, CSF). HIV can also be transmitted through the placenta (intrauterine transmission), perinatally, and through breast milk.

HIV primarily infects macrophages and CD4+ T cells. Macrophages are thought to play a key role in primary HIV-1 infection. Infection of and replication in monocytes/macrophages results in the spread of HIV to other tissues.

- Viral entry to **CD4+ T cells** and macrophages is **initiated** through **interaction** of the envelope glycoproteins (**gp120**) with **CD4** molecules of target cells.
- Fusion with target cells is further facilitated through their own chemokine receptors (**CCR5** or **CXCR4**). CXCR4 is located on T cells, and CCR5 is located on macrophages.
- HIV invades CD4+ T cells, impairing both the humoral and cell-mediated arms of the immune system (Figure 5-73).

PRESENTATION

The hallmarks of initial infection with HIV are an abrupt drop in the CD4+ T-cell count and rapid viral replication (increased **viral load**). Typical course of an HIV-infected individual is as follows (Figure 5-74):

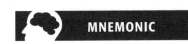

KEY FACT

gp24 and gp120 are primary target antigens for early detection.

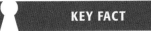

MNEMONIC

Time course of HIV infection: 4 **Fs:**
Flulike (acute), **F**eeling fine (latent), **F**alling count, **F**inal crisis

KEY FACT

Although 40–70% of infected patients experience symptoms in the acute stage, the symptoms are rather nonspecific; most HIV cases are not detected at this time.

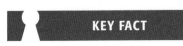

KEY FACT

The clinical latency varies greatly, lasting from a few weeks to over 20 years, depending on the patient.

KEY FACT

Mutations in **CCR5** can lead either to immunity (homozygous) or to slower progression to AIDS (heterozygous).
Mutations in **CXCR4** lead to rapid progression to AIDS.

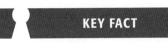

CLINICAL CORRELATION

HIV-positive patients are said to be at risk for developing **candidiasis** (thrush) and **tuberculosis** once their **CD4+** T-cell count drops **below 400.** These are AIDS-defining conditions.

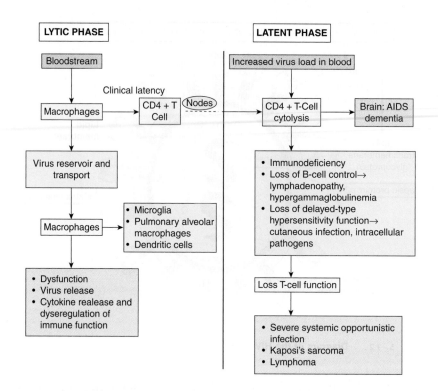

FIGURE 5-73. **HIV/AIDS cycle and evasion.**

- **Primary infection; acute HIV syndrome (CDC category A):** Patients may experience mononucleosis-like syndrome, which usually occurs 4–8 weeks after initial infection. Major symptoms include, but are not limited to, **fever, generalized lymphadenopathy, headache, myalgia,** and **pharyngitis.**

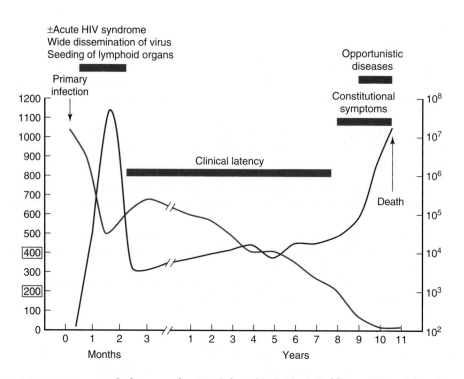

FIGURE 5-74. **Typical course of an HIV-infected individual.** Red line = CD4+ T lymphocyte count (cells/mm³); blue line = HIV RNA copies per mL plasma.

- **Clinical latency stage:** CD4+ T-cell count rebounds, and most symptoms of the acute infection subside. However, lymphadenopathy can be present throughout the entire course of an HIV infection. During the latent phase, virus replicates in lymph nodes.
- **Disease progression and later stages (AIDS):** Dictated by the number of viable CD4+ T cells. As they decline over time, patients have an increased risk of acquiring common and not so common infections (**CDC category B and C**). These conditions are summarized in Table 5-32.

DIAGNOSIS

- **ELISA** tests for initial screening (sensitive, high false-positive rate, RULE OUT test): detects antibodies to viral antigens **p24, p17, gp120,** and **gp41.**
- **Western blot:** Warranted if ELISA test yields positive results (specific, high false-negative rate, RULE IN test). **HIV infection is confirmed if antibodies to** at least two HIV antigens **are** positive. ELISA/Western blot are often falsely negative in the first few months of HIV infection and falsely positive initially in babies born to infected mothers (anti-gp120 crosses placenta).
- **HIV DNA–PCR:** Helpful for monitoring effects of drug therapy on viral load. Also used to screen for HIV infection in newborns of HIV-positive mothers.
- **CD4+ T-cell count:** Assess treatment progress. AIDS diagnosis with 200 or less CD4+ cells/mm^3 (normal: 500–1500). Considered HIV-positive if AIDS-defining condition is present or CD4/CD8 ratio < 1.5.

TREATMENT

Patients are usually placed on highly active antiretroviral therapy (**HAART**).

- HAART includes at least two reverse transcriptase inhibitors combined with a protease inhibitor (Figure 5-75).
- Pregnant women are prescribed zidovudine (AZT), which has been shown to prevent perinatal transmission of the virus.

PROGNOSIS

There is no cure for AIDS. All patients with HIV/AIDS eventually die from complications of the disease or from opportunistic infections.

NEGATIVE (SINGLE)-STRANDED RNA VIRUSES—SS (–) RNA

GENERAL CHARACTERISTICS

Negative, single-stranded RNA viruses have the largest variety in structure (Table 5-33). All are enveloped and replicate in the host cell cytoplasm with the exception of orthomyxoviruses, which along with retroviruses, are unique in that they replicate in the nucleus. The capsid shape varies from icosahedral to helical. There are also linear, circular, segmented, and nonsegmented genomes among the negative single-stranded RNA viruses.

Paramyxoviridae

GENERAL CHARACTERISTICS

Large, enveloped, ss (–) RNA, nonsegmented.

Major cause of diseases of upper respiratory tract (URT), lower respiratory tract (LRT; parainfluenza and respiratory syncytial virus [RSV]), and systemic diseases (measles, mumps). Paramyxoviruses are the most important causes of

---

> **KEY FACT**

Antigen p24 is detectable shortly after initial infection, so it is often used as an early sign of HIV infection.

> **KEY FACT**

Definitive diagnosis of HIV infection can be made only when there are antibodies to at least two viral antigens, as confirmed by Western blot analysis.

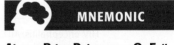 **MNEMONIC**

Always Bring Polymerase Or Fail Replication

Arenaviridae
Bunyaviridae
Paramyxoviridae
Orthomyxoviridae
Filoviridae
Rhabdoviridae
Negative-sense RNA viruses require RNA-dependent RNA polymerase in order to replicate.

TABLE 5-32.   Commonly Encountered HIV-Associated Infections

	Condition	Key Point	Causative Agent
Neoplasm	Hairy leukoplakia	Often on lateral tongue	EBV
	Non-Hodgkin's lymphoma	Often on oropharynx (Waldeyer ring)	
	Primary CNS lymphoma	More likely to have multiple lesions than in immunocompetent population	
	Squamous cell carcinoma	Often in anus (gay male) or cervix (female)	HPV
Skin/ mucosa	Fluffy white, "cottage-cheese" lesions	Often on buccal mucosa	*Candida albicans*
	Superficial vascular proliferation	Biopsy reveals neutrophilic inflammation	*Bartonella henselae*—causes bacillary angiomatosis
	Superficial, neoplastic proliferation of vasculature	Biopsy reveals lymphocytic inflammation	HHV-8—causes Kaposi sarcoma
Systemic	Low-grade fevers, cough, hepatosplenomegaly	Oval yeast cells within macrophages; seen when CD4+ < 100 cells/mm^3	*Histoplasma capsulatum*—causes only pulmonary symptoms in immunocompetent hosts
GI	Chronic, watery diarrhea	Acid-fast cysts seen in stool; seen when CD4+ < 200 cells/mm^3	*Cryptosporidium* or *Isospora belli*
	Chronic ulcers or esophagitis	Candida esophagitis seen when CD4+ < 100 cells/mm^3	HSV (also causes bronchitis/ pneumonitis)
CNS	Meningitis	India ink stain reveals narrow-based budding	*Cryptococcus neoformans*—may also cause encephalitis
	Progressive multifocal leukoencephalopathy	Due to reactivation of a latent virus; results in demyelination	JC virus (Polyomavirus)
	HIV encephalitis/AIDS dementia complex	Virus gains CNS access via infected macrophages	Occurs late in course of HIV infection; microglial nodules with multinucleated giant cells
	Abscesses	Many ring-enhancing lesions on imaging. Seen when CD4+ < 100 cells/mm^3	*Toxoplasma gondii*
	Retinitis	Cottonwool spots on funduscopic exam or blindness; Seen when CD4+ < 50 cells/mm^3	Cytomegalovirus
Respiratory	Interstitial pneumonia	Biopsy reveals cells with intranuclear and cytoplasmic inclusion bodies	
	Invasive aspergillosis	Pleuritic pain, hemoptysis, infiltrates on imaging	*Aspergillus fumigatus*
	Pneumonia	Seen when CD4+ < 200 cells/mm^3	*Pneumocystis jiroveci*
	Tuberculosis-like disease	Seen when CD4+ < 50 cells/mm^3	Disseminated *Mycobacterium avium-intracellulare*

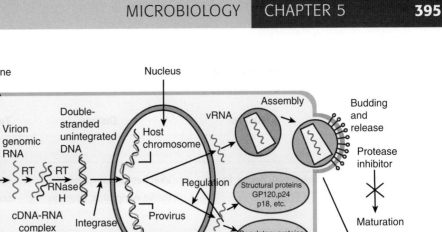
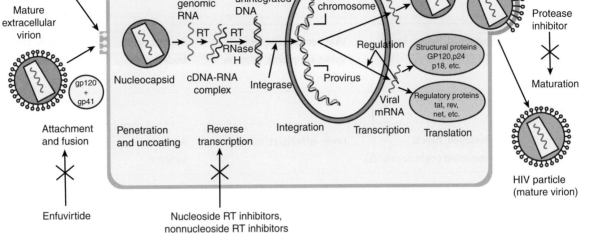

FIGURE 5-75. **Replicative cycle of HIV-1 showing the sites of action of available antiretroviral agents.** Available antiretroviral agents are shown in blue; cDNA, complementary DNA; gp120 + gp41, extracellular and intracellular domains, respectively, of envelope glycoprotein; mRNA, messenger RNA; RNase H, ribonuclease H; RT, reverse transcriptase. (Modified with permission from Brunton LL, Parker KL, Buxton ILO, Blumenthal DK. *Goodman & Gilman's The Pharmacological Basis of Therapeutics*, 11th ed. New York: McGraw-Hill, 2006: 1274.)

TABLE 5-33. **Negative-Stranded RNA Viruses**

FAMILY	STRUCTURE	DISEASE	ROUTE OF TRANSMISSION	IMPORTANT FACTS
Paramyxoviridae				
Parainfluenza	Enveloped, helical, linear.	Croup, bronchiolitis, pneumonia.	Aerosol/ airborne.	Self-limiting disease.
Measles	Enveloped, helical, linear.	Cough, coryza, conjunctivitis, rash.	Aerosol/ airborne.	Symptoms due to immune response.
Mumps	Enveloped, helical, linear.	Aseptic meningitis, meningoencephalitis, parotitis, unilateral nerve deafness, orchitis.	Aerosol/ airborne.	Infection confers lifelong immunity.
Respiratory syncytial virus	Enveloped, helical, linear.	Bronchiolitis, pneumonia.	Aerosol/ airborne.	Can be deadly to infants.
Rhabdoviridae				
Rabies	Enveloped, bullet/helical, linear.	Fever, nausea, hydrophobia, delirium, paralysis, and coma.	Animal bite.	Evidence of infection, including symptoms and the detection of antibody; does not occur until too late for intervention.

(continues)

TABLE 5-33. Negative-Stranded RNA Viruses *(continued)*

FAMILY	STRUCTURE	DISEASE	ROUTE OF TRANSMISSION	IMPORTANT FACTS
Filoviridae				
Ebola/Marburg viruses	Enveloped, helical, linear.	Viral hemorrhagic fevers, flulike symptoms, death in ~90%.	Contact with body fluids.	Most deadly hemorrhagic fevers.
Orthomyxoviridae				
Influenza	Enveloped, helical, segmented (eight segments).	Fever, arthralgias, malaise.	Aerosol/airborne.	Undergoes antigenic shift and antigenic drift.
Deltaviridae				
HDV "delta agent"	Enveloped, helical, circular.	Can confect or superinfect with HBV to worsen its prognosis. Chronic disease (carriers).	Same as HBV.	Defective virus that requires HBsAg as its envelope.
Bunyaviridae				
Hantavirus	Enveloped, helical, linear → circular, segments.	Hantavirus renal disease (HVRD), HV cardiopulmonary syndrome (HVCPS).	Inhale rodent feces.	Treat with ribavirin.
Rift Valley fever virus	Enveloped, helical, linear → circular, segments.	Acute febrile illness (saddle-back fever), myalgias, low back pain, headache, anorexia, retroorbital pain.	Tick-borne.	Most common in sub-Saharan Africa, or in military personnel on tours of duty.
La Crosse virus	Enveloped, helical, linear → circular, segments.	Viral encephalitis.	Mosquito vector.	Most important cause of insect encephalitis in the Midwest.
California encephalitis	Enveloped, helical, linear → circular, segments.	Viral encephalitis.	Mosquito vector.	
Crimean-Congo hemorrhagic fever	Enveloped, helical, linear → circular, segments.	Hemorrhagic viral encephalitis.	Mosquito vector.	
Arenaviridae	Ambisense.			
Lymphocytic choriomeningitis virus (LCMV)	Enveloped, helical, circular, segmented.	Aseptic meningitis or encephalitis; asymptomatic to mild febrile illness most common.	Rat.	No human–human transmission except mother to fetus.

TABLE 5-33. **Negative-Stranded RNA Viruses *(continued)***

Family	Structure	Disease	Route of Transmission	Important Facts
Lassa fever	Enveloped, helical, circular, segmented.	Hemorrhagic fever, multisystem involvement, often including encephalitis and facial swelling.	Rat.	High death rates in pregnant women in 3rd trimester and fetuses (~95% mortality rate). *Complications:* Most common is deafness in ~1/3 of cases.

respiratory infections in infants and young children (younger than 5 years). Typical virus organization is depicted in Figure 5-76.

Membrane fusion and hemolysin activities are carried out by **F,** fusion glycoprotein. It exists as inactive **F0,** which is cleaved to the active **F1** form by cellular proteases. Also responsible for large syncytia formation in cells infected with paramyxoviruses by causing respiratory epithelial cells to fuse.

Parainfluenza

CHARACTERISTICS

Primarily affects young children (3–8 years of age), manifesting through URT **(common cold)** and LRT infections. Parainfluenza viruses (PIVs) are also a

> **MNEMONIC**
>
> **PaRaMyxovirus**
> **P**arainfluenza (croup)
> **R**SV (bronchiolitis in babies; Rx Ribavirin)
> **M**easles or **M**umps

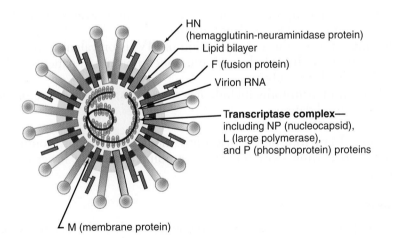

FIGURE 5-76. **Schematic diagram of a paramyxovirus showing major components (not drawn to scale).** The lipid bilayer is shown as the yellow concentric circle; underlying the lipid bilayer is the viral matrix protein (*maroon concentric circle*). Inserted through the viral membrane are the hemagglutinin-neuraminidase (HN) attachment glycoprotein and the fusion (F) glycoprotein. (Not all paramyxoviruses possess hemagglutinin and neuraminidase activities; those glycoproteins are designated H or G.) Inside the virus is the negative-strand virion RNA, which is encased in the nucleocapsid protein (N/NP). Associated with the nucleocapsid are the L and P proteins, and together this complex has RNA-dependent RNA transcriptase activity. (Modified with permission from Brooks GF, Carroll KC, Butel JS, Morse SA. *Jawetz, Melnick, & Adelberg's Medical Microbiology,* 24th ed. New York: McGraw-Hill, 2007: 549.)

PIV-1 = croup in children ages 6 months to 5 years; prevalent in autumn.

PIV-3 = second only to (RSV) as a cause of **pneumonia** and **bronchiolitis** in infants (younger than 6 months).

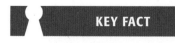

CLINICAL CORRELATION

Most common conditions associated with PIVs:

- Common cold with fever
- Croup
- Bronchiolitis and pneumonia

FLASH BACK

The same drug used to treat hepatitis C (ribavirin) is also sometimes used in severe cases of RSV or in PIV infections in the seriously immunocompromised.

KEY FACT

Because of its high potency and prolonged intramuscular half-life, dexamethasone is the preferred anti-inflammatory drug for croup.

common cause of community-acquired respiratory tract infections in adults. Reinfection with PIV can occur throughout life, with elderly and immuno-compromised persons being at a greater risk of serious complications of infections.

PATHOGENESIS

Disease is airborne, and virus invades the mucosa of the URT. It may progress to the lower segments and does not disseminate.

CLINICAL SYMPTOMS

Clinical manifestations include:

- **Common cold:** Upper respiratory infection, may last 2–3 days to 1 week. Disease has an acute onset and subsides after 7–10 days if uncomplicated.
    - **Symptoms** include runny nose, nasal congestion, and sneezing. In addition, sore throat, cough, and headache are not uncommon. Adults and older children with colds generally have minimal to no fever. Young children, however, may have fever of 38–39°C.
- **Croup:** Affects the larynx, trachea, and bronchi (laryngotracheobronchitis). Mild cold usually persists for several days before the barking "seal-like" cough becomes evident.
    - **Symptoms** include fever, hoarse barking cough, laryngeal obstruction, and inspiratory stridor.
- **Bronchiolitis:** Begins as a mild upper respiratory infection that, over a period of 2–3 days, can develop into increasing respiratory distress with wheezing and a **tight, wheezy cough.** The peak incidence of bronchiolitis is during the first year of life, it dramatically declines until it virtually disappears by school age.
    - **Signs and symptoms** include fever, expiratory wheezing, tachypnea, retractions, crackles, and air trapping.
- **Pneumonia** is usually a complication of PIV, is prevalent in infants, very young children, the elderly, and immunocompromised patients. It is associated with all viral subtypes:
    - **Signs and symptoms** include fever, crackles, and evidence of pulmonary consolidation.

In addition, **PIVs routinely cause** otitis media, pharyngitis, conjunctivitis, and coryza, occurring separately or in combination with a lower respiratory infection.

TREATMENT

Mainly supportive. Antivirals and antibiotics as needed. No vaccine available.

- **Ribavirin** aerosol or systemic therapy has been used to treat PIV infections in children and adults who are severely immunocompromised. Broader use at this time is of uncertain clinical benefit.
- **Antibiotics** are used only when bacterial complications (eg, otitis, sinusitis) develop.
- **Corticosteroids** and **nebulizers** are used to treat respiratory symptoms and to help reduce the inflammation and airway edema of croup.

Respiratory Syncytial Virus (RSV)

CHARACTERISTICS

Acute viral infection with short incubation period and recovery occurring within 7–12 days. RSV is the most important cause of LRT disease in young children. Almost all children have been infected with RSV by the age of 2.

PATHOGENESIS

Disease is airborne, transmitted via aerosols. The virus invades the mucosa of the URT and replicates only within respiratory epithelium. RSV does not have HN or NA attachment proteins; only F (fusion) glycoprotein.

CLINICAL SYMPTOMS

In most infants, the virus causes **symptoms resembling** those of the **common cold.** In infants born prematurely or those with chronic disease, RSV can cause a severe or even life-threatening disease.

- **Signs and symptoms** include low-grade fever, cough, tachypnea, cyanosis, retractions, wheezing, and crackles.
- Most common **complications** are ear infections. Less common, but serious complications include pneumonia (0.5–1%) and respiratory failure (2%).

TREATMENT

Mostly supportive with airway management (most important). **Ribavirin** is a nucleoside analog and is the only antiviral approved for use. However, it is not used routinely. Its main use is in infants at serious risk for LRT infections.

- **Prevention: Palivizumab (Synagis),** monoclonal anti-F-reactive antibody, is indicated for the **prevention** of serious LRT disease caused by RSV in pediatric patients and prematurely born infants (at < 32 weeks' gestation).
- **No vaccine available.** Strict hygiene and contact precautions with diseased individuals are imperative.

Measles (Rubeola)

CHARACTERISTICS

Highly infectious **childhood febrile exanthem.** Has long incubation period of about 2 weeks followed by a classic viral prodrome and virus-specific immune response. Complete recovery ensues 7–10 days after onset of measles rash. The clearance of virus coincides approximately with fading of the rash. A differential diagnosis of rubeola with other common "red rashes of childhood" can be found in Table 5-34.

PATHOGENESIS

Disease is airborne, transmitted by aerosolized particles. It infects the respiratory tract and replicates locally in the respiratory epithelium before spreading to regional lymphatic tissue (further replication). Ultimately, viremia develops, and the virus disseminates throughout the body.

CLINICAL SYMPTOMS

Clinical picture develops in relation to above-described pathogenic characteristics (Figure 5-77):

- **Classic viral prodrome** occurs following the incubation period. It is commonly referred to as the **3 C's: Cough, Coryza, and Conjunctivitis** with photophobia.
    - Pathognomonic **Koplik spots** typically arise on the buccal, gingival, and labial mucosae within 2–3 days of initial symptoms. The Koplik spots are 1- to 2-mm blue-gray macules on an erythematous base (Figure 5-78).
    - **Giant-cell pneumonia,** characterized by **Warthin-Finkeldey cells** (multinucleated giant cells with eosinophilic nuclear and cytoplasmic

KEY FACT

Measles: ssRNA, linear, enveloped, helical.

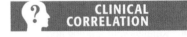

CLINICAL CORRELATION

Patients with compromised cell-mediated immunity do not develop rash, but can develop measles giant-cell pneumonia.

TABLE 5-34. "Lots of Spots": Red Rashes of Childhood

CONDITION	DESCRIPTION
Rubella (German measles, 3-day measles)	A Rubivirus; rash begins at head and moves down; postauricular tenderness
Rubeola (measles)	A paramyxovirus; beginning at head and moving down; rash preceded by cough, coryza, conjunctivitis, and blue-white (Koplik) spots on buccal mucosa
Varicella (chickenpox)	A herpesvirus (VZV); rash begins at chest, spreads to face and extremities with lesions of different age
Roseola (exanthem subitum, sixth disease)	A herpesvirus (HHV-6/HHV-7); macular truncal rash appearing suddenly after defervescence of high fever; usually affects infants and young children
Erythema infectiosum (fifth disease)	A parvovirus (B19); "Slapped cheek" rash on face which later appears over body in reticular, "lace-like" pattern
Streptococcus pyogenes (scarlet fever)	Erythematous, sandpaper-like rash with fever and sore throat
Variola (smallpox)	A poxvirus, thankfully eradicated, but potential bioterrorist threat
Hand-foot-mouth disease	A coxsackievirus (type A); Rash on palms and soles, ulcers in oral mucosa

CLINICAL CORRELATION

Measles may also cause:
- Croup
- Pneumonia
- Diarrhea with protein-losing enteropathy
- Keratitis with scarring and blindness
- Encephalitis
- Hemorrhagic rashes (black measles) in malnourished children with poor medical care

inclusion bodies) found in the lungs and sputum. Rare condition found only in the immunosuppressed.
- Additional **prodromal symptoms** may include fever, malaise, myalgias, photophobia, and periorbital edema.
- **Virus-specific immune response** is characterized by the appearance of the **rash.** Measles rash is a maculopapular erythematous rash.
  - Rash typically begins at the hairline and spreads caudally over the next 3 days as the prodromal symptoms resolve.
  - Lasts 4–6 days and then fades from the head downward. Lesion density is greatest above the shoulders, where macular lesions may coalesce.
  - Desquamation may be present but is generally not severe.
- **Complete recovery** from measles generally occurs within 7–10 days from onset of the rash.

TREATMENT

Mainly supportive care; IV hydration, antipyretics. Secondary infections such as pneumonia and otitis media should be treated with antibiotics.

- **Postexposure prophylaxis** with immune globulin may be given within 6 days of exposure to high-risk patients such as immunocompromised children and pregnant women.

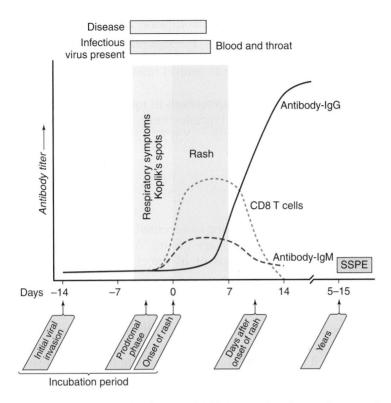

FIGURE 5-77. Natural history of measles infection. Viral replication begins in the respiratory epithelium and spreads to monocyte-macrophages, endothelial cells, and epithelial cells in the blood, spleen, lymph nodes, lung, thymus, liver, and skin and to the mucosal surfaces of the gastrointestinal, respiratory, and genitourinary tracts. The virus-specific immune response is detectable when the rash appears. Clearance of virus is approximately coincident with fading of the rash. SSPE, subacute sclerosing panencephalitis. (Modified with permission from Brooks GF, Carroll KC, Butel JS, Morse SA. *Jawetz, Melnick, & Adelberg's Medical Microbiology*, 24th ed. New York: McGraw-Hill, 2007: 559.)

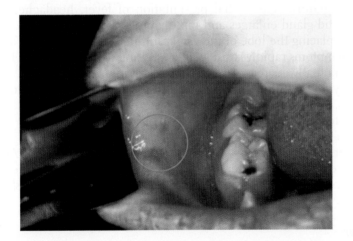

FIGURE 5-78. Koplik spots. The spots manifest as white or bluish lesions with an erythematous halo on the buccal mucosa. They usually occur in the first 2 days of measles symptoms and may briefly overlap the measles exanthem. The presence of the erythematous halo differentiates Koplik spots from Fordyce spots (ectopic sebaceous glands), which occur in the mouths of healthy individuals. (Image courtesy of CDC's Public Health Image Library.)

- **Prevention:** There is one serotype worldwide; all cases are clinically apparent. The **MMR vaccine (3-in-1)** protects against measles, mumps, and rubella and consists of live attenuated virus. Infection produces lifelong immunity. Maternal antibody can protect newborns.
- **Complications:**
  - **Common:** Respiratory complications in up to 15% of cases.
  - **Uncommon and severe:** Postinfectious encephalomyelitis, subacute sclerosing panencephalopathy (SSPE), and bacterial superinfection due to immunosuppression.

Mumps

CHARACTERISTICS

A systemic infection usually affecting unvaccinated children between the ages 2 and 12, but can occur in other age groups. Mumps usually spreads from person to person by saliva droplets or by direct contact with contaminated articles.

PATHOGENESIS

The URT is the point of initial entry via the inhalation of respiratory droplets. The virus then spreads to draining lymph nodes and replicates in lymphocytes, after which it disseminates hematogenously to the salivary gland, as well as other glands.

- Long incubation period (an average of 16–18 days).
- No clinical indication of infection in approximately one-third of infected individuals; however, they can still transmit the disease.
- The period of communicability (transmissibility) is usually from 9 days before onset of parotid edema to 1–2 days after onset of swelling and occasionally lasting as long as 7 days after swelling.

CLINICAL SYMPTOMS

- **Parotid glands:** After initial presentation of fever, headache, and otitis, the parotid gland enlarges and rapidly progresses to maximum size in 1–3 days, displacing the lobe of the ear, resulting in increased pain and tenderness. Symptoms rapidly subside after swelling reaches its peak. The parotid gland gradually decreases in size in 3–7 days.
- **Epididymo-orchitis** is the second most common manifestation of adult mumps. Symptoms include:
  - Acute onset of fever, chills, nausea, vomiting, and lower abdominal pain following parotitis.
  - After the acute syndrome, the testes begin to swell rapidly. As the fever decreases, the pain and edema subside. A loss of turgor demonstrates atrophy. Impaired fertility is uncommon, but is a greater risk when the infection occurs after puberty.

TREATMENT

Supportive.

PREVENTION

There is only one serotype worldwide. Infection confers lifelong immunity (both humoral and cell-mediated immune response are induced). Infants are protected for approximately 6 months by maternal antibodies. The MMR vaccine is used as described previously.

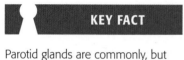

KEY FACT

Mumps: ssRNA, linear, enveloped, helical.

KEY FACT

Parotid glands are commonly, but not always, affected by mumps.

KEY FACT

Postpubertal males who develop mumps have a 15–20% risk of developing orchitis.

COMPLICATIONS

Mumps infection can invade the epithelial cells of multiple organs, including the testes, ovaries, pancreas, meninges, kidneys, thyroid, bladder, and kidney.

- **Meningoencephalitis** is the most common complication in children and results from a primary infection of the neurons or postinfection encephalitis with demyelination.
- **Aseptic meningitis** is usually indistinguishable from other causes. The mumps virus can be isolated in the CSF.
- **Unilateral deafness,** permanent or transient, is uncommon. However, mumps is the leading cause of deafness worldwide.
- **Pancreatitis** is a severe but fortunately rare manifestation.
    - **Elevated amylase** is seen, regardless of the presence of pancreatitis.
    - **Lipase** is a more specific indicator of pancreatic involvement and should be tested if this complication is suspected.

Orthomyxoviridae (Influenza A, B, and C Viruses)

GENERAL CHARACTERISTICS

Large, enveloped, ss (–) RNA, segmented. Unlike most RNA viruses, influenza **replicates** in the host cell's **nucleus** (recall that Orthomyxoviridae and Retroviridae are the only two RNA viruses to do this). However, it acquires its envelope from the host cell membrane through budding. It has several important structural proteins (Table 5-35). Notably, HA promotes viral entry, whereas NA promotes progeny virion release, and M2 membrane protein promotes viral uncoating. These three proteins are especially relevant because they serve as targets for anti-influenza drugs.

There are three known serotypes of influenza viruses: A, B, and C.

- Types A and B exhibit continual antigenic changes; type C does not.
- Influenza A has human and zoonotic hosts (aquatic birds, chickens, ducks, pigs, horses, and seals), whereas B and C types have human hosts only. Type A viruses are the most virulent and cause the most disease among humans.

TABLE 5-35. Selected Structural and Functional Proteins of Influenza Viruses

ENCODED PROTEIN	FUNCTION
HA (hemagglutinin)	- Mediator of viral attachment to host cells
	- Binds to sialic acid
	- Fusion activity at acid pH
	- Host range determinant
	- Vaccine/drug target; 95% of outer spikes
NA (neuraminidase)	- Cleaves sialic acid from HA–host cell complex; promotes virus release from cells
	- Vaccine/drug target (zanamivir/oseltamivir); 5% of outer spikes
M2 (membrane protein)	- Essential for virus uncoating, drug target (amantadine/rimantadine)

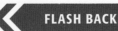
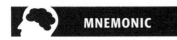
PATHOGENESIS

Influenza causes protracted illness with short incubation period (1–4 days) and exhibits both respiratory and systemic symptoms. It spreads by respiratory droplets or contact with contaminated surfaces and hands. It colonizes the respiratory epithelium and replicates locally. There is no viremia; systemic symptoms are ascribed to interferon and cytokines produced by the host. Antigenic variants of influenza virus are caused by **antigenic shift** and **antigenic drift** (Figure 5-79).

CLINICAL SYMPTOMS

Major cause of local infections of respiratory tract with constitutional symptoms.

- Uncomplicated influenza typically presents with cough, sore throat, runny or stuffy nose, fever, muscle aches and pains, headache, and fatigue.
- GI symptoms such as nausea, vomiting, and diarrhea also can occur but are more common in children than in adults.

TREATMENT

- **Amantadine** (24–48 hours after onset of symptoms) and **rimantadine** target the M2 ion channel responsible for the alteration of pH required for viral uncoating and assembly. Both are specific for **influenza A** virus.
- **Zanamivir (Relenza)** and **oseltamivir phosphate (Tamiflu)** are neuraminidase inhibitors for **both** influenza **A** and **B.**

VACCINE

Natural immunity toward a **single** influenza **strain** is long lasting and is provided by IgA of the respiratory tract. The single best way to prevent the flu is the flu vaccine. The flu vaccine is contraindicated for those with severe egg allergy, although in some cases it may still be safely given under the supervision of an allergist. There are two types of vaccines:

- Intramuscular **flu shot** is an inactivated vaccine. It contains three influenza strains (2A's and 1B), and is approved for use in individuals older than 6 months of age, both healthy people and those with chronic medical conditions.

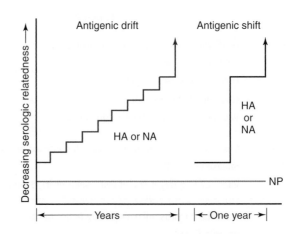

FIGURE 5-79. **Antigenic drift and antigenic shift account for antigenic changes in the two surface glycoproteins (HA and NA) of influenza virus.** Changes in HA and NA occur independently. Internal proteins of the virus, such as the nucleoprotein (NP), do not undergo antigenic changes. (Modified with permission from Brooks GF, Carroll KC, Butel JS, Morse SA. *Jawetz, Melnick, & Adelberg's Medical Microbiology,* 24th ed. New York: McGraw-Hill, 2007: 537.)

- The **nasal-spray** flu vaccine is a live, attenuated flu virus. It is approved for use in healthy people 5 years to 49 years of age who are not pregnant.

Antibodies develop within approximately 2 weeks following vaccination. Flu vaccines do not protect against flulike illnesses caused by noninfluenza viruses.

COMPLICATIONS

Rare, affects specific populations.

- **Pneumonia:** Young children, immunocompromised patients and elderly people in nursing homes are particularly susceptible. In some epidemics (depending on the viral strain), pregnant women are at high risk as well.
- Can be primary influenza, bacterial, or a combination of the two. Infection with *Staphylococcus aureus* is common.
- **Reye syndrome.**

Rhabdoviridae (Rabies)

CHARACTERISTICS

Simple negative-sense enveloped ssRNA virus. The key differentiating characteristic is its **bullet-shaped** capsid.

PATHOGENESIS

The virus is secreted in the animal's saliva, and infection results from a bite of the rabid animal. More commonly acquired from bat, raccoon, and skunk bites than from dogs in the United States. Following local inoculation, the virus progresses to the peripheral nervous system and reaches the central nervous system by way of **retrograde axonal transport.** The incubation period may be 3 months or longer; hence, the rabies virus is considered a **slow virus.**

CLINICAL SYMPTOMS

The initial symptoms of rabies are fever, malaise, headache, pain or paresthesia at the bite site, GI symptoms, fatigue, and anorexia. After the initial "flulike" syndrome, the patient develops **hydrophobia,** seizures, disorientation, and hallucinations. The final symptoms are paralysis, which may lead to respiratory failure, and coma. Unfortunately, rabies cannot be diagnosed until it is too late to treat. **Negri bodies** in the cytoplasm of affected neurons are the hallmark diagnostic finding.

TREATMENT

Postexposure prophylaxis (PEP) is used to prevent overt clinical illness in affected persons. The wound is cleaned and the patient is administered human rabies immunoglobulin and the rabies vaccination, which is a killed-virus vaccine.

DOUBLE-STRANDED RNA VIRUSES

Double-stranded RNA viruses (ie, the Reoviruses) all lack an envelope and have an icosahedral capsid and segmented genome (Table 5-36). The segmented genome allows for switching of various segments among viruses within the same family. This is called **antigenic shift.**

FLASH FORWARD

Reye syndrome: Hepatoencephalopathy resulting from the use of salicylates in children with upper respiratory infections, influenza A or B, or varicella.

TABLE 5-36. Overview of Double-Stranded RNA Viruses

FAMILY	STRUCTURE	DISEASE	ROUTE OF TRANSMISSION	IMPORTANT FACTS
Reoviridae				
Reovirus	Naked, icosahedral, segmented	Causes mild, self-limiting infections of the upper respiratory or GI tracts.	Aerosol and fecal-oral.	Very stable and have been detected in sewage and river water.
Colorado tick fever virus	Naked, icosahedral, segmented	Causes serious hemorrhagic disease due to vascular endothelial infection. Symptoms of acute disease include fever and muscle/joint pain; can have subclinical cases.	Transmitted by wood tick *Dermacentor andersoni.*	Found in western and northwestern United States, as well as western Canada.
Rotavirus	Naked, icosahedral, segmented	Diarrhea.	Fecal-oral.	Most common agent of infantile diarrhea worldwide, #1 cause of fatal diarrhea in children.

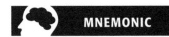

MNEMONIC

ROTA = **R**ight **O**ut **T**he **A**nus.
Diarrhea in Children: If the child is old enough to **walk,** it's more likely Nor**walk;** otherwise, it's more likely Rotavirus.

Rotavirus

CHARACTERISTICS

This double-stranded segmented RNA virus is a common agent of diarrhea in children. Human disease is caused by group A and, occasionally, group B and C rotaviruses. Commonly found in the winter and in kindergartens/day care centers.

PATHOGENESIS

The virus is spread via the fecal-oral route and possibly the respiratory route. The mechanism is intestinal villous destruction and atrophy with decreased reabsorption of sodium and water, with consequent copious osmotic diarrhea.

CLINICAL SYMPTOMS

The major clinical findings are vomiting, diarrhea, fever, and dehydration. Because most patients have large quantities of virus in stool, the direct detection of viral antigen is the method of choice for diagnosis.

TREATMENT

Supportive care. The **RotaTeq (PRV) vaccine** is a pentavalent human–bovine reassortment and is currently recommended for infants in the United States. The previous version, RotaShield, was removed from the market after being linked to **intussusception in children.**

SLOW VIRUSES AND PRION DISEASES

Slow Viruses

These viruses are etiologically associated with diseases that exhibit slow and progressive course, spanning months to years. Many involve the central nervous system and ultimately lead to death. An example is subacute sclerosing panencephalitis (SSPE), a chronic, progressive, incurable, and ultimately fatal illness caused by a rare persistent infection of the measles virus (a paramyxovirus).

Prion Diseases

Prion diseases are a related group of rare, fatal brain diseases that affect animals and humans. These diseases were previously classified as slow virus diseases. The term *prion* is an abbreviation for *proteinaceous infectious particle* (PrP). PrP exists in two known conformations. The first is a nonpathogenic cellular type that is predominantly alpha-helical in secondary structure (PrPc). Its normal function in biological tissues remains uncertain. The second conformation is a pathogenic variant that consists of mostly β-pleated sheet (PrPsc). This is the form of PrP that produces disease in animals and humans by inducing normal proteins in the infected host organism to misfold, thus propagating itself in a manner analogous to viruses.

Prion diseases are also known as **transmissible spongiform encephalopathies (TSE)** and include bovine spongiform encephalopathy (BSE, or mad cow disease) in cattle, Creutzfeldt-Jakob disease (CJD) in humans, and scrapie in sheep (Table 5-37). TSEs can be sporadic, inherited, or acquired.

TABLE 5-37. **Overview of Prion Diseases**

FAMILY	STRUCTURE	DISEASE	ROUTE OF TRANSMISSION	IMPORTANT FACTS
Animal Disease				
Scrapie	Proteinaceous infectious particle (PrP).	Sheep: Chronic, progressive fatal ataxia and pruritus.	Digesting prions, contact with infected tissue or contaminated medical equipment.	Name came from sheep scraping their hind legs.
Bovine spongiform encephalopathy (BSE)	PrP.	Mad cow disease.	Same as above.	Attributed to feeding cows parts of sheep that have scrapie.
Human Disease				
Creutzfeldt-Jakob disease (CJD)	PrP.	Spongiform encephalitis, usually sporadic.	Same as above.	Rapidly progressive and often fatal dementia, with spongiform change in gray matter. Reactive astrocytosis, amyloid plaques.
Kuru	PrP.	Spongiform encephalitis in cannibals.	Same as above.	Ataxia and shivering with spongiform change in gray matter. Reactive astrocytosis, amyloid plaques.
Gerstmann-Sträussler-Scheinker syndrome	PrP.	Spongiform encephalitis, usually familial.	Same as above.	Dysarthria and ataxia, followed by progressive memory loss and death.

Microbiology: Systems

NORMAL FLORA

Although bacteria are commonly associated with infection, even healthy individuals harbor a variety of organisms, as described in Table 5-38. In fact, the average person's body contains 10 times more bacterial cells than human cells. This symbiosis begins when membrane rupture allows flora from the vagina and surrounding environment to migrate into the previously sterile fetus. Neonates delivered by caesarian section have no flora but are rapidly colonized after birth. *Normal flora* are permanently resident microorganisms found in all people, whereas *colonization* indicates a temporary or long-term presence of certain organisms not considered part of the normal flora.

Beneficial Effects

By competing with pathogens, indigenous flora play an important role in **defense against infection.** Anaerobic bacteria in the intestines are a major source of **vitamin K,** help make **B vitamins,** and break down cellulose to aid digestion. The normal flora are essential for normal immune system development and probably have other significant functions still undiscovered.

Role in Infection

Although usually harmless in their native environment, normal flora can cause infection if they migrate to otherwise sterile locations in the body or

> **KEY FACT**
>
> Vitamin K is essential for the production of clotting factors II, VII, IX, and X, as well as the anticoagulant proteins C and S.

TABLE 5-38. Location of Normal Flora and Potential Associated Pathogens

LOCATION	NORMAL FLORA	POTENTIAL PATHOGENS
Skin	*Staphylococcus epidermidis, Propionibacterium, Corynebacterium.*	*Staphylococcus aureus*
Nasopharynx	Viridans streptococci (group D), *Neisseria, S epidermidis.*	*Streptococcus pneumoniae* *N meningitides* *Haemophilus influenzae* Group A streptococci *S aureus* (found in anterior nares of 25–30% of healthy people)
Mouth/oropharynx	Viridans streptococci, *Fusobacterium.*	*Candida albicans*
Dentition	*Prevotella melaninogenica.*	*Streptococcus mutans*
Colon	96-99% are anaerobic. *Bacillus fragilis, Fusobacterium, Clostridium* >> *Escherichia coli, Enterococcus.*	*E coli, B fragilis, Klebsiella, Enterococcus, Enterobacter, Clostridium*
Vagina	*Lactobacillus acidophilus.* May be colonized by *E coli* and group B streptococci. Prepubertal and postmenopausal: *S epidermidis* (skin flora).	*Candida*
Upper urinary tract and bladder	Normally sterile.	*E coli*

areas to which they are not indigenous. If the overall composition of the normal flora is altered, as by antibiotic use or immune deficiency, overgrowth of particular organisms can lead to disease. Chronic carriers harbor significant numbers of pathogenic organisms that can infect other persons.

- **Urinary tract infections** (UTIs) in sexually active women are often caused by intestinal *E coli* that spreads to the urinary bladder.
- **Endocarditis** can occur when viridans streptococci enter the bloodstream following dental procedures and lodge on susceptible heart valves.
- **Peritonitis** can occur when ruptured viscera from conditions such as appendicitis, diverticulitis, or a penetrating abdominal wound introduce mixed fecal bacteria into the peritoneal cavity.
- *Clostridium difficile* **(pseudomembranous) colitis** can develop when the composition of the normal flora of the GI tract is altered by **antibiotic therapy.** This leads to overgrowth of the opportunistic pathogen *C difficile,* whose toxin causes illness.
- **Candidiasis** is a fungal infection, commonly caused by *Candida albicans.* Vaginal candidiasis is a common complication of antibiotic therapy in women. Oral candidiasis (thrush) may be an early sign of an immune deficiency, such as HIV/AIDS.

MICROBIAL DISEASES OF THE RESPIRATORY TRACT

Upper Respiratory Infections

Infections of the upper respiratory tract (URIs) result from invasion of the oral and nasal cavities, sinuses, pharynx, and tonsils. Middle respiratory tract infections involve the larynx, epiglottis, and trachea. Viruses are the most common cause of URIs. Bacteria may secondarily infect these tissues as a complication of a viral infection. Except for group A streptococcal pharyngitis, antibiotics are rarely indicated for URIs and should **not** be prescribed.

- **Dental caries** are caused by *S mutans.*
- **Periodontal disease** is associated with anaerobic bacteria such as *Bacteroides, Actinomyces,* and *Prevotella.*
- **Rhinitis** is most often caused by viruses such as adenovirus, rhinovirus, coxsackievirus A, echovirus, coronavirus, influenza, and respiratory syncytial virus (RSV).
- **Sinusitis** can be acute or chronic. Acute sinusitis is usually caused by *Streptococcus pneumoniae* or *Haemophilus influenzae.* Chronic sinusitis is more likely to involve anaerobic organisms.
- **Pharyngitis** is most often caused by viruses such as adenovirus, rhinovirus, coronavirus, influenza, and Epstein-Barr virus. "Strep throat" is caused by *Streptococcus pyogenes* (group A). Key clinical manifestations of strep throat include a **sore erythematous throat, fever, tonsillar exudates, and tender cervical lymphadenopathy.** Patients typically have **no cough.** Treatment of strep throat with antibiotics is important because of the potential for dangerous sequelae, such as rheumatic fever.
- **Epiglottitis** is becoming less common since the implementation of vaccine programs for *H influenzae,* formerly the most common cause of epiglottitis in children. Today, this potentially life-threatening inflammatory disease of the epiglottis is more likely to be caused by *S aureus.* The young patient usually prefers to sit upright with neck extended to ease breathing. Plain film of the lateral cervical spine reveals a swollen epiglottis, dubbed the "thumbprint sign" (Figure 5-80).

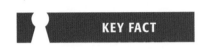

KEY FACT

Glucocorticoids cause dose-dependent immunosuppression by blocking cytokine production and release, preventing leukocyte migration, impairing T-cell function, and inducing T-cell apoptosis.

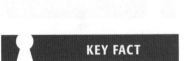

KEY FACT

In a young adult with pharyngitis, consider infectious mononucleosis caused by Epstein-Barr virus (EBV). A positive monospot (heterophile antibody) test is diagnostic. If the test is negative and the disease is prolonged, check for IgM and IgG against the viral capsid antigen (VCA) and IgG to nuclear antigen (EBNA).

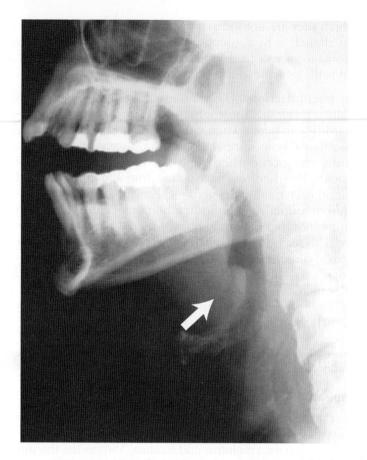

FIGURE 5-80. **Radiographic "thumbprint sign" of epiglottitis in a child.** (Reproduced with permission from Tintinalli JE, Kelen DG, Stapczynski JS. *Tintinalli's Emergency Medicine: A Comprehensive Study Guide*, 6th ed. New York: McGraw-Hill, 2004: 1497.)

Lower Respiratory Infections

Infections of the lower respiratory tract involve the bronchi, bronchioles, alveoli, and extra-alveolar lung tissues. Bronchitis and bronchiolitis are, like URIs, more commonly caused by viruses than bacteria.

- **Laryngotracheal bronchitis (croup)** is most often caused by parainfluenza virus. It classically manifests in a child who presents with a seal-like **barking cough**.
- **Pneumonia** is most often caused by bacteria and viruses, but fungi, mycobacteria, and parasites may also cause infection. Clues to the causative organism can be found in the patient's age (Table 5-39), where the infection was acquired (ie, community vs. hospital), the patient's immune status, and other risk factors.

COMMUNITY-ACQUIRED PNEUMONIA

Causes of **"typical"** pneumonia include:

- *Streptococcus pneumoniae*
- *Haemophilus influenzae*
- *Moraxella catarrhalis*

Causes of **"atypical"** pneumonia include:

- *Mycoplasma pneumoniae* ("walking pneumonia")
- *Chlamydophila pneumoniae*

KEY FACT

Typical community-acquired pneumonia is heralded by an abrupt onset of fever, chills or rigors, respiratory distress, and purulent or bloody sputum. Radiographs often demonstrate **lobar consolidation** (Figure 5-81) and the patient may have pleuritic chest pain.

KEY FACT

Atypical organisms cause diffuse interstitial disease, rather than lobar disease, and are characterized by the subacute onset of dry cough, malaise, myalgias, sore throat, fever, and headache. The chest film is usually either normal or shows diffuse rather than localized infiltrates.

TABLE 5-39.   Causes of Pneumonia by Age Group

Age Group	Most Likely Pathogen	Other Causes
Neonates (0–6 wk)	*Streptococcus agalactiae* (group B)	*E coli* *Chlamydia trachomatis*
Children (6 wk–18 yr)	Viruses like respiratory syncytial virus (RSV), influenza, and parainfluenza	*Mycoplasma pneumoniae* *Chlamydophila pneumoniae* *Streptococcus pneumoniae*
Young adults (18–40 yr)	*M pneumoniae* Viruses	*C pneumoniae* *Streptococcus pneumoniae*
Older adults (40–65 yr)	*Streptococcus pneumoniae* Viruses	*H influenzae* *M pneumoniae*
Elderly (> 65 yr)	*Streptococcus pneumoniae* Viruses	*H influenzae* Gram-negative rods *Moraxella catarrhalis* *Mycobacterium tuberculosis* (reactivation)

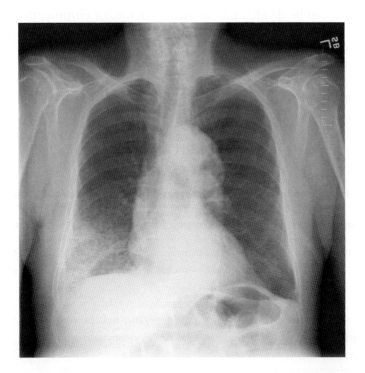

FIGURE 5-81.   Right lobar pneumococcal pneumonia. Right-sided infiltrate localized to the right lower lobe in a 32-year-old man with a history of HIV. (Reproduced with permission from Fauci AS, Braunwald E, Kasper DL, et al. *Harrison's Principles on Internal Medicine*, 17th ed. New York: McGraw-Hill, 2008: Fig. 128-1A.)

- *Legionella* (associated with contaminated aerosolized water, classically in air-conditioning systems)
- Viruses

Hospital-acquired (nosocomial) pneumonia is most likely to be caused by *S aureus* as well as *Pseudomonas aeruginosa* and other gram-negative rods.

Some population-specific agents of pneumonia are summarized in Table 5-40.

MICROBIAL DISEASES OF THE CARDIOVASCULAR SYSTEM

Infective Endocarditis

Infective endocarditis occurs when endothelial damage allows circulating microorganisms to colonize as a focal collection of platelets and fibrin on heart valves or other cardiac surfaces. Colonization leads to **vegetation** and subsequent inflammatory, embolic, and immunologic complications. Clinical manifestations can include fever, heart murmur, and signs of systemic embolization such as painful indurated nodules on the fingers and toes (**Osler nodes**), painless erythematous macules on the palms and soles (**Janeway lesions**), red linear lesions in the nailbeds (**splinter hemorrhages**), retinal hemorrhages with clear centers (**Roth spots**) (Figure 5-82), and strokes.

CLASSIFICATION OF ENDOCARDITIS

Endocarditis can be divided into **acute, subacute,** or **chronic,** depending on the virulence of the causative organism and the progression of the disease if no treatment is initiated (Table 5-41). The microbiology of native and prosthetic valve endocarditis is significantly different.

SPECIAL POPULATIONS

IV drug users tend to get **right-sided** endocarditis, with vegetations on the **tricuspid** valve. Typical organisms in this population include *S aureus*, enterococci, gram-negative enteric bacilli, and *C albicans*.

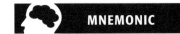

MNEMONIC

HACEK

***H**aemophilus aphrophilus,*
H parainfluenzae, and
H paraphrophilus
***A**ggregatibacter* (formerly
Actinobacillus)
actinomycetemcomitans
***C**ardiobacterium hominis*
***E**ikenella corrodens*
***K**ingella kingae*

TABLE 5-40. Common Pneumonial Pathogens Associated with Specific Populations

POPULATION AFFECTED	COMMON PATHOGENS CAUSING PNEUMONIA
Aspiration	Anaerobes (*Bacteroides, Fusobacterium, Peptostreptococcus*) admixed with aerobes (*Streptococci, S aureus, H influenzae, P aeruginosa*)
Immunocompromised hosts, including organ transplant recipients	*Staphylococcus*, gram-negative rods, fungi, viruses, *Aspergillus, Cryptococcus,* tuberculosis, cytomegalovirus (CMV)
HIV/AIDS	*Pneumocystis jiroveci* (previously *P carinii* or PCP)
Cystic fibrosis	*P aeruginosa, Burkholderia cepacia, S aureus*
Alcoholics/IV drug users	*Streptococcus pneumoniae, Klebsiella pneumoniae, S aureus*
Postviral infections	*S aureus, H influenzae, S pneumoniae*

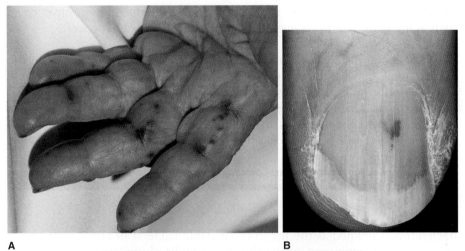

A   B

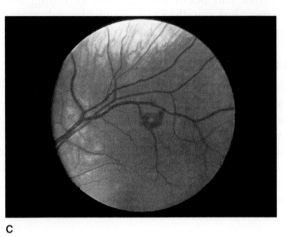

C

FIGURE 5-82. **Infective endocarditis.** (A) Janeway lesions; (B) splinter hemorrhage; (C) Roth spot. (Parts A and B reproduced with permission from Wolff K, Johnson RA, Suurmond D. *Fitzpatrick's Color Atlas & Synopsis of Clinical Dermatology*, 5th ed. New York: McGraw-Hill, 2005: 636 and 1010. Part C courtesy of William E. Cappaert, MD as printed in Knoop KJ, Stack LB, Storrow AB. *Atlas of Emergency Medicine*, 2nd ed. New York: McGraw-Hill, 2002: 80.)

TABLE 5-41. **Types of Endocarditis**

TYPE OF ENDOCARDITIS	INCUBATION TIME	MOST COMMON CAUSE
Acute	Days to weeks	*Staphylococcus aureus;* beta-hemolytic streptococci; gram-negative rods
Subacute	Weeks to months	Viridans *streptococci*; *Enterococcus*; occasionally fungi
Prosthetic valve	Varies	Coagulase-negative staphylococci and corynebacteria, in addition to the organisms associated with native-valve endocarditis

Prosthetic-valve endocarditis is usually associated with gram-positive cocci such as *S aureus*, coagulase-negative staphylococci, and enterococci.

HACEK organisms are a group of gram-negative bacilli that are part of the normal oropharyngeal flora. They are slow-growing (mean and median time to detection of 3.4 and 3 days, respectively) and have a tendency to be involved in endocardial infections. These organisms cause infections in IV drug users who contaminate the needle or injection site with saliva, as well as in patients with poor dental hygiene or preexisting valvular damage.

MICROBIAL DISEASES OF THE BLOODSTREAM

Bacteremia

Bacteremia is defined as the presence of viable bacteria in circulating blood. Transient bacteremia can occur during tooth brushing, menstruation, and other daily activities, but usually resolves quickly and asymptomatically secondary to leukocyte clearance of the bacteria.

KEY SOURCES OF BACTEREMIA

Except in endocarditis and the transient daily bacteremias mentioned earlier, bacteremia is usually associated with a significant, localized infection elsewhere in the body. A common risk factor for bacteremia is an indwelling urinary catheter, which provides easy access for *E coli* to invade via the urinary tract. The microbiology of bacteremia reflects that of the underlying disease; bacteremia associated with pneumonia is caused by pneumonia pathogens (eg, *S pneumoniae*); bacteremia associated with abdominal trauma tends to be caused by colonic flora such as *E coli* and anaerobes.

Sepsis

Sepsis is defined as a systemic inflammatory state associated with either laboratory-confirmed bloodstream infection or an obvious source of contamination (eg, an open wound). Four clinical criteria define the *systemic inflammatory response syndrome* (SIRS):

- Temperature, either $> 38.5°C$ or $< 35°C$
- Heart rate, > 90 beats per minute
- Respiratory rate, either > 20 breaths per minute or measurement of the arterial CO_2 concentration < 32 mm Hg
- White blood cell count, either $> 12,000$ cells/mm^3, $< 4,000$ cells/mm^3, or $> 10\%$ immature band forms

When two or more of these clinical criteria are present the patient is said to have SIRS, which can result from noninfectious causes, and when SIRS is accompanied by infection the patient has *sepsis*. This life-threatening condition can progress to *severe sepsis*, **septic shock,** and *refractory septic shock*. The immediate goal in clinical management of sepsis is support of respiratory and cardiovascular function, followed by rapid administration of appropriate antimicrobial therapy.

Gastrointestinal malignancy is often associated with bacteremia caused by *S bovis* and *Clostridium septicum*.

MICROBIAL DISEASES OF THE GI TRACT

Food-Poisoning Syndromes

Caused by eating food contaminated with bacterial toxins (Table 5-42) or live organisms (Table 5-43). Symptoms may include nausea, vomiting, abdominal cramps, diarrhea, fever, chills, weakness, and headache. Onset of symptoms varies with cause—from as few as 2–6 hours to 1 or 2 days after ingestion.

Bacterial Causes of Diarrhea Not Associated With Food

Cholera is an acute disease of the small intestine caused by *Vibrio cholerae*. This gram-negative curved or "comma-shaped" bacillus is spread by the fecal-oral route, usually via **contaminated water.** The bacteria attach to intestinal epithelial cells and release the cholera toxin, which activates **adenylate cyclase,** increasing intracellular cAMP and stimulating **hypersecretion** of Na^+, K^+, Cl^-, HCO_3^- and water. This produces secretory "**rice water**" diarrhea, with volume depletion, normal-gap metabolic acidosis, and hypokalemia. Treatment is supportive, including oral rehydration solutions.

Shigella is spread by the fecal-oral route, usually from hand-to-hand contact. Bacteria invade the epithelial cells lining the colon and release Shiga toxin, which destroys the cells by **inhibiting the 60S ribosome.** The disease is characterized by fever, abdominal pain, and inflammatory diarrhea that may contain specks of bright red blood and pus. A very small number of organisms can lead to widespread infection; thus the median infective dose (ID_{50}) is very low. Treatment is with ciprofloxacin.

Clostridium difficile (**pseudomembranous**) **colitis** occurs iatrogenically in 60 of every 100,000 hospital patients as a result of **antibiotic** administration, which alters the intestinal flora and allows overgrowth of *C difficile*. The bacteria produce an enterotoxin and a cytotoxin, leading to the formation of creamy to greenish exudates (pseudomembranes) in the colon (Figure 5-15). Clinical manifestations include fever, cramping, and severe diarrhea that may or may not involve bleeding. Diagnosis is with **toxin assay of stool.** Treatment is with metronidazole or oral vancomycin.

Yersinia enterocolitica is another cause of bloody diarrhea associated with outbreaks in day care centers. Can also cause fever, leukocytosis, and abdomi-

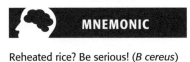

MNEMONIC

Reheated rice? Be serious! (*B cereus*)

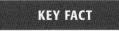

KEY FACT

Cholera is endemic to the developing nations of Africa and Asia; fewer than 100 cases occurred in the United States over the past decade, and most were acquired overseas.

Bacterial dysentery, mostly from *Shigella* infection, is extremely common with nearly half a million cases annually in the United States, and more than 150 million cases worldwide with a million associated deaths.

TABLE 5-42. **Food-Poisoning Syndromes Caused by Preformed Toxins**

ORGANISM	ASSOCIATED FOOD	POINTS TO REMEMBER
Staphylococcus aureus	Potato salad, custard, mayonnaise, meats left at room temperature.	Severe vomiting and diarrhea appear 2–6 hours after ingestion.
Bacillus cereus	Reheated rice and other starchy foods, undercooked meat or vegetables.	May cause emetic or diarrheal disease. Both *S aureus* and *B cereus* start and end relatively quickly.
Clostridium botulinum (adults)	Inadequately preserved canned foods (bulging cans).	Neurotoxin binds synaptic vesicles in cholinergic nerves, blocks acetylcholine release, causes paralysis and death.

TABLE 5-43. Food-Poisoning Syndromes Caused by Bacterial Infection

ORGANISM	ASSOCIATED FOOD	POINTS TO REMEMBER
Salmonella enteriditis	Poultry, meat, fish, eggs.	Most common cause of noninvasive food poisoning in the United States; may cause watery or mucous diarrhea. Flagellar motility. Gallbladder is an important reservoir for organisms, thus cholecystectomy is indicated for asymptomatic carriers.
Campylobacter jejuni	Poultry, milk, contaminated water.	Most common invasive bacterial enterocolitis; produces crypt abscesses and ulcers resembling ulcerative colitis, causes explosive diarrhea with blood and/or mucus, may cause Guillain-Barré syndrome. Growth at 42°C (***Camp**ylobacter* likes the hot **camp**fire).
Clostridium perfringens	Meat that is unrefrigerated or cooled too slowly.	Causes cramps and watery diarrhea lasting 24 hours. Can also cause "gas gangrene."
Clostridium botulinum (infants)	Honey.	Spores contaminate honey and germinate in infant's GI tract; neurotoxin blocks acetylcholine release, causes constipation and "floppy baby."
Enterohemorrhagic *E coli* (EHEC) strain O157:H7	Hamburger meat, spinach.	Shiga-like toxin causes severe inflammatory diarrhea; can lead to hemolytic uremic syndrome.
Vibrio parahaemolyticus, V vulnificus	Raw or undercooked seafood (usually oysters).	Causes vomiting and watery diarrhea that are self-limited. *V vulnificus* can also cause wound infections from contact with contaminated shellfish.
Listeria monocytogenes	Deli meats, unpasteurized milk and cheese.	Occurs sporadically, and rarely. Limited to pregnant and immunocompromised patients, though high mortality rate.

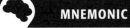

MNEMONIC

Entero**path**ogenic *E coli* is **path**etic.
Entero**aggre**gative *E coli* **aggre**gates along the intestinal wall.
Entero**t**oxigenic *E coli* is the most common cause of **t**raveler's diarrhea.
Entero**in**vasive *E coli* **in**vades and **in**flames the colon.

nal pain localized to the right lower quadrant that is often mistaken for appendicitis; this is known as the "pseudoappendicitis" syndrome.

Escherichia coli gastroenteritis occurs when this component of the normal intestinal flora acquires virulence factors (Table 5-44).

Parasitic Causes of Diarrhea

Amebiasis is an infection caused by amoebae; *Entamoeba histolytica* is the primary pathogenic amoeba of humans. It is spread by cysts in fecally contaminated food and can lead to asymptomatic passage of cysts, nondysenteric infection characterized by watery diarrhea, or dysenteric infection characterized by **bloody diarrhea** and tenesmus, especially in malnourished or immunocompromised persons. This also causes right upper quadrant pain resulting from liver abscesses, with "flask-shaped" lytic lesions elsewhere in the GI tract.

Giardiasis is caused by the protozoan parasite *Giardia lamblia*, which is a single-celled parasite with a prominent ventral sucking disk and flagella (Figure 5-83). Patients may ingest cysts from **open water**, including clear-running mountain streams, since many animal species harbor pathogenic *Giardia*. In the small intestine, each cyst develops into two trophozoites that use their sucking disks to attach themselves to the columnar cells of the duodenum,

TABLE 5-44. **Types of *Escherichia coli* Causing Gastroenteritis**

ORGANISM	VIRULENCE FACTOR	CLINICAL FEATURES
Enteropathogenic *E coli*	Bacteria adhere to intestinal epithelial cells and prevent fluid absorption.	Secretory diarrhea associated with epidemics in infants.
Enteroaggregative *E coli*	Aggregates of bacteria adhere to intestinal epithelial cells and prevent fluid absorption.	Secretory diarrhea—one cause of traveler's diarrhea.
Enterotoxigenic *E coli*	Heat-stable enterotoxin activates guanylate cyclase, inhibiting intestinal fluid uptake; heat-labile enterotoxin activates adenylate cyclase, stimulating hypersecretion of fluids (just like cholera toxin).	Secretory diarrhea (up to 20 L/day), most common cause of traveler's diarrhea.
Enterohemorrhagic *E coli*	Shiga-toxin positive, often type O157:H7. Has a very low ID_{50} (10–100 organisms). Causes HUS in up to 10% of infected kids. Recognition of EHEC is critical, as antibiotic therapy causes **increased** morbidity and mortality.	Inflammatory diarrhea and dysentery and HUS.
Enteroinvasive *E coli*	Bacteria invade the epithelial cells lining the colon, then replicate and destroy the cells; also produces small amounts of Shiga-like toxin.	Inflammatory diarrhea.

HUS = hemolytic-uremic syndrome.

mechanically impairing duodenal function. Many patients remain asymptomatic; however, symptomatic disease can range from a self-limited acute diarrhea to severe chronic diarrhea. Treatment is with metronidazole.

Cryptosporidiosis is caused by protozoa of the genus *Cryptosporidium*, predominantly *C parvum* and *C hominis*. Ingestion of oocysts from fecally contaminated water results in infection of the brush border of the intestine, leading to a self-limited diarrheal illness in immunocompetent patients. In immunocompromised patients, however, the diarrhea is often severe and unrelenting. In HIV-infected patients HAART should be initiated to boost immunity; nitazoxanide or paromomycin can be used if the diarrhea does not resolve.

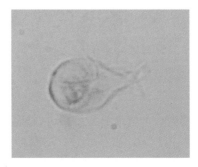

FIGURE 5-83. ***Giardia lamblia* trophozoites.** Wet mount stained with iodine. (Image courtesy of CDC's Public Health Image Library; content provider Dr. Mae Melvin.)

Viral Causes of Diarrhea

Viral gastroenteritis is spread via the fecal-oral route. Viruses cause diarrhea by invading the intestinal epithelial cells and multiplying intracellularly. As they subvert host cell metabolism, fluid transport is disrupted, and cell destruction occurs, leading to decreased fluid reabsorption. The resulting nausea, vomiting, and watery diarrhea are usually self-limited but can lead to life-threatening dehydration in patients who are very young, malnourished, or immunocompromised.

- **Rotavirus** is the most common cause of diarrhea in children. Its incidence increases during the winter. Stool antigen testing may aid the diagnosis.
- **Norwalk virus** is a common cause of diarrheal outbreaks among adults and children, particularly on cruise ships, in nursing homes, and at camps.
- **Astrovirus** is an important cause of diarrhea in children younger than 1 year.
- **Cytomegalovirus** is an important cause of colitis, which produces chronic watery diarrhea in patients with HIV/AIDS and other profoundly immunosuppressed patients.

MNEMONIC

SSEEK PP

Serratia marcescens
Staphylococcus saprophyticus
E coli
Enterobacter cloacae
Klebsiella pneumoniae
Pseudomonas aeruginosa
Proteus mirabilis

MICROBIAL DISEASES OF THE URINARY AND REPRODUCTIVE SYSTEMS

Infections commonly occur as a result of fecal contamination, sexual transmission, or as a complication of medical instrumentation (eg, catheterization).

Urinary Tract Infections (UTIs)

Defined by the presence of bacteria in the urine (bacteriuria) in combination with symptoms such as dysuria, urgency, and frequency, as well as suprapubic pain and WBCs (but not WBC casts) in the urine. The urinary tract is normally sterile, but infection is frequently caused by ascension of coliform bacteria such as *E coli* into the bladder via the urethra. Any cause of urinary stasis, such as a tumor, stone, enlarged prostate, neurogenic bladder, catheterization, diabetes, recent kidney surgery, or the presence of a foreign body can predispose to UTI. Common causative organisms are listed in Table 5-45.

A urine sample should be obtained **midstream** after the initial urine in the urethra has been voided. Bacterial counts are highest in the first morning void as the bacteria have multiplied overnight and the sample is likely to be relatively concentrated. Classically, a value of 10^5 colony-forming units (CFU) of *E coli* per milliliter is considered the cutoff to establish infection, but in samples collected by suprapubic aspirate CFUs as low as 10^2 are associated with symptoms. In the typical well-collected, midstream urine sample, a useful rule of thumb is that a single isolate in a concentration of 10^4–10^5 may be pathogenic; at a concentration $> 10^5$ it's probably pathogenic.

Women, especially sexually active young women, are at risk for developing UTIs because of the short length of the female urethra and the presence of fecal bacteria in female perineal flora. UTIs are 10 times more common in women than in men. Uncomplicated UTIs in the outpatient setting can be

TABLE 5-45. **Bacteria Causing Urinary Tract Infections**

ORGANISM	DISTINCTIVE FEATURES
Serratia marcescens	Some strains produce a red pigment (marcescens red like a maraschino cherry); often nosocomial and drug-resistant.
Staphylococcus saprophyticus	Second leading cause of community-acquired urinary tract infection (UTI) in sexually active women.
E coli	Leading cause of UTI in otherwise healthy outpatients; colonies have a metallic sheen on EMB (eosin–methylene blue) agar.
Enterobacter cloacae	Often nosocomial and drug-resistant.
Klebsiella pneumoniae	Often nosocomial and drug-resistant; may have a large mucoid capsule and viscous colonies.
Pseudomonas aeruginosa	Blue-green pigment and fruity odor; usually nosocomial and drug-resistant.
Proteus mirabilis	Motility causes "swarming" on agar; produces urease; associated with high urine pH and struvite calculi.

treated empirically with trimethoprim-sulfamethoxazole (TMP-SMX) or fluo-roquinolones. Causative organisms include:

- Uropathogenic *E coli* (70–95%)
- *Staphylococcus saprophyticus* (10–15%)
- *Klebsiella pneumoniae* and other gram-negative rods; occasionally yeasts.

Hospitalized patients are at increased risk for developing UTIs, typically secondary to the presence of Foley catheters. This is the most common hospital-acquired infection. *E coli* remains the most common causative organism, but other causative organisms, such as *Proteus, Klebsiella, Serratia, Pseudomonas, Enterobacter, Enterococcus*, and yeasts, are seen much more frequently than in outpatients. Urine culture should be performed in hospitalized patients to determine the specific bacteria causing the infection.

Pregnancy is frequently associated with asymptomatic bacteriuria both from pelvic compression by the fetus causing urinary stasis as well as high circulating levels of progesterone causing urinary tract dilation. Bacteriuria during pregnancy is a risk factor for pyelonephritis and also increases the risk for preterm labor and low birth weight. Because of these risks, bacteriuria in pregnant women is considered a true UTI, whereas bacteriuria in another person without symptoms is presumed to represent normal flora or colonization. Pregnant women should be screened for bacteriuria early in pregnancy and should always be treated, regardless of the presence of symptoms.

Children with recurrent UTIs should be evaluated for vesicoureteral reflux and other congenital abnormalities. Frequent UTIs or other pelvic infections in children raise the concern for child abuse. UTIs in otherwise healthy men are also often associated with urinary tract pathology.

Sexually Transmitted Infections

Sexually transmitted infections (STIs) are among the most common infectious diseases in the United States today. Because they share a common mechanism of transmission, it is not uncommon for a patient to present with more than one infection simultaneously. In many cases, individuals are asymptomatic while carrying (and transmitting) these infections. Women in particular are at risk for developing serious complications, such as pelvic inflammatory disease (PID), from even asymptomatic STIs. These infections are summarized in Table 5-46.

Chlamydia is the most commonly reported STI in the United States and is a leading cause of infertility in women. The causative organism, *C trachomatis*, is an obligate intracellular bacterium with 15 immunotypes. Immunotypes D-K cause genital tract infections and immunotypes L1–L3 cause genital ulcers (lymphogranuloma venereum). Most cases of chlamydia infection are **asymptomatic,** but the disease may cause dysuria and mucopurulent discharge from the urethra as well as subacute PID.

Gonorrhea is a common STI characterized by acute **purulent urethral discharge** and painful or difficult urination. In contrast to chlamydia, gonorrheal PID is typically acute and associated with high fever. It is caused by *Neisseria gonorrhoeae*, aerobic gram-negative cocci that are characteristically coffee bean-shaped in pairs. Because coinfection with *C trachomatis* is common, patients diagnosed with gonorrhea should also be treated for chlamydia infection.

TABLE 5-46.   Sexually Transmitted Infections

DISEASE	ORGANISM	CLINICAL FEATURES	TREATMENT
Chlamydia	*Chlamydia trachomatis* (D–K)	Urethritis, cervicitis, conjunctivitis, pelvic inflammatory disease (PID), infertility, reactive arthritis (Reiter syndrome).	Doxycycline for 7 days or single-dose azithromycin.
Lymphogranuloma venereum	*C trachomatis* (L1–L3)	Ulcers, lymphadenopathy, rectal strictures.	Doxycycline for 21 days.
Gonorrhea	*Neisseria gonorrhoeae*	Urethritis, cervicitis, PID, prostatitis, epididymitis, arthritis, creamy purulent discharge.	Ceftriaxone (also treat for possible *Chlamydia*).
Primary syphilis	*Treponema pallidum*	Painless chancre.	Single dose of benzathine penicillin G IM.
Secondary syphilis	*T pallidum*	Rash (affecting palms and soles), fever, lymphadenopathy, condylomata lata.	Single dose of benzathine penicillin G IM.
Tertiary syphilis	*T pallidum*	Gummas, aortitis. Meningitis, tabes dorsalis, general paresis, Argyll-Robertson pupils.	Three doses of benzathine penicillin G IM. 10–14 days of aqueous crystalline penicillin G IV.
Genital herpes	Herpes simplex virus (usually HSV-2)	Painful penile, vulvar, or cervical ulcers; can cause systemic symptoms such as fever, headache, myalgia.	Acyclovir, famciclovir, or valacyclovir.
Trichomoniasis	*Trichomonas vaginalis*	Vaginitis, frothy vaginal discharge, "strawberry cervix."	Metronidazole (for patient and partners).
AIDS	Human immunodeficiency virus (HIV)	Opportunistic infections, Kaposi's sarcoma, lymphoma.	Highly active antiretroviral therapy (HAART).
Condylomata acuminata	Human papillomavirus (HPV), types 6 and 11	Genital warts.	Cryotherapy or surgical excision.
Cervical cancer	Human papillomavirus (HPV), types 16, 18, and others		
Hepatitis B	Hepatitis B virus	Jaundice, liver failure.	INF-α, lamivudine, adefovir, or entecavir.
Chancroid	*Haemophilus ducreyi*	Painful genital ulcer, inguinal lymphadenopathy.	Azithromycin, ceftriaxone, or ciprofloxacin.
Granuloma inguinale (donovanosis)	*Klebsiella granulomatis*	Small papule or painless beefy red ulcer with rolled edges that bleed easily.	Doxycycline for 3–5 weeks until lesions resolve.
Bacterial vaginosis	*Gardnerella vaginalis*, anaerobes	Noninflammatory, clue cells, malodorous discharge (fishy smell); positive whiff test.	Metronidazole or clindamycin.

Pelvic inflammatory disease (PID) can be a serious complication of STIs in women. Chlamydia infection and gonorrhea are the most common primary causes, either alone or in combination. Organisms infecting the vagina and cervix ascend the female genital tract and cause disease in the uterus, fallopian tubes, and ovaries. The infection progresses to form scar tissue and adhesions. Sequelae can include **ectopic pregnancy, hydrosalpinx, tubo-ovarian abscess (TOA), infertility,** and **chronic pelvic pain.** Another complication is **Fitz-Hugh–Curtis syndrome** resulting from peritoneal spread of infection to the liver capsule with characteristic "violin string" adhesions of parietal peritoneum to liver. Serious PID is often polymicrobial in origin, when normal urogenital flora proliferate within the fallopian tubes and ovaries behind scarring and blockage associated with chlamydia or gonorrhea.

Vaginal Infections

Vaginitis often manifests with symptoms such as itching, burning, irritation, and abnormal discharge. The three most common vaginitides are bacterial vaginosis, candidiasis, and trichomoniasis, which together account for more than 90% of cases. Several diagnostic criteria used to differentiate these infections are listed in Table 5-47.

Bacterial vaginosis is the most common cause of vaginitis. It is caused by an overgrowth of organisms such as *Gardnerella vaginalis, Mobiluncus, Mycoplasma hominis,* and *Peptostreptococcus.* It can manifest with a thin, white, adherent vaginal discharge, which releases a fishy odor when mixed with KOH (positive whiff test). Diagnosis is confirmed by saline wet mount showing epithelial cells covered in bacteria (**clue cells**), as seen in Figure 5-22.

Candidiasis is a fungal infection that can be associated with antibiotic use or immune deficiency.

Trichomoniasis is an STI that produces a frothy vaginal discharge and a characteristic "strawberry cervix" due to punctate petechial hemorrhages dotting the cervix. This is a flagellated organism with "corkscrew" motility on wet prep. The bacterium can be isolated from up to 80% of male partners of infected women; therefore, both the patient and her partner(s) should be treated.

TABLE 5-47. Diagnostic Characteristics of Common Vaginal Infections

	NORMAL	**BACTERIAL VAGINOSIS**	**CANDIDIASIS**	**TRICHOMONIASIS**
Complaints	None	Discharge, odor	Discharge, **itching**	Frothy discharge, itching, odor
Discharge	White, clear, flocculent	Thin, adherent, white-gray, homogeneous	White, curd-like	White to yellow-green, frothy
Amine odor	Absent	Present (fishy)	Absent	Variable
Microscopic	Lactobacilli	Clue cells, cocci	Budding yeast and pseudohyphae	Trichomonads
Vaginal pH	3.8–4.2	> 4.5	< 4.5	> 4.5

TORCH

***T**oxoplasma*—Avoid domestic cats and cat litter in pregnancy.

Other infections: *HIV*—Screen with ELISA antibody test using an "opt-out" approach; treat with antiretroviral drugs to reduce transmission. *Syphilis*—Screen with VDRL or RPR; confirm with FTA-Abs or MHA-TP.

***R**ubella*—Screen for IgG immunity; vaccinate postpartum if nonimmune.

***C**ytomegalovirus*—Amniocentesis for PCR if confirmed primary maternal infection.

***H**erpes*—deliver by Cesarean section if the mother has active lesions in the birth canal.

Infections During Pregnancy

A number of infections can cause severe congenital problems if a patient contracts them during pregnancy. The acronym TORCH (toxoplasmosis; other infections; rubella; cytomegalovirus; herpes simplex virus) identifies infectious diseases commonly screened for during pregnancy. Nonspecific findings common to many of these infections include hepatosplenomegaly, jaundice, thrombocytopenia, and growth retardation.

Toxoplasmosis is a parasitic disease contracted by eating undercooked meat or being exposed to aerosolized cat feces. It is usually asymptomatic or causes a mild flulike illness in healthy adults; however, when transmitted to the neonate, it can result in the classic "triad" of chorioretinitis, hydrocephalus, and intracranial calcification, often accompanied by mental retardation and/or or seizures.

Other infections includes syphilis, and infections with parvovirus B19, hepatitis B virus, varicella-zoster virus, and HIV. HIV should be screened for in all pregnant patients. Antiretroviral therapy with zidovudine greatly reduces the likelihood that the virus will be transmitted to the fetus during pregnancy and delivery (from 25% to approximately 8%). HIV-positive women should be counseled not to breast-feed their babies.

Rubella is a viral infection typically transmitted via respiratory droplets that causes a mild rash and flulike illness in healthy adults. During the first trimester of pregnancy, however, it can lead to miscarriage, stillbirth, or serious birth defects. Congenital rubella syndrome includes the classic "triad" of **heart malformations** (most often patent ductus arteriosus or pulmonary hypoplasia), deafness, and cataracts. Other common manifestations include mental retardation and a "blueberry muffin" rash.

Cytomegalovirus (CMV) infection can be transmitted during delivery or via breast milk. Usually asymptomatic or producing a heterophile-negative mononucleosis-like illness in adults; infected neonates may develop hearing loss, seizures, and mental retardation.

Herpes is a common viral infection causing painful mucosal ulcers. A neonate typically becomes infected while passing through the birth canal during an active maternal outbreak. This leads to an often fatal neonatal encephalitis with widespread herpetic (vesicular) lesions of the skin and eye.

Syphilis is an STI with a wide variety of clinical manifestations in adults. During pregnancy, treponemes can pass through the placenta to the fetus. Approximately 50% of these fetuses are aborted or stillborn. The remainder may present with the **Hutchinson triad** of notched teeth, eighth cranial nerve deafness, and interstitial keratitis. Infected infants may also present with other syphilitic stigmata such as a saddle nose, short maxilla, saber shins, and severe hydrops fetalis.

MICROBIAL DISEASES OF THE BONES, JOINTS, AND SKIN

Osteomyelitis

INFECTION OF THE BONE

Osteomyelitis can occur as a result of trauma, postsurgical infection, hematogenous spread of bacteria into the bone, invasion of the bone from a contiguous source of infection, or skin breakdown in the setting of vascular insufficiency. Direct spread from a soft tissue infection is most common in adults, whereas hematogenous spread is more common in children. Osteomyelitis is far more common in children. The most common cause of osteomyelitis overall is S *aureus*, although certain populations may be predisposed to infection with other organisms.

- **Sexually active patients** may rarely present with osteomyelitis caused by N *gonorrhoeae*, although septic arthritis is a much more common manifestation of this infection.
- **Diabetics and drug addicts** may present with osteomyelitis caused by P *aeruginosa*.
- **Sickle cell disease** is associated with *Salmonella* osteomyelitis.
- **Prosthetic joint replacements** are associated with osteomyelitis due predominantly to staphylococcal organisms, such as S *aureus* or *coagulase-negative staphylococci*.
- **Cat** and **dog bites** are associated with *Pasteurella multocida* osteomyelitis.
- **Tuberculosis** can lead to **vertebral** osteomyelitis (Pott disease).

Infectious Arthritis

Bacterial invasion of a joint. S *aureus* and N *gonorrhoeae* are the first and second most common causes, respectively, of infectious arthritis in adults. The disease typically affects a single large joint, producing pain, tenderness, warmth, and erythema. The synovial fluid is thick and cloudy with many white blood cells, although bacteria may not be evident on Gram stains or cultures.

Lyme disease is another significant cause of septic arthritis in endemic areas. The arthritis of Lyme may be mono- or polyarticular, and Gram stains and cultures are negative.

Cellulitis

Cellulitis is an acute, spreading infection of the skin extending into the subcutaneous tissues. Group A streptococci and S *aureus* are the most common causes.

Erysipelas is a superficial cellulitis with prominent lymphatic involvement. It most commonly manifests on the legs with lesions that are bright red, edematous, and indurated with a sharp, raised border. It is almost always caused by group A streptococci.

Erythrasma is a superficial infection caused by *Corynebacterium*. Scaly plaques are present between the toes, and erythematous plaques are found in the intertriginous areas. Diagnosis is confirmed with the Wood's lamp.

Erythema Chronicum Migrans (ECM); Lyme Disease

This characteristic target-shaped rash is indicative of **Lyme disease,** caused by the spirochete *Borrelia burgdorferi* and transmitted by *Ixodes* ticks in the United States. The rash may be accompanied by nonspecific constitutional symptoms in the first stage. Later manifestations include migratory arthralgias, meningitis, facial nerve palsy, atrioventricular nodal block, and arthritis. The diagnosis of Lyme disease at the ECM stage (prior to the development of antibody) is clinical, based on exposure history and the characteristic rash. The organism is difficult to culture and culturing is not routinely performed. For systemic syndromes consistent with Lyme disease, serology is the mainstay of diagnosis; IgM antibody appears within a month of infection, and IgG persists for many years. Despite a great deal of controversy in the popular literature, scientific evidence supports Lyme serology as a reliable diagnostic test, similar to other serodiagnostic methods. In addition, there is no evidence that prolonged antibiotic therapy, as given by some practitioners, provides benefit in chronic Lyme disease.

MICROBIAL DISEASES OF THE EYE AND EAR

Conjunctivitis

Children and neonates are particularly susceptible to conjunctivitis. Neonatal conjunctivitis can be classified according to its temporal presentation after birth:

- **Day 1:** Silver nitrate susceptibility.
- **Days 1–4:** *Neisseria gonorrhoeae*. Manifests with **hyperpurulent exudates**.
- **Days 3–10:** *Chlamydia trachomatis*. Manifests with purulent exudates. Microscopic evaluation reveals **inclusion bodies** in cells. This infection may progress to blindness if left untreated.

POSTNEONATAL AND CHILDHOOD

Purulent exudates suggest infection with *H influenzae* or *S pneumoniae*. Watery exudates and sore throat with recent swimming pool exposure suggest adenovirus ("pink eye"), a nonenveloped virus resistant to chlorination.

- **Contact lens wearers** can develop conjunctivitis after leaving contacts in their eyes for long periods of time (*Pseudomonas*) or from using homemade saline (*Acanthamoeba*).
- **Parasitic causes** of conjunctivitis include *Trypanosoma cruzi* (Chagas disease) and *Trichinella*. Both are uncommon in the United States and more typically manifest with systemic illness rather than isolated conjunctivitis.
- **Conjunctivitis with vision loss** may be caused by *C trachomatis*, types A, B, and C. These immunotypes are uncommon in the United States, but chronic infection commonly causes corneal scarring and blindness in less developed countries.

Otitis

Otitis externa is most commonly caused by *P aeruginosa* and *S aureus*, though many cases are polymicrobial. It causes severe tenderness and pain. Swimmers and diabetics are at increased risk for this infection. Treatment is with antibiotic drops (typically an aminoglycoside or fluoroquinolone), with or without steroids.

Otitis media is an exceedingly common infection in children under the age of 6 years. It usually arises as a complication of a viral upper respiratory infection. Secretions and inflammation cause a relative obstruction of the eustachian tubes. As the mucosa of the middle ear absorbs air that cannot be replaced because of this obstruction, negative pressure is generated, and a serous effusion develops. This provides a fertile medium for bacterial growth. Common causal organisms include *S pneumoniae*, *H influenzae*, and *Moraxella*, and viruses.

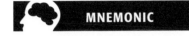

MNEMONIC

In chronologic order of presentation—

Some Neonates Can Hardly See Anything

Silver nitrate susceptibility
Neisseria gonorrhoeae
Chlamydia trachomatis
Haemophilus influenzae
Streptococcus pneumoniae
Adenovirus

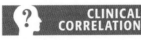

CLINICAL CORRELATION

Children older than six months can be observed without treatment if the illness is mild; severe illness or age younger than six months are indications for antibiotic therapy. Antibiotics reduce the duration of symptoms by 1 day in ~10% of kids, and antibiotics also cause side effects in ~10% of kids.

TABLE 5-48   Causes of Meningitis by Age Group

AGE GROUP	MOST COMMON PATHOGENS	OTHER CAUSES
Newborn (0–6 months)	Group B streptococci *E coli*	*Listeria*
Children (6 mo–6 yr)	*Streptococcus pneumoniae*	*Neisseria meningitides* *Haemophilus influenzae* type B Enteroviruses
6–60 yr	*N meningitidis* *S pneumoniae*	Enteroviruses Herpes simplex virus
Elderly (> 60 yr)	*S pneumoniae*	Gram-negative rods *Listeria*

MICROBIAL DISEASES OF THE NERVOUS SYSTEM

Meningitis

Inflammation of the leptomeninges and underlying CSF. Symptoms include headache; fever; nuchal rigidity; and neurologic abnormalities including altered mental status, cranial nerve dysfunction, and seizures. As with pneumonia, the common causes of meningitis can be grouped according to the age of the patient (Table 5-48). The incidence of *H influenzae* type B meningitis, formerly the most common cause of meningitis in children, has declined significantly with the introduction of vaccine programs in the past 10–15 years. Bacterial, viral, and fungal causes of meningitis can be differentiated by characteristic patterns of the patient's CSF, as summarized in Table 5-49.

HIV/AIDS is associated with meningitis and other CNS manifestations caused by opportunistic pathogens such as *Cryptococcus*, *Toxoplasma*, cytomegalovirus (CMV), and JC virus (progressive multifocal leukoencephalopathy). *Toxoplasma* infection is often complicated by temporal lobe necrosis or abscess.

NOSOCOMIAL INFECTIONS

Table 5-50 summarizes the pathogens commonly associated with various hospital-related risk factors.

CLINICAL CORRELATION

Bacterial meningitis is more common from late fall to early spring.

KEY FACT

Using two drugs that are both either bactericidal or bacteriostatic is often **synergistic** (eg, penicillin/ aminoglycoside or trimethoprim-sulfonamide).
Using a bacteriostatic drug with a bactericidal drug is often **antagonistic** (eg, penicillin/ tetracycline).

TABLE 5-49.   Cerebrospinal Spinal Fluid Findings in Meningitis

CAUSE	PRESSURE	CELL TYPE	PROTEIN	GLUCOSE
Bacterial	↑	↑ PMNs	↑	↓
Fungal/TB	↑	↑ Lymphocytes	↑	↓
Viral	Normal/↑	↑ Lymphocytes	Normal/↑	Normal

PMNs = polymorphonuclear leukocytes.

TABLE 5-50. Risk Factors and Associated Pathogens Implicated in Nosocomial Infections

RISK FACTOR	PATHOGEN
Newborn nursery	Cytomegalovirus, respiratory syncytial virus
Urinary catheterization	*E coli, Proteus mirabilis*
Respiratory therapy equipment	*P aeruginosa*
Work in renal dialysis unit	Hepatitis B virus
Hyperalimentation	*C albicans*
Water aerosols	*Legionella*

Antimicrobials

ANTIBACTERIAL DRUGS

Antibacterial drugs are commonly classified as either bactericidal or bacteriostatic, meaning that they actively kill bacteria or prevent the bacteria from replicating. Bacteriostatic drugs that prevent replication help the body by giving the immune system time to mobilize and destroy the infective agents. Table 5-51 lists the site and mechanism of action of the major antibacterial drugs. It categorizes the drugs as either bactericidal or bacteriostatic, which is important for understanding the action of individual drugs as well as the synergistic or antagonistic effects of certain drug combinations. It is important to remember that exceptions exist where a drug that is usually -cidal (or -static) may act as a -static (or -cidal) when used against certain bacteria or in certain organs. Figures 5-84 and 5-85 illustrate the sites of action of the drugs in the cell.

β-Lactams

Bacterial cell walls contain peptidoglycans, which are repeating disaccharides with amino acid side chains. The amino acid side chains are cross-linked with one another via covalent bonds, thus strengthening the cell wall.

MECHANISM

Bactericidal. These compounds are so named because they have a β-lactam ring (Figure 5-86), which binds to and irreversibly inactivates the bacterial **transpeptidase** enzyme responsible for peptidoglycan cross-linking. The inhibition of transpeptidase (**penicillin-binding protein**) in turn inhibits cross-linking, leading to the arrest of cell wall synthesis, thus killing the dividing bacteria. Transpeptidase inhibition also results in the activation of **autolytic enzymes** that dissolve the cell wall.

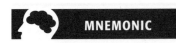

MNEMONIC

Bactericidal antibiotics are in the cell wall **FAM**ily: β-Lactams, **F**luoroquinolones, **A**minoglycosides, **M**etronidazole.

TABLE 5-51. Antibiotics: Site of Action and Mechanism

SITE OF ACTION	MECHANISM OF ACTION	BACTERICIDAL	BACTERIOSTATIC
Cell wall	Inhibit peptidoglycan cross-linking.	β-Lactams (penicillins, cephalosporins, aztreonam, imipenem)	
	Inhibit peptidoglycan polymerization.	Vancomycin, bacitracin	
	Inhibits cell wall synthesis by binding PBP3.	Aztreonam	
Outer membrane	Disrupt outer membrane in gram-negative bacteria.	Polymyxins	
Nucleotide synthesis	Inhibit dihydropteroate synthetase.		Sulfonamides
	Inhibit dihydrofolate reductase.	Trimethoprim/sulfamethoxazole	Trimethoprim, pyrimethamine
DNA	Inhibit type II topoisomerase.	Fluoroquinolones (ciprofloxacin)	
	Inhibit mRNA synthesis.	Rifampin	
50S Ribosomal subunit	Block initiation complex formation.		Linezolid
	Block release of nascent peptides from the ribosome.	Quinupristin/dalfopristin	
	Block peptide bond formation and peptide release from the ribosome.		Clindamycin
	Inhibit peptide bond formation.		Chloramphenicol
	Block release of nascent peptides from the ribosome.		Macrolides (erythromycin)
30S Ribosomal subunit	Cause miscoding of mRNA and incorrect amino acid linking for peptide formation, blocking normal protein synthesis.	Aminoglycosides (gentamicin)	
	Block binding of tRNA and addition of amino acids to the peptide chain.		Tetracyclines
Various	Toxic metabolites.	Metronidazole	
Other	Unknown.		Nitrofurantoin

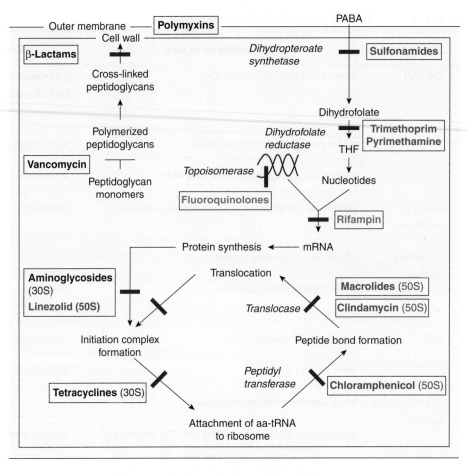

FIGURE 5-84. **Mechanism of action of major antibacterials.**

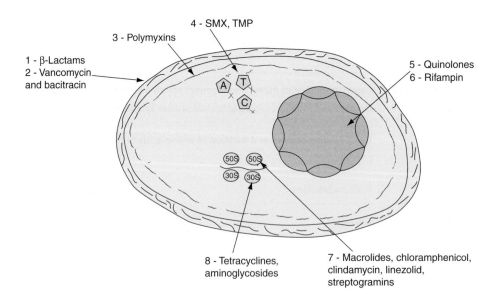

FIGURE 5-85. **Cellular targets of major antibacterials.** (Reproduced with permission from Le T, et al. *First Aid for the USMLE Step 1*, 19th ed. New York: McGraw-Hill, 2009: 178.)

RESISTANCE

Bacteria have evolved different ways of protecting themselves from β-lactam drugs.

- **Inactivation via β-lactamase:** Both gram-positive and gram-negative bacteria have enzymes that cleave the C–N bond in the β-lactam ring, thereby inactivating the antibiotic.
- **Changes in drug target through mutation of binding site:** Through mutations, bacteria can develop forms of transpeptidase to which β-lactams cannot bind.
- **Decreased permeability, restricting drug entry, drug efflux pumps:** Because of their size or charge, some β-lactam drugs are unable to pass through the outer membrane of gram-negative bacteria, and some bacteria actually have the capability of pumping drug out. Note that this is not a mechanism of resistance for gram-positive bacteria because they do not have outer membranes.

CLASSES

Listed are the four clinically available classes of β-lactams, which differ in their susceptibility to bacterial β-lactamase, spectrum of coverage, and side effect profiles.

- Penicillins
- Cephalosporins and cephamycins
- Monobactams
- Carbapenems

PENICILLIN

USES

- Narrow-spectrum; primarily effective against gram-positive bacteria and fastidious gram-negative bacteria. Not penicillinase resistant.
- *Neisseria meningitidis.*
- *Clostridia.*
- Most anaerobes except *B fragilis* group.
- Spirochetes: Drug of choice for syphilis.

SIDE EFFECTS

Hypersensitivity (urticaria, pruritus, fever, anaphylaxis, nephritis, joint swelling); rash; hemolytic anemia (Coombs-positive).

OXACILLIN, NAFCILLIN, CLOXACILLIN, DICLOXACILLIN, METHICILLIN

RESISTANCE

β-Lactamase-resistant because of their bulky R groups and therefore can be used without clavulanic acid.

USES

- Narrow-spectrum gram-positive coverage. Also referred to as the "antistaphylococcal penicillins" because of good activity against many strains of *S aureus*. Methicillin-resistant *S aureus* (MRSA) is a major nosocomial and community-acquired pathogen. Oxacillin is the most commonly used member of this group. Dicloxacillin is available orally.
- Particularly effective for organisms that produce β-lactamase.

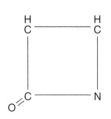

FIGURE 5-86. **The β-lactam ring, the chemical structure that inhibits peptidoglycan cross-linking.**

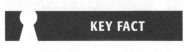

Clavulanic acid, a β-lactam-like molecule, binds to and inactivates β-lactamase → confers broader activity to β-lactamase-susceptible penicillins.

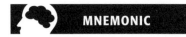

Pencillin G is given IM or IV; pencillin V is given PO.

MNEMONIC

Unlike other penicillins, **N**afcillin is **N**ot susceptible to β-lactamase.

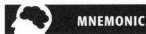

Am**O**xicillin is an **O**ral form of ampicillin.

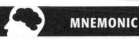

Ampicillin/amoxicillin coverage—

HELPS Slaughter *Enterococcus*

***H**aemophilus influenzae*
***E** coli*
***L**isteria*
***P**roteus mirabilis*
***S**almonella*
***S**higella*
***E**nterococcus*

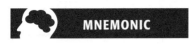

Piperacillin is powerful against *Pseudomonas.*

KEY FACT

Other antipseudomonal antibiotics include third- and fourth-generation cephalosporins, aztreonam, and imipenem.

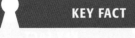

Organisms covered by first-generation cephalosporins—

PECK

***P**roteus mirabilis*
***E**scherichia **C**oli*
***K**lebsiella*

SIDE EFFECTS

Hypersensitivity; interstitial nephritis (especially methicillin when used in combination with aminoglycosides—thus methicillin is no longer used).

AMPICILLIN, AMOXICILLIN (AMINOPENICILLINS)

RESISTANCE

β-Lactamase-sensitive.

USES

- Moderate-spectrum gram-positive and gram-negative coverage.
- Drug of choice for some gram-positive organisms, enterococcus and *Listeria.*
- When used in combination with clavulanic acid, provides extended coverage to gram-negative rods, *H influenzae, E coli, P mirabilis, Salmonella, Shigella.*
- Amoxicillin is second-line treatment for Lyme disease.

SIDE EFFECTS

Hypersensitivity; rash; pseudomembranous colitis.

TICARCILLIN, CARBENICILLIN, PIPERACILLIN

RESISTANCE

β-Lactamase-sensitive.

USES

- Extended spectrum for gram-negative rods, including *Pseudomonas.*
- Synergistic with aminoglycosides against *Pseudomonas* (both are bactericidal).

SIDE EFFECTS

Hypersensitivity; interference with platelet function can cause bleeding. Most commonly used in combination with β-lactamase inhibitors such as ticarcillin-clavulanic acid and piperacillin-tazobactam.

CLAVULANIC ACID, SULBACTAM, TAZOBACTAM

MECHANISM

Binds to β-lactamase and prevents its binding and destruction of the β-lactam ring on susceptible penicillins.

USES

- Expands the spectrum of activity for antibiotics that are susceptible to β-lactamases.
- Used in combination with penicillin, ampicillin, piperacillin, and ticarcillin.
- Expands activity against gram-positive cocci (eg, *S aureus*), anaerobes (eg, *B fragilis*), and gram-negative rods (eg, *H influenzae* and *Klebsiella*).

SIDE EFFECTS

None.

CEPHALOSPORINS

MECHANISM

Same as penicillin.

USE

- First-generation (**cefazolin, cephalexin**): Gram-positive cocci; *P mirabilis*, *E coli*, *K pneumoniae*. β-Lactamase-sensitive.
- Second-generation (**cefotetan, cefuroxime**): Gram-positive cocci; extended gram-negative coverage includes *H influenzae, Enterobacter, Neisseria, P mirabilis, E coli, Klebsiella, S marcescens*. Moderate β-lactamase resistance.
- Third-generation (**cefoperazone, ceftazidime, ceftriaxone**): Broad-spectrum gram-negative coverage; most cross blood-brain barrier and are commonly used for treatment of meningitis and sepsis.
- Ceftazidime for *Pseudomonas*.
- Ceftriaxone for gonorrheal infections.
- Fourth-generation (**cefepime**): Increased activity against *Pseudomonas* and gram-positive cocci due to increased resistance to β-lactamase.

SIDE EFFECTS

Hypersensitivity; 5–10% of patients with penicillin allergy have cross-reactivity with cephalosporins; increases aminoglycoside nephrotoxicity; cephalosporins containing a methylthiotetrazole group (cefotetan, cefoperazone) can cause disulfiram-like reaction with ethanol and increased risk of bleeding; cefaclor and cephalexin can cause a serum sickness–like reaction; vitamin K deficiency.

AZTREONAM (MONOBACTAMS)

USES

- Gram-negative rods, including *Pseudomonas*.
- No activity against gram-positive organisms or anaerobes.
- β-Lactamase-resistant.
- Reserved for infections that are resistant to other antibiotics and for patients who cannot tolerate pencillins or aminoglycosides.
- Safe in pregnancy. No penicillin cross-reactivity.

SIDE EFFECTS

Usually nontoxic; occasional rash, GI distress, fever, phlebitis.

IMIPENEM/CILASTATIN, MEROPENEM (CARBAPENEMS)

USES

- Broad-spectrum against gram-positives, gram-negatives, and anaerobes.
- Drugs of choice for *resistant gram-negative infections*.
- The broadest spectrum β-lactam drugs available; but they do not cover MRSA, vancomycin-resistant enterococci (VRE), or cell wall-deficient organisms such as the rickettsiae and *Chlamydia*.
- β-Lactamase–resistant, but carbapenemases are an increasing problem.
- Imipenem must be used with **cilastatin**, a renal dehydropeptidase inhibitor that prevents the metabolism of imipenem in the kidneys.

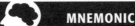

MNEMONIC

Organisms covered by second-generation cephalosporins—

HEN PECKS

Haemophilus influenzae
Enterobacter
Neisseria
Proteus mirabilis
Escherichia **C**oli
Klebsiella
Serratia marcescens

KEY FACT

Enterococci are resistant to all cephalosporins.

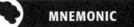

MNEMONIC

Make imipenem **EVER LASTIN'** with ci**LASTATIN.**

SIDE EFFECTS

- Hypersensitivity and rash; GI distress; drug fever; seizures at high serum levels, especially in patients with renal dysfunction; cross-reactivity with penicillin.
- **Meropenem** is not degraded by renal dehydropeptidase and presents a reduced risk of seizures.

Peptidoglycan Synthesis Inhibitors

VANCOMYCIN

MECHANISM

Bactericidal for most target bugs. Prevents polymerization of peptidoglycans by binding D-alanyl-D-alanine moiety of cell wall precursors and preventing the addition of murein units to the growing polymer chain.

RESISTANCE

Acquisition of an enzyme that changes D-alanyl-D-alanine precursors to D-alanyl-D-lactate precursors. This is the mode of resistance in VRE.

USES

- Effective against nearly all gram-positives but reserved for multidrug-resistant bacteria such as MRSA.
- Used orally for pseudomembranous colitis caused by *C difficile*, along with metronidazole.

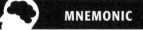

MNEMONIC

The **Red Man** in the **Van: Van**comycin causes flushing.

SIDE EFFECTS

Generally well tolerated. Flushing "red man syndrome" caused by rapid infusion due to histamine release (can be largely prevented by slow infusion and pretreatment with antihistamines); nephrotoxicity; ototoxicity; thrombophlebitis. Decreased dosage is needed for patients with renal dysfunction.

BACITRACIN

MECHANISM

Inhibits peptidoglycan precursors from being transported across the bacterial cell membrane.

USES

- Topical antibiotic for wound irrigation.
- Covers gram-positive bacteria.

SIDE EFFECTS

Nephrotoxicity prevents systemic use.

Drugs That Disrupt the Bacterial Cell Membrane

POLYMYXIN

MECHANISM

Polymyxins are basic proteins that act like detergents. They bind to and disrupt the cell membrane of gram-negative bacteria: "**MYX**ins **MIX** up Membranes."

USES

- Resistant gram-negative infections.
- Resistant *Pseudomonas* in cystic fibrosis.

SIDE EFFECTS

When given systemically: nephrotoxicity (acute tubular necrosis) and neurotoxicity.

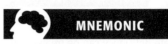

Nucleotide Synthesis Inhibitors

SULFONAMIDES (SULFAMETHOXAZOLE, SULFADIAZINE, SULFADOXINE, TRISULFAPYRIMIDINES)

MECHANISM

Bacteriostatic: Synergistic with trimethoprim and pyrimethamine. PABA analogs inhibit **dihydropteroate synthetase,** the enzyme essential for synthesis of folate in bacteria. As a result, synthesis of purines, thymidine, and certain amino acids is impaired (Figure 5-87).

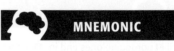

USES

- Treatment in combination for *Nocardia*.
- *Toxoplasma*.
- Used with trimethoprim (TMP-SMX) for uncomplicated UTIs, *Salmonella*, *Shigella*, *Serratia*, *P jiroveci* (PCP).
- Sulfadiazine—silver ointment for burn infection.

SIDE EFFECTS

Hemolytic anemia in glucose-6-phosphate dehydrogenase (G6PD) deficiency; kernicterus in neonates; hypersensitivity (including Stevens-Johnson syndrome); photosensitivity; interstitial nephritis.

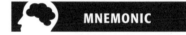

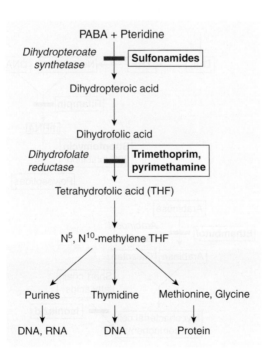

FIGURE 5-87. **Inhibitors of the folate pathway.** PABA, *para*-aminobenzoic acid.

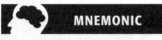
TRIMETHOPRIM, PYRIMETHAMINE

MECHANISM

Bacteriostatic, synergistic with sulfonamides. Folic acid analog that inhibits dihydrofolate reductase (**DHFR**) and decreases synthesis of purines, thymine, and certain amino acids (Figure 5-88).

USES

- Trimethoprim: See Sulfonamides. Widely used as a combination agent for a variety of infections.
- Pyrimethamine: Used with sulfadiazine to treat parasitic infections such as toxoplasmosis.

SIDE EFFECTS

Bone marrow suppression; GI distress; pruritus; rash.

DNA Topoisomerase Inhibitors

FLUOROQUINOLONES (CIPROFLOXACIN, NORFLOXACIN, OFLOXACIN, GATIFLOXACIN, MOXIFLOXACIN)

MECHANISM

Bactericidal. Inhibit DNA gyrase (topoisomerase II) and topoisomerase IV, two bacterial enzymes that unwind, sever, and reanneal DNA during replication and transcription. Good oral bioavailability, but must not be taken with antacids, which inhibit absorption.

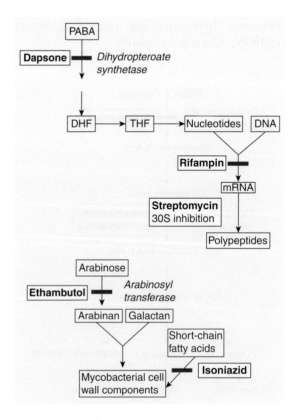

FIGURE 5-88. **Antimycobacterial drugs.**

USES

- Gram-negative rods that cause UTIs and gastroenteritis (including *Pseudomonas*).
- *Neisseria gonorrhoeae*.
- Mycobacteria.
- Atypicals such as *Mycoplasma* and *Legionella*.
- Some gram-positive bacteria. Drug of choice for anthrax.

SIDE EFFECTS

GI distress; rash; superinfections; CNS effects (headaches, seizures, and/or insomnia); mild photosensitivity; prolonged QT interval; contraindicated in pregnant women and children because it may cause cartilage damage, with symptoms of leg cramps and myalgias; may cause tendinitis and tendon rupture in adults.

Protein Synthesis Inhibitors at the 50S Ribosomal Subunit

CHLORAMPHENICOL

MECHANISM

Bacteriostatic. Binds to 50S ribosomal subunit and blocks the proper positioning of tRNA and the addition of new amino acids to the polypeptide chain.

USES

- Meningitis caused by meningococcus, pneumococcus, *H influenzae* in individuals with penicillin allergy.
- Used topically for eye infections.

SIDE EFFECTS

Idiosyncratic aplastic anemia (1 in 30,000 doses); reversible bone marrow suppression; gray baby syndrome (seen in premature infants who lack hepatic UDP-glucuronyl transferase). Limited use because of multiple severe toxicities. Crosses blood-brain barrier and placenta.

MACROLIDES (ERYTHROMYCIN, AZITHROMYCIN, CLARITHROMYCIN)

MECHANISM

Bacteriostatic. Binds reversibly to the 23S rRNA of the 50S ribosomal subunit and blocks the translocation step.

USES

Broad spectrum of action. STIs (*Chlamydia*, *N gonorrhea*); pneumonia (*Mycoplasma*, *Legionella*); streptococcal infection in patients allergic to penicillin; *C diphtheriae*; nontuberculous mycobacteria.

SIDE EFFECTS

Prolonged QT interval (especially erythromycin); GI distress; acute cholestatic hepatitis; allergy—fever, eosinophilia, rashes; P450 inhibition (increases levels of warfarin, others).

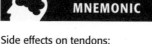

MNEMONIC

Side effects on tendons:
Fluoroquino**LONES** hurt
attachments to your **BONES**.

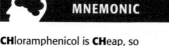

MNEMONIC

CHloramphenicol is **CH**eap, so it is used widely by public health professionals in developing nations—**MPH**s use chloramphenicol to treat meningitis caused by **M**eningococcus, **P**neumococcus, **H** *influenzae*.

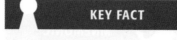

KEY FACT

Azithromycin is safe to use in pregnancy.

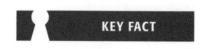

KEY FACT

Linezolid is a drug of choice for VRE.

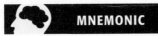

MNEMONIC

Site of action of protein synthesis inhibitors—

Buy AT 30, CELL at 50

Aminoglycosides and **T**etracyclines inhibit the **30**S ribosomal subunit.
Chloramphenicol, **E**rythromycin, **L**inezolid, and C**L**indamycin inhibit the **50**S ribosomal subunit.

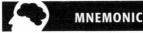

MNEMONIC

Acronym for the aminoglycosides—

GNATS

Gentamicin
Neomycin
Amikacin
Tobramycin
Streptomycin

KEY FACT

Aminoglycosides:
- Ineffective against anaerobes since O_2 is needed for drug uptake.
- The only protein synthesis inhibitors that are bactericidal.

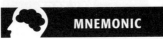

MNEMONIC

Organisms covered by tetracyclines—

VACUUM your BedRooM Tonight

Vibrio cholerae
Acne
Chlamydia
Ureaplasma **U**realyticum
Mycoplasma pneumoniae
Borrelia burgdorferi
Rickettsia
Multidrug-resistant **M**alaria
(Plasmodium falciparum)
Tularemia

CLINDAMYCIN, LINCOMYCIN

MECHANISM

Bacteriostatic. Binds the 50S ribosomal subunit and inhibits the aminoacyl translocation step by blocking the growth and release of the growing peptide chain.

USES

- Narrow spectrum, covers anaerobes in mixed infections.
- Implicated as a causative agent in pseudomembranous colitis due to *C difficile* infection.
- Drug of choice for anaerobic infections above the diaphragm (*B fragilis* and *C perfringens*).
- Safe in pregnancy.

SIDE EFFECTS

Pseudomembranous colitis (*C difficile* superinfection); GI distress.

LINEZOLID

MECHANISM

Bacteriostatic. Binds to 50S ribosomal subunit and inhibits initiation complex formation.

USES

Effective against MRSA and VRE.

SIDE EFFECTS

Same as clindamycin; bone marrow suppression may be treatment-limiting; ocular and peripheral neuritis.

QUINUPRISTIN/DALFOPRISTIN

MECHANISM

Bactericidal. This combination of streptogramin antibiotics binds to the 50S ribosomal subunit and inhibits protein synthesis at two successive steps.

USES

MRSA and VRE.

SIDE EFFECTS

Phlebitis; hyperbilirubinemia.

Protein Synthesis Inhibitors at the 30S Ribosomal Subunit

AMINOGLYCOSIDES (GENTAMICIN, NEOMYCIN, AMIKACIN, TOBRAMYCIN, STREPTOMYCIN)

MECHANISM

Bactericidal. Enter bacteria via an O_2-dependent transporter. Exert effect by:

- Inhibiting formation of initiation complex.
- Causing misreading of mRNA, resulting in the creation of aberrant proteins.
- Preventing all protein synthesis at high concentrations.
- Causing breakup of polysomes.

USES

- Serious gram-negative rod infections; often used in combination with a β-lactam.
- Used with β-lactams or vancomycin for synergistic effect to treat serious gram-positive infections.
- Neomycin—given in the setting of bowel surgery and hepatic encephalopathy.
- Streptomycin—mycobacteria.
- Spectinomycin—second-line treatment for gonorrhea.

SIDE EFFECTS

Contraindicated in renal insufficiency due to reversible nephrotoxicity (especially when used with cephalosporins); irreversible ototoxicity (especially when used with loop diuretics); nondepolarizing neuromuscular blockade at high concentrations; contraindicated in pregnancy owing to teratogenicity; Fanconi syndrome (dysfunction of renal electrolyte reabsorption); neomycin—GI malabsorption and superinfection.

TETRACYCLINES (TETRACYCLINE, DOXYCYCLINE, MINOCYCLINE, DEMECLOCYCLINE) AND GLYCYLCYCLINE (TIGECYCLINE)

MECHANISM

Bacteriostatic. Inhibit the 30S ribosomal subunit by preventing attachment of the aminoacyl-tRNA to the ribosome. Must be imported through the inner cytoplasmic membrane via an energy-dependent active transport system present in bacteria but not humans. Must not be taken with milk, antacids, or iron-containing agents because the presence of divalent cations inhibits proper absorption in the gut. Limited CNS penetration.

USES

- Broad-spectrum: *V cholerae*, acne, *Chlamydia*, *Ureaplasma urealyticum*, *Mycoplasma pneumoniae*, *Borrelia burgdorferi*, *Rickettsia*, multidrug-resistant malaria (*P falciparum*), tularemia. Tigecycline is a new drug used to treat gram-negative infections resistant to other agents.
- Second line after penicillin for syphilis.

SIDE EFFECTS

- GI distress; tooth discoloration and bone growth abnormalities in young children; photosensitivity; fatty liver disease in women. Drugs past expiration date can cause Fanconi syndrome.
- Minocycline—reversible vestibular toxicity.
- Demeclocycline—used to treat syndrome of inappropriate antidiuretic hormone (SIADH) because it causes nephrogenic diabetes insipidus as an ADH antagonist.

Drugs That Act Via Toxic Metabolites

METRONIDAZOLE

MECHANISM

Bactericidal. Bioactivation of the drug in anaerobic environments produces toxic metabolites that react with bacterial DNA, protein, and bacterial and protozoal cell membranes.

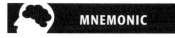

MNEMONIC

Antiprotozoal coverage—

GET GAP on the metro(nidazole)

Giardia
Entamoeba
Trichomonas
Gardnerella vaginalis
Anaerobes (*Bacteroides, Clostridium*)
H **P**ylori (used with bismuth and amoxicillin or tetracycline for "triple therapy")

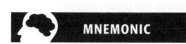

MNEMONIC

Helicobacter pylori *treatment—*

BAM! Use these three drugs and *H pylori* is gone!

Bismuth
Amoxicillin
Metronidazole

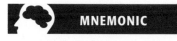

MNEMONIC

Antibiotics contraindicated in pregnancy—

SAFe Moms Take Really Good Care

Sulfonamides—kernicterus
Aminoglycosides—ototoxicity
Fluoroquinolones—cartilage damage
Metronidazole—teratogenic
Tetracyclines—fatty liver in mother; impaired bone growth, and tooth discoloration in baby
Ribavirin (antiviral)—teratogenic
Griseofulvin (antifungal)—teratogenic
Chloramphenicol—gray baby syndrome

USES

- Drug of choice for pseudomembranous colitis (due to *C difficile*).
- Anaerobic infections below the diaphragm.
- Antiprotozoal: *Giardia, Entamoeba, Trichomonas.*
- Used with bismuth and amoxicillin (or tetracycline) for *H pylori* "triple therapy."

SIDE EFFECTS

Headache, nausea, metallic taste in mouth, disulfiram-like reactions with ethanol, teratogen. Patients should be cautioned not to drink alcohol while taking metronidazole.

Antibacterial Coverage

Table 5-52 illustrates the spectrum of coverage for the antibacterial drugs. It is provided as a reference and is not meant to be memorized! Unless otherwise noted, all drugs within the same class have roughly the same coverage. For example, nafcillin has the same coverage as oxacillin.

Antimycobacterial Drugs

Other than dapsone, which is used to treat leprosy and *Pneumocystis jiroveci* (PCP), all antimycobacterial agents in this section are used to treat tuberculosis. Isoniazid is used for prophylaxis in addition to treatment of active infection. Figure 5-87 illustrates the mechanism of action of the antimycobacterial drugs, with the exception of pyrazinamide.

DAPSONE

MECHANISM

Dapsone is an analog of *para*-aminobenzoic acid (PABA) that inhibits dihydropteroate synthase. Humans don't synthesize folate de novo, so this drug is highly specific for microorganisms.

USES

- *Mycobacterium leprae* (leprosy), as a component of combination therapy with rifampin and clofazimine.
- *P jiroveci* pneumonia (PCP) prophylaxis and treatment.

SIDE EFFECTS

Hemolysis in patients with G6PD deficiency; methemoglobinemia.

RIFAMPIN

MECHANISM

Bactericidal against both intracellular and extracellular bacteria. Blocks mRNA synthesis by inhibiting DNA-dependent RNA polymerase.

USES

- *Mycobacterium tuberculosis*, as component of combination therapy (NEVER used alone).
- *Mycobacterium leprae*, as component of combination therapy with dapsone and clofazimine.
- Prophylaxis for *H influenzae* and *N meningitidis*.

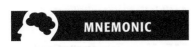

KEY FACT

Dapsone has the same mechanism of action as the sulfonamides.

MNEMONIC

Drugs for tuberculosis—

RIPES

Rifampin—always used in combination therapy
Isoniazid
Pyrazinamide
Ethambutol
Streptomycin

MNEMONIC

4 R's of Rifampin:

RNA polymerase inhibitor
Red/orange body fluids
Rapid resistance if used alone
Ramps up P450 system

TABLE 5-52. Antibiotic Coverage

Drugs	S epidermidis	S aureus	Listeria	Group B strep	Enterococcus	S pneumoniae	Group A strep	N meningitidis	H influenzae	E coli	Klebsiella	Enterobacter	Serratia	Pseudomonas	Mouth	Gut	B fragilis
				Gram-Positive Bacteria						**Gram-Negative Bacteria**						**Anaerobes**	
Penicillin			■	■	■	■	■	■							■		
Nafcillin		■	■	■	■	■	■	■									
Ampicillin			◆	■	◆	■	■	■	■								
Ticarcillin				■	■	■	■	■	■	■	■	■	■	■	■	■	■
Cephalosporins (1st gen.)	■	■	■	■	■	■	■	■	■	■	■	■					
Cephalosporins (2nd gen.)	■	■	■	■	■	■	■	■	■	■	■	■			*	*	*
Cephalosporins (3rd gen.)	■	■	■	■	■	■	■	■	■	■	■	■	■	■			
Cephalosporins (4th gen.)	■	■	■	■	■	■	■	■	■	■	■	■	■	■			
Aztreonam											■	■		■			
Imipenem		■	■	■	■	■	■	■	■	■	■	◆	■	■	■		■
Vancomycin	■	■	■	■	■	■	■									■	
Gentamicin					■					■	■	■	■	■			
Tobramycin					■					■	■	■	■	■			
Amikacin										■	■	■	■	■			
Erythromycin	■	■	■	■		■	■										
Clindamycin	■	■	■			■	■								◆	■	◆
Azithromycin	■	■	■	■		■	■	■	■						■	■	■
Tetracycline				■		■	■		■	■	■	■		■			
Chloramphenicol						■		■	■								■

■, coverage; ◆, drug of choice; *Cefotetan.

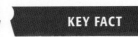

SIDE EFFECTS

Hepatotoxicity; turns urine and tears orange-red.

ISONIAZID (INH)

MECHANISM

Mycobactericidal. Following activation by mycobacterial catalase-peroxidase enzyme KatG, INH inhibits an enzyme needed for the synthesis of mycolic acid, a component of the mycobacterial cell wall.

USES

- *Mycobacterium tuberculosis.*
- Only drug that can be used alone as prophylaxis against TB.
- Given with pyridoxine (vitamin B_6) to prevent peripheral neuropathy.

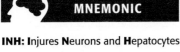

SIDE EFFECTS

Hepatitis; hemolysis in G6PD-deficient individuals; systemic lupus erythematosus (SLE)-like syndrome; peripheral neuropathy.

PYRAZINAMIDE

MECHANISM

Mycobactericidal. A prodrug that is activated by a mycobacterial enzyme. It inhibits the synthesis of fatty acid precursors of mycolic acid.

USE

Mycobacterium tuberculosis.

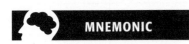

SIDE EFFECTS

Hepatitis; asymptomatic hyperuricemia; arthralgias.

ETHAMBUTOL

MECHANISM

Mycobacteriostatic. Inhibits arabinosyl transferase, an enyzme required for synthesis of arabinogalactan, a component of the mycobacterial cell wall.

USES

Used in combination to treat *M tuberculosis* and *M avium-intracellulare.*

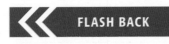

SIDE EFFECTS

Hepatotoxicity; optic neuritis with red-green color blindness.

ANTIFUNGALS

Antifungal drugs target several sites critical to fungal viability and replication (Figure 5-89 and Table 5-53).

Azoles (Ergosterol Synthesis Inhibitors)

MECHANISM

Disrupt permeability of the fungal membrane by inhibiting ergosterol synthesis and incorporation into fungal membranes. Ergosterol, which is unique to fungi, is a cholesterol-like molecule necessary for membrane stability.

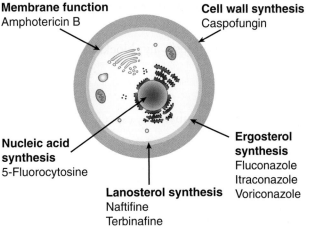

Membrane function
Amphotericin B

Cell wall synthesis
Caspofungin

Nucleic acid synthesis
5-Fluorocytosine

Ergosterol synthesis
Fluconazole
Itraconazole
Voriconazole

Lanosterol synthesis
Naftifine
Terbinafine

FIGURE 5-89. **Fungal components targeted by antifungals.** DHF, dihydrofolate; PABA, *para*-aminobenzoic acid; THF, tetrahydrofolate.

USES

Systemic mycoses.

- Clotrimazole and miconazole are topical and, thus, used for fungal skin infections.
- Fluconazole is used to treat cryptococcal meningitis in AIDS patients and many *Candida* infections, but some *Candida* species are inherently resistant, and some can develop resistance during therapy.
- Ketoconazole is now rarely used to treat fungal infections.
- Newer azoles such as voriconazole and posaconazole have significant activity against *Aspergillus* species.

SIDE EFFECTS

Ketoconazole inhibits androgen and cortisol synthesis in the adrenal cortex, leading to gynecomastia in men, liver dysfunction secondary to inhibition of the cytochrome P450 system (drug interactions).

TABLE 5-53.   Antifungal Drugs

DRUG	MECHANISM	INDICATIONS FOR USE	SIDE EFFECTS
Azoles	Ergosterol synthesis inhibitors.	Systemic mycoses.	Inhibition of cytochrome P450.
Terbinafine	Blocks fungal cell wall synthesis.	Dermatophytoses.	Diarrhea, headache, indigestion, taste changes.
Flucytosine	Antimetabolite.	Used with amphotericin to treat systemic mycoses.	Bone marrow suppression.
Amphotericin, nystatin	Pore-forming.	Systemic mycoses, oral candidiasis.	Nephrotoxicity.
Caspofungin and other micafungin	Cell wall synthesis inhibitors.	Invasive aspergillosis.	GI upset, flushing.
Griseofulvin	Mitosis inhibitor.	Dermatophytoses.	Teratogenic, bone marrow suppression.

Terbinafine (Fungal Squalene Epoxidase Inhibitor)

MECHANISM

Blocks fungal cell wall synthesis by blocking synthesis of precursor to ergosterol.

USES

Preferred treatment of dermatophytoses, especially onychomycosis because it accumulates in nails.

SIDE EFFECTS

Not metabolized by P450 and therefore little potential for drug interactions.

Flucytosine (Antimetabolite)

MECHANISM

Inhibits DNA synthesis by conversion to fluorouracil, which competes with uracil.

USES

Treatment of systemic mycoses in combination with amphotericin B.

SIDE EFFECTS

Bone marrow suppression, leading to leukopenia and thrombocytopenia, is a common side effect of antimetabolites.

Amphotericin B, Nystatin (Pore-Forming)

MECHANISM

Bind to ergosterol, thereby disrupting the fungal membrane and generating pores that allow leakage of electrolytes and disruption of homeostasis, causing lysis. Nystatin is too toxic for systemic use.

USES

- Amphotericin B—systemic mycoses. May sometimes be administered intrathecally for fungal meningitis (crosses the blood-brain barrier inefficiently).
- Nystatin—swish and swallow for oral candidiasis (there is no oral absorption).
- May be used topically for diaper rash or vaginal candidiasis.

SIDE EFFECTS

"Shake and bake" fever and chills; IV phlebitis ("amphoterrible"); nephrotoxicity measured as a reversible increase in blood urea nitrogen (BUN):creatinine ratio, along with increased excretion of metabolites (less when using lipid variant) that is reversible with hydration; arrhythmias.

Echinocandins: Caspofungin, Micafungin, Anidulofungin (Cell Wall Synthesis Inhibitors)

MECHANISM

Inhibits cell wall synthesis by inhibiting synthesis of β-glucan.

USES

Invasive aspergillosis, *Candida* infections, other mycoses.

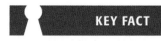

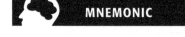

SIDE EFFECTS

GI upset, flushing.

Griseofulvin (Mitosis Inhibitors)

MECHANISM

Inhibits growth of dermatophytes by interfering with microtubule function, thereby disrupting mitoses. The drug concentrates in the stratum corneum in keratin-containing tissues (eg, nails).

USES

Oral treatment of superficial infections. Represents a slow cure because it relies on keratin cells to divide—the fungus is shed along with the keratinized stratified squamous epithelium.

SIDE EFFECTS

Teratogenic, carcinogenic, increased warfarin metabolism (resulting in decreased international normalized ratio [INR]), and bone marrow suppression.

ANTIPARASITICS

Although the antiparasitics are a large and heterogeneous group of drugs, their spectrum of activity somewhat relates to the taxonomy of the parasites, that is, antinematode, antihelminth, antimalarial (Table 5-54).

Antihelminthics

ALBENDAZOLE

MECHANISM

Prevents polymerization of parasite microtubules by inhibiting fumarate reductase.

USES

Cestode (tapeworm) infections in which the patient is an intermediate host (parasite in larval state migrates through patient)—*Taenia solium* neurocysticercosis, *Echinococcus* hydatid disease. Also a second-line agent in some nematode infections.

SIDE EFFECTS

Headache, abnormal liver function tests, mild GI side effects.

PRAZIQUANTEL

MECHANISM

Blocks voltage-gated calcium channels, increasing calcium influx into the helminth, which causes severe spasms and paralysis of the worms' muscles.

USES

Cestode, trematode (flukes) infections in which the patient is a definitive host (sexually mature helminth-laying eggs). Examples include *Taenia solium* contracted by ingesting undercooked pork tapeworm, schistosomiasis, clonorchiasis, *Paragonimus westermani*.

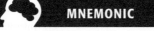

MNEMONIC

Griseofulvin: A greasy ol' fulcrum that prys the nail dermatophytes off.

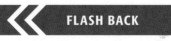

FLASH BACK

Recall that drugs that inhibit growth but do not primarily kill organisms are referred to as bacteriostatic drugs. Griseofulvin is an example.

KEY FACT

Corticosteroids must be given with albendazole in the treatment of cysticercosis to reduce symptoms resulting from the degenerating cysts, which typically elicit a strong host immune response.

TABLE 5-54. **Antiparasitic Agents**

Drug Name	Mechanism	Indications	Side Effects
Albendazole	Inhibits polymerization of parasitic microtubules.	Neurocysticercosis, echinococcus (hydatid disease), some cestodes.	Headache.
Praziquantel	Blocks voltage-gated calcium channels.	Cestodes, trematodes.	Cramps and diarrhea.
Mebendazole/pyrantel pamoate	Blocks glucose absorption, paralyzes worms.	Intestinal nematode.	Diarrhea, abdominal pain.
Thiabendazole	Blocks mitochondrial fumarate reductase.	*Strongyloides*, trichinosis.	Hallucinations, severe diarrhea, nausea/vomiting, numbness/tingling of hands or feet.
Ivermectin	Paralyzes and kills offspring of adult nematode.	Filariasis and other nematode infections, sometimes in combination with thiabendazole.	Arthralgias.
Diethylcarbamazine	Effective against microfilarial diseases.	Bancroft's filariasis, loiasis, onchocerciasis, toxocariasis.	Swelling/itching face, loss of vision and arthralgias with long-term use.
Metronidazole	Forms toxic metabolites in anaerobic cells, making it parasiticidal.	*Gardnerella vaginalis* (bacterial vaginitis), giardiasis, *E histolytica* (amebic dysentery), *T vaginalis*, anaerobes (*Bacteroides, Clostridium*).	Disulfiram-like reaction with alcohol, headache, metallic taste.
Chloroquine	Generates toxic heme by-products that kill the parasite within infected RBCs.	Prophylaxis and treatment of malaria.	Severe hemolysis in G6PD-deficient patients, blurred vision.
Quinine	Depresses oxygen uptake and intercalates into DNA.	Prophylaxis and treatment of malaria.	Cinchonism (tinnitus, deafness), proarrhythmic, hemolysis in G6PD-deficient patients; hypoglycemia.
Mefloquine	Unknown.	Prophylaxis and treatment of malaria, chloroquine-resistant malaria.	Mood changes, suicidality, unusual dreams.
Atovaquone and proguanil	Proguanil has synergy with atovaquone.	Prophylaxis and treatment of malaria, chloroquine-resistant malaria; treatment of *P jiroveci* pneumonia.	Fever, skin rash.
Nifurtimox	Formation of free radicals.	Chagas disease caused by *Trypanosoma cruzi*.	Hypersensitivity, GI complaints, neuropathy.

TABLE 5-54. Antiparasitic Agents *(continued)*

Drug Name	Mechanism	Indications	Side Effects
Suramin, melarsoprol	Act to deplete *T gambiense* and *T rhodanese* of energy by inactivating pyruvate kinase causing inhibition of ATP synthesis leading to their death.	African sleeping sickness (suramin when in blood, melarsoprol when in CNS); suramin also for river blindness.	Suramin: Urticaria, nausea and vomiting, adrenal cortical damage Melarsoprol: Exceptionally toxic, should be used only by experienced providers.
Sodium stibogluconate/ pentavalent antimony	Unknown.	Leishmaniasis.	Phlebitis of injected veins, pancreatitis, cardiac conduction abnormalities, GI disturbances.
Artemether, artesunate	Unknown mechanism of action.	Antimalarial; may have antihelminthic activity as well but not well-studied for that indication.	Usually well-tolerated.
Sulfadiazine + pyrimethamine	Pyrimethamine interrupts folate synthesis by inhibiting dihydrofolate reductase synergizing with sulfadiazine inhibition of dihydropteroate synthetase, thereby preventing DNA, RNA synthesis.	Toxoplasmosis, malaria.	Folate deficiency; therefore, add leucovorin to drug regimen (folate supplement that does not rely on dihydrofolate reductase).

RBC = red blood cell; CNS = central nervous system.

SIDE EFFECTS

Abdominal cramps, diarrhea, sometimes bloody.

MEBENDAZOLE/PYRANTEL PAMOATE

MECHANISM

Mebendazole prevents glucose absorption by the nematode, eventually causing loss of energy and death of the worm. Pyrantel pamoate paralyzes the nematodes.

USES

Intestinal nematode infections.

- **Fecal-oral transmission**—*Enterobius vermicularis* (pinworm), trichuriasis (whipworm).
- **Fecal-oral + lung migration**—*Ascaris lumbricoides* (giant roundworm).
- **Skin penetration + lung migration**—*Ancylostoma duodenale* (hookworm).

SIDE EFFECTS

GI complaints.

MNEMONIC

The "**thi**gh" (**thi**abendazole) is (used to treat) the **strong**est muscle (***Strongyloides***). No need for corticosteroids prior to treatment of ***Strongyloides*** with thiabendazole.

THIABENDAZOLE

MECHANISM

Thiabendazole inhibits the helminth-specific mitochondrial fumarate reductase.

USES

Skin penetration + lung migration.

- *Strongyloides stercoralis* infections.
- Trichinosis (pork worms), *Toxocara canis* (cutanea larval migrans) and toxocariasis (visceral larval migrans).

SIDE EFFECTS

Hallucinations, severe diarrhea, nausea/vomiting, numbness/tingling in hands or feet.

IVERMECTIN

MECHANISM

Acts to paralyze and kill offspring of adult nematodes.

USES

In combination with thiabendazole for strongyloidiasis, onchocerciasis (river blindness).

SIDE EFFECTS

Arthralgias, painful glands in the neck and groin, tachycardia, ocular irritation.

DIETHYLCARBAMAZINE

MECHANISM

Uncertain mechanism but effective against microfilaria. Only available through the Centers for Disease Control and Prevention (CDC).

USES

- Filariasis
- Loiasis
- Onchocerciasis (river blindness).
- Toxocariasis

SIDE EFFECTS

Swelling/itching face, loss of vision, and arthralgias with long-term use.

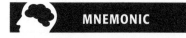

MNEMONIC

RIVER blindness is treated with **IVER**mectin.

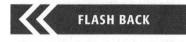

FLASH BACK

Bismuth and **A**moxicillin/tetracycline are used with **M**etronidazole as part of "triple therapy" for *H pylori*—**BAM!**

ANTIPROTOZOALS

Metronidazole

MECHANISM

Forms toxic metabolites in cell of anaerobic pathogens.

USES

Gardnerella vaginalis (bacterial vaginitis), giardiasis, *E histolytica* (amebic dysentery), *T vaginalis*, anaerobic bacteria.

SIDE EFFECTS

Disulfiram-like reaction with alcohol, headache, metallic taste, teratogenic.

Other Antiprotozoal Drugs

BENZNIDAZOLE, NIFURTIMOX

MECHANISM

Generates superoxide free radicals that cause lipid membrane peroxidation, enzyme inactivation, and DNA damage.

USES

Chagas disease caused by *T cruzi*; nifurtimox is also used in combination with eflornithine for African sleeping sickness.

SIDE EFFECTS

Hypersensitivity, GI complaints, neuropathy.

SURAMIN, MELARSOPROL, EFLORNITHINE

MECHANISM

Inactivate pyruvate kinase, which inhibits ATP synthesis. This depletes *T gambiense* and *T rhodiense* of energy, leading to their death. Eflornithine inhibits parasite ornithine decarboxylase.

USES

African sleeping sickness (suramin used for blood-based infections, melarsoprol for CNS infections). Suramin is also used for river blindness. Eflornithine is useful only for the Gambian strain of the African trypanosome.

SIDE EFFECTS

- Suramin: Urticaria, nausea and vomiting, adrenal cortical damage.
- Melarsoprol: Exceptionally neurotoxic, should be used only by experienced providers.

SODIUM STIBOGLUCONATE/PENTAVALENT ANTIMONY

USES

Leishmaniasis.

SULFADIAZINE + PYRIMETHAMINE

MECHANISM

Pyrimethamine interrupts folate synthesis by inhibiting dihydrofolate reductase. Synergistic with sulfadiazine inhibition of dihydropteroate synthetase, thereby preventing DNA and RNA synthesis.

USES

Toxoplasmosis, malaria.

SIDE EFFECTS

Folate deficiency; therefore leucovorin (folate supplement that does not rely on dihydrofolate reductase) is added to drug regimen.

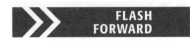

KEY FACT

Disulfiram-like reactions may also occur with chloramphenicol, third-generation cephalosporins, procarbazine, and first-generation sulfonylureas.

FLASH FORWARD

Recall that sulfonamides, isoniazid, aspirin, ibuprofen, nitrofurantoin, and fava beans also cause hemolysis in **G6PD**-deficient patients by increasing oxidative stress in RBCs.

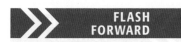
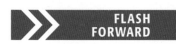
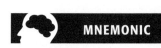
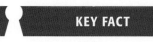
ANTIMALARIALS

Chloroquine

MECHANISM

Generates toxic heme by-products that kill the parasite within infected RBCs.

USES

Prophylaxis and treatment of malaria. Widespread resistance limits use to parts of the Caribbean and Latin America.

SIDE EFFECTS

Severe hemolysis in G6PD-deficient patients, blurred vision.

Primaquine

MECHANISM

Disrupts mitochondria and binds to DNA.

USES

Prevent relapse caused by *Plasmodium vivax* and *P ovale* hypnozoites latent in hepatocytes.

SIDE EFFECTS

Nausea, vomiting, abdominal cramps.

Quinine

MECHANISM

Depresses oxygen uptake and intercalates into DNA.

USES

Prophylaxis and treatment of malaria. Used by some elderly people to relieve leg cramps (not FDA-approved).

SIDE EFFECTS

Cinchonism (tinnitus, deafness), proarrhythmic, hemolysis in G6PD-deficient patients, hypoglycemia.

Mefloquine

USES

Prophylaxis and treatment of malaria, chloroquine-resistant malaria.

SIDE EFFECTS

Mood changes, suicidality, unusual dreams.

Atovaquone and Proguanil

MECHANISM

Proguanil has synergy with atovaquone.

USES

Prophylaxis and treatment of malaria, chloroquine-resistant malaria, treatment of *P jiroveci* pneumonia.

SIDE EFFECTS

Fever, skin rash.

The Artemisinins: Artemether and Artesunate

MECHANISM

Not well understood.

USES

Treatment of malaria, chloroquine-resistant malaria; ideally employed as part of combination therapy. Extremely effective novel drugs. Short half-life limits effectiveness as prophylaxis.

SIDE EFFECTS

Rare allergic reactions, generally well tolerated.

ANTIVIRALS

Knowing which sites are critical to viral activity will help in understanding both viral function and how the antiviral agents disrupt viral infection and replication (Table 5-55 and Figure 5-90).

Anti-influenza

AMANTADINE

MECHANISM

Blocks viral penetration/uncoating, may buffer pH of endosome. Causes the release of dopamine from intact nerve terminals. Resistance occurs from mutation of M2 protein; because resistance is so widespread (90% of influenza A strains), it is rarely used.

USES

Prophylaxis and treatment for influenza A; Parkinson disease.

SIDE EFFECTS

Ataxia, dizziness, slurred speech, hallucinations (exacerbated by anticholinergics).

ZANAMIVIR, OSELTAMIVIR

MECHANISM

Inhibits influenza neuraminidase, decreasing viral release.

USES

Shortens symptoms of influenza A and B infection by 1–2 days.

RIBAVIRIN

MECHANISM

Inhibits synthesis of guanine nucleotides by competitively inhibiting inosine monophosphate (IMP) dehydrogenase.

USES

RSV, chronic hepatitis C (in combination with IFN-α).

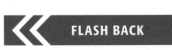
FLASH BACK

Recall that neuraminidase cleaves neuraminic acid to disrupt the mucin barrier in the URT. Removal of the mucin coat exposes sialic acid receptors for hemagglutinin binding, promoting viral adsorption.

FLASH BACK

Remember that influenza A undergoes antigenic *shift* and infects humans, mammals (swine), and birds, whereas influenza B infects only humans and therefore undergoes only antigenic *drift*.

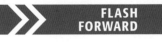
FLASH FORWARD

IFN-α is a leukocyte product that inhibits viral replication.

TABLE 5-55.   Antiviral Drugs

Drug Name	Mechanism	Indications for Use	Side Effects
Amantadine	Blocks viral penetration/ uncoating, may buffer pH of endosome.	Prophylaxis and treatment for influenza A; Parkinson disease.	Ataxia, dizziness, slurred speech, hallucinations (exacerbated by anticholinergics).
Zanamivir, oseltamivir	Inhibits influenza, neuraminidase.	Shortens symptoms from influenza A and B infection by 1–2 days.	
Ribavirin	Inhibits synthesis of guanine nucleotides by competitively inhibiting inosine monophosphate dehydrogenase.	RSV, chronic hepatitis C (in combination with IFN-α).	Hemolytic anemia, severe teratogen.
Acyclovir	Preferentially inhibits viral DNA polymerase when phosphorylated by viral thymidine kinase.	HSV, VZV, EBV. Relieves pain and discomfort of mucocutaneous and genital herpes lesions but does not eradicate the virus. Prophylaxis in immunocompromised patients and prevents recurrent genital herpes infections.	Delirium, tremor, nephrotoxicity by crystallizing in renal tubules.
Ganciclovir	Phosphorylation by viral kinase, preferentially inhibiting CMV DNA polymerase.	CMV (especially in immunocompromised patients—AIDS, bone marrow transplant patients).	Leukopenia, neutropenia, thrombocytopenia— pancytopenia; renal toxicity; more toxic to host enzymes than acyclovir, affecting rapidly dividing cells.
Protease inhibitors: saquinavir, ritonavir, indinavir, nelfinavir, amprenavir	Inhibit assembly of new virus by blocking HIV protease.		GI intolerance (nausea, diarrhea), hyperglycemia, lipid abnormalities, thrombocytopenia (indinavir).
Nucleosides: zidovu**dine,** (AZT), didanosine (**d**dI), zalcitabine (**d**dC), stavudine (**d**4t), lamivudine (3tc), abacavir	Inhibit DNA elongation.		Lactic acidosis, peripheral neuropathy (d's), megaloblastic anemia (AZT).
Nonnucleosides: nevirapine, efavirenz, delavirdine	Induce conformational change in HIV-1 reverse transcriptase.		Rash.
Entry inhibitor: enfuvirtide	Prevents HIV-1 fusion to gp41.		Injection-site reactions.

TABLE 5-55. **Antiviral Drugs** *(continued)*

DRUG NAME	MECHANISM	INDICATIONS FOR USE	SIDE EFFECTS
Integrase inhibitor: raltegravir	Prevents HIV-1 integrase from inserting viral DNA into host cell genome.		Myopathy.
IFN-α	Leukocyte product that inhibits viral replication.	Chronic hepatitis B and C, Kaposi sarcoma (HHV-8).	All interferons may cause neutropenia.
IFN-β	Fibroblast product that inhibits viral replication.	Relapsing multiple sclerosis.	
IFN-γ	Released by T_H1 cells to stimulate macrophage to destroy phagocytosed contents.	NADPH oxidase deficiency.	

CMV = cytomegalovirus; EBV = Epstein-Barr virus; HSV = herpes simplex virus; NADPH = reduced form of nicotinamide adenine dinucleotide; RSV = respiratory syncytial virus; VSV = varicella-zoster virus.

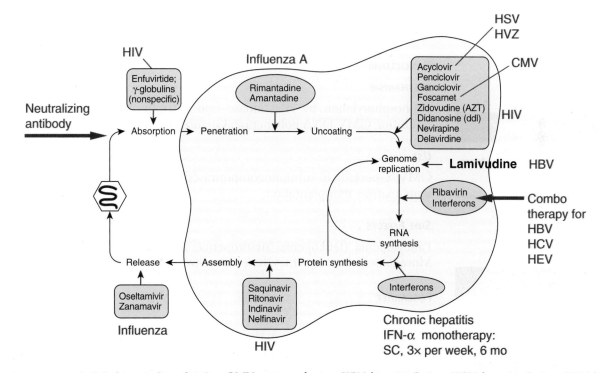

FIGURE 5-90. **Antiviral agent sites of action.** CMV, cytomegalovirus; HBV, hepatitis B virus; HCV, hepatitis C virus; HEV, hepatitis E virus; HSV, herpes simplex virus; HVZ, herpes varicella-zoster; IFN, interferon; SC, subcutaneously.

SIDE EFFECTS

Hemolytic anemia, severe teratogen.

Antiherpes

ACYCLOVIR

MECHANISM

Preferentially inhibits viral DNA polymerase when phosphorylated by viral thymidine kinase into a triphosphate form that causes chain termination. Guanosine analog.

USES

HSV, VZV. Relieves pain and discomfort of mucocutaneous and genital herpes lesions but does not eradicate the virus. Also used for encephalitis. Used for prophylaxis in immunocompromised patients, prevents recurrent genital herpes infections. Famcyclovir is required for herpes zoster.

Recall that CMV lacks thymidine kinase, rendering acyclovir ineffective against CMV infection because it requires activation by viral thymidine kinase.

SIDE EFFECTS

Usually well tolerated; may cause delirium or tremor if dose not adjusted to compensate for renal failure; rare nephrotoxicity by crystallizing in renal tubules.

GANCICLOVIR

MECHANISM

5′-Phosphorylation by viral kinase into a triphosphate form, preferentially inhibiting CMV DNA polymerase. Guanosine analog.

USE

CMV, especially in immunocompromised patients such as those with AIDS, bone marrow transplantation.

SIDE EFFECTS

Pancytopenia (leukopenia, neutropenia, thrombocytopenia). Renal toxicity. More toxic to host enzymes than is acyclovir. Impacts rapidly dividing cells.

FOSCARNET

MECHANISM

Viral DNA polymerase inhibitor binding to pyrophosphate-binding site of enzyme. Resistance occurs through mutation of DNA polymerase to no longer permit binding. Does not require activation by viral kinase, unlike acyclovir and gancyclovir.

USE

Second-line treatment for CMV retinitis in immunocompromised patients if ganciclovir fails, or HSV if acyclovir fails.

SIDE EFFECTS

Highly nephrotoxic.

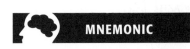

KEY FACT

Because ribavarin may cause a hemolytic anemia, it should be avoided in patients with hematologic disorders such as sickle cell anemia and thalassemia major.

MNEMONIC

Never (**-navir**) tease a pro—**pro-tease** inhibitors all end in -navir.

KEY FACT

AZT as well as multiagent antiretroviral therapies are used during pregnancy to reduce risk of fetal transmission by first treating the mother, then the baby following delivery. Transmission depends on the viral load of the patient and the degree of blood transfer. Breast-feeding is another potential source of transmission and should be discouraged in HIV-positive mothers unless no alternative exists.

HIV Therapy

USE

Highly active antiretroviral therapy (HAART) entails a combination therapy using protease inhibitors and reverse transcriptase inhibitors. Initiated when patients have low CD4 counts (< 350 cells/mm^3) or high viral load. The scheduling of initation of HAART is a subject of active debate, and the recent trend has been to initiate therapy earlier in disease.

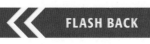

FLASH BACK

The HIV structure and life cycle are key to understanding the action of antiretroviral therapy!

PROTEASE INHIBITORS (SAQUINAVIR, RITONAVIR, INDINAVIR, NELFINAVIR, AMPRENAVIR)

MECHANISM

Inhibit maturation of new virus by blocking HIV protease in virions.

SIDE EFFECTS

GI intolerance (nausea, diarrhea), hyperglycemia, lipid abnormalities, thrombocytopenia (indinavir).

REVERSE TRANSCRIPTASE INHIBITORS

MECHANISM

Preferentially inhibit reverse transcriptase of HIV, thereby preventing incorporation of viral genome into host DNA.

SIDE EFFECTS

Bone marrow suppression (neutropenia, anemia) is common to both nucleosides and nonnucleosides. Granulocyte-macrophage colony-stimulating factor (GM-CSF) and erythropoietin can be used to reduce bone marrow suppression.

NUCLEOSIDES (ZIDOVUDINE [ZDV, FORMERLY AZT], DIDANOSINE [DDI], ZALCITABINE [DDC], STAVUDINE [D4T], LAMIVUDINE [3TC], ABACAVIR)

MECHANISM

These drugs become incorporated into the proviral DNA but because they lack hydroxyl groups further nucleosides cannot be added and DNA elongation is stopped.

SIDE EFFECTS

Lactic acidosis, peripheral neuropathy (ddl, ddC, d4T), megaloblastic anemia (ZDV).

NONNUCLEOSIDES (NEVIRAPINE, EFAVIRENZ, DELAVIRDINE)

MECHANISM

Induce conformational change in HIV-1 reverse transcriptase by binding to a site distant from the catalytic site.

SIDE EFFECT

Rash.

Fusion Inhibitor (Enfuvirtide)

MECHANISM

Binds to gp41 to prevent conformational change required for viral fusion with the host CD4 cell membrane, thus preventing viral entry and replication. Active against HIV-1 but not HIV-2.

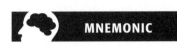

SIDE EFFECT

Subcutaneous injection site reaction, hypersensitivity reaction, increased risk of bacterial pneumonia.

Integrase Inhibitor (Raltegravir)

MECHANISM

Blocks the catalytic site of HIV-1 integrase, thereby preventing it from inserting viral DNA into host cell genome.

SIDE EFFECT

Myopathy.

Interferons

SIDE EFFECT

Neutropenia.

INTERFERON-α

MECHANISM

Leukocyte product that inhibits viral replication.

USES

Chronic hepatitis B and C, Kaposi sarcoma (HHV-8).

INTERFERON-β

MECHANISM

Fibroblast product that inhibits viral replication.

USE

Relapsing multiple sclerosis.

Interferon-γ

MECHANISM

Released by T_H1 cells to stimulate macrophages to destroy phagocytosed contents.

USE

NADPH oxidase deficiency.

See Tables 5-56 through 5-59.

TABLE 5-56. Inhibition of Cell Wall Synthesis (Peptidoglycan/PG Biosynthesis) Antibiotic

	Binding Site	Mechanism of Action	Bactericidal or Bacteriostatic	Bacteria Affected	Advantages	Disadvantages
Inhibition of soluble enzymes located in cytoplasm (must get inside the bacteria to work) blocking PG formation						
Fosfomycin	Active site of pyruvoyl transferase.	PEP structural analog. Blocks PG synthesis (UDP-MurNAc formation).	Bactericidal	Broad-spectrum.		High-frequency, single dose resistance. Limited to UTIs.
D-Cycloserine	Active site of alanine racemase and D-alanine synthetase.	Competitive inhibitor of alanine racemase and D-alanine synthetase. Blocks PG synthesis (UDP-MurNAc pentapeptide formation).	Bacteriostatic	Broad-spectrum.	Rigid ring structure causes high-affinity bonding to enzymes.	Neurotoxic side effects. Limited to TB.
Inhibition of membrane-bound enzymes (must get through peptidoglycan layer to work) blocking transpeptidation (cross-linking) of PG						
Vancomycin	D-Alanyl-D-alanine residues on pentapeptide.	Blocks GCL formation. Steric hindrance prevents precursor binding to synthetase. Binding occurs on **outer face,** after GCL translocation across membrane.	Bactericidal	Gram-positive (esp. staphylococci and enterococci).	NOT degraded by β-lactamase.	Resistance emerges when target (D-ala-D-ala) residue is modified.
Bacitracin	Lipid pyrophosphate of GCL-PP.	Blocks GCL formation on **outer face.** Final step of GCL synthesis (blocks dephosphorylation of GCL-PP → GCL-P).	Bactericidal	Gram-positive (esp. staphylococci).	Not degraded by β-lactamase.	Topical use only.

(continues)

TABLE 5-56.   Inhibition of Cell Wall Synthesis (Peptidoglycan/PG Biosynthesis) Antibiotic *(continued)*

	BINDING SITE	MECHANISM OF ACTION	BACTERICIDAL OR BACTERIOSTATIC	BACTERIA AFFECTED	ADVANTAGES	DISADVANTAGES
β-Lactam antibiotics	Terminal D-ala-D-ala-COOH region of pentapeptide.	Inhibit transpeptidases.	Bactericidal	Older: Narrow-spectrum, gram-positive.	Very effective acylating agents for active sites of multiple transpeptidase enzymes (penicillin binding proteins or PBPs).	Kills only growing cells (ie, when cross-linking in progress).
Penicillins Cephalosporins Cephamycins Carbapenems Monobactams		Substrate analogs of terminal D-ala-D-ala-COOH region of pentapeptide.		Newer: Broad-spectrum, gram-negative and *Pseudomonas aeruginosa*.	Activates autolytic enzymes that degrade old peptidoglycan.	Can cause hypersensitivity reactions (anaphylaxis). Degraded by β-lactamase (penicillinase); cleavage of β-lactam ring inactivates drug. Often administered with a β-lactamase inhibitor.

Bacteriostatic → microorganisms can overcome inhibition of cell wall synthesis by using an excess of D-alanine.

Murein is the principle PG layer, forming the rigid cell wall of most bacteria (except *Mycoplasma,* rickettsia and related organisms, and l-form mutants).

GCL is a carrier molecule that anchors intermediates to the cytoplasmic membrane and facilitates their translocation from the cytoplasmic face of membrane to the outer face. Blocking its formation prevents the cell from completing synthesis of the cell wall.

GCL = glycosyl carrier lipid; PBP = penicillin-binding protein; PEP = phosphoenolpyruvate; PG = peptidoglycan; TB = tuberculosis; UP-MurNAc = uridine-*N*-acetylmuramic acid; UTI = urinary tract infection.

TABLE 5-57. Inhibition of Protein Synthesis

Antibiotic	Binding Site	Mechanism of Action	Bactericidal or Bacteriostatic	Bacteria Affected	Advantages and Basis for Selectivity	Disadvantages and Sources of Resistance
Inhibition of recognition step in polypeptide chain synthesis—all drugs act on 30S subunit						
Streptomycin and aminoglycosides (gentamicin, tobramycin, kanamycin, etc).	Specific proteins on 30S subunit. Strep. = S12 (no common site). Newer aminoglycosides target two proteins (30S & 50S).	**Misreading** of mRNA due to distortions of codons in recognition region of A-site. Cyclic polysomal blockade → kills by *destabilizing* 70S initiation complex (does not block formation).	Bactericidal	Broad-spectrum (esp. gram-negative but also gram-positive).	Target binding sites absent in host. Streptomycin actively transported into bacterial cells and *not* human cells (selective toxicity). Newer aminoglycosides less susceptible to resistance (can't occur in single step).	*Older aminoglycosides:* High-frequency, single-dose resistance develops when target protein mutates. Nephrotoxicity and ototoxicity. Ineffective against intracellular bacteria (*Chlamydia, Rickettsia*). Ineffective against anaerobes (transport into microbe requires O_2).
Tetracyclines.	30S subunit (specific target not known).	Inhibits aa-tRNA binding to A-site.	Bacteriostatic	Broad spectrum (*Chlamydia, Mycoplasma, Rickettsia,* other select gram +/−).	Active transport into bacterial cells and *not* human cells (some still gets in). Useful against intracellular microorganisms (hydrophobic).	Resistance develops by decreased entry into microbe, **active efflux** out, or **elongation factor** proteins that protect 30S subunit.
Spectinomycin.	30S subunit.	Formation of unstable 70S complex only.	Bacteriostatic	Narrow-spectrum.		Treat **gonorrhea** only.

(continues)

TABLE 5-57.   Inhibition of Protein Synthesis *(continued)*

Antibiotic	Binding Site	Mechanism of Action	Bactericidal or Bacteriostatic	Bacteria Affected	Advantages and Basis for Selectivity	Disadvantages and Sources of Resistance
Inhibition of peptidyl transfer step in polypeptide chain synthesis—both drugs act on 50S subunit						
Chloramphenicol.	50S subunit. Preformed polysomes.	Alters P-site tRNA, blocking peptidyl transfer.	Bacteriostatic	Broad-spectrum.	Unable to enter mitochondria (host).	Resistance by plasmid-encoded acetylation of tRNA or porin mutation.
Lincomycin and clindamycin.	50S subunit. Only ribosomes w/*very short* polypeptide chains.	Similar to chloramphenicol (blocks peptidyl transfer).	Bacteriostatic	Narrow-spectrum. Gram-positive bacteria (both). Clindamycin w/ staphylococci and anaerobic gram-negative bacteria.	Esp. effective against *Bacteroides* genus. Effective against anaerobic bacteria.	Resistance develops owing to methylation of 23S ribosomal RNA (also causes resistance to erythromycin).
Drugs that inhibit translocation step in polypeptide chain synthesis						
Erythromycin and other macrolides (azithromycin, clarithromycin).	50S subunit. L15 and L16 proteins.	Prevents ejection of tRNA from P-site after transfer. Prevents peptidyl-tRNA from returning to P-site from A-site.	Bacteriostatic	Medium spectrum (esp. for *Legionella*, *Chlamydia*, *Campylobacter*) as well as Staphylococcus and Streptococcus strains.		Resistance develops owing to methylation of 23S ribosomal RNA (also causes resistance to clindamycin). Hydrolysis of macrolide lactone ring and active efflux.

TABLE 5-58.   Inhibition of Nucleic Acid Synthesis

Antibiotic	Binding Site	Mechanism of Action	Bactericidal or Bacteriostatic	Bacteria Affected	Advantages and Basis for Selectivity	Disadvantages and Sources of Resistance
Drugs that inhibit precursor synthesis						
Sulfonamides	Active site of dihydropteroic acid synthetase.	Competitive inhibitor of dihydropteroic acid synthetase (inhibits folate synthesis). Structural analog of PABA.	Bacteriostatic	Broad-spectrum. Bacterial and some parasitic infections.	Synergistic when used with trimethoprim.	Inhibits only new synthesis of tetrahydrofolic acid. Inhibition can be overcome by excess of *para*-aminobenzoic acid (PABA).
Trimethoprim	Active site of dihydrofolate reductase.	Competitive inhibitor of dihydrofolate reductase (inhibits folate synthesis). Structural analog of pteridine ring of dihydrofolic acid.	Bacteriostatic	Broad-spectrum.	Synergistic when used with sulfonamides. Bacterial enzyme has much higher affinity for drug than for host.	Inhibits only utilization of *existing* pools of dihydrofolate.
Para-Aminosalicylic acid (PAS)		Akin to sulfonamide. Competitive inhibitor of dihydrofolate reductase (inhibits folate synthesis).	Bacteriostatic	Broad, but different from sulfonamides. Effective against *M tuberculosis.*		
Drugs that inhibit RNA synthesis						
Rifampin and rifabutin	β-Subunit of DNA-dependent. RNA polymerase.	Inhibits mRNA synthesis. Inhibits *initiation* of transcription (but not ongoing transcription).	Bactericidal	Narrow-spectrum (gram-positive bacteria, *Neisseria,* mycobacteria). Rifabutin for *M avium* infection.	Host RNA polymerase not sensitive to drug. Mitochondria RNA-sensitive but impermeable.	Does not inhibit transcription already in progress. Resistance develops rapidly when used as monotherapy. Never use alone!
Drugs that inhibit DNA synthesis						
Quinolones (ciprofloxacin, norfloxacin, etc)	DNA gyrase (topoisomerase).	Inhibit DNA gyrase (topoisomerase) of prokaryotic organisms only.	Bactericidal	Newer quinolones broad-spectrum and *Pseudomonas.*		Resistance by altering gyrase subunit structure. Resistance by altering porins of gram-negative bacteria.

TABLE 5-59. Alteration of Cell Membranes

Antibiotic	Binding Site	Mechanism of Action	Bactericidal or Bacteriostatic	Bacteria Affected	Advantages and Basis for Selectivity	Disadvantages and Sources of Resistance
Polymyxins and colistin (polymyxin E)	Hydrophobic tail inserts into cell membranes. Hydrophilic head (a cyclic polypeptide) binds PE and LPS.	Binding disrupts cytoplasmic membrane, causes loss of inner components and cell death. Pore also creates leak in cells.	Bactericidal	Narrow-spectrum (gram-negative).	UTIs and other infections caused by multiresistant gram-negative bacteria that do not respond to other antibiotics. Active against growing *and* nongrowing cells. Host cells do not have PE and LPS in their membranes.	Resistance by altering cell membrane (lipid A moiety of LPS).
Amphotericin B and nystatin (polyene antibiotics).	Hydrophobic portion binds ergosterols in fungal membrane.	Inserts into fungal membranes forming a channel/pore into cell.	Fungicidal (*not* effective against bacteria!)	Opportunistic mycoses (ie, *Candida, Aspergillus,* etc).	IV treatment of systemic mycoses and ointments. Ergosterol targets not in host membranes.	Absorbed poorly in gut. Toxicity (still binds cholesterol, but to lesser extent). Include nausea, anemia, vomiting, diarrhea, nephrotoxicity.

LPS = lipopolysaccharides; PE = phosphatidylethanolamine; UTIs = urinary tract infections.

Immunology

Principles of Immunology

The immune system distinguishes foreign molecules and potential **pathogens** from the body's own cells and removes these pathogens from the body. Cells of the immune system respond to **antigens**, molecular structures (eg, peptides) capable of producing an immune response. Infection or autoimmune disease can result from the failure of these processes.

CONCEPTS OF IMMUNITY

Immune processes can be divided into those that are present at birth (**innate immunity**) and those that require antigen exposure before forming a precise response (**adaptive immunity**).

Innate Immunity

Innate immunity is composed of rapid, nonspecific immunologic processes that recognize and destroy certain common antigens. The protein receptors (eg, Toll-like receptors) involved in recognizing these antigens are germline encoded, so they do not require prior exposure for shaping the response. Some components of innate immunity include:

- Physical barriers, such as skin and mucous membranes
- Cells, such as **neutrophils, macrophages,** and **dendritic cells**
- The **complement** system

Adaptive Immunity

Adaptive immunity encompasses those highly specific immune processes that are much slower than innate immunity on first exposure. This response has the capacity for memory. Cells of adaptive immunity have the ability to undergo genetic rearrangements, resulting in a highly specific and powerful response to pathogens. Key components of adaptive immunity include:

- Cellular components, such as T lymphocytes (**cell-mediated immunity**), also referred to as T cells.
- Antibody-producing B lymphocytes (**humoral immunity**), also referred to as B cells.

Apart from classifying immunity based on how the body detects and responds to insults, immune processes can be classified based on how immune protection is acquired, that is, **passive immunity or active immunity.**

Passive Immunity

Passive immunity is provided by preformed antibodies from a source outside the body. Exposure to virulent pathogens or toxins can result in serious illness or death if the body's own immune system is unable to mount an adequate response. Preformed antibodies can be administered therapeutically to quickly neutralize the pathogens. While exhibiting antigen specificity, the antibodies are short-lived, and the body is unable to respond to a subsequent exposure (ie, lack of immune memory). Some examples of passive immunity include:

- Antibodies in mothers' milk for breast-fed infants
- Administered **antitoxins** for tetanus or botulinum toxins
- Administered **antibodies** to the hepatitis B or rabies virus

---

KEY FACT

The innate immune system uses nonspecific markers to prime the body for an adaptive response. Subsequently, lymphocytes are responsible for the two key features of adaptive immunity: specificity and memory.

TABLE 6-1. **Subsets of Immunity**

	INNATE	ADAPTIVE	PASSIVE	ACTIVE
Source	Within the body	Within the body	Outside the body	Within the body
Speed of protection	Rapid	Slow on first exposure, faster on subsequent exposures	Rapid	Slow on first exposure, faster on subsequent exposures
Specificity	Nonspecific	Specific	Specific	Specific
Memory	No	Yes	No	Yes

Active Immunity

Active immunity is the body's intrinsic mechanism to fight infection. In general, active immunity has a slower onset than does passive immunity, but it has the capacity for immune memory, which results in a rapid response to a second exposure to a pathogen. Some important components of active immunity include:

- **Lymphocytes** and other immune cells
- Lymphoid organs

Table 6-1 summarizes the characteristics of each subset of immunity.

ANATOMY OF THE IMMUNE SYSTEM

The immune system is composed of both primary and secondary lymphoid organs, as summarized in Table 6-2. The primary or central lymphoid organs include the bone marrow and thymus and are involved in lymphocyte production and development. The spleen and lymph nodes are considered secondary, or peripheral, lymphoid organs and are important sites of antigen interaction with cells of the immune system.

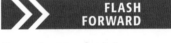
FLASH FORWARD

Chemotherapy or radiation treatment may result in leucopenia (low white blood cell count) and therefore immunosuppression due to bone marrow damage.

Bone Marrow

The bone marrow is the location of **hematopoiesis,** or production of white and red blood cells. In addition, the **maturation of B cells** occurs in the bone marrow. Some immunodeficiency syndromes can be treated by bone marrow transplantation, thus providing a source of functional cells to protect the body.

TABLE 6-2. **Organs of the Immune System**

	ORGAN	FUNCTION
Primary	Bone marrow	Production immune cells, maturation of B cells.
	Thymus	Maturation of T cells.
Secondary	Spleen	Interaction of immune cells with antigen.
	Lymph nodes	Interaction of immune cells with antigen.

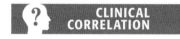
Thymus

This encapsulated primary lymphoid organ is located in the anterior mediastinum. The thymus is derived from the third branchial pouch during development and is the site of **T-cell differentiation**, maturation, and selection. The thymus increases in size until adolescence, when it begins to atrophy and accumulate fat.

Following production in the bone marrow, immature T cells migrate to the thymic **cortex** early in their development to undergo positive and negative selection (see section on Anergy and Tolerance later in chapter). Selection begins in the cortex as the cells reach the **corticomedullary junction** and continues as the T cells move into the inner **medulla**. Mature T cells are finally released into the bloodstream and travel to peripheral sites (Figure 6-1).

Microscopically, the cortex stains darkly owing to the density of lymphocytes. The medulla is lighter, with fewer lymphocytes and a higher concentration of dendritic and epithelial reticular cells.

Spleen

The spleen is a secondary lymphoid organ located in the upper left quadrant of the peritoneal cavity. It contains many blood-filled sinuses that filter antigens and cells from the blood. Microscopically, the splenic parenchyma is divided into the red and white pulp. The **red pulp** is the location of red blood cell storage and turnover; it contains rich vasculature with splenic cords (cords of Billroth) and fenestrated capillaries (sinusoids), The sinusoid structure allows blood cells to freely pass through capillary walls.

The **white pulp** is the location of immune cell interaction. Blood flows into the white pulp through the central arteriole, which is surrounded by the **periarterial lymphatic sheath (PALS)** of T cells. Follicles of B cells are found more distant from the central arteriole; they have pale germinal centers when B cells are activated. The marginal zone surrounds both the PALS and lymphocytic follicle, in addition to separating the white and red pulp. Antigen-presenting cells (**APCs**) in the marginal zone ingest pathogens by phagocytosis and present them to nearby lymphocytes. Blood is drained through the **marginal sinus** located within the marginal zone. The microscopic structure of the spleen is shown in Figure 6-2.

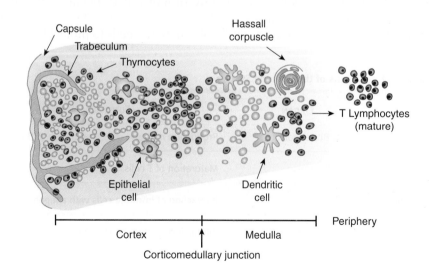

FIGURE 6-1. **Microscopic structure of the thymus.**

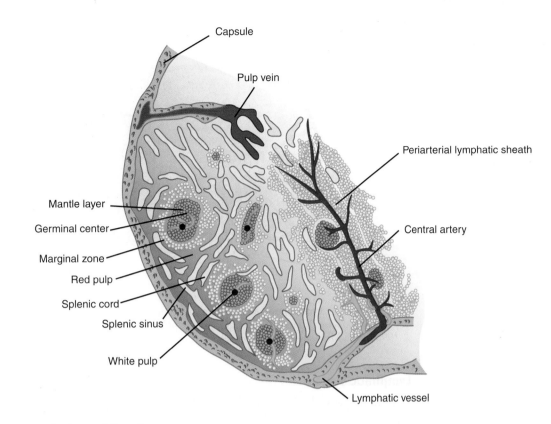

Capsule

Pulp vein

Periarterial lymphatic sheath

Mantle layer

Germinal center

Marginal zone

Red pulp

Splenic cord

Splenic sinus

White pulp

Central artery

Lymphatic vessel

FIGURE 6-2. **Anatomy of the spleen.**

Lymph Nodes

Lymph nodes are encapsulated secondary lymphoid organs that receive lymph from multiple afferent vessels, providing the opportunity for interaction between the stored immune cells and the lymphatic fluid. The fluid is returned to the lymphatic ducts through the efferent vessel after the antigens and pathogenic cells contained in the fluid encounter APCs, B cells, and T cells.

The tissue architecture of lymph nodes is maximized for antigen recognition and response, as shown in Figure 6-3.

- Primary, or inactive, follicles are dense with stored lymphocytes awaiting antigen presentation.
- Secondary, or active, follicles have pale **germinal centers** within the cluster of lymphocytes. Here, B cells proliferate and produce antibodies in response to antigens.

T cells are found in the **paracortex** between the follicles and the medulla. The paracortex may become enlarged in severe infections, such as viral infections, that result in a cellular immune response.

Lymph nodes are supplied by their own capillary system. B and T lymphocytes enter and exit lymph nodes via **high endothelial venules** located in the paracortex. The medullary sinus drains cells and fluid in the medulla into the efferent lymphatic duct. APCs within the sinus filter the lymph by engulfing pathogens and presenting them to lymphocytes.

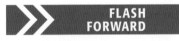

FLASH FORWARD

Painful, tender lymphadenopathy is indicative of an inflammatory process, whereas nonpainful, nontender lymphadenopathy is often associated with a neoplasm.

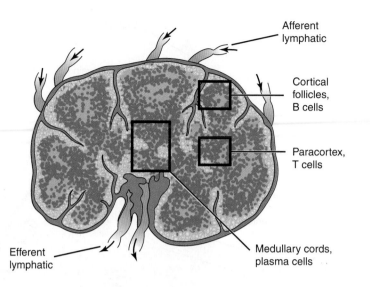

FIGURE 6-3. **Lymph node architecture.** (Modified with permission from Chandrasoma P, Taylor CR. *Concise Pathology*, 3rd ed. Originally published by Appleton & Lange. Copyright © 1998 by the McGraw-Hill Companies, Inc.)

Lymphatic System

Lymphatic vessels drain fluid from the body, filter it through lymph nodes, and return it to the circulatory system. A summary of lymphatic drainage sites is presented in Table 6-3. The **right lymphatic duct** drains the right arm and right half of the head and neck, whereas the **thoracic duct** drains all other body parts. The fluid from the thoracic duct and right lymphatic duct is returned to the left and right subclavian veins, respectively.

TABLE 6-3. **Lymphatic Drainage Sites**

Area of Body	Primary Lymph Node Drainage Site
Upper limb, lateral breast	Axillary
Stomach	Celiac
Duodenum, jejunum	Superior mesenteric
Sigmoid colon	Colic (drains to inferior mesenteric)
Rectum (lower), anal canal above pectinate line	Internal iliac
Anal canal below pectinate line	Superficial inguinal
Testes	Para-aortic
Scrotum	Superficial inguinal
Thigh (superficial)	Superficial inguinal
Lateral side of dorsum of foot	Popliteal

Peripheral Lymphoid Tissue

Collections of lymphocytes outside the spleen and lymph nodes that are at prime locations for antigen interaction are termed peripheral lymphoid tissue. Some examples of peripheral lymphoid tissue include:

- Gut-associated lymphoid tissue (GALT), which includes the tonsils, appendix, and Peyer patches of the intestines.
- Mucosal-associated lymphoid tissue (MALT).
- Bronchial-associated lymphoid tissue (BALT).

CELLS AND MOLECULES OF THE IMMUNE SYSTEM

Innate Immunity

PHAGOCYTIC CELLS

Phagocytic cells engulf pathogens and debris and include:

- **Neutrophils** are myeloid cells present in acute inflammatory responses. These cells contain multilobed nuclei and abundant cytoplasmic myeloperoxidase granules for killing pathogens. Myeloperoxidase is notable for its ability to catalyze the production of hypochlorite ions (bleach). Neutrophils are short-lived.
- **Macrophages** are differentiated myeloid cells present in both pathologic and normal physiologic responses. These cells are large, amorphous, and have high phagocytic capacity and a longer life span than neutrophils. Macrophages are derived from monocytes that leave the bloodstream and differentiate in response to cytokines.
- **Dendritic cells** are differentiated myeloid cells that engulf antigen in the epithelia of the skin, gastrointestinal, and respiratory tracts. Before antigen exposure, they can be identified by long, fingerlike processes of cytoplasm. After taking up antigen and becoming activated, they travel to lymph nodes where they present antigen to T cells.

ANTIGEN-PRESENTING CELLS

APCs process engulfed pathogens and express the resulting antigens to other immune cells. Some examples of APCs include:

- Dendritic cells
- Macrophages
- B cells

Following phagocytosis of extracellular pathogens, APCs digest the pathogen into peptides within phagolysosomes. The peptides are loaded on to a major histocompatibility complex (MHC) II molecule within an endosome, which fuses with the cell membrane so the MHC II–antigen complex may be presented to T cells. In this way, APCs provide a link between innate and adaptive immunity.

NATURAL KILLER (NK) CELLS

Natural killer cells contain lytic granules that attack and kill virus-infected or cancerous cells that lack MHC I. Unlike lymphocytes, NK cells lack specific antigen receptors. Binding of the antibody constant region to NK cell surface receptors also triggers the release of lytic granules in a process known as **antibody-dependent cellular cytotoxicity (ADCC).**

A summary of the cells of the innate immune system is provided in Table 6-4.

TABLE 6-4. Cells of the Innate Immune System

CATEGORY	CELL TYPES	FUNCTION	MECHANISMS
Phagocytes	Neutrophils, macrophages, dendritic cells.	Engulf foreign particles.	Phagocytosis.
Antigen-presenting cells	Dendritic cells, macrophages, B cells.	Present particles to T cells (ie, to adaptive immune system).	Complexing antigen with MHC II.
Natural killer cells	Natural killer cells.	Destroy virus-infected and tumor cells.	Detects down-regulation of MHC I, antibody-dependent cellular cytoxicity.

MHC = major histocompatibility complex.

THE COMPLEMENT SYSTEM

The complement system comprises a cascade of proteins, C1 through C9, that result in the lysis of pathogenic cells, as shown in Figure 6-4. The complement system links innate immunity and the humoral branch of adaptive immunity. The complement cascade can be activated in three ways:

- The **classic pathway** is activated when C1 recognizes and binds the constant fragment of either IgG or IgM in an antigen-antibody complex, thus linking the innate and adaptive immune systems.
- The **alternative pathway** is triggered when activated C3 recognizes certain nonspecific antigens on microbial surfaces.
- The **lectin pathway** is activated when mannose-binding lectin, a serum protein, recognizes carbohydrate antigens on the surface of microorganisms such as encapsulated bacteria or viruses.

The three activation pathways converge on the generation of **C3 convertase,** an enzyme that remains associated with the pathogen surface to trigger cleavage of other complement proteins. C3 convertase breaks down C3 molecules to the enzymatically active **C3b** and the **anaphylatoxin** C3a, which mediates a local inflammatory response. C3b is also important in triggering phagocytosis of pathogens.

Binding of C3b to C3 convertase creates **C5 convertase,** which cleaves C5 into C5a (another anaphylatoxin) and C5b, which is inserted into the cell membrane of the pathogen. The binding of C6, C7, C8, and C9 to C5b follows, forming the **membrane attack complex (MAC),** which perforates the pathogen's cell membrane and causes major damage to the cell.

A summary of the functions of complement proteins is shown in Table 6-5.

As with the coagulation system, the formation of a few active enzymes can lead to rapid activation and amplification of the complement cascade. Therefore, regulatory proteins are important in maintaining control of the cascade:

- **C1 esterase inhibitor** (C1INH) breaks apart the C1 enzyme, thus limiting its activation. Deficiency of C1INH results in **hereditary angioedema,** in which tissue edema occurs because of uncontrolled activation of the clas-

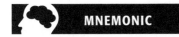

MNEMONIC

GM makes **classic** cars: Ig**G** and Ig**M** are part of the **classic** complement pathway.

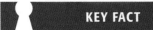

KEY FACT

C3a and C5a function as anaphylotoxins and are responsible for the recruitment of inflammatory cells. C5a also functions as a neutrophil chemotactic factor.

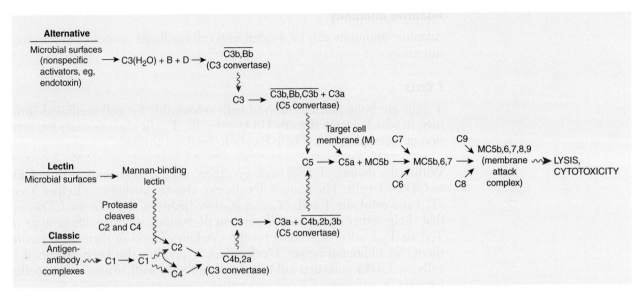

FIGURE 6-4. **The complement system.** (Modified with permission from Levinson W. *Medical Microbiology and Immunology: Examination and Board Review*, 8th ed. New York: McGraw-Hill, 2004: 432.)

sic pathway and a resulting increase in C2 kinin. In addition, absence of C1INH leads to overproduction of bradykinin by kallikrein.

- **Decay-accelerating factor** (DAF, also CD55) disrupts formation of C3 convertase, thus halting the complement cascade. In **paroxysmal nocturnal hemoglobinuria**, the protein that associates DAF with the red blood cell membrane is abnormal, thus making the RBCs more susceptible to complement-induced lysis.

TABLE 6-5. **Complement System Proteins**

	FUNCTION	PATHWAYS INVOLVED	DEFICIENCY RESULTS
C1	Recognize antigen-antibody complexes.	C	
C2	Part of C3 convertase.	C, L	
C3a	Anaphylatoxin.	C, A, L	Recurrent pyogenic infections (respiratory tract).
C3b		C, A, L	
C4a	Anaphylatoxin.	C, L	
C5a	Anaphylatoxin, neutrophil chemotaxis.	C, A, L	
C5b, C6, C7, C8, C9	Cytolysis (MAC).	C, A, L	Recurrent *Neisseria* infections (C6–C8).

MAC = membrane attack complex; C = classical pathway; A = alternative pathway; L = lectin pathway.

Adaptive Immunity

Adaptive immunity can be divided into cell-mediated immunity and humoral immunity.

T Cells

T cells are bone marrow–derived cells responsible for **cell-mediated immunity,** in which T cells directly kill target cells. T cells also stimulate the activation of macrophages and help B cells to produce antibody.

Within the thymus, T cells undergo differentiation to become mature CD4+ or CD8+ T cells. The mature T cells can also be divided into **helper T cells** (T_H) and **cytotoxic T cells** (T_C), as seen in Table 6-6. T_H cells are CD4+ cells that "help" other immune cells perform their functions; they differentiate into $T_H 1$ or $T_H 2$ cells, depending on the cytokines found in their local environment. An additional helper T cell subset, $T_H 17$, has also been described. T_C cells are CD8+ cells that kill target cells infected with viruses or intracellular bacteria. A summary of T-cell maturation is presented in Figure 6-5.

B Cells

B lymphocytes are bone marrow–derived cells involved in **humoral immunity.** Their main function is to recognize extracellular pathogens and differentiate into **plasma cells** that produce antibodies to target pathogens for elimination from the body.

Antibodies

Antibodies are proteins composed of two **heavy (H) chains** and two **light (L) chains.** Both heavy and light chains have a **constant (C_H or C_L) region** that is identical for all antibodies of the same **isotype,** or class, as well as a **variable region (V_H or V_L)** that has been designed by the B cell to specifically recognize an antigen. This general structure is shown in Figure 6-6.

Antibodies can be broken into fragments by enzymatic digestion. In the presence of the protease papain, the antibody molecule is broken into two anti-

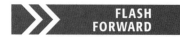

FLASH FORWARD

A systemic accumulation of immunoglobulin light chains (eg, in multiple myeloma) is responsible for Bence Jones proteinuria and amyloidosis AL.

TABLE 6-6. Major Classes of T Cells

T Cell Type	Cluster Differentiation (CD) Marker	Cytokine Requirements for Activation	Function
$T_H 1$	CD4	IL-12	Activate macrophages and T_C via IL-2 and IFN-γ.
$T_H 2$	CD4	IL-4	Stimulate immunoglobulin production by B cells via IL-4 and IL-5.
$T_H 17$	CD4	IL-6, TGF-β	Produce IL-17 and IL-22 in response to extracellular bacteria and fungi.
T_C	CD8	IL-2, IFN-γ	Kill cells infected with virus or intracellular bacteria.

IFN = interferon; IL = interleukin.

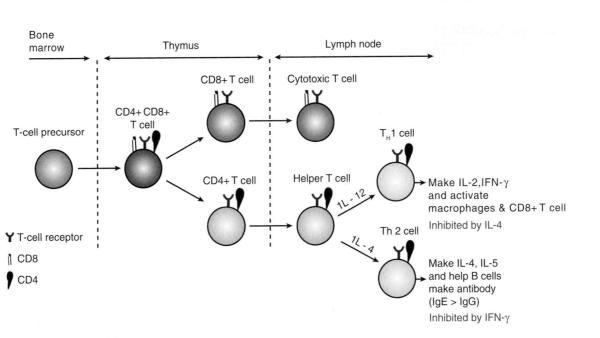

FIGURE 6-5. **T-cell maturation.**

gen-binding fragments (**Fab**) and one constant fragment (**Fc**). The Fab fragments are each composed of one light chain and one N-terminal end of the heavy chain, which are normally attached to each other by disulfide bonds. The Fc fragment is composed of the two C-terminal ends of the heavy chains.

Antibodies have four major functions:

- **Opsonization:** Binding of immunoglobulin, particularly **IgG,** to microbial surfaces enhances phagocytosis by phagocytes. Phagocytes have cell surface receptors that bind the Fc portion of antibodies.
- **Neutralization:** Binding to microbial surfaces can prevent adherence to and infection of host tissues. Furthermore, binding to antigens or inflammatory molecules can prevent an excessive immune response (eg, in passively administered anti-TNF-α antibodies).

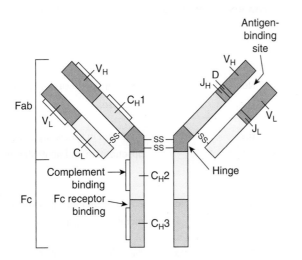

FIGURE 6-6. **Antibody structure.** (Modified with permission from Ganong WF. *Review of Medical Physiology*, 22nd ed. New York: McGraw-Hill, 2005: 528.)

Allotype: Ig epitope that differs among members of the same species (polymorphism)

Isotype: Ig epitope common to a single class of Ig—determined by heavy chain (eg, IgG, IgA, etc)

Idiotype: Ig epitope determined by antigen-binding site (specific for given antigen)

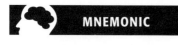

MNEMONIC

GAMma globulin is the most abundant antibody in human serum: Ig**G** > Ig**A** > Ig**M**

- **Complement activation:** Binding of IgG or IgM to antigens activates the complement system, leading to phagocytosis, anaphylaxis, and cytolysis, as previously described.
- **Antibody-dependent cellular cytotoxicity (ADCC):** Binding of antibodies to cell surface receptors on NK cells and eosinophils causes the release of cytotoxic granules, as previously described.

Immunoglobulins with similar structures belong to the same class, or **isotype** ("same" type). There are five immunoglobulin isotypes, as determined by their heavy-chain constant regions. See Table 6-7 for a summary.

ANTIBODY DIVERSITY

Although B cells contain a limited number of antibody-encoding genes, they can produce a diverse number of antibody molecules by four mechanisms:

- **Somatic recombination of VJ or VDJ genes:** Each B cell in an individual contains a given set of genes to transcribe and translate into antibody molecules. However, these genes have multiple exon segments in various regions (V and J regions for light chains and V, D, and J regions for heavy chains) that can be differentially spliced together. In this way, B cells can produce antibodies with different amino acid sequences, and thus different antigen specificities. This is also known as "combinatorial diversity."
- **Genetic recombination:** During VJ or VDJ recombination, various DNA segments are cut out of the genome. To repair the strand breaks, the enzyme **terminal deoxynucleotidyl transferase (TdT)** adds nucleotides to the sticky ends of the DNA strands.
- **Random combinations of heavy and light chains:** The differentially spliced heavy- and light-chain genes must then combine to form a functional antibody molecule.
- **Somatic hypermutation:** Once B cells have been activated (following the binding of their BCR [B-cell receptor] to antigen), the variable regions of the immunoglobulin genes are subject to a high rate of random point

TABLE 6-7. **Immunoglobulin Isotypes**

	EXPRESSED BY	STRUCTURE	COMPLEMENT FIXATION	CROSSES PLACENTA	FUNCTION
IgM	Mature B cell (surface or secreted).	Monomer or pentamer (with J-chain)	Yes	No	Primary response.
IgD	Mature B cell (surface).	Monomer	No	No	Functions as B-cell receptor for early immune response.
IgG	Plasma cells (secreted; high concentration in serum).	Monomer	Yes	Yes	Important in secondary responses; opsonization and neutralization.
IgA	Plasma cells (secreted).	Monomer or dimer (with J-chain)	No	No	Prevents pathogen attachment to mucous membranes; found in secretions.
IgE	Plasma cells (secreted; low concentration in serum).	Monomer	No	No	Type I hypersensitivity (induces mast cell degranulation); worm immunity.

mutations. At some point, these mutations result in an antibody that is more specific to the initial antigen than was the original antibody molecule; these B cells are selected to differentiate into plasma cells in a process known as **affinity maturation.**

Cell Surface Proteins

In addition to their normal functions, cell surface proteins function as useful identifying markers of immune system components. Through flow cytometry, lymphocytes and other cells can be separated based on their cell surface components. This is useful when attempting to count the number of T or B lymphocytes in a patient or to determine the level of differentiation of a population of cells (eg, when evaluating for immunodeficiency or lymphoid cancers).

T-Cell Receptors

T-cell receptors (TCRs) are two-component cell surface receptors responsible for T cell signaling on binding antigen. TCR components have both a constant region and a variable region that binds a particular antigen. Most TCRs have one α chain and one β chain (α:β TCR), but some are γ:δ.

TCRs interact with MHC molecules, as shown in Figure 6-7.

B-Cell Receptors

B-cell receptors (BCRs) are membrane-bound antibody (IgM or IgD) that has been designed by the B cell for antigen recognition. Once the BCR binds antigen, and the appropriate costimulation is received, the B cell differentiates into an antibody-producing plasma cell that is capable of generating antibodies of all isotypes.

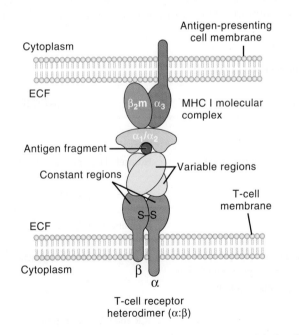

FIGURE 6-7. **T-cell and antigen-presenting cell interaction.** (Modified with permission from Ganong WF. *Review of Medical Physiology,* 22nd ed. New York: McGraw-Hill, 2005: 527.)

MAJOR HISTOCOMPATIBILITY COMPLEXES

Major histocompatibility complexes (MHCs) are surface proteins responsible for communication with T cells and NK cells. The **human leukocyte antigen (HLA) genes** encode the MHC proteins. The characteristics of MHC I and II molecules are listed in Table 6-8.

MHCs are the most important molecules pertaining to organ and tissue transplantation. **HLA matching** allows for the determination of suitability of donor tissue for transplantation and the likelihood of rejection by the recipient. There are multiple types of tissue grafting:

- **Autografts:** Transfer of an individual's own tissue to another location. Skin autografts are used when transferring healthy skin to a burned or damaged location on the same individual.
- **Syngeneic grafts:** A transfer of tissue between genetically identical members of the same species, such as between identical twins.
- **Allografts (homografts):** Transfer of tissue between genetically different members of the same species. These grafts are commonly used for organ and tissue transplantation.
- **Xenografts (heterografts):** Transfer of tissue between different species. For example, some heart valve replacements are performed with modified porcine valves.

Even with meticulous HLA matching and proper drug therapy, tissue transplantation may not be fully accepted by the recipient. The body can undergo **transplant rejection** in a variety of ways, as presented in Table 6-9.

CLUSTERS OF DIFFERENTIATION

Clusters of differentiation (CDs) are surface protein complexes widely found on cells of the immune system. There are hundreds of known CDs, with a wide variety of functions. The most common and well-characterized CDs will be presented here.

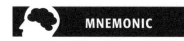

MNEMONIC

Understanding tissue grafting is as easy as understanding prefixes:
Auto = self (self-tissue)
Syn = same (same genetic tissue)
Allo = similar (similar tissue from same species)
Xeno = stranger ("stranger" tissue from different species)

MNEMONIC

CD**4** × MHC **2** = **8** = CD**8** × MHC **1**

TABLE 6-8. Characteristics of Major Histocompatibility Complexes (MHCs)

	MHC I	MHC II
Expressed by	All nucleated cells.	APCs.
Present	Intracellular peptides (self- and viral peptides).	Extracellular peptides (engulfed pathogens).
Acquires peptide in	Rough ER.	Vesicles, after fusion with acidic endosomes.
Associated with	β_2–Microglobulin.	Invariant chain (before transport to cell surface).
Encoded by	α Chain: HLA-A, -B, and -C genes.	HLA-DR, -DP, and -DQ genes.
	β Chain: Chromosome 15 (β_2^- microglobulin).	
Binds to	TCR and CD8 coreceptor.	TCR and CD4 coreceptor.

APC = antigen-presenting cell; ER = endoplasmic reticulum; HLA = human leukocyte antigen; TCR = T cell receptor.

TABLE 6-9. **Categories of Transplant Rejection**

Category	Features
Hyperacute	Occurs due the presence of preformed antidonor antibodies in the recipient (eg, ABO blood type antibodies). Seen within minutes of transplantation.
Acute	Occurs due to T_C reaction with foreign MHCs and is reversible with immunosuppressants. Seen within weeks of transplantation.
Chronic	Occurs due to antibody-mediated damage of vasculature (fibrinoid necrosis) and is irreversible. Seen within months to years of transplantation.
Graft vs. host disease	Occurs in an irradiated immunocompromised host. Grafted immunocompetent T cells recognize the body as "foreign," causing widespread organ dysfunction. Common symptoms are rash, jaundice, and diarrhea.

T CELLS

Mature T cells express CD3 and either CD4 or CD8. **CD3** is associated with the TCR and is required for signal transduction through the TCR. **CD4** on T_H cells is a coreceptor for MHC II molecules on APCs. CD4 is also the receptor for human immunodeficiency virus (HIV). **CD8** on T_C cells is a coreceptor for MHC I molecules on cells expressing abnormal intracellular peptides (typically virus-infected cells).

T cells also express CD40 ligand, or **CD40L,** which is important in antibody isotype switching, and **CD28,** which is important in T cell activation.

B CELLS

In addition to the BCR, **CD19** and **CD20** are markers for B lymphocytes. Another surface protein, **CD21,** is involved in the complement pathway and is the receptor for Epstein-Barr virus (EBV). B cells also express **CD40,** which binds CD40L of helper T cells. This interaction is a crucial costimulatory signal for B cells, stimulating differentiation and isotype switching.

A summary of the most common cell surface proteins is found in Table 6-10.

Cytokines

Cytokines are intercellular communication signals that are crucial in immune system function. Some important classes of cytokines include interleukins, chemokines, interferons, and tumor necrosis factors.

INTERLEUKINS

A family of secreted proteins with a diversity of actions. The most common interleukins are summarized in Table 6-11.

INTERFERONS

Interferons are secreted proteins from virus-infected cells that promote the transition of local cells to an antiviral state. Interferons bind to interferon receptors on the target cell surface, signaling the uninfected cell to degrade viral mRNA and increase antigen presentation. Interferons also activate

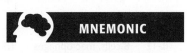

MNEMONIC

HOT T-BONE stEAk:

IL-1 (**HOT** fever)
IL-2 (**T** cells)
IL-3 (**BONE** marrow)
IL-4 (Ig**E**)
IL-5 (Ig**A**)

MNEMONIC

"Clean up on **aisle 8**": Neutrophils are recruited to clear infections by chemotactic factor **IL-8.**

TABLE 6-10. Summary of Cell Surface Proteins

	CELL-SPECIFIC SURFACE PROTEINS	ADDITIONAL SURFACE PROTEINS
T cells	CD3, TCR	CD28
Helper T cells	CD4	CD40L
Cytotoxic T cells	CD8	
B cells	IgM, CD19, CD20	MHC II, B7, CD21, CD40
Macrophages	–	MHC II, CD14, Fc receptors, C3b receptors
Natural killer cells	CD56	CD16
Nucleated cells	–	MHC I

MHC = major histocompatibility complex; TCR = T-cell receptor.

TABLE 6-11. Functions of Interleukins

	SECRETED BY	ACTS UPON	RESULTS IN
IL-1	Macrophages	T cells, B cells, neutrophils, fibroblasts, epithelial cells, hepatocytes.	Growth, differentiation of cells; endogenous pyrogen; production of acute phase proteins.
IL-2	T_H cells	T_H and T_C cells.	Growth of cells.
IL-3	Activated T cells	Bone marrow stem cells.	Growth and differentiation of cells.
IL-4	T_H2 cells	B cells.	Growth of cells; class switching of IgE and IgG.
IL-5	T_H2 cells	B cells, eosinophils.	Differentiation/activation of eosinophils; class switching of IgA.
IL-6	T_H cells, macrophages	Hepatocytes, B cells.	Production of acute phase proteins and immunoglobulins; endogenous pyrogen.
IL-8	Macrophages	Neutrophils.	Chemotaxis.
IL-10	T_H2 cells	T_H2 and T_H1 cells.	Turns off immune response; helps attenuate response to prevent autoimmunity.
IL-12	B cells, macrophages	NK and T_H1 cells.	Activation of cells.
IL-13	T_H2 cells	Eosinophils.	Activation of eosinophils.

IL = interleukin; NK cell = natural killer cell.

NK cells and stimulate them to kill infected cells. There are three types of interferons:

- **IFN-α** and **IFN-β** signal a cell to produce a protein that degrades viral (but not host) mRNA.
- **IFN-γ** signals for increased expression of MHC I and MHC II, thus increasing antigen presentation in all cells that receive the signal. IFN-γ is also secreted by helper T cells to stimulate phagocytosis by macrophages.

TUMOR NECROSIS FACTORS

TNF-α, a protein secreted by macrophages and T cells, is a key mediator of the inflammatory response during infection and autoimmune disease (Figure 6-8).

Immune System Interactions

T-CELL ACTIVATION

Naïve T cells are not activated until they receive stimulation from an APC. The TCR binds antigen presented on the MHC molecule of the APC (the **primary signal**). A **secondary (costimulatory) signal** is also required for T-cell activation; one example is the binding of the B7 surface glycoprotein of the APC to CD28 on the T cell. These two interactions result in clonal expansion of the T cell. A summary of this process is shown in Figure 6-9.

ISOTYPE SWITCHING

Naïve (mature but inactive) B cells express IgM on their surface but do not secrete antibody until activation and **isotype switching** occurs. Once IgM binds antigen, antigenic peptides are presented via MHC II. The binding of MHC II to the TCR and CD4 of T$_H$ cells, along with the binding of the appropriate costimulatory molecules (CD40 on the B cell and CD40L on the T cell), triggers the T cell to produce cytokines. These cytokines induce isotype switching, which results in the production of various immunoglobulin isotypes via changes in expression of the constant region of heavy-chain genes.

? CLINICAL CORRELATION

Infliximab and adalimumab are anti-TNF-α antibodies that are used to reduce inflammation in autoimmune diseases such as rheumatoid arthritis and Crohn disease. Etanercept, a decoy TNF-α receptor, is used for similar purposes.

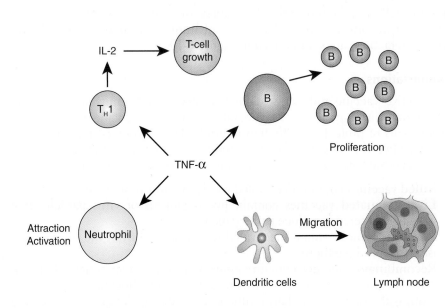

FIGURE 6-8.   Functions of tumor necrosis factor (TNF)-α.

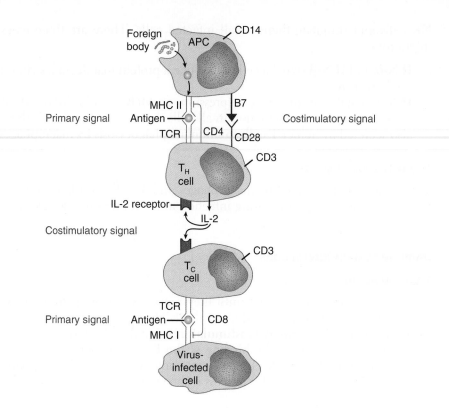

FIGURE 6-9. **T-cell activation.** Two signals are required for T-cell activation: Signal 1 (primary signal) and Signal 2 (costimulatory signal). Helper T-cell (T_H) activation: (1) Foreign body is phagocytosed by antigen-presenting cells (APC); (2) Foreign antigen is presented on major histocompatability (MCH) II and recognized by T-cell receptor (TCR) on T_H cell (Signal 1); (3) "Costimulatory signal" is given by interaction of B7 and CD28 (Signal 2); (4) T_H cell activated to produce cytokines. Cytotoxic T-cell (T_C) activation: (1) Endogenously synthesized (viral or self) proteins are presented on MHC I and recognized by TCR on T_C cell (Signal 1), (2) Interleukin 2 (IL-2) from T_H cell activates T_C cell to kill virus-infected cell (Signal 2).

SUMMARY

Immune cells and the molecules they express or secrete are significantly interconnected to form a coordinated, efficient immune response to pathogens. These interactions are summarized in Figure 6-10.

Immunizations

An effective vaccine induces sustained, protective immunity in the recipient without causing illness. In general, an effective vaccine must provide several years of protection, although multiple doses (boosters) may be necessary. Effective vaccines stimulate the production of neutralizing antibodies or induce cell-mediated immunity. There are multiple types of vaccines:

- **Killed vaccines** contain inactivated whole organisms or viruses.
- **Live attenuated vaccines** contain live organisms or virus particles that have been altered to reduce pathogenicity.
- **Toxoid vaccines** contain inactivated toxins isolated from the microorganisms that produce them.
- **Recombinant vaccines** contain engineered protein components that can stimulate production of protective antibodies to a pathogen.
- **Conjugate vaccines** contain synthetic compounds designed to induce a stronger immune response than the original pathogen or compound. For example, carbohydrates are weakly antigenic, but when combined with a

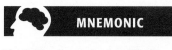

MNEMONIC

The Sal**K** polio vaccine is a **K**illed vaccine.

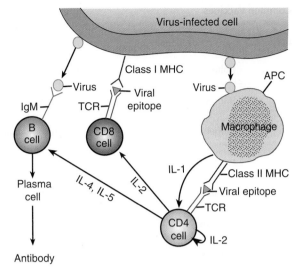

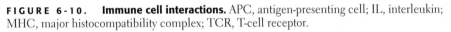

FIGURE 6-10. **Immune cell interactions.** APC, antigen-presenting cell; IL, interleukin; MHC, major histocompatibility complex; TCR, T-cell receptor.

protein fragment, the resulting compound is better able to stimulate the production of protective antibodies.

Important vaccines are listed in Table 6-12.

ANERGY AND TOLERANCE

Because T- and B-cell specificity is determined by random recombination events to create a large repertoire of antigen receptors, some developing immune cells react with self-antigen. These cells must be removed by one of the mechanisms discussed below to prevent autoimmune disease.

T Cells

CLONAL SELECTION

T cells undergo both positive and negative selection during development (Figure 6-11). **Positive selection** occurs in the cortex of the thymus when T cells bind self-MHC. Positive selection ensures that T cells that do not recognize self-MHC do not survive in the periphery. **Negative selection** occurs next, in the thymic medulla, as T cells that react to self-antigens are deleted. T cells then proceed to the periphery. Clonal selection ensures that the mature T-cell population can react with foreign antigen (presented by MHC I and MHC II), but does not react with self-antigen.

PERIPHERAL TOLERANCE

Inevitably, some self-antigens are expressed at very low levels (or not at all) in the thymus, so that T cells reacting to these antigens do not undergo negative selection. These cells are released to the periphery (Figure 6-12), where they must be controlled through the following processes:

- **Clonal deletion:** A T cell that binds repeatedly (eg, because of a high concentration of self-antigen) undergoes programmed cell death.
- **Anergy:** Anergic T cells recognize self-antigen but remain inactive owing to a lack of the costimulatory molecules (CD80/CD86) required for activation of the T cell.

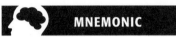

MNEMONIC

Killed vaccines–

RIP Always

Rabies
Influenza
Salk **P**olio
H**A**V

TABLE 6-12. Common Vaccines

Type of Vaccine	Prevents	Protects From
Killed	Polio[a]	Poliovirus
	Rabies	Rhabdovirus
	Influenza	An orthomyxovirus
	Hepatitis A	Hepatitis A virus (HAV)
	Cholera	*Vibrio cholerae*
Live attenuated	Measles[b]	A paramyxovirus
	Mumps[b]	A paramyxovirus
	Rubella[b]	A togavirus
	Polio[c]	Poliovirus
	Chickenpox	Varicella-zoster virus (VZV)
	Yellow fever	A flavivirus
	Smallpox	A poxvirus
	Pharyngitis, pneumonia	Adenovirus
	Tuberculosis (BCG)[d]	*Mycobacterium tuberculosis*
	Salmonellosis	*Salmonella typhi*
	Tularemia	*Francisella tularensis*
Toxoid	Diphtheria[e]	*Corynebacterium diphtheriae*
	Tetanus[e]	*Clostridium tetani*
	Whooping cough[e]	*Bordetella pertussis*
Recombinant	Hepatitis B	Hepatitis B virus (HBV)
	Cervical cancer	Human papillomavirus (HPV)
Conjugate	Meningitis	*Haemophilus influenzae* type b
	Meningitis	*Neisseria meningitidis*
	Pneumonia	*Streptococcus pneumoniae*

[a]The Salk intramuscular polio vaccine (IPV) contains inactive poliovirus.

[b]The measles, mumps, and rubella vaccines are often combined (MMR).

[c]The Sabin oral polio vaccine (OPV) contains mutated poliovirus.

[d]The bacillus Calmette-Guérin (BCG) vaccine contains a different strain of the bacteria that causes tuberculosis. This vaccine is not used in the United States but is widely used in other countries.

[e]The diphtheria, tetanus, and pertussis vaccines are often combined (DTP or DTaP).

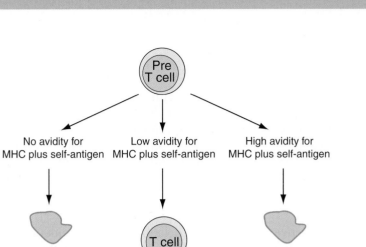

FIGURE 6-11. **Central T-cell tolerance.** MHC, major histocompatibility complex.

■ **Active suppression:** Self-reactive T cells are kept nonfunctional when self-antigen is presented at low levels. The cells reacting at low levels differentiate into regulatory cells, which secrete regulatory cytokines to prevent other cells from reacting to that antigen. This is the most common mechanism for controlling peripheral T cells. Regulatory T cells (T suppressor cells) are recognized by their coexpression of both CD4 and CD25.

■ **Ignorance:** Like any other T cell, if a self-reactive T cell never encounters its antigen, it will die from lack of stimulation.

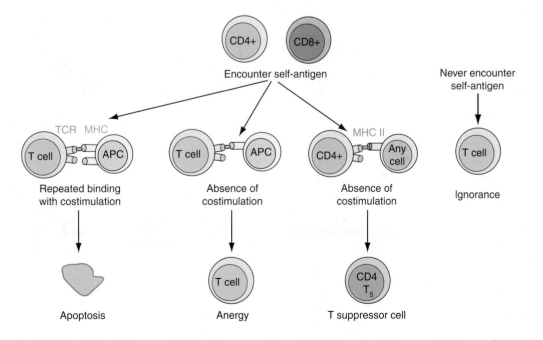

FIGURE 6-12. **Peripheral T-cell tolerance.** APC, antigen-presenting cell; MHC, major histocompatibility complex; TCR, T-cell receptor.

B Cells

CLONAL DELETION

B cells that react with self-antigen can either be deleted or undergo receptor editing of the light chain during their development in the bone marrow. Receptor editing changes the antigen specificity of the cell with the goal of preventing recognition and binding to self-proteins. This receptor-editing event serves as the last chance for the autoreactive B cell to escape deletion. Failing this, the cell is deleted. This process is termed **negative selection.**

ANERGY

Sometimes self-reactive B cells escape deletion and are accidentally released to the periphery. When these self-reactive cells encounter the antigen they recognize in the absence of costimulatory molecules, they are stimulated to become permanently **anergic.** Costimulatory molecules are activation signals expressed on APCs stimulated by the inflammatory response of the innate immune system (see Figure 6-13).

CLONAL IGNORANCE

Other B cells bind only weakly to self-antigen and so escape detection and deletion. These B cells are usually nonfunctional (since their binding is weak), but can become activated if the concentration of their antigen is unusually high.

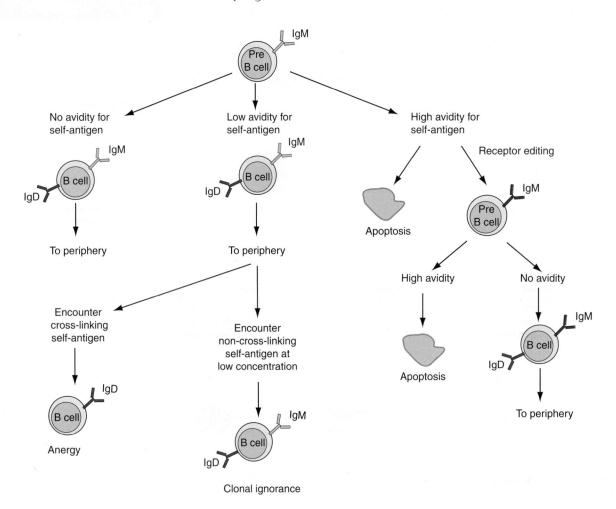

FIGURE 6-13. **B-cell anergy and tolerance.** Ig, immunoglobulin.

TABLE 6-13. Summary of Anergy and Tolerance in B Cells and T Cells

	ANTIGEN REACTIVITY	LOCATION	OUTCOME	REACTIVATION?
T cells				
Clonal selection	Normal signaling.	Thymus	Positive and negative selection.	---
Clonal deletion	Strong and repeated reaction to self-antigen.	Periphery	Cell death.	No
Anergy	Normal recognition of self-antigen.	Periphery	Cell nonfunctional, lack of costimulation.	Yes
Active suppression	Low-frequency recognition of self-antigen.	Periphery	Cell differentiates to a regulatory T cell.	No
Ignorance	Never encounters self-antigen.	Periphery	Cell death from lack of stimulation.	No
B cells				
Clonal deletion	Strong reaction to self-antigen.	Bone marrow	Light-chain rearrangement or deletion.	No
Anergy	Strong reaction to self-antigen.	Periphery	Cell nonfunctional, lack of costimulation.	No
Clonal ignorance	Weak reaction to self-antigen.	Periphery	Cell nonfunctional, weak binding.	Yes

Anergy and tolerance are very similar in T cells and B cells. Table 6-13 summarizes the key points related to each and allows for comparison between the two.

Pathology

HYPERSENSITIVITY

There are four types of hypersensitivity, as seen in Table 6-14. Types I through III are antibody mediated, whereas type IV is mediated by T cells. The general

TABLE 6-14. Hypersensitivity

Type I	Anaphylactic IgE-mediated	First and fast.
Type II	Cytotoxic IgM, IgG-mediated	Cy-**2**-toxic.
Type III	Immune complex	**3** things in an immune complex: antigen-antibody-complement. Includes **serum sickness** (mostly due to drugs) and **Arthus reaction.**
Type IV	Cell-mediated (delayed type)	Delayed = **4th** and last. **4 Ts = T** lymphocytes, **T**ransplant rejections, **T**B skin tests, **T**ouching (contact dermatitis).

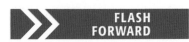

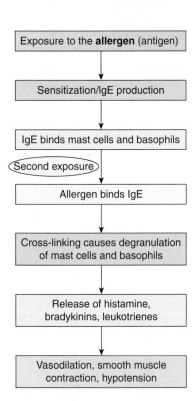

FIGURE 6-14. **Pathogenesis of type I hypersensitivity.**

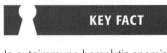

effector mechanism of all four types is immune-mediated damage to otherwise normal, healthy tissue.

Type I: IgE-Mediated

Also called **immediate hypersensitivity,** the type I response can be **anaphylactic** (systemic) or **atopic** (local). After being sensitized to an antigen, the patient experiences an immune response to low concentrations of that same antigen. Genetic susceptibility plays a role in this reaction.

PATHOGENESIS

Figure 6-14 outlines the pathogenesis of type I hypersensitivity.

Common manifestations include urticaria, allergic rhinitis, and asthma. All three are characterized by local effects, and patients generally have consistently high circulating levels of IgE.

- **Urticaria,** or hives, is the mildest form of atopy. Histamine release causes vasodilation and a visible wheal and flare.
- **Allergic rhinitis** and **asthma** result from inhalation of allergens. This can cause inflammation of either the nasal mucosa, leading to rhinitis, or of the lower bronchi, resulting in bronchial constriction and air trapping (asthma).
- **Anaphylaxis** is the most severe form of type I hypersensitivity and occurs when histamine and other mediators are released systemically. Widespread vasodilation and increased vessel permeability can result in hypotension and shock, accompanied by bronchoconstriction.

Type II: Antibody-Mediated (Cytotoxic)

Antibody-mediated hypersensitivity occurs when antibodies are directed to cell surface antigens.

PATHOGENESIS

- Circulating antibody binds to an antigen on the pathogen.
- Complement is activated.
- Outcomes include:
  - Opsonization, followed by phagocytosis.
  - Antibody-dependent cell-mediated cytotoxicity (**ADCC**).
  - Cell death mediated by NK or T cells.
  - Immune response–mediated damage to healthy tissue.

Incompatible **blood transfusions** are a common example. The recipient has preformed antibodies to the donor's major RBC antigens, resulting in rapid destruction of the infused red blood cells.

Erythroblastosis fetalis results from an Rh mismatch between mother and fetus. Rh antibodies (from a sensitized Rh– mother) pass transplacentally and attack fetal (Rh+) erythrocytes. The by-products of RBC destruction can cause brain damage. The mother is treated with anti-Rh IgG antibody (RhoGAM), which binds the fetal Rh+ erythrocytes, thus removing them from circulation before the mother's immune system can respond to and mount an anti-Rh response, and preventing the formation of Rh antibodies.

Goodpasture syndrome is caused by antiglomerular basement membrane antibodies (anti-GBM), which bind to type IV collagen. The antibody forms complexes in the kidney and lungs, resulting in glomerulonephritis and pulmonary hemorrhage.

Type III: Immune Complex–Mediated

Soluble antigen-antibody complexes form when antigen is abundant. Complex deposition in tissues causes type III hypersensitivity.

PATHOGENESIS

- Clearance of infections creates antigen-antibody complexes.
- Normally, the complexes aggregate into clusters that activate the complement system, which triggers an inflammatory response to clear the infection.
- Certain smaller complexes escape detection and are deposited in the walls of blood vessels. They accumulate on the endothelium and synovium of joints, leading to:
  - Complement activation resulting in tissue inflammation, which manifests as vasculitis (endothelium) or arthritis (synovium).
  - Chemotaxis of neutrophils that cause significant tissue damage or arthritis.

Systemic lupus erythematosus (SLE) is associated with antibodies to self-proteins known as antinuclear antibodies (**ANAs**). Kidney disease is a major consequence of SLE because the immune complexes are deposited in the glomerulus and cause inflammation and tissue damage.

Serum sickness occurs when serum or antibodies, such as horse antivenom for a snakebite victim, are administered to a patient. Approximately 1 week following the treatment, antibodies are formed to the foreign proteins, leading to lymphadenopathy and systemic inflammatory symptoms such as fever, arthralgias and urticarial plaques.

The **Arthus reaction** is a local swelling at the site of injection of an antigen to which the patient has been immunized. The reaction occurs quickly and can be cleared within 24 hours. It is now most often seen at the site of desensitization allergy shots.

Type IV: Cell-Mediated (Delayed Type)

T cells are primed as effector cells specific to intracellular antigens or aberrant cells (foreign or mutated).

PATHOGENESIS

Initial exposure to an antigen or infection causes production of memory immune cells, among them effector T cells. On repeated exposure, effector T cells are drawn to the site, where they proliferate and activate a macrophage response to clear the infection (Figure 6-15). This process generally takes 1–2 days.

The **tuberculin skin test** uses hypersensitivity to determine whether a person has been previously exposed to *Mycobacterium tuberculosis*. Tuberculin purified protein derivative (**PPD**) is injected in the skin. If a T cell has been previously sensitized to the PPD antigen, its proliferation results in erythematous induration at the site of injection, indicating previous exposure. It is important to note that with certain T-cell immunodeficiencies (ie, HIV), induration may not be seen despite previous exposure.

Contact dermatitis results from a similar reaction, except that the T cells are sensitized to topical antigens such as urushiol from poison ivy. These reactions generally involve both CD4+ and CD8+ T cells and can be as wide-

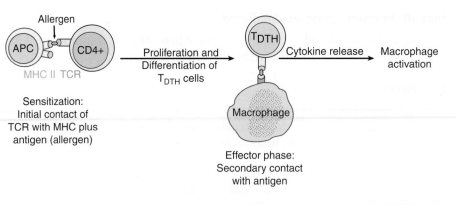

FIGURE 6-15. Delayed-type hypersensitivity. APC, antigen-presenting cell; TCR, T-cell receptor; T_{DTH}, delayed-type hypersensitivity helper T cells.

spread as the area of contact. Exposure to a large volume of antigen increases the magnitude of the immune response, which consequently can cause severe local tissue damage, and in some cases, systemic responses.

IMMUNODEFICIENCY

B-Cell Deficiencies

TRANSIENT HYPOGAMMAGLOBULINEMIA (OF INFANCY)

A naturally occurring deficiency of B-cell-secreted immunoglobulins occurring in infants 3–6 months of age. At this age, maternal IgG is disappearing, but the infant's B cells are not yet producing sufficient quantities of antibodies to suppress infections. Although this occurs in all infants, some display a more profound depression of antibody levels and require treatment.

PRESENTATION

Recurrent and potentially severe bacterial infections.

DIAGNOSIS

Measure circulating antibody levels and confirm that the level is lower than for age-matched standards.

TREATMENT

If the infections are threatening, intravenous immunoglobulin (IVIG) can be given to boost the immune response.

PROGNOSIS

Most infants eventually develop normal circulating immunoglobulin levels and have no lasting sequelae.

BRUTON AGAMMAGLOBULINEMIA

An X-linked defect in Bruton tyrosine kinase (Btk), which functions in B-cell differentiation, maturation, and signaling. B cells fail to develop normally past the pre-B-cell stage, resulting in low levels of all classes of immunoglobulins after 6 months of age.

PRESENTATION

Recurrent extracellular pyogenic and enterovirus infections.

MNEMONIC

The 3 B's:

Bruton agammaglobulinemia is seen in young **B**oys that are especially susceptible to **B**acterial infections.

DIAGNOSIS

B cells are absent on peripheral smear, immunoglobulin levels are low to undetectable, and the patient lacks tonsils. Lymph node biopsy showing lack of germinal centers is confirmatory.

TREATMENT

IVIG from adult donors.

DYSGAMMAGLOBULINEMIA (SELECTIVE IMMUNOGLOBULIN DEFICIENCY)

Lack of any immunoglobulin class due to defective B-cell class switching or activation. The most common type is circulating IgA deficiency, affecting as many as 1 in 600 people. Affected individuals have decreased mucosal immunity and potentially increased susceptibility to autoimmune disease.

PRESENTATION

Often asymptomatic and diagnosed incidentally in patients with chronic lung disease. Common associated conditions include milk allergy, diarrhea, and chronic sinus infections.

DIAGNOSIS

Decreased serum titers of IgA.

TREATMENT

Antibiotics are given to symptomatic patients to help clear infections.

PROGNOSIS

IgA deficiency is not known to cause any significant morbidity or mortality.

See Table 6-15 for a summary of B-cell-related immunodeficiencies.

T-Cell Deficiencies

THYMIC APLASIA (DIGEORGE SYNDROME)

DiGeorge syndrome is characterized by the triad of hypocalcemia, tetany, and the absence of T cells. The defect is caused by defective formation of the third and fourth pharyngeal pouches early in gestation. Thymic aplasia is associated

> **CLINICAL CORRELATION**
>
> Some patients with IgA deficiency can have circulating anti-IgA IgG antibodies. If they are transfused with either blood or IVIG containing IgA, they are at risk for a transfusion reaction.

TABLE 6-15. Summary of B-Cell Immunodeficiency Syndromes

	IMMUNE DEFECT	COMMON INFECTIONS
Transient hypogammaglobulinemia	Uniformly decreased immunoglobulins.	Recurrent bacterial sinopulmonary infections (ie, otitis media, pneumonia, and sinusitis).
Bruton agammaglobulinemia	Loss of Btk tyrosine kinase leads to complete absence of B cells.	
Dysgammaglobulinemia	Defective class switching leads to decrease of immunoglobulin, most commonly IgA.	

with 22q11 chromosomal microdeletions. The syndrome results in a nondeveloping thymus and a lack of parathyroid glands, which cause T-cell and calcium deficiencies, respectively.

PRESENTATION

Neonatal tetany and recurrent opportunistic viral and fungal infections. A velocardiofacial syndrome (VCFS), infants often also show facial abnormalities or cardiac malformations (or both).

DIAGNOSIS

Patients generally present with **cyanosis** or **tetany** due to the cardiac disease or hypocalcemia, respectively. Fluorescent in situ hybridization can be used to detect the 22q11 chromosomal deletion. Chest radiographs shows absent or greatly reduced thymic shadow. Low to undetectable circulating T cells are seen, as well as low circulating levels of immunoglobulin (due to lack of B cell activation by T cells).

TREATMENT

If the patient possesses any fragments of thymus, immunomodulatory agents can be given to stimulate thymic growth. If not, fetal thymic transplantation can be performed if the patient remains symptomatic.

PROGNOSIS

Given proper treatment of cardiac disease and hypocalcemia, patients with thymic aplasia have a good prognosis. Many even survive without thymic transplantation, although the reason for this is unknown.

CHRONIC MUCOCUTANEOUS CANDIDIASIS

A selective lack of T-cell reactivity to *Candida* species.

PRESENTATION

Recurrent *Candida* infections on skin and mucosal areas.

DIAGNOSIS

Laboratory studies show normal levels and functioning of both B and T cells. Diagnosis is made on highly specific T-cell challenge.

TREATMENT

Antimycotic agents can aid the patient in clearing the infection, but avoidance of potential sources of infection is more effective.

PROGNOSIS

The prognosis for this condition is quite good, as the *Candida* infections rarely become systemic.

ACQUIRED IMMUNODEFICIENCY SYNDROME (AIDS)

The sequelae of infection with HIV, which directly infects and kills CD4+ helper T cells. This immunosuppression manifests as a loss of cell-mediated immunity and can lead to opportunistic infections (Table 6-16) and malignancies. HIV and AIDS are discussed in greater detail in Chapter 5 (Microbiology).

TABLE 6-16. **Most Common Opportunistic Infections in Untreated AIDS Patients**

Protozoa	▪ *Toxoplasma gondii*
	▪ *Isospora belli*
	▪ *Cryptosporidium* spp.
Fungi	▪ *Candida albicans*
	▪ *Cryptococcus neoformans*
	▪ *Coccidioides immitis*
	▪ *Histoplasma capsulatum*
	▪ *Pneumocystis jiroveci*
Bacteria	▪ *Mycobacterium avium-intracellulare*
	▪ *Mycobacterium tuberculosis*
	▪ *Listeria monocytogenes*
	▪ *Nocardia asteroides*
	▪ *Salmonella* spp.
	▪ *Streptococcus* spp.
Viruses	▪ Cytomegalovirus
	▪ Herpes simplex virus
	▪ Varicella zoster virus
	▪ Adenovirus
	▪ Polyomavirus
	▪ JC virus
	▪ Hepatitis B virus
	▪ Hepatitis C virus

PRESENTATION

General wasting and constitutional symptoms (fever, weight loss, etc). Affected individuals also have increased occurrence of opportunistic infections and rare malignancies, such as the virally mediated Kaposi sarcoma.

DIAGNOSIS

HIV seropositivity is initially determined by enzyme-linked immunosorbent assay (**ELISA**) (highly sensitive), and then confirmed with Western blot (highly specific). A low peripheral blood CD4+ T cell count is an indicator that an HIV-positive patient is progressing to AIDS.

TREATMENT

Control viral replication with highly active antiretroviral therapy (**HAART**) including reverse transcriptase inhibitors or protease inhibitors (or both). Treat infections with appropriate antibiotics. Broad-spectrum antibiotics are often given prophylactically to decrease the occurrence of opportunistic infections.

PROGNOSIS

With the development of more advanced medications, the survival time of newly infected patients has increased drastically in the developed world. However, in resource-poor areas, the median survival time after infection is only about one decade.

See Table 6-17 for a summary of T-cell-related immunodeficiencies.

TABLE 6-17. **Summary of T-Cell Immunodeficiency Syndromes**

	IMMUNE DEFECT	PRESENTATION
DiGeorge syndrome	Thymic aplasia due to defective formation of 3rd/4th pharyngeal pouches.	Cyanosis and/or tetany.
Chronic mucocutaneous candidiasis	Decreased T-cell reactivity to *Candida* spp.	Recurrent *Candida* infections.
Acquired immunodeficiency syndrome	HIV-induced depletion of CD4+ T cells.	Opportunistic infections (see Table 6-16).

Combined Deficiencies

SEVERE COMBINED IMMUNODEFICIENCY (SCID)

Class of inherited disorders leading to malfunctioning of both B and T cells. Enzyme deficiencies in **adenosine deaminase (ADA)** or purine nucleotide phosphorylase can cause accumulation of toxic metabolites in the purine degradation pathways of lymphocytes. **X-linked SCID** is the most common and results from a defect in the common gamma chain, which is shared by many cytokine receptors.

PRESENTATION

Failure to thrive and chronic infections (of all types) in an infant with low lymphocyte counts.

DIAGNOSIS

Flow cytometry indicating lack of lymphocytes. More specific diagnosis is made by gene mutation analysis.

TREATMENT

Bone marrow transplantation, prophylactic antibiotics. There are also several experimental gene therapy treatments for SCID that utilize viral-mediated delivery of the defective gene to bone marrow cells.

PROGNOSIS

In the absence of treatment, death occurs within 1 year of birth.

WISKOTT-ALDRICH SYNDROME

An X-linked defect occurs in Wiskott-Aldrich syndrome protein (WASP), causing cellular defects in the actin cytoskeleton. This affects all hematopoietic cells, especially platelets and T cells. T cells lose the ability to stimulate B cells in response to capsular polysaccharides present on some bacteria.

PRESENTATION

Pyogenic infections, bleeding diathesis, and eczema. Affected individuals also have an increased incidence of autoimmune disorders and lymphoma.

DIAGNOSIS

Low serum IgM with normal levels of IgG and IgA, abnormally small platelets on peripheral smear.

TREATMENT

Bone marrow transplantation.

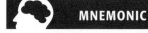

MNEMONIC

Wiskott-Aldrich syndrome can be summed up by the mnemonic **WIPE:**

Wiskott-Aldrich
Recurrent pyogenic **I**nfections
Thrombocytopenic **P**urpura
Eczema

PROGNOSIS

In the absence of treatment, most patients do not live beyond adolescence.

HYPER-IgM SYNDROME

This syndrome is caused by an X-linked defect in T cell CD40-ligand. The CD40-CD40 ligand interaction is required for full activation of B cells as well as antibody class switching.

PRESENTATION

Recurrent bacterial infections. Individuals may also have increased susceptibility to autoimmune disorders or lymphoma.

DIAGNOSIS

Serum antibody titers reveal increased IgM and decreased IgA and IgG.

TREATMENT

Bone marrow transplantation. If no donor, immune function is augmented with IVIG and the administration of appropriate antibiotics to treat infections.

PROGNOSIS

Varies, but is significantly better with early diagnosis or bone marrow transplantation.

ATAXIA-TELANGIECTASIA

Ataxia-telangiectasia is an autosomal recessive defect in the ATM protein that leads to insufficient cellular responses to DNA damage. Lymphocytes are targeted because of high rates of proliferation and the need to rapidly divide. It is associated with IgA deficiency and malignancies.

PRESENTATION

Cerebellar ataxia and oculocutaneous telangiectasias in early childhood; increased susceptibility to mucosal infections.

DIAGNOSIS

Clinical presentation in addition to identified genetic defects on both alleles of ATM.

TREATMENT

Antibiotics for infection.

PROGNOSIS

Most patients die of infections, cancer, or advanced neurodegenerative disease in their mid-20s.

See Table 6-18 for a summary of the combined immunodeficiencies.

Phagocyte Deficiencies

LEUKOCYTE ADHESION DEFICIENCY SYNDROME

This syndrome occurs due to an autosomal recessive mutation in the LFA-1 integrin receptor, which is responsible for phagocyte binding to endothelium. This prevents phagocytic infiltration at the site of infection or injury.

TABLE 6-18. **Summary of Combined Immunodeficiency Syndromes**

	CAUSE	PRESENTATION	TREATMENT
Severe combined immunodeficiency	Multiple genetic associations; see text.	Failure to thrive in infancy.	Bone marrow transplantation
Wiskott-Aldrich syndrome	X-linked defective *WASP* gene.	Pyogenic infections, bleeding diathesis, eczema.	
Hyper-IgM syndrome	X-linked defect in T-cell CD40 ligand.	Recurrent bacterial infections.	
Ataxia-telangiectasia	Autosomal recessive defect in *ATM* gene.	Cerebellar ataxia, oculocutaneous telangiectasia, mucosal infections.	Antibiotics for infections

PRESENTATION

Increased frequency of **bacterial infections** in the first year of life with an absence of pus, often preceded by delayed separation of the umbilical cord.

DIAGNOSIS

Leukocytosis, flow cytometric analysis of integrins, or phagocyte functional studies.

TREATMENT

Bone marrow transplantation is the only treatment with documented benefit. Other options include prophylactic administration of antibiotics and regular leukocyte transfusions.

PROGNOSIS

Without treatment, patients die within a few years. Success varies with treatments.

CHRONIC GRANULOMATOUS DISEASE

Chronic granulomatous disease (CGD) is caused by a defective NADPH oxidase system (mutation in any of the four enzymes). It impairs the production of reactive oxygen intermediates required for the killing of phagocyted pathogens. As a result, phagocytes can internalize bacteria but are unable to kill certain classes. This malfunction causes accumulations of immune cells in granulomas, which form at the site of infection.

PRESENTATION

Severe infections with catalase-positive bacteria (eg, *Staphylococcus aureus*, *Escherichia coli*, *Aspergillus*) or fungal infections, especially of the skin; hepatosplenomegaly; and lymphadenopathy.

DIAGNOSIS

Phagocyte function is determined using a test of the ability to reduce nitroblue tetrazolium dye. The specific defect is determined by genetic testing.

TREATMENT

Bone marrow transplantation can be curative. IFN-γ and prophylactic antibiotics are the current standard of care.

PROGNOSIS

Depends on severity of disease; highest mortality is seen in children.

CHÉDIAK-HIGASHI SYNDROME

This autosomal recessive mutation in lysosomal trafficking regulator (LYST) causes a failure of vesicle fusion in neutrophils (impaired phagosome-lysosome fusion), platelets, and melanocytes, among others.

PRESENTATION

Recurrent infections (especially *Streptococcus* and *Staphylococcus*), hair with a silvery metallic sheen, diffuse hypopigmentation of the skin with occasional acral (ears, nose) hyperpigmentation, prolonged bleeding times, and widespread lymphoproliferation. Peripheral neuropathy may also be seen.

DIAGNOSIS

Microscopic analysis of peripheral blood shows large granules in leukocytic cells.

TREATMENT

Bone marrow transplantation ameliorates all symptoms except peripheral neuropathy.

PROGNOSIS

Death resulting from infection or excess lymphoma-like states usually occurs within the first decade of life. See Table 6-19 for a summary of phagocyte immunodeficiencies.

AUTOANTIBODIES AND ASSOCIATIONS

Although autoimmune disease is discussed in detail in the Pathology section, it is important to note key autoantibody associations, as found in Table 6-20.

HLA ASSOCIATIONS

HLA associations are important when considering familial inheritance of disease or disease susceptibility. Table 6-21 lists important HLA-linked disorders.

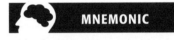

MNEMONIC

Antibodies that cross the placenta—

TAP D3

Anti-**T**SH receptor
Anti-**A**ch receptor, Anti-**P**latelet
Anti-**D**esmoglein-**3**

TABLE 6-19. Summary of Major Phagocyte Deficiency Syndromes

	DEFECT	PRESENTATION	TREATMENT
Leukocyte adhesion deficiency	Autosomal recessive defect in LFA-1.	Recurrent pyogenic infections, delayed wound healing.	Bone marrow transplantation.
Chronic granulomatous disease	Mutation in any of 4 NADPH oxidase enzymes.	Catalase + bacterial infections.	
Chédiak-Higashi disease	Autosomal recessive mutation in LYST.	Recurrent infections, partial albinism.	

TABLE 6-20.   Autoantibodies and Their Associations

DISEASE	ANTIBODY	COMMENTS
Autoimmune hemolytic anemia	Anti-RBC	Rh and I antigens are the targets.
Autoimmune hepatitis	Antismooth muscle	
Celiac disease	Antigliadin Antitissue transglutaminase	For diagnosis, antitissue transglutaminase IgG and IgA (both) are key.
Crohn disease	Antidesmin	
Goodpasture syndrome	Antibasement membrane	Antigen is type IV collagen; found in the kidney and lungs.
Graves disease	Antithyroid-stimulating hormone receptor	Crosses placenta; antibody is stimulatory at the receptor.
Hashimoto thyroiditis	Antithyroid peroxidase, Antithyroglobulin	
Multiple sclerosis	Antimyelin	
Myasthenia gravis	Anti-acetylcholine receptor	Crosses placenta, antibody is inhibitory at the nicotinic ACh-receptor.
Pemphigus vulgaris	Antidesmoglein-3	Crosses placenta.
Pernicious anemia	Anti-intrinsic factor, Antiparietal cell	Results in vitamin B_{12} deficiency.
Polymyositis, dermatomyositis	Anti-Jo-1	
Primary biliary cirrhosis	Antimitochondrial Antiactin	
Rheumatoid arthritis	Anti-IgG (rheumatoid factor)	Also found in 30% of SLE.
Progressive systemic sclerosis (scleroderma)	Anticentromere Anti-Scl-70 (topoisomerase)	Associated with CREST syndrome (calcinosis, Raynaud phenomenon, esophageal dysmotility, sclerodactyly, telangiectasia). Diffuse, specific.
Sjögren syndrome	Anti-Ro (SS-A) and Anti-La (SS-B)	
Systemic lupus erythematosus (SLE)	Antinuclear (ANA) Anti-dsDNA, Anti-Smith Antihistone	Thought to be microbially induced. Specific and diagnostic. Only seen in drug-induced cases.
Thrombocytopenic purpura	Antiplatelet	Crosses placenta.
Type I diabetes mellitus	Anti-islet cell Anti-insulin	

TABLE 6-20.   Autoantibodies and Their Associations *(continued)*

DISEASE	ANTIBODY	COMMENTS
Vasculitis	Antineutrophil (C-ANCA, P-ANCA)	Found in Wegener granulomatosis, microscopic polyangiitis, and Churg-Strauss syndrome, among others.
Miscellaneous	Antimicrosomal	Found in SLE, rheumatoid arthritis, Sjögren syndrome, and Hashimoto thyroiditis, among others.

GENERAL AUTOIMMUNE PATHOLOGY

Under ordinary circumstances, the body is able to distinguish between its own normal cells and abnormal cells, or in other words, self and nonself. Immature B cells that strongly react to self-antigens in the bone marrow are either destroyed or undergo alteration of receptor specificity. Mature B lymphocytes encounter high concentrations of self-antigens in the peripheral lymphoid tissues, learn to recognize these antigens and do not mount an immune response against them. If these natural mechanisms of immunologic tolerance to self fail, then autoimmune pathology may develop. This development can be influenced by a number of factors, including genetics and infections.

Genes may predispose individuals to particular autoimmune diseases. **HLA genes** are an important type of gene frequently associated with autoimmunity. Individuals who inherit certain HLA alleles are at an increased risk of devel-

TABLE 6-21.   HLA-Linked Disorders

HLA TYPE	ASSOCIATED DISEASE
A1	Graves disease, dermatitis herpetiformis.
B8	Graves disease, celiac disease, autoimmune hepatitis, primary sclerosing cholangitis, dermatitis herpetiformis.
B27	Psoriasis, ankylosing spondylitis, inflammatory bowel disease, reactive arthritis, acute anterior uveitis.
DR2	Goodpasture syndrome, multiple sclerosis, systemic lupus erythematosus (SLE), hay fever, narcolepsy.
DR3	Celiac disease, myasthenia gravis, SLE, Graves disease, type I DM, autoimmune hepatitis, primary sclerosing cholangitis, dermatitis herpetiformis.
DR4	Rheumatoid arthritis, type I DM, pemphigus vulgaris, giant-cell (temporal) arteritis, autoimmune hepatitis.
DR5	Hashimoto thyroiditis, pernicious anemia.
DR7	Steroid-responsive nephrotic syndrome.
DR8	Primary biliary cirrhosis.

oping certain autoimmune diseases. However, autoimmune diseases are not *caused* by HLA alleles, and the majority of patients with a particular allele associated with disease never develop that disease. The exact mechanism of autoimmunity is frequently unknown, but it has been hypothesized that particular HLA alleles may be inefficient at displaying self-antigens or may fail to stimulate T cell regulation. Non-HLA genes may also be associated with particular autoimmune diseases.

Infections may activate self-reactive lymphocytes, leading to an autoimmune response. Many mechanisms can be involved in this activation; an infection may induce a local immune response and promote the survival of self-reactive T lymphocytes, infections may injure tissues and release self-antigens that are normally isolated from the immune system, or infectious organisms may produce peptides that are similar to self-antigens and trigger an autoimmune response via cross-reactivity (**molecular mimicry**).

SYSTEMIC AUTOIMMUNE DISEASES

Systemic Lupus Erythematosus (SLE)

SLE is a chronic inflammatory autoimmune disorder characterized by immunologic abnormalities, such as the presence of **ANAs**. ANAs are polyclonal IgG, IgM, and IgA autoantibodies that are reactive with antigens in the cell nucleus. They are not organ-specific and are not cytotoxic to intact, viable cells. However, they are deposited as immune complexes, thus triggering inflammatory changes and tissue damage. ANAs are found in the serum of patients with SLE, but they may also be seen with other autoimmune disorders, such as rheumatoid arthritis (RA) and systemic sclerosis. Ninety percent of patients with SLE are females between the ages of 14 and 45. The disease is most common and severe in black females.

PRESENTATION

Many manifestations of SLE are possible. Symptoms often wax and wane over time. **Arthritis** and muscle pain are the most common complaints. The arthritis associated with SLE is symmetrical and affects the small joints of the hands, feet, wrists, knees, and elbows. Other common findings in this disease can include:

- **Malar rash,** butterfly-shaped erythematous patches or plaques on the cheeks, as shown in Figure 6-16.
- **Discoid rash,** erythematous plaques with overlying hyperkeratosis and scale, often leading to atrophic scarring.
- **Nephritis** (occurring in half of all patients), which can lead to nephrotic syndrome, renal failure, and death. As the renal disease progresses, a characteristic "wire loop" pattern can be seen on biopsy caused by the thickening of the capillaries.
- **Hematologic abnormalities,** such as anemia (due to both chronic disease and circulating anti-RBC antibodies), thrombocytopenia (due to antiplatelet antibodies), and recurrent thromboses (particularly in association with antiphospholipid syndrome).
- **Cardiac manifestations,** such as pericarditis, myocarditis, valvulitis, or characteristic vegetations affecting both sides of cardiac valves (**Libman-Sacks endocarditis**).
- **Neurologic disturbances,** such as strokes and seizures.
- **Pulmonary abnormalities,** such as fibrosis and pulmonary hypertension.
- **Mucositis,** with ulcers in the nose and mouth.
- **Photosensitivity,** a rash that develops after exposure to sunlight.

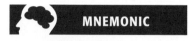

KEY FACT

The presence of antiphospholipid antibodies in patients with SLE may result in false-positive results on syphilis tests (rapid plasma reagin [RPR] and venereal disease research laboratory [VDRL]).

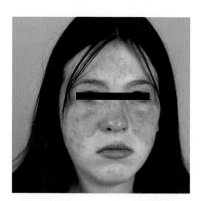

FIGURE 6-16. **Malar rash in young woman with systemic lupus erythematosus.** (Reproduced with permission from Wolff K, Johnson RA, Suurmond D. *Fitzpatrick's Color Atlas & Synopsis of Clinical Dermatology,* 5th ed. New York: McGraw-Hill, 2005: 385.)

MNEMONIC

I'M DAMN SHARP

Immunologic disorder
Malar rash
Discoid rash
Antinuclear antibodies
Mucositis
Neurologic disturbances
Serositis (pleuritis, pericarditis)
Hematologic abnormalities
Arthritis
Renal disorders
Photosensitivity

DIAGNOSIS

- Diagnostic criteria for SLE include a history of at least four of the findings summarized by the mnemonic **I'M DAMN SHARP.**
- Laboratory tests may be useful for confirming the diagnosis. ANA is over 95% *sensitive* for SLE, but not very specific. Antibodies to double-stranded DNA (**anti-dsDNA**) are very *specific* and are associated with a poor prognosis. Anti-Smith (**anti-Sm**) antibodies are also very *specific* for SLE, but not prognostic. **Antihistone** antibodies can be seen in certain cases of drug-induced lupus.

TREATMENT

The treatment for lupus depends on its manifestations. Nonsteroidal anti-inflammatory drugs (NSAIDs) are the typical treatment for arthritis, and sunscreen can be used for photosensitivity. **Systemic steroids** are often given if there is major organ involvement, but chronic use carries a risk of avascular necrosis, osteoporosis, diabetes, and ocular disease. Hydroxychloroquine is used for skin disease and arthritis. The cytotoxic agent cyclophosphamide and the antimetabolites mycophenolate mofetil and azathioprine are particularly useful for treating lupus nephritis.

PROGNOSIS

SLE is an unpredictable disease, and outcomes vary drastically. It is typical for patients to experience a series of relapses and remissions, although symptom-free periods may last for years. Prognosis is improved with early detection and treatment for kidney disease. Death can occur secondary to renal failure, infection, stroke, or other complications.

Progressive Systemic Sclerosis (Scleroderma)

A generalized rheumatologic disorder of connective tissue, progressive systemic sclerosis is characterized by degenerative and inflammatory changes leading to fibrosis and collagen deposition. The disease is more common in women and typically manifests between the ages of 30 and 50 years. The overall cause is unknown, but several pathogenic mechanisms have been proposed, including endothelial cell injury, fibroblast activation, and immunologic derangement. T cells sensitized to collagen and other skin antigens infiltrate the skin of patients with systemic sclerosis. **Antitopoisomerase** (formerly anti-Scl-70) antibodies are associated with diffuse systemic sclerosis and **anticentromere** antibodies are associated with limited systemic sclerosis (CREST syndrome).

PRESENTATION

Skin involvement is almost universal in patients with progressive systemic sclerosis. Skin may be edematous or indurated early in the disease, but progresses to sclerosis with hair loss, decreased sweating, and loss of the ability to make a skin fold. This gives the skin a characteristic tight and shiny appearance. Other common manifestations of the disease include:

- **Raynaud phenomenon,** episodic attacks of vasospasm, which cause tingling and color change in the digits, progressing from white to blue to red (Figure 6-17). This phenomenon can be precipitated by cold temperature, emotional upset, and cigarette smoking.
- **Telangiectasias,** punctate macular lesions representing dilated small vessels just beneath the dermis. These can be seen on the face, palms, and digits (Figure 6-18).

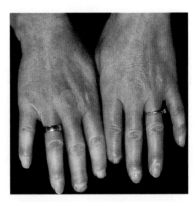

FIGURE 6-17.   Hands of a patient with systemic sclerosis showing sclerodactyly and Raynaud phenomenon. (Reproduced with permission from Wolff K, Johnson RA, Suurmond D. *Fitzpatrick's Color Atlas & Synopsis of Clinical Dermatology*, 5th ed. New York: McGraw-Hill, 2005: 399.)

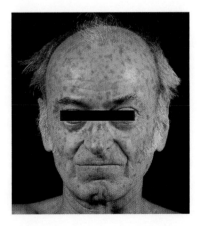

FIGURE 6-18.   Telangiectasias covering the face of a man with CREST syndrome. (Reproduced with permission from Wolff K, Johnson RA, Suurmond D. *Fitzpatrick's Color Atlas & Synopsis of Clinical Dermatology*, 5th ed. New York: McGraw-Hill, 2005: 401.)

In the GI tract, systemic sclerosis can manifest with dilation and impaired motility of the lower esophagus, atony of the small bowel with bacterial overgrowth and malabsorption, or dilation of the large intestine with formation of pseudodiverticula. In the lungs, pulmonary interstitial fibrosis and pulmonary hypertension can occur. Patients with rapidly progressive disease may experience the sudden onset of malignant hypertension leading to acute renal failure.

There are multiple subtypes of progressive systemic sclerosis, with differing manifestations and prognoses.

- **Diffuse systemic sclerosis** is characterized by widespread skin involvement, rapid progression, and early visceral involvement. Skin changes appear rapidly following the development of Raynaud's phenomenon. This subtype of systemic sclerosis is associated with antitopoisomerase antibodies (formerly anti-Scl-70).
- Limited systemic sclerosis, or **CREST syndrome,** is associated with a clinical course characterized by **calcinosis, Raynaud phenomenon, esophageal dysmotility, sclerodactyly,** and **telangiectasia.** Skin changes typically appear years after Raynaud phenomenon and are often limited to the face and distal extremities. This subtype of systemic sclerosis is associated with anticentromere antibodies.
- **Localized scleroderma,** or morphea, is confined to the skin, with no visceral involvement.

DIAGNOSIS

History and physical evaluation are typically the basis for a diagnosis of scleroderma. Serologic testing for antitopoisomerase or anticentromere antibodies can be used to support the diagnosis but not exclude it. ANAs are present in about 95% of patients. Skin biopsy specimen demonstrating atrophy and thinning of the epidermis, fibrosis, and focal collections of lymphocytes in the deep dermis, and loss of dermal appendages such as hair follicles and sweat glands can be helpful in some cases.

TREATMENT

There are no FDA-approved treatments for systemic sclerosis. D-Penicillamine may be used to treat the skin manifestations. Severe Raynaud's phenomenon may be treated with calcium channel blockers. Angiotensin-converting enzyme (ACE) inhibitors are used to treat hypertension and prevent progression to renal crisis. Cyclophosphamide may be used for fulminant presentations or in cases of active alveolitis.

PROGNOSIS

Diffuse systemic sclerosis is a serious disease with a 10-year survival rate of about 20%. Prognosis is improving with increased use of ACE inhibitors to prevent renal crisis, which was formerly the leading cause of death. Pulmonary involvement is now the primary cause of mortality.

CREST syndrome is a more benign disease with a 10-year survival rate of > 70%.

Sjögren Syndrome

A chronic autoimmune disorder, Sjögren syndrome is characterized by lymphocytic infiltration of the exocrine glands. It is the second most common rheumatologic disorder (after RA) and is much more common in women than in men. It can occur either as a primary disease or secondary to other autoimmune disorders, such as RA and SLE. The pathogenesis of the disease involves circulating autoantibodies that cause activated T and B cells to accumulate around blood vessels and ducts, particularly in the salivary and lacrimal glands. These autoantibodies target the **muscarinic acetylcholine receptor,** chronic stimulation of which ultimately causes parenchymal tissue to lose the ability to produce fluid (eg, saliva and tears). As the disease progresses, it may affect other major organ systems and can rarely evolve into malignant lymphoma.

PRESENTATION

The hallmark symptoms of Sjögren syndrome are dry mouth (**xerostomia**) and dry eyes (**xerophthalmia**). This combination of symptoms can lead to difficulty chewing, dysphagia, dental caries, periodontal disease, keratoconjunctivitis, impairment in vision, and corneal ulcerations. Parotid gland enlargement is common. Other symptoms can include arthralgias, myalgias, Raynaud's phenomenon, and nonthrombocytopenic purpura.

DIAGNOSIS

The damaged corneal epithelium can be visualized using the Rose Bengal stain. Both ANA and rheumatoid factor (RF) are usually present. **Anti-Ro (SS-A)** and **anti-La (SS-B)** are associated with earlier onset, longer duration, and more extraglandular manifestations. Salivary gland biopsy reveals a **lymphocytic infiltrate.**

TREATMENT

Treatment of Sjögren syndrome focuses on relieving symptoms and includes artificial tears, lozenges, and oral hygiene.

PROGNOSIS

Primary Sjögren syndrome generally has a good prognosis unless significant extraglandular manifestations develop. The prognosis for secondary disease depends on the primary autoimmune disorder. Patients have a small risk of developing lymphoma.

Reactive Arthritis

Reactive arthritis is an autoimmune disease characterized by urethritis, conjunctivitis, arthritis, and mucocutaneous lesions. Also known by its older name, Reiter syndrome, this disease occurs in two forms. The **postvenereal** (endemic) form is triggered following urethritis or cervicitis, usually caused by *Chlamydia trachomatis* or *Mycoplasma pneumoniae.* The **postdysenteric** (epidemic) form is triggered following infectious diarrhea, usually due to *Shigella flexneri, Salmonella,* or *Yersinia.* The postvenereal form occurs almost exclusively in males, whereas the postdysenteric form affects both sexes equally. HLA-B27 is present in 80% of patients.

PRESENTATION

Symptoms generally appear 1–3 weeks after the inciting episode of urethritis/cervicitis or diarrhea. **Urethritis** ultimately occurs regardless of the inciting infection. **Arthritis** mainly affects the lower extremities and is asymmetrical. **Conjunctivitis** is usually accompanied by mucopurulent discharge, lid edema, and anterior uveitis. **Mucocutaneous lesions** can include painless superficial ulcers of the palate and buccal mucosa, painless ulcers on the penis (balanitis circinata), and a hyperkeratotic rash affecting the soles, palms, scrotum, trunk, and scalp (keratoderma blennorrhagica).

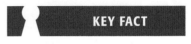

KEY FACT

The combination of xerostomia and xerophthalmia is known as the **sicca complex.**

KEY FACT

The **seronegative spondyloarthropathies** are a group of related inflammatory joint diseases associated with HLA-B27. These include the **PAIR** diseases:
- **P**soriatic arthritis
- **A**nkylosing spondylitis
- **I**nflammatory bowel disease with enteropathic arthritis
- **R**eactive arthritis

Serologic testing for RF is typically negative in these diseases.

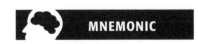

MNEMONIC

Reactive arthritis:
Hurts to see (conjunctivitis)
Hurts to pee (urethritis)
Hurts to climb a tree (arthritis)

DIAGNOSIS

History and physical evaluation are sufficient to make the diagnosis of reactive arthritis. Aspirates of joint fluid are usually sterile, and examination of biopsy specimen of the rash is indistinguishable from that for psoriasis.

TREATMENT

NSAIDs are the mainstay of treatment for joint symptoms. Sulfasalazine is an alternative for patients who have a contraindication to or do not experience relief from NSAIDs.

PROGNOSIS

The disease is usually self-limited, lasting between 2 and 6 months. Symptoms recur in about 50% of patients, but permanent joint damage is uncommon.

Sarcoidosis

Sarcoidosis is a multisystemic disorder characterized by an exaggerated cellular immune response to an unknown antigen, leading to the formation of **noncaseating, "naked" granulomas** in affected tissues. It is most common in black females between the ages of 20 and 40.

PRESENTATION

Sarcoidosis can occur in any organ system, but most commonly affects the lungs and lymph nodes. It is asymptomatic in about 50% of patients and is often diagnosed incidentally after radiographic imaging for other reasons. **Dyspnea** is the most common complaint. Patients may also present with vague constitutional symptoms such as fever, malaise, weight loss, and fatigue.

DIAGNOSIS

Chest radiography is an important tool in differentiating sarcoidosis from other granulomatous diseases involving the lungs, as described in Table 6-22. Definitive diagnosis is made by biopsy, often requiring 5–10 samples from the lung parenchyma. Histologic characteristics of sarcoidosis in comparison with other granulomatous diseases are described in Table 6-23.

TREATMENT

Steroids are the mainstay of therapy for patients with symptomatic sarcoidosis, although exact regimens vary drastically according to the location and severity of the disease.

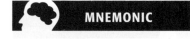

MNEMONIC

The major features of sarcoidosis can be remembered with the mnemonic **GRAIN:**

Gammaglobulinemia
Rheumatoid arthritis
ACE increase
Interstitial fibrosis
Noncaseating granulomas

TABLE 6-22. **Differentiating Granulomatous Diseases by Chest Film**

	SARCOIDOSIS	**TUBERCULOSIS**	**HYPERSENSITIVITY PNEUMONITIS**
Hilar adenopathy	Bilateral	Unilateral	Absent
Parenchymal infiltrate	Lower/middle fields	Localized or miliary	Diffuse
Cavity formation	Rare	Common	Rare
Pleural effusion	Unusual	Common	Absent

TABLE 6-23. Differentiating Granulomatous Diseases by Histology

	SARCOIDOSIS	TUBERCULOSIS	HYPERSENSITIVITY PNEUMONITIS
Caseation	Absent	Present	Rare
Necrosis	Rare	Present	Rare
Inclusions	Present (70%)	Rare	Rare
Eosinophils	Present	Minimal	Prominent
Bronchiolitis	Rare	Rare	Present

PROGNOSIS

Most cases of sarcoidosis resolve spontaneously, usually over a period of about 2–5 years. One-third of cases persist for longer than 5 years, and 5% result in death. Pulmonary fibrosis and extrapulmonary manifestations such as chronic iritis, lupus pernio (violaceous plaques on the face [nose, ears, cheeks] or digits), and tracheal involvement are associated with a less favorable prognosis.

OTHER AUTOIMMUNE DISEASES

Autoimmune diseases associated with specific organ systems are covered in greater detail elsewhere, but autoantibody targets and clinical features are summarized in Table 6-24.

TABLE 6-24. Autoantibody Targets and Clinical Features of Autoimmune Diseases

DISEASE	AUTOANTIBODY TARGET(S)	CLINICAL FEATURES
Systemic Autoimmune Diseases		
Systemic lupus erythematosus	Cell nucleus (ANA), double-stranded DNA, Smith, histone.	Arthritis, malar rash, nephritis, serositis, photosensitivity.
CREST syndrome	Centromere.	Calcinosis, Raynaud phenomenon, esophageal dysmotility, sclerodactyly, telangiectasias.
Sjögren syndrome	Ro/SSA, La/SSB).	Xerostomia, xerophthalmia, parotid enlargement.
Reactive arthritis	Unknown.	Urethritis, conjunctivitis, arthritis, mucocutaneous lesions.
Sarcoidosis	Unknown.	Dyspnea, constitutional symptoms, incidental finding on chest film.
Diseases of the Vascular System		
Vasculitis (multiple)	Neutrophil cytoplasm components (eg, C-ANCA, P-ANCA).	Hemoptysis (lung involvement), hematuria and proteinuria (renal involvement), palpable purpura (skin involvement).

(continues)

TABLE 6-24. Autoantibody Targets and Clinical Features of Autoimmune Diseases *(continued)*

Disease	Autoantibody Target(s)	Clinical Features
Diseases of the Endocrine System		
Diabetes mellitus type I	Pancreatic islet cells, insulin.	Thirst, polyuria, hyperglycemia, retinopathy, nephropathy, neuropathy, ketoacidosis.
Graves disease	Thyroid-stimulating hormone receptor, thyroid peroxidase.	Hyperthyroidism, proptosis, pretibial myxedema.
Hashimoto thyroiditis	Thyroid peroxidase, thyroglobulin.	Hypothyroidism with episodes of hyperthyroidism.
Diseases of the Gastrointestinal System		
Celiac disease (nontropical sprue)	Tissue transglutaminase, gliadin, endomysium.	Ingestion of **gluten** causes diarrhea, steatorrhea, nausea, vomiting.
Primary biliary cirrhosis	Mitochondria.	Pruritus, jaundice, hepatomegaly, xanthelasma, transaminitis, hypercholesterolemia.
Primary sclerosing cholangitis	Neutrophil cytoplasm components (P-ANCA).	Pruritus, jaundice, hepatomegaly, **"beading" of bile ducts** on ERCP.
Autoimmune hepatitis	Smooth muscle, liver-kidney-microsome.	Jaundice, ascites, spider angiomata, esophageal varices, transaminitis.
Diseases of the Blood		
Autoimmune hemolytic anemia	Red blood cells.	Pallor, fatigue.
Pernicious anemia	Parietal cells, intrinsic factor.	Cobalamin (vitamin B_{12}) deficiency, **megaloblastic anemia, atrophic glossitis,** neuropathic pain and paresthesias, myelopathy.
Idiopathic thrombocytopenic purpura	Platelet membrane glycoproteins (eg, glycoprotein IIb/IIIa).	Petechiae, ecchymoses, epistaxis, easy bruisability.

TABLE 6-24. Autoantibody Targets and Clinical Features of Autoimmune Diseases *(continued)*

DISEASE	AUTOANTIBODY TARGET(S)	CLINICAL FEATURES
Diseases of the Musculoskeletal System		
Rheumatoid arthritis	Fc portion of IgG (rheumatoid factor).	Symmetrical arthritis, swan-neck and boutonniere deformities, morning stiffness.
Diseases of the Skin		
Pemphigus vulgaris	Desmoglein-3 and desmoglein-1.	Oropharyngeal erosions, flaccid cutaneous vesicles and bullae.
Pemphigus foliaceus	Desmoglein-1.	Crusts and occasionally, delicate flaccid cutaneous vesicles and bullae.
Epidermolysis bullosa acquisita	Type VII collagen (anchoring fibrils).	Tense vesicles and bullae leading to erosions on extensor surfaces of hands, elbows, knees, and ankles.
Bullous pemphigoid	BPAg1, BPAg2 (type XVII collagen).	Intensely pruritic urticarial patches followed by tense vesicles bullae on the trunk and extremities.
Cicatricial pemphigoid	Epiligrin, BPAg2, BPAg1.	Ocular lesions causing red eye, itching, and burning leading to scarring. Oral and genital erosions.
Linear IgA bullous dermatosis	BPAg2.	Vesicles and bullae on trunk and extremities, ocular lesions causing pain and discharge.
Dermatitis herpetiformis	Epidermal transglutaminase-3.	Pruritic vesicles and crusts on elbows, knees, and buttocks (associated with celiac disease).
Diseases of the Nervous System		
Myasthenia gravis	**Postsynaptic** nicotinic acetylcholine receptors.	Facial muscle weakness that spreads to the trunk and limbs.
Lambert-Eaton myasthenic syndrome	Voltage-gated calcium channels on the **presynaptic** motor nerve terminal.	Proximal muscle weakness of the lower extremities, autonomic dysfunction (dry mouth, constipation, pupillary constriction, sweating).
Multiple sclerosis	Myelin.	Fatigue, paresthesias, tremor, optic neuritis.
Autoimmune inner ear disease	Various inner ear antigens.	Bilateral sensorineural hearing loss.
Diseases of the Renal System		
Goodpasture syndrome	Glomerular basement membrane, pulmonary basement membrane.	Oliguria, nephritic syndrome, pulmonary hemorrhage.

C-ANCA = circulating antineutrophilic cytoplasmic antibody; ECRP = endoscopic retrograde cholangiopancreatography; P-ANCA = perinuclear antineutrophilic cytoplasmic antibody.

NOTES

Pathology

NEOPLASIA

Neoplasia refers to an abnormal and unregulated growth of cells within the body that typically arises from clonal proliferation of a single cell. These cells are unresponsive to normal cell regulation and continue to divide and grow beyond the normal needs of the organism. The word *neoplasia* is derived from the Greek *neo* (new) and *plasia* (growth). Before a tissue becomes neoplastic, other cellular changes are usually detected, as listed below.

Definitions

- **Hyperplasia:** Increase in the **number** of cells (reversible). *Hyper-* = excessive.
- **Metaplasia:** Replacement of one adult cell type by another (can be reversible). Often secondary to irritation or environmental exposure (eg, squamous metaplasia in the trachea and bronchi of smokers). *Meta-* = transformation.
- **Dysplasia:** Abnormal growth with loss of cellular orientation, shape, and size compared with normal tissue maturation. Commonly preneoplastic (can be reversible). *Dys-* = abnormal.
- **Anaplasia:** Abnormal cells that are undifferentiated and resemble primitive cells of the original tissue. *Ana-* = backward.

Cell Types

Neoplasms usually consist of cells of **epithelial** or **mesenchymal** origin. Epithelial tissues are derived from either the embryological ectoderm or endoderm. Mesenchymal tissues derived from embryological mesoderm include blood cells, vessels, smooth muscle, skeletal muscle, bone, and fat. Tumors consisting of cells derived from all three germ layer are called **teratomas.**

Nomenclature

- **Prefix:** The prefix of the term used for a neoplasm depends on the tissue type, as seen in Table 7-1.

TABLE 7-1. Tumor Nomenclature by Cell Type and Type of Neoplastic Process

CELL TYPE	BENIGN	MALIGNANT
Epithelium	▪ Adenoma. ▪ Papilloma.	▪ Adenocarcinoma ▪ Papillary carcinoma
Blood cells	All blood cell neoplasms are malignant.	▪ Leukemia ▪ Lymphoma
Blood vessels	Hemangioma.	Angiosarcoma
Smooth muscle	Leiomyoma.	Leiomyosarcoma
Skeletal muscle	Rhabdomyoma.	Rhabdomyosarcoma
Bone	Osteoma.	Osteosarcoma
Fat	Lipoma.	Liposarcoma
> 1 Cell type	Mature teratoma.	Immature teratoma

- **Suffix, benign neoplasm:** The suffix *-oma* is generally used for benign neoplastic processes.
- **Suffix, malignant neoplasm:** Malignant neoplasms of epithelial origin end in *-carcinoma*, whereas those of mesenchymal origin end in *-sarcoma*.
- **Exception:** Few malignant neoplasms have names that end in *-oma* (eg, melanoma, mesothelioma, immature teratoma, lymphoma).

Neoplastic Progression

Cancerous cells pass through several stages as the disease progresses. Cells in more advanced stages are more poorly differentiated, as outlined in Figure 7-1.

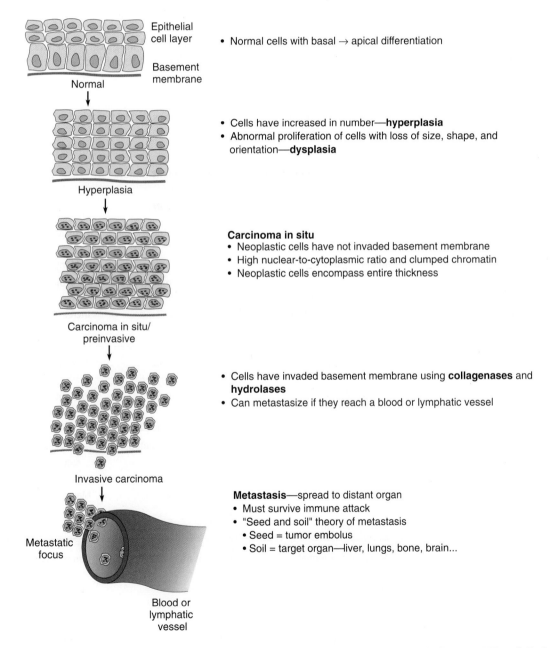

FIGURE 7-1. **Neoplastic progression.** (Modified with permission from McPhee S, Lingappa VR, Ganong WF, et al. *Pathophysiology of Disease: An Introduction to Clinical Medicine*, 3rd ed. New York: McGraw-Hill 2000: 84.)

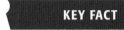
Tumor Grade and Stage

GRADE

Classification system that describes the degree of differentiation of tumor cells based on histologic characteristics.

- Usually graded I–IV based on the degree of differentiation and number of mitoses per high-power field.
- Higher grade = more advanced tumor.

STAGE

- Greater prognostic value than grade.
- Indicates the spread of tumor in a specific patient.
- Based on the site and size of the primary lesion, spread to regional lymph nodes, and the presence or absence of metastases.
- A commonly used staging system is **TNM staging**: **T** for size of **T**umor, **N** for lymph **N**ode involvement, and **M** for **M**etastases.

Characteristics of Neoplastic Cells

Benign and malignant cells have features that distinguish them from each other, as seen in Table 7-2.

TABLE 7-2. Properties of Benign and Malignant Tumors

PROPERTY	BENIGN	MALIGNANT
Differentiation	Well-differentiated	Usually poorly differentiated
Mitotic figures	▪ Few ▪ No atypical mitotic figures	▪ Many ▪ Atypical mitotic figures
Nuclear-to-cytoplasm (N:C) ratio	Normal	Increased
Pleomorphism	Absent or minimal	Present
Hyperchromasia	Absent or minimal	Present
Circumscription and encapsulation	▪ Well-circumscribed ▪ May be encapsulated	▪ Poorly circumscribed ▪ Irregular ▪ Not encapsulated
Homogeneity	Homogeneous	May be heterogeneous
Rate of growth	Usually slow	Rapid
Metastatic potential	Does not metastasize	Can metastasize
Necrosis	No necrosis	May have necrosis/hemorrhage
Physical examination findings	▪ Mobile ▪ Well-defined	▪ Fixed ▪ Irregular; poorly defined

Metastasis

Malignant neoplasms have the potential to metastasize to distant sites. Other than metastasis to regional lymph nodes, the lung, liver, brain, and bone are the most common sites.

METASTASIS TO LIVER

- Metastatic disease of the liver is much more common than primary liver neoplasms.
- Primary neoplasms that metastasize to the liver, in order of decreasing frequency:
    - Colon
    - Stomach
    - Pancreas
    - Breast
    - Lung

METASTASIS TO BRAIN

- Approximately half of brain malignancies are due to metastatic disease from primary neoplasms located elsewhere.
- Primary neoplasms that metastasize to brain:
    - Lung
    - Breast
    - Skin (melanoma)
    - Kidney (renal cell carcinoma)
    - GI tract

METASTASIS TO BONE

- Metastatic disease of bone is much more common than primary bone tumors.
- The most common primary sites are breast and prostate.
- Primary neoplasms that metastasize to bone:
    - Lungs
    - Kidney
    - Thyroid
    - Prostate
    - Testes
    - Breast

DIRECT (LOCAL) EFFECTS OF TUMOR GROWTH

- Destruction of normal architecture (**infiltration**).
    - **Nonhealing ulcers** from destruction of epithelial surfaces, such as those of the stomach, colon, mouth, or bronchus.
    - **Hemorrhage** from ulcerated areas or eroded vessels.
    - **Pain** due to involvement of any site with sensory nerve endings. Most tumors are initially painless.
    - **Seizures and increased intracranial pressure** from space-occupying brain tumors.
    - **Perforation** of a visceral ulcer can lead to **peritonitis** (inflection and inflammation of the peritoneum, the serous membrane that lines the abdominal cavity and the viscera) and **free air (air in the abdominal cavity)**.
    - **Bone involvement** can lead to pathologic fractures.
    - **Inflammation** of a serosal surface leads to **pleural effusion, pericardial effusion**, and **ascites**.

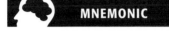

MNEMONIC

Cancer Sometimes Penetrates Benign Liver:

Colon
Stomach
Pancreas
Breast
Lung

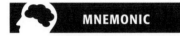

MNEMONIC

Lots of Bad Stuff Kills Glia:

Lung
Breast
Skin
Kidney
GI tract

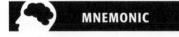

MNEMONIC

Live and Kicking Tumors Penetrate The Bone:

Lung
Kidney
Thyroid
Prostate
Testes
Breast
Alternative: The **K**ids **P**refer **BLT**s.

- Local neurologic deficits: Loss of sensory or motor function caused by nerve compression or destruction (eg, recurrent laryngeal nerve involvement by lung or thyroid cancer results in hoarseness).
- Pressure effects on normal organs or systems (can also occur through infiltration).
- **Obstruction:**
  - Obstructed bronchus → **pneumonia**
  - Obstructed biliary tree → **jaundice**
  - Obstructed intestines → **constipation, strangulation**
  - Obstructed venous or lymphatic drainage → **edema, superior vena cava syndrome**

Paraneoplastic Effects

Various signaling molecules may be secreted by tumors without regulation, leading to systemic effects, as seen in Table 7-3.

Carcinogenesis

Genetic damage can disturb the normal mechanisms that regulate cell proliferation and DNA repair. One genetic disruption often leaves cells vulnerable to others. Damage accumulating over time results in a process called **tumor progression.** Progression often leads to more aggressive tumor cells.

Cancer-related genes can be described under two separate categories:

TABLE 7-3.   **Paraneoplastic Effects of Tumors**

NEOPLASM	MEDIATORS	EFFECT
Squamous cell lung carcinoma.	Parathyroid hormone–related peptide.	Hypercalcemia (most common endocrine paraneoplastic syndrome).
Renal cell carcinoma.	TGF-α.	
Breast carcinoma. Multiple myeloma. Bone metastasis.	TNF-α. Interleukin-2.	Cachexia, fever, inflammation.
Small-cell lung carcinoma.	ACTH or ACTH-like peptide.	Cushing syndrome.
Small-cell lung carcinoma. Intracranial neoplasms.	Antidiuretic hormone or atrial natriuretic peptide.	SIADH.
Renal cell carcinoma.	Erythropoietin.	Polycythemia.
Thymoma. Bronchogenic carcinoma.	Antibodies against presynaptic Ca^{2+} channels at the neuromuscular junction.	Lambert-Eaton myasthenic syndrome.
Carcinoid tumors. Small-cell lung carcinomas.	Gonadotropin-releasing hormone. Growth hormone.	Acromegaly.

ACTH = adrenocorticotropic hormone; SIADH = syndrome of inappropriate antidiuretic hormone secretion; TGF-α = transforming growth factor alpha; TNF-α = tumor necrosis factor alpha.

PROTO-ONCOGENES

- **Action:** Cause cells to grow and proliferate.
- **How they lead to cancer:** Mutations or translocations lead to **activation/overexpression** of these genes, and growth continues in an uncontrolled manner through excessive proliferation or inadequate apoptosis. Associated diseases are listed in Table 7-4.
- **Required hits:** Cancerous growth can occur with a single gene mutation.

TUMOR SUPPRESSOR GENES/ANTIONCOGENES

- **Action:** Regulate normal cell growth and differentiation by inhibiting cell cycle, mediating DNA repair, or initiating apoptosis when too much cell damage has occurred.
- **How they lead to cancer:** Mutations or translocations **inactivate** these genes, leading to genetic instability or unchecked cell proliferation. See Table 7-5 for associated cancers.
- **Required hits:** Usually cause cancer only if both genes are inactivated; "two-hit" hypothesis.

Carcinogenic Agents

Genetic damage can be inherited or can result from exposure to chemicals, radiation, and viruses/microbes.

- **Chemicals:** The diseases associated with chemical exposure are listed in Table 7-6.
  - **Initiators** are chemicals that lead to irreversible damage to a cell's DNA.
  - **Promoters** do not affect the DNA, but promote cell growth and differentiation by other methods; their effects are usually reversible.
- **Radiation:** Penetrant high-energy waves can directly damage DNA.
  - **Ultraviolet (UV) rays** lead to squamous cell carcinoma, basal cell carcinoma, and melanoma in the skin.
  - **UVB rays** specifically lead to the formation of **pyrimidine dimers** in DNA. Usually, the nucleotide excision repair pathway repairs these dimers, but the damage can exceed the cell's ability to repair itself.

KEY FACT

The following can lead to cancer:
Proto-oncogenes: Turned ON
Tumor suppressor genes: Turned OFF

TABLE 7-4.   Proto-Oncogenes and Their Associated Tumor

GENE	ASSOCIATED TUMOR	ACTION
abl	Chronic myelogenous leukemia.	Signal transduction
c-myc	Burkitt's lymphoma.	Transcriptional activator
bcl-2	Follicular and undifferentiated lymphomas.	Inhibits apoptosis
erb-B2/Her-2	Breast, ovarian, and gastric carcinomas.	Growth factor receptor
ras	Colon carcinoma.	Signal transduction
L-*myc*	**L**ung tumor.	Transcriptional activator
N-*myc*	**N**euroblastoma.	Transcriptional activator
ret	Multiple endocrine neoplasia I and II.	Growth factor receptor

TABLE 7-5. **Tumor Suppressor Genes and Associated Tumors**

Gene	Chromosome	Associated Tumor	Action
Rb	13q	▪ Retinoblastoma ▪ Osteosarcoma	Regulation of the cell cycle.
BRCA1 and BRCA2	17q, 13q	Breast and ovarian cancer	DNA repair.
p53	17p	▪ Most human cancers ▪ Li-Fraumeni syndrome	Regulation of the cell cycle and apoptosis after DNA damage.
p16	9p	Melanoma	Cell cycle control/DNA repair.
APC	5q	Colorectal cancer	Inhibition of signal transduction.
WT1	11q	Wilm tumor	Nuclear transcription.
NF1	17q	Neurofibromatosis type 1	Inhibition of ras signal transduction.
NF2	22q	Neurofibromatosis type 2	Signaling and cytoskeletal regulation.
DPC	18q	Pancreatic cancer	Cell surface receptor.
DCC	18q	Colon cancer	Cell surface receptor.

TABLE 7-6. **Chemical Carcinogens**

Toxin	Associated Cancer
Aflatoxins	Hepatocellular carcinoma.
Vinyl chloride	Angiosarcoma of the liver.
CCl_4	Centrilobular necrosis and fatty change of the liver.
Nitrosamines	Esophageal and gastric cancer.
Cigarette smoke	Carcinoma of the larynx and lung.
Asbestos	Mesothelioma and bronchogenic carcinoma.
Arsenic	Squamous cell carcinoma of the skin.
Naphthalene (aniline) dyes	Transitional cell carcinoma.
Alkylating agents	Leukemia.
Alcohol	Hepatocellular carcinoma.
Benzene	Acute leukemia.
Diethylstilbestrol (DES)	Clear cell adenocarcinoma of the vagina in offspring of mothers given the drug during pregnancy.

- **Ionizing radiation** predominantly causes single- and double-stranded breaks. It is associated with a variety of cancers, including **leukemia** in those exposed to atomic blasts, **thyroid cancers** in those who have had previous head and neck radiation, and **osteosarcoma** in watch-dial workers who are exposed to radium.
- **Viruses and microbes:** Can cause cellular or direct DNA damage and thus predispose to cancer, as seen in Table 7-7.

CLINICAL CORRELATION

In **xeroderma pigmentosum,** an autosomal recessive disease, the nucleotide excision repair pathway itself is dysfunctional. Those affected have a high incidence of skin cancer.

Tumor Immunity

Affected cells often display tumor antigens that can stimulate the immune system. Tumor antigens may be specific (tumor-specific antigens [**TSAs**]) if expressed only in tumor cells or associated (tumor-associated antigens [**TAAs**]) if expressed in both normal and tumor cells. These antigens may also be used clinically to confirm the diagnosis, monitor for tumor recurrence, and monitor the response to therapy (Table 7-8). Because these antigens are not expressed by normal tissues or are expressed at relatively low amounts, **cytotoxic T lymphocytes** and **natural killer cells** can recognize and destroy the neoplastic cells. The cancer cells can also escape the immune system through many mechanisms, including:

- Selection for cells that do not express TSAs, TAAs, human leukocyte antigen (HLA), or costimulatory receptors.
- Immunosuppression.

TABLE 7-7. **Viruses and Microbes, Associated Cancers, and Mechanisms**

VIRUS/ MICROBE	ASSOCIATED CANCER	MECHANISM
HPV 16,18	Cervical, vulvar, penile, and anal carcinoma	E7 inactivates *Rb*; E6 disables *p53*.
HTLV-1	Adult T-cell leukemia	The *tax* gene leads to a high rate of proliferation of T cells, which are subsequently vulnerable to mutations and translocations.
HBV, HCV	Hepatocellular carcinoma	Causes chronic liver injury and regenerative hyperplasia, which can increase vulnerability to transformation.
EBV	■ Burkitt lymphoma ■ Nasopharyngeal carcinoma	Leads to proliferation of B cells; high rate of mutations and translocations.
HHV-8	■ Kaposi's sarcoma ■ B-cell lymphoma	Common in immunocompromised patients.
Helicobacter pylori	Gastric cancer	Chronic inflammation.

EBV = Epstein-Barr virus; HBV = hepatitis B virus; HCV = hepatitis C virus; HHV = human herpesvirus; HPV = human papillomavirus; HTLV = human T-lymphotropic virus.

TABLE 7-8. Tumor Antigens and Associated Cancers

ANTIGEN	ASSOCIATED CANCER
Prostatic acid phosphatase	▪ Prostatic carcinoma ▪ Used for screening
Carcinoembryonic antigen	▪ Colorectal, pancreatic, gastric, and breast cancers ▪ Nonspecific
α-Fetoprotein	▪ Hepatocellular carcinomas ▪ Nonseminomatous germ cell tumors of the testis (ex-yolk sac tumor)
β-hCG	▪ Hydatidiform moles ▪ Choriocarcinomas ▪ Gestational trophoblastic tumors
CA-125	Ovarian malignant epithelial tumors
S-100	▪ Melanoma ▪ Neural tumors ▪ Astrocytomas
Alkaline phosphatase	▪ Metastases to bone ▪ Obstructive biliary disease ▪ Paget disease of bone
Bombesin	▪ Neuroblastoma ▪ Lung and gastric cancer
Tartrate-resistant acid phosphatase	Hairy cell leukemia

β-hCG = beta human chorionic gonadotropin.

Epidemiology

Cancer is the second leading cause of death in the United States (after heart disease). For this reason, it is important to understand the epidemiology of cancer.

Common cancers are listed below from most to least common. See also Table 7-9 for cancer incidence and death rates.

▪ **Males:** Prostate, lung, and colorectal.
▪ **Females:** Breast, lung, and colorectal.

Highest mortality rate (from most to least common):

▪ **Males:** Lung, prostate.
▪ **Females:** Lung, breast.

Note: Lung cancer deaths are decreasing in males, but increasing in females.

TABLE 7-9. Cancer Incidence and Death Rates[a] for All Cancer Sites Combined, by Race/Ethnicity and Sex, United States, 2006

	INCIDENCE		DEATH	
	MALE	**FEMALE**	**MALE**	**FEMALE**
All Races	538.8	407.9	221.1	153.7
White	531.0	412.4	218.7	153.4
Black	585.9	381.1	287.8	176.9
American Indian/Alaska Native	282.9	254.5	137.0	108.9
Asian/Pacific Islander	313.3	269.3	128.2	93.3
Hispanic	404.7	317.9	145.4	101.4

[a]Rates are per 100,000 population and age-adjusted to the 2000 U.S. standard population. (*Source:* United States Cancer Statistics: 1999–2006 Incidence and Mortality Web-based Report Pre-release Data.)

These cancers are common in the population at large, but other cancers are associated with particular diseases, as shown in Tables 7-10 and 7-11.

CELL DEATH

There are two major forms of cell death: **apoptosis** and **necrosis.** Apoptosis occurs physiologically, but either type of cell death can occur in pathologic situations. Each type of cell death results in a distinct morphologic appearance.

Apoptosis

Apoptosis is also known as **programmed cell death** because it occurs via a series of distinct and highly regulated steps that all cells can perform. Intracellular enzymes are activated to degrade DNA and proteins. The resulting apoptotic bodies can be cleared by phagocytosis. Because the cellular contents are not released, apoptosis does *not* result in an **inflammatory response** (Figure 7-2).

CAUSES

Apoptosis may be physiologic, usually induced by specific activation of death receptors or loss of growth factors:

- **Programmed tissue removal** during embryogenesis (eg, webbings between the digits).
- Tissue loss in an adult, usually hormone dependent.
- **Cell turnover,** as in intestinal epithelia.
- Death of a host cell after its function has been fulfilled (ie, the end of an immune response).
- Lymphocyte selection.
- Death induced by cytotoxic T cells.

TABLE 7-10. Diseases and Associated Neoplasms

Condition	Neoplasm
Down syndrome	▪ Acute lymphoblastic leukemia ▪ Acute myelogenous leukemia
Albinism	▪ Melanoma ▪ Basal and squamous cancer of the skin
Chronic atrophic gastritis	Gastric adenocarcinoma
Pernicious anemia	
Postsurgical gastric remnants	
Tuberous sclerosis	▪ Astrocytoma ▪ Cardiac rhabdomyoma
Actinic keratosis	Squamous cell carcinoma of the skin
Barrett esophagus/chronic gastroesophageal reflux	Esophageal adenocarcinoma
Plummer-Vinson syndrome	Squamous cell carcinoma of the esophagus
Cirrhosis (alcoholic; hepatitis B or C)	Hepatocellular carcinoma
Ulcerative colitis	Colonic adenocarcinoma
Paget disease of bone	▪ Osteosarcoma ▪ Fibrosarcoma
Immunodeficiency	Malignant lymphomas
AIDS	▪ Aggressive malignant lymphomas (non-Hodgkin) ▪ Kaposi sarcoma
Autoimmune disease (eg, Hashimoto thyroiditis, myasthenia gravis)	Benign and malignant thymomas
Acanthosis nigricans	Visceral malignancy (stomach, lung, breast, uterus)
Dysplastic nevus	Malignant melanoma

Apoptosis can also occur pathologically as a response to cellular damage, usually resulting from more mild injuries in which fewer cells are injured. Common examples include:

▪ **DNA damage** from radiation or cytotoxic drugs.
▪ Certain viral infections (eg, hepatitis).
▪ Pathologic atrophy.
▪ Tumor cell regression or turnover.

TABLE 7-11.   **Inherited Diseases Associated with Cancers**

SYNDROME	INHERITANCE	ASSOCIATED CANCER
Retinoblastoma	Autosomal dominant.	Retinoblastoma.
Familial adenomatous polyposis coli	Autosomal dominant.	Colon adenocarcinoma.
Multiple endocrine neoplasia	Autosomal dominant.	▪ I: Thyroid, parathyroid, adrenal cortex, pancreas, pituitary. ▪ II: Pheochromocytoma, medullary carcinoma of the thyroid. ▪ III: Pheochromocytoma, medullary carcinoma, mucocutaneous neuromas.
Neurofibromatosis	Autosomal dominant.	▪ Neurofibromas. ▪ Pheochromocytomas. ▪ Wilms tumor. ▪ Rhabdomyosarcoma. ▪ Leukemia.
Von Hippel–Lindau syndrome	Autosomal dominant.	▪ Hemangioblastoma. ▪ Adenomas. ▪ Renal cell carcinoma.
Xeroderma pigmentosa	Autosomal recessive (DNA repair).	▪ Melanoma. ▪ Squamous and basal cell carcinoma of the skin.
Ataxia-telangiectasia	Autosomal recessive (DNA repair).	Lymphomas (sensitivity to ionizing radiation).
Bloom syndrome	Autosomal recessive (DNA repair).	Leukemia/lymphoma.
Fanconi anemia	Autosomal recessive (DNA repair).	Myelodysplastic syndrome/leukemia (sensitivity to mitomycin C).
Hereditary nonpolyposis colon cancer syndrome	Autosomal recessive (DNA repair).	Colon, breast, and ovarian cancers.

MORPHOLOGY

The distinctive features of apoptotic cells allow for easily identification by electron microscopy. These include:

- **Cell shrinkage** with dense cytoplasm.
- **Condensation of chromatin** at the periphery of the nuclear membrane.

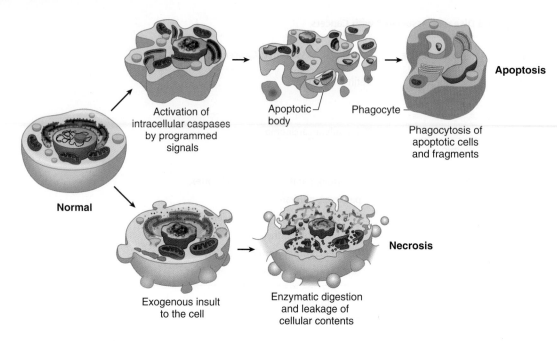

FIGURE 7-2. **Comparison of apoptosis and necrosis.**

- Membrane **cytoplasmic blebs** and cellular fragmentation into apoptotic bodies.
- **Phagocytosis** of apoptotic cells or bodies.

Typically, the plasma membrane remains intact and prevents the cellular contents (eg, lysosomal enzymes) from damaging adjacent tissue or stimulating an inflammatory response. On histologic section, apoptotic cells appear **strongly eosinophilic** with dense chromatin, and are generally found in small groups.

MECHANISMS OF APOPTOSIS

Apoptosis occurs when signals activate **caspases,** which are a family of cysteine proteases. The activated caspases cleave the cellular cytoskeleton proteins. They also activate DNAses, which fragment the nuclear DNA into 50- to 300-kilobase pieces. This is seen as a **DNA ladder** when extracted DNA is run on gel electrophoresis. Apoptotic cells also flip **phosphatidylserine** from the inner to the outer layer of their plasma membrane, which targets the cell for clearance by macrophages.

Apoptosis can be induced by two separate pathways, as seen in Figure 7-3: Extrinsic (death receptor–initiated) or intrinsic (mitochondrial).

- The **extrinsic pathway** is activated when **death receptors,** such as the type 1 tumor necrosis factor receptor, or Fas, on the cell surface are stimulated. Cross-linking of these death receptors leads to signaling that activates caspase-8. This pathway of apoptosis is blocked by a protein called FLIP.

The **intrinsic pathway** involves the release of proteins, including **cytochrome c,** from a leaky mitochondrion. These proteins activate caspase-9. Intrinsic apoptosis is regulated by a balance between proapoptotic cellular molecules Bak, Bax, and Bim, and antiapoptotic molecules Bcl-2 and Bcl-x.

Both of these pathways converge on the same cascade of activated caspases. Each caspase exists as a zymogen, or inactive proenzyme, and is activated through cleavage by the previous caspase in the cascade. Caspases, including

CLINICAL CORRELATION

In follicular lymphoma, a type of non-Hodgkin's lymphoma, translocation of chromosomal arms of 14 and 18 results in uncontrolled Bcl-2 expression, which prevents apoptosis and leads to uncontrolled cell growth.

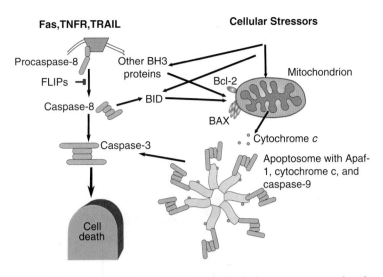

Fas,TNFR,TRAIL

Cellular Stressors

Procaspase-8

Other BH3 proteins

FLIPs

Bcl-2

Mitochondrion

Caspase-8

BID

BAX

Cytochrome c

Caspase-3

Apoptosome with Apaf-1, cytochrome c, and caspase-9

Cell death

FIGURE 7-3. **Two major pathways of apoptosis.** Both the intrinsic (mitochondrion-based) and extrinsic (death receptor) signaling pathways are shown. Apaf, apoptotic proteinase-activating factor; BAX, Bcl-2 associated X protein; Bcl-2, BH3. Bcl-2 homology domain; BID, Bcl-2 interacting domain; FLIP, FLICE inhibitory protein; TNFR, tumor necrosis factor receptors, TRAIL, TNF-related apoptosis-inducing ligand. (Modified with permission from Lichtman M, Beutler E, Kipps T, et al. *Williams Hematology*, 7th ed. New York: McGraw-Hill, 2006: 153.)

caspase-3 and caspase-6, function as "ultimate executioners" and promote protein cleavage and DNA breakdown within the cell.

Necrosis

Necrosis is uncontrolled degradation of cells in living tissues following irreparable cellular damage. The plasma membrane is often disrupted, releasing cellular contents into the surrounding area; this results in tissue damage and an inflammatory response. Debris is enzymatically digested and ultimately phagocytosed. If necrotic cells are not removed, they promote mineral deposition, leading to **dystrophic calcification.**

CAUSES

Necrosis is generally considered to be due to irreversible exogenous injury that exceeds the body's ability to repair itself. This can have many forms:

- **Ischemia/hypoxia** is the most common type of cell injury.
- **Ischemia/reperfusion injury** can occur when blood flow returns to ischemic tissue, causing free radical formation.
- Chemical injuries.

MORPHOLOGY

The appearance of damaged cells lies on a continuum between reversibly injured and necrotic cells. Several hallmarks are visible on histologic sections (Figure 7-4):

- Increased eosinophilia.
- **Myelin figures** replace dead cells.
- Breakdown of nuclear DNA leads to **karyolysis,** or loss of chromatin basophilia.
- Alternatively, DNA may condense into a shrunken mass, seen as **pyknosis.**
- A pyknotic nucleus may fragment, in a process called **karyorrhexis;** ultimately, the nucleus disappears.

KEY FACT

Irreversible injuries occur when the cell cannot reverse the disturbances in mitochondrial and membrane function.

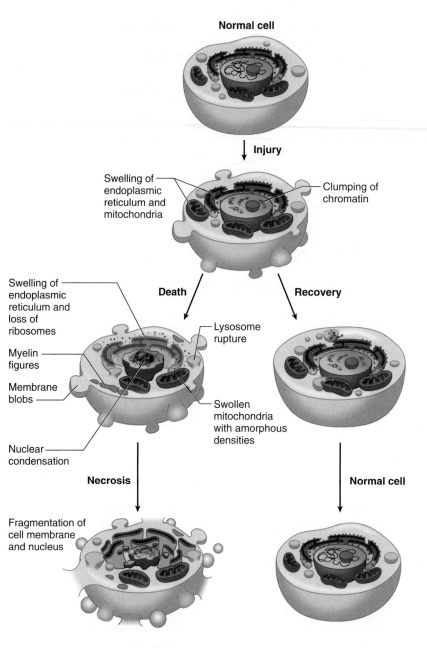

FIGURE 7-4. **Processes of cell injury.**

TYPES OF NECROSIS

Necrosis can take multiple forms, based on the type of injured tissue and mechanism of injury.

- **Coagulative necrosis** is thought to occur when injury causes acidosis and denatures degradative enzymes. The outline of the cell is maintained. Coagulative necrosis results in two types of infarction: (1) pale type, which is found in dense tissues and prevents RBCs from diffusing through the necrotic tissue (eg, heart) and (2) hemorrhagic type, which is found in tissues such as the lungs where RBCs can diffuse through the necrotic tissue (Figure 7-5).
- Bacterial and some fungal infections cause **liquefactive necrosis.** Cell outlines are lost due to enzymatic digestion. Liquefactive necrosis is also observed following hypoxic injury to the central nervous system (CNS).

- **Caseous necrosis** is usually found in granulomas following infection with tuberculosis. The appearance is often described as white and "cheesy." Cells are amorphous, and tissue architecture is completely degraded.
- **Fat necrosis** is not a strict morphologic pattern of necrosis, but refers to necrotic destruction of large areas of fat. Usually due to acute pancreatitis, in which activated pancreatic enzymes degrade adipocytes. Released fat from adipocytes combine with calcium, resulting in **fat saponification.**

Any form of necrosis can result in the release of cellular contents, with subsequent inflammation.

Inflammation

Inflammation is the immune system's response to toxic agents or damaged tissues. This response can be divided into **vascular and cellular reactions,** involves the **secretion of mediators,** and is followed by attempted tissue repair.

Vascular Reaction

Changes in the vasculature allow immune cells and mediators to migrate from the blood vessel to the site of injury. Changes occur in the following order:

- Ultra-short neurogenic reflex of vasoconstriction lasting seconds.
- **Vasodilation** in the arterioles and capillary beds mainly due to the action of histamine and nitric oxide on vascular smooth muscle resulting in increased blood flow to the injured area (causing redness and heat).
- Histamine-mediated **permeability** of the vessel wall along with increased hydrostatic pressure from increased blood flow, resulting in loss of protein-rich fluid into the extracellular tissues (causing swelling).
- Loss of fluid results in increased cellular concentrations in the blood, so flow is slowed, causing **stasis.**
- Stasis allows for increased leukocyte migration through the endothelium.

Cellular Reaction

Leukocytes, particularly neutrophils and macrophages, are responsible for the removal of offending agents and damaged tissue. They are often the first responders at the site of injury. Leukocytes must travel from the blood vessel lumen to the interstitial tissue in a process called **extravasation** (Figure 7-6). This has three steps:

- **Margination, rolling,** and **adhesion** to the endothelium. Endothelium is specially activated to bind cells in inflammatory states.
- **Transmigration (diapedesis)** across the vessel wall.
- **Migration** within the interstitial tissue to the site of injury.

The specific molecules which mediate the steps above are discussed later in this chapter.

On arrival, leukocytes attempt to remove the microbe or other agent via **phagocytosis** and release substances such as lysosomal enzymes, reactive oxygen intermediates, and prostaglandins. These mediators can damage the endothelium and surrounding tissues. Many acute and chronic human diseases result from an excessive inflammatory response.

Chemical Mediators of Inflammation

Mediators are produced in response to microbial products or host proteins activated by microbes or damaged tissues. These chemicals can be activated

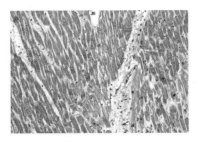

FIGURE 7-5.   Necrosis. High magnification micrograph of a myocardial infarction showing prominent contraction band necrosis with karyolysis (loss of the nuclei), edema and an inflammatory infiltrate consistent of monocytes and lymphocytes. (Image courtesy of Wikipedia; permission granted under the GNU Free Documentation License and Creative Commons Attribution ShareAlike 3.0 license.)

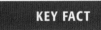

KEY FACT

Remember the five cardinal signs of inflammation:
Rubor = Redness
Tumor = Swelling
Calor = Heat
Dolor = Pain
Function laesa = Loss of function

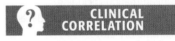

CLINICAL CORRELATION

Defects in leukocyte function compromise the immune response. **Chronic granulomatous disease** is a congenital disorder in which leukocytes cannot generate superoxide, necessary for bacterial killing. This disease results from defects in the genes encoding the reduced form of nicotinamide adenine dinucleotide phosphate (NADPH) oxidase.

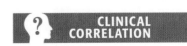

CLINICAL CORRELATION

Leukocyte-induced injury is responsible for both acute diseases (eg, septic shock and vasculitis) and chronic diseases (including arthritis).

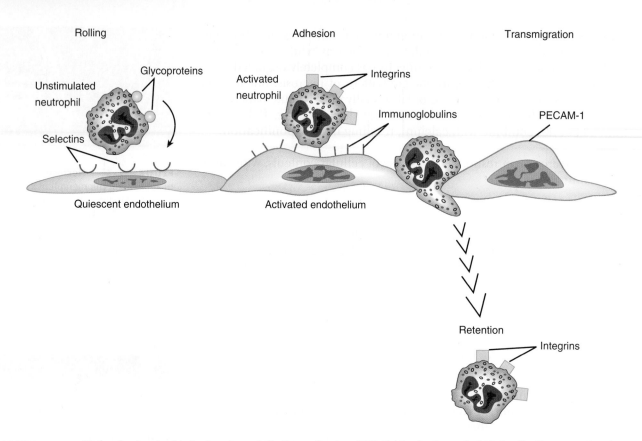

FIGURE 7-6. **Molecules involved in leukocyte-endothelium adhesion.** PECAM-1, platelet endothelial cell adhesion molecule 1.

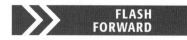

FLASH FORWARD

Many drugs target mediators of inflammation, including antihistamines and nonsteroidal anti-inflammatory drugs.

from precursors in plasma or may be newly produced by cells. Mediators are generally short-lived once they are activated, which helps limit the damage caused by inflammation. They fall into several categories (Table 7-12).

The roles of these mediators in inflammation are summarized in Table 7-13.

Laboratory findings associated with inflammation are summarized in Table 7-14.

Acute Inflammation

Acute inflammation is a rapid vascular and cellular response to an agent causing tissue damage. Onset occurs in seconds to minutes, and the reaction lasts for several hours or days.

STIMULI

Acute inflammatory responses can have multiple causes:

- Microbial infections or toxins.
- Tissue necrosis from any cause (eg, hypoxia).
- Physical (trauma, frostbite) or chemical damage.
- Foreign bodies.
- Hypersensitivity reactions.

MAJOR CELLS INVOLVED

Neutrophils are recruited to the site of injury and are responsible for clearing the area. Other cell types produce inflammatory mediators.

TABLE 7-12. Inflammatory Mediators

Compound	Source	Function
Histamine/ serotonin	Stored preformed in mast cells, platelets, and enterochromaffin cells.	▪ Dilates arterioles. ▪ Increases permeability of venules.
Complement cascade (C3a, C5a)	Plasma.	▪ Functions in innate and adaptive immunity. ▪ Increases vascular permeability.
Coagulation system	Thrombin found in plasma.	Promotes vascular permeability and leukocyte migration.
Kinin system	Plasma.	Release of bradykinin causes contraction of smooth vessel and dilation of blood vessels.
Prostaglandins/ leukotrienes	Many cells.	Contributes to pain and fever during inflammation.
Cytokines	Many cells.	Systemic acute-phase responses (eg, fever, loss of appetite, neutrophilia).
Nitric oxide	Constitutively expressed or induced by cytokine activation.	▪ Potent vasodilator. ▪ Reduces platelet aggregation. ▪ Microbicidal.
Lysosomal enzymes	Leukocytes.	▪ Microbicidal. ▪ Destructive to endothelium and surrounding tissues.
O_2-derived free radicals	Leukocytes (NADPH oxidative system).	▪ Microbicidal. ▪ Destructive to endothelium and surrounding tissues.

NADPH, reduced form of nicotinamide adenine dinucleotide phosphate.

TABLE 7-13. Functions of Chemical Mediators in Inflammation

Sign	Reaction	Mediators
Redness	Vasodilation	Histamine, prostaglandins, nitric oxide (NO).
Heat	Vasodilation, fever	Histamine, prostaglandins, NO, interleukin-1, tumor necrosis factor (TNF).
Swelling	Increased vascular permeability	Histamine, serotonin, bradykinin, leukotrienes.
Pain	Release of mediators	Prostaglandins, bradykinin.
Loss of function	Tissue damage	NO, lysosomal enzymes, O_2-derived free radicals.

TABLE 7-14.　**Associated Lab Findings in Inflammation**

Lab	Findings	Mechanism/Significance
WBC	Leukocytosis; left shift; toxic granulation	IL-1 and TNF mediates leukocytosis, resulting in presence of premature WBCs.
ESR	Elevated ESR	Inflammatory factors promote RBC rouleaux formation, resulting in prolongation of the rate of RBC settling in a vertical tube.
CRP	Elevated; an acute phase reactant	Sensitive indicator of acute inflammation. May be used as a marker to monitor disease states and therapy.
Albumin	Decreased	Due to catabolic action of inflammation. The liver synthesizes acute-phase reactants from albumin breakdown. Prealbumin is not affected by inflammation and may be a better marker of protein nutritional state.
LFTs	Elevated	LFTs such as AST and ALT may be elevated in inflammatory states secondary to cellular damage in the liver.

ALT = alanine aminotransferase; AST = aspartate aminotransferase; CRP = C-reactive protein; ESR = erythrocyte sedimentation rate; IL = interleukin; LFTs = liver function tests; TNF = tumor necrosis factor.

MORPHOLOGIC FEATURES

Major patterns of acute inflammation are dictated by the location, duration, and cause of inflammation.

- **Serous inflammation** is marked by a thin fluid, similar to that seen in a blister, surrounding the injured area.
- **Fibrinous inflammation** results from more serious injuries that allow the larger molecule fibrin to pass through the vessel wall. The fibrinous exudates may organize to form scar tissue if not removed by macrophages. This pattern is characteristic of inflammation of body cavity linings, such as the pericardium, pleura, and meninges.
- **Purulent inflammation** is marked by the production of pus, an exudative fluid (protein-rich) containing neutrophils and necrotic cells. A contained area of purulent inflammation is referred to as an **abscess,** and is commonly seen in bacterial infections.
- When a sufficient amount of necrotic inflammatory tissue is removed from the skin or any mucosal surface, a local defect, which reveals the dermis or the lamina propria, respectively, is formed. This is what is known as an **ulcer.** Mucosal ulcers occur most commonly in the gastrointestinal tract (eg, after prolonged aspirin use). Skin ulcers, on the other hand, are commonly the result of poor blood circulation (such as in the case of diabetic patients).

OUTCOMES

Acute inflammation has three possible outcomes:

- **Progression** to chronic inflammation.
- **Resolution,** resulting in clearance of the harmful stimulus and rebuilding of injured tissue. The tissue regains its normal function.
- **Fibrosis,** in which the damaged tissue is replaced with scar tissue. The tissue loses its function permanently.

Chronic Inflammation

Inflammation, tissue destruction, and tissue repair proceed simultaneously for a longer duration.

CAUSES OF CHRONIC INFLAMMATION

- **Persistent microbial and viral infection:** Characteristically caused by tuberculosis, syphilis, or particular viral, fungal, or parasitic infections. Organisms evoke a delayed-type hypersensitivity reaction from the host. Incomplete clearance of the organism leads to chronic inflammation.
- **Ongoing exposure to a toxic agent:** May be exogenous, as in silicosis due to long-term inhalation of silica, or endogenous, such as the reaction to plasma lipids in atherosclerosis.
- **Autoimmune diseases,** in which the inflammatory response to autoantigens results in tissue damage.

MAJOR CELLS INVOLVED

Chronic inflammation is marked by infiltration of mononuclear cells, especially **macrophages.** Macrophages promote fibrosis and angiogenesis through their production of growth factors and cytokines but also cause tissue damage by releasing reactive oxygen species and proteases. Lymphocytes, plasma cells, eosinophils, and mast cells may also be involved.

MORPHOLOGIC FEATURES

Generally, chronic inflammation is characterized by the presence of mononuclear cells, damaged tissue, and tissue repair. Repair is visible as fibrosis (formation of connective tissue) and angiogenesis (growth of new blood vessels).

Granulomatous inflammation is a distinctive type of chronic inflammation. Causes of granulomatous inflammation include: (1) **infectious** (eg, tuberculosis, histoplasmosis) and (2) **noninfectious** (eg, sarcoidosis, Crohn disease). Granulomatous inflammation is characterized by the formation of granulomas, focal sites of inflammation consisting of **central caseous necrosis** surrounded by macrophages, some of which form giant cells with multiple nuclei at the periphery (**Langhans-type giant cells**), as seen in Figure 7-7. The periphery of the granuloma is surrounded by lymphocytes and the occasional plasma cell. Granulomas can also have **noncaseous necrosis,** usually in response to foreign bodies or in sarcoidosis. In these cases, giant cells have nuclei scattered throughout the cell (foreign body–type giant cell).

OUTCOMES

Chronic inflammation causes fibrosis, with resultant loss of function.

CELL ADHESION

The inflammatory response requires migration of leukocytes to the site of inflammation. This occurs via an interaction between various specific adhesion molecules within the **selectin, integrin, mucin-like glycoprotein,** and **immunoglobulin families on endothelial cells and other leukocytes.** Surface expression and avidity of these molecules can be modulated by chemical mediators, such as cytokines.

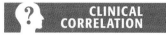

CLINICAL CORRELATION

The delayed-type hypersensitivity reaction in tuberculosis is the basis for the purified protein derivative (PPD) skin test.

KEY FACT

Caseous necrosis indicates an infectious disease, prototypically tuberculosis. Noncaseous necrosis is found in sarcoidosis and Crohn disease.

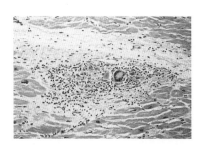

FIGURE 7-7. Sarcoidosis. Photomicrograph shows a noncaseating granuloma with a multinucleated giant cell (H&E, ×40). (Reproduced with permission from Fuster V, Alexander RW, O'Rourke RA. *Hurst's The Heart,* 11th ed. New York: McGraw-Hill, 2004: 1963.)

The different families are involved in distinct steps of the leukocyte response (Figure 7-6).

- **Rolling:** Leukocytes migrate to the vessel periphery and move along the endothelium.
  - The endothelium increases expression of **selectins**.
  - Selectins bind with low affinity to leukocyte **sialyl-Lewis X glycoproteins**.
- **Adhesion:** Leukocytes bind firmly to endothelial cells:
  - The endothelium expresses immunoglobulin members vascular cell adhesion molecule 1 (**VCAM-1**) and intercellular adhesion molecule 1 (**ICAM-1**).
  - VCAM-1 and ICAM-1 bind with high affinity to **integrins** on the leukocyte surface.
- **Transmigration:** Leukocytes pass through the endothelium into tissue. Immunoglobulin **platelet endothelial cell adhesion molecule (PECAM-1)** or **CD31** in the interendothelial space facilitates movement.
- **Retention in tissue:** Leukocytes remain in the extracellular space.
- **Integrins** on the leukocyte surface bind to matrix proteins at the site of inflammation.

HLA ASSOCIATIONS

Major histocompatibility complex (MHC) alleles associated with autoimmune diseases are primarily located within the classical MHC II loci. MHC II presents antigen to CD4+ T cells, which in turn activate B cells to produce antibody. Therefore, the binding specificities of these alleles are directly linked to the capacity of MHC II to bind self-antigen and initiate an autoimmune disease.

HLA Genes

In humans there are four **HLA genes** known as *HLA-A, HLA-B, HLA-C,* and *HLA-D. HLA-A, HLA-B,* and *HLA-C* produce MHC class I molecules, which are expressed by most all nucleated cells. They allow immune cells to monitor the cytoplasmic contents of each cell, especially during intracellular infections.

HLA-D, on the other hand, produces MHC class II molecules, which are only expressed by specialized cells (such as B cells, macrophages, dendritic cells, and other "antigen presenters") which display material acquired from extracellular spaces (eg, bacterial proteins). *HLA-D* is now recognized to contain three separate genes known as *HLA-DP, HLA-DQ,* and *HLA-DR,* with *HLA-DR* being the most extensively studied and related to certain human diseases.

HLA Polymorphism and Disease Risk

Each HLA gene is highly **polymorphic,** which is to say that there are many variants or alleles in the human population. Each variant is given a different number, such as *HLA-B8, HLA-B27, HLA-DR2,* or *HLA-DR3.* (Note that a single individual can, at most, have two variants for any particular HLA gene, one from his or her mother and the other from his or her father.)

Because HLA molecules are in the business of presenting antigens, it is thought that they may be able to bind self-proteins and elicit autoimmunity. Some alleles predispose to certain autoimmune diseases, whereas others are associated with increased incidence and severity as summarized in Table 7-15.

TABLE 7-15. **HLA-Associated Diseases**

HLA Type	Disease Association
B8	▪ Graves disease ▪ Celiac sprue
B27	▪ Ankylosing spondylitis ▪ Reactive arthritis ▪ Reiter syndrome ▪ Acute anterior uveitis ▪ Psoriasis ▪ Inflammatory bowel disease
DR2	▪ Goodpasture syndrome ▪ Multiple sclerosis ▪ Narcolepsy ▪ SLE ▪ Hay fever ▪ *Protective* in type 1 diabetes mellitus (type 1 DM)
DR3	▪ Celiac disease ▪ Myasthenia gravis ▪ SLE ▪ Graves disease ▪ Type 1 DM ▪ Idiopathic Addison disease
DR4	▪ Rheumatoid arthritis ▪ Type 1 DM ▪ Pemphigus vulgaris
DR5	▪ Hashimoto thyroiditis ▪ Pernicious anemia
DR7	Steroid-responsive nephritic syndrome
DR11	▪ Hashimoto thyroiditis ▪ Celiac disease
Dw3	Sjögren syndrome
Dw4	Rheumatoid arthritis

SLE = systemic lupus erythematosus.

AUTOANTIBODIES

Autoantibodies are antibodies targeted to self; they generally bind portions of nucleic acid and protein. These antibodies can be used to **establish a diagnosis** of an autoimmune disease, **classify the disease,** or **indicate its prognosis or activity.** For example, one criterion for the diagnosis of systemic lupus erythematosus (SLE) is the presence of antinuclear antibody (ANA). However, this antibody is also seen in Sjögren syndrome, systemic sclerosis, and rheumatoid arthritis. Therefore, more specific antibodies, such as anti-dsDNA and anti-Smith, are used to verify the diagnosis of SLE.

Autoantibodies are also used to classify disease. For instance, drug-induced SLE is almost uniformly associated with the presence of antihistone antibodies.

Finally, autoantibodies may be used as prognostic factors and to indicate disease activity. The presence of antibodies to cyclic citrullinated peptide in rheumatoid arthritis indicates a high likelihood of developing the more severe, erosive form of the disease. In active disease, increased levels of circulating rheumatoid factor (RF) are seen, hence RF allows for an indirect measurement of the disease activity. For more information on autoantibodies and their specific disease associations, see Table 6-20.

CHAPTER 8

General Pharmacology

Pharmacodynamics

Pharmacodynamics describes a drug's mechanism of action and its physiologic effects—in other words, what the drug does and how it does it.

AGONISTS AND ANTAGONISTS

Drugs can be broadly classified as agonists or antagonists depending on their action at a target site or receptor. A single drug can have multiple actions; it may act as an agonist at one type of receptor and an antagonist at another.

Agonists

Agonists bind to a receptor and stabilize it in an active conformation.

- **Full agonists:** Produce a maximum response after binding to the receptor.
- **Partial agonists:** Produce a less-than-maximum response after binding to the receptor.
- When both full agonists and partial agonists are present in a system, the overall response may be less than the response to full agonists. Depending on the binding affinity, partial agonist molecules may preferentially bind to receptors and prevent full agonists from binding to the same receptors and exerting a maximum response. Thus, partial agonists may also be called **partial antagonists** or **mixed agonist-antagonists.**

Antagonists

Antagonists inhibit the action of an agonist, but have no effect in the absence of the agonist. They are broadly categorized as receptor antagonists or nonreceptor antagonists (Figure 8-1).

- **Nonreceptor antagonists:** Do not bind to receptors but inhibit the ability of the agonist to initiate its action.
- **Receptor antagonists:** Bind to either the active site or an allosteric site.

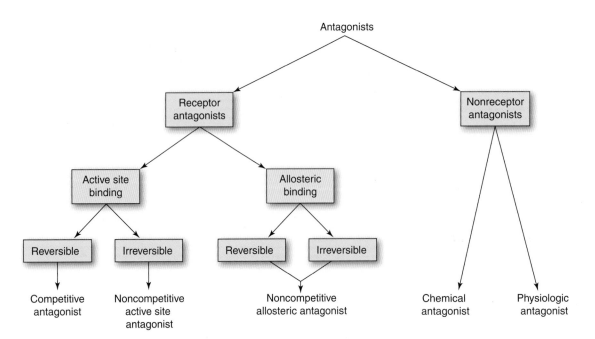

FIGURE 8-1. Antagonists categories.

The active site is where agonists bind to produce a response. **Allosteric sites** are sites other than the active site that are involved in receptor activation. In both cases, binding of the antagonist prevents agonists from activating the receptor; active site antagonist prevents agonist binding, whereas an allosteric site antagonist prevents receptor activation without preventing agonist binding.

NONRECEPTOR ANTAGONISTS

- Inhibit agonists directly or affect the downstream pathway of the agonist.
- Divided into **chemical antagonists** or **physiologic antagonists.**
    - Chemical antagonists inactivate the agonist directly. Examples are antibodies or protamine, which bind heparin directly to inactivate heparin.
    - Physiologic antagonists mediate a response opposite to that of the agonist receptor. An example is atropine, which is a type of muscarinic adrenergic antagonist that produces mydriasis.

COMPETITIVE ANTAGONISTS

- Compete with agonists for the same active site and bind reversibly.
- By occupying the active site, the competitive antagonist blocks agonists from binding and activating the receptor.
- Antagonist effects can be overcome by flooding the system with another molecule (ie, an agonist) that binds to the same site, thereby outnumbering and outcompeting the competitive antagonist.

NONCOMPETITIVE ANTAGONISTS

- Bind to an allosteric site on the receptor.
- Exert effect by changing the conformation of the receptor such that agonists cannot activate the receptor, even if they can bind to the active site.
- Effect cannot be overcome by flooding the system with an agonist molecule.

IRREVERSIBLE ANTAGONISTS

- Bind irreversibly to either the active site or to an allosteric site on the receptor.
- Bind to the site with very high affinity; their antagonist effects cannot be overcome either by saturating the system with an agonist molecule or by washing the antagonist out of the system.

DOSE RESPONSE

Dose-response curves represent the elicited response as a function of drug dose.

Affinity

- A measure of how tightly a drug binds to a receptor.
- Inversely related to K_d, the dissociation constant for the drug-receptor complex.

Potency

- Measured by the concentration of drug required for 50% or half-maximal response.
- Drug A is more **potent** than drug B if a lower concentration of drug A is required for a 50% response.

CLINICAL CORRELATION

Naloxone is an opioid receptor antagonist used to reverse life-threatening opioid overdose. Buprenorphine is a partial mu opioid receptor agonist used for opioid addiction treatment. Because it is a partial agonist, it produces a morphine-like analgesia but with milder euphoric symptoms.

Efficacy

- Measured by the **maximal response** that can be achieved by the drug.
- Two drugs are equally efficacious if they can achieve the same maximal response at the highest possible doses.

Figure 8-2 shows the dose-response curve of an agonist alone and when an agonist is combined with a competitive antagonist and a noncompetitive antagonist, respectively. The x-axis is a log scale of agonist dose, and the y-axis is the percent response at each dose of agonist.

Competitive Antagonism

- Antagonists bind reversibly to the same site as the agonist (**active site**).
- The maximum response is the same as with the agonist alone.
- Produces a right shift of the curve, such that the agonist dose needed to achieve a certain response is higher in the presence of a competitive antagonist (decreased potency).
- **Summary:** A higher dose of the agonist is needed to achieve a given response (decreased potency, increased K_d), but the maximum response is unchanged (same efficacy).

Noncompetitive Antagonism

- Antagonists bind to a site other than the active site that reduces the function of the receptor (**allosteric site**).
- The maximum response in the presence of the antagonist is less than with the agonist alone.
- The agonist dose needed to achieve a certain percentage of the maximum response does not change in the presence of a noncompetitive antagonist (no change in potency), but the maximum response is reduced (decreased efficacy).
- **Summary:** The dose needed to achieve a certain percentage of the maximum response is unchanged (same potency, same K_d), but the maximum response is reduced (decreased efficacy). Noncompetitive antagonism cannot be overcome by increasing the agonist dose.

Table 8-1 shows a comparison of competitive antagonists, noncompetitive antagonists, and partial agonists.

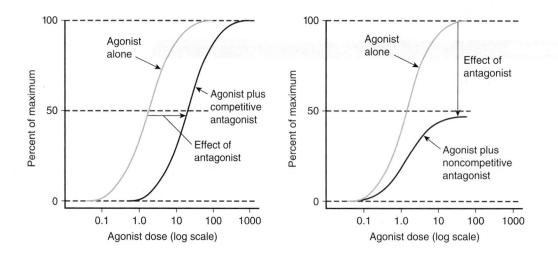

FIGURE 8-2. **Dose-response curve with antagonists.** (Modified with permission from Katzung BG, Trevor AJ. *Pharmacology: Examination & Board Review*, 5th ed. Stamford, CT: Appleton & Lange, 1998: 13, 14.)

TABLE 8-1.   Properties of Drug-Receptor Interaction Antagonists

Antagonist Type	Effect on Potency	Effect on Efficacy	Reversibility
Competitive antagonist.	Decreased	No change.	Reversible by adding agonist.
Noncompetitive antagonist.	No change	Decreased.	Cannot be reversed by adding agonist.
Partial agonist (mixed agonist-antagonist).	Decreased	Decreased or no change.	May or may not be reversible by adding full agonist, depending on relative binding affinities and concentrations of the full and partial agonists.

Spare Receptors

- Not all receptors have to be occupied for maximal response.
- In the presence of spare receptors, maximal response occurs at a lower agonist dose than that required for receptor saturation.
- Less than 50% of receptors need to be bound to achieve half-maximal response, such that potency $< K_d$.

Therapeutic Index

- Important clinical tool for measuring the dose-related toxicity of a drug.
- TD_{50}—drug dose at which 50% of patients experience **adverse effects.**
- ED_{50}—drug dose at which 50% of patients experience **desired therapeutic effects.**
- **Therapeutic index**—ratio of the drug dose at which 50% of patients experience side effects to the drug dose at which 50% of patients experience therapeutic effects (Figure 8-3).

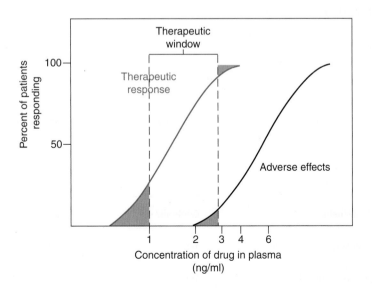

FIGURE 8-3.   Therapeutic index. (Reproduced with permission from Brunton LL, Lazo JS, Parker KL. *Goodman & Gilman's The Pharmacological Basis of Therapeutics*, 11th ed. New York: McGraw-Hill, 2006: Fig. 5-5.)

Therapeutic index $= TD_{50}/ED_{50} =$ median toxic dose/median effective dose

Lithium carbonate is an effective cationic medication used for the treatment of bipolar disorder that exerts numerous effects at the cellular level. Although the medication is effective, it has a narrow therapeutic index, that is, the difference in dose of TD_{50} and the ED_{50} is very close. Therefore, serum lithium monitoring is an important aspect of therapy.

Pharmacokinetics–

ADMET

Absorption
Distribution
Metabolism
Excretion
Toxicity

Pharmacodynamics is what a drug does to the body.
Pharmacokinetics is what the body does to a drug.

■ **High therapeutic index** drugs—those that achieve therapeutic doses well before causing toxicity and are relatively safe.
■ Drugs with a **low or narrow therapeutic index** have a smaller dosing margin that separates desired effects from toxicity.

Therefore, drugs with a low therapeutic index must be used precisely and serum levels should be monitored closely.

Pharmacokinetics

Pharmacokinetics describes the movement and metabolism of drugs into, out of, and within the body. In other words, pharmacokinetics details how the body processes the drugs that enter it. It can also be known by the acronym ADMET.

ENTRY

A drug can enter the body by one of several different routes.

■ Enteral (oral)
■ Parenteral: By injection
■ Intravenous/intra-arterial
■ Intramuscular
■ Subcutaneous
■ Intrathecal: Into the subarachnoid space
■ Across a mucous membrane: For example, sublingual, rectal, vaginal
■ Transdermal: Across the skin

Each of these routes of administration has advantages and disadvantages in terms of cost, convenience, pain, risk of infection, rate of onset, and the ability of drugs to cross the barrier. Table 8-2 compares the two most common routes of administration: oral and parenteral.

Bioavailability

■ The fraction of the administered drug that reaches the systemic circulation and ultimately, the target organ.

TABLE 8-2. Oral Versus Parenteral Administration

ATTRIBUTE	ORAL	PARENTERAL
Convenient	Yes	No
Risk of infection	No	Yes
Bioavailability	Generally < 1	1
GI absorption required	Yes	No
First-pass metabolism	Yes	No
Onset of action	Generally slow	Generally fast

GI = gastrointestinal.

- By definition, IV drugs are administered directly into the circulation and have a bioavailability of 1.
- Other routes of administration may have incomplete absorption or undergo first-pass metabolism, in which case bioavailability < 1 (Figure 8-4).

DISTRIBUTION

- Once a drug reaches the systemic circulation, it has easy access to nearly every target organ in the body.
- The exceptions are the brain and the testes, which are relatively protected from the general systemic circulation by physiologic barriers.
- The drug can then spread or distribute from the bloodstream into nonvascular organs and tissues, such as muscle, fat, and bone.
- The extent to which a drug distributes among the various compartments in the body depends on multiple factors, including the chemical nature of the drug, the volume of the individual compartments, and the number of drug receptors in those compartments.

Volume of Distribution

- A theoretical calculation of the fluid volume that would be needed to contain the total amount of absorbed drug at the concentration of drug found in the plasma at steady state.
- Drugs that are largely taken up by nonvascular compartments, such as fat, have a high volume of distribution because they have low plasma concentration. This is due to the fact that nonvascular tissues must usually be saturated before the plasma concentration reaches steady state. For example, drugs that have a lipophilic or nonpolar structure are readily taken up by adipose tissue. The adipose tissue serves as a "sink," and it is only after this

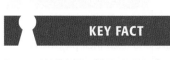

KEY FACT

The bioavailability of drugs administered intravenously is 1.0 or 100%.
Bioavailability = quantity of drug reaching systemic circulation/ quantity administered.

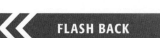

KEY FACT

Drugs administered intravenously can reach the systemic circulation and target organ before modification by the liver.

FLASH BACK

Both the **blood-brain barrier** and the **blood-testis barrier** are formed by the presence of **tight junctions,** which exquisitely restrict the passage of substances dissolved in the blood. Tight junctions are composed of proteins from the claudin and occludin families and exist between endothelial cells or other specialized cells surrounding the endothelium.

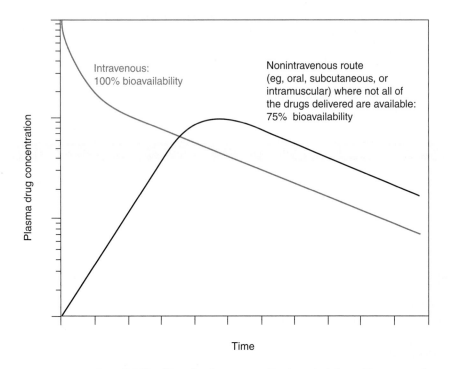

FIGURE 8-4. Bioavailability. Note that because medication administered intravenously has a 100% bioavailability, its plasma drug concentration starts high and then declines as it undergoes metabolism. This is in contrast to nonintravenous route of administration where the plasma drug concentration takes time to build up as the medication is being absorbed.

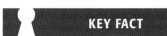
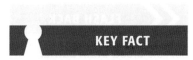
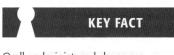
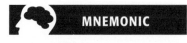
sink is filled that the concentration of the drug in the blood can begin to rise. The equation takes into account tissues that act as sinks, and therefore the calculated volume of distribution may be many times the actual fluid volume in the body.

- Drugs with a large volume of distribution often require a higher initial dose to achieve a therapeutic concentration than drugs with a small volume of distribution.

Protein Binding

- Binding to plasma proteins keeps drugs in the vascular compartment, thus reducing the ability of the drug to diffuse from the blood into the tissues.
- Drugs can interact with their target receptors only when they are free or unbound.
- Protein-bound drugs are inactive.
- Drugs that are highly protein-bound have a low volume of distribution.
- **Albumin** is the most important plasma-binding protein.
- When plasma drug levels are measured, the measurement is usually of the total drug concentration, which includes both free and protein-bound components.
- Theoretically, competition for binding sites on albumin and other proteins can produce drug-drug interactions. However, no such clinically relevant examples have been documented.

First-Pass Metabolism

- All orally ingested drugs are first metabolized by the liver before they enter the systemic circulation; this is called **first-pass metabolism.**
- First-pass metabolism is important to keep in mind when calculating drug dosage.
- Drugs that are not administered orally are not subject to first-pass metabolism.
- Orally administered drugs enter the GI system: GI → portal circulation → liver → hepatic vein → inferior vena cava → heart → systemic circulation → target organs.
- First-pass metabolism is affected by the cytochrome P450 system in the liver. It is classified into two types of biotransformation reaction: (1) oxidation/reduction reaction (phase I) and (2) conjugation/hydrolysis reaction (phase 2).

CYTOCHROME P450 SYSTEM

- A superfamily of enzymes found mainly in the smooth endoplasmic reticulum of hepatocytes.
- In the liver, these enzymes catalyze the metabolism of both exogenous drugs and toxins and endogenous compounds.
- Hydrophobic drugs are metabolized in a two-phase reaction.

Phase I Reaction

Enzymes add or unmask a polar moiety in the drug to make it more soluble via oxidation/reduction reactions.

Phase II Reaction

- Conjugation reactions add more soluble moieties to the polar moiety from phase I to make the drug metabolite more soluble and, thus, able to be renally excreted.

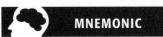

- Drugs are usually detoxified after phase II, although in some cases metabolites are more toxic than the parent compound. Acetaminophen is one such example.

In addition to being metabolized by the cytochrome P450 system, many drugs also either induce or inhibit the system. This in turn affects the metabolism of other drugs and forms the basis for many clinically important drug-drug interactions. Table 8-3 lists some commonly tested drugs that induce and inhibit the cytochrome P450 system. As with the Common Drug Reactions that appears later in the chapter, this list is not meant to be comprehensive.

EXCRETION

Just as drugs can enter the body via several different routes, they can also be excreted by the body in several ways.

Renal Excretion

- **Urinary/renal excretion** is the most common mechanism of drug elimination.
- Drugs that are eliminated via this route are **hydrophilic** (water-soluble), or have been made water soluble by P450 reactions.
- Renal excretion is affected by factors such as the glomerular filtration rate (GFR—which determines how *quickly* the drug can be filtered), the pro-

MNEMONIC

P450 inhibitors—

Inhibitors Stop Cyber-Kids from Eating Ripe Grapefruits And Flying Very Quickly to Distant Metropolis City

Isoniazid
Sulfonamides
Cimetidine
Ketoconazole
Erythromycin
Ritonavir
Grapefruit juice
Amiodarone
Fluoxetine
Verapamil
Quinidine
Disulfiram
Metronidazole
Ciprofloxacin

TABLE 8-3. P450 Inducers and Inhibitors

INDUCERS	INHIBITORS
Barbiturates	Isoniazid
Phenytoin	Sulfonamides
Cigarette smoke	Cimetidine
Ethanol	Ketoconazole
Rifampin	Erythromycin
Griseofulvin	Ritonavir
Carbamazepine	Grapefruit juice
Omeprazole	Amiodarone
Gemfibrozil	Fluoxetine
Doxorubicin	Verapamil
Nefazodone	Quinidine
Valproic acid	Disulfiram
Zileuton	Metronidazole
	Ciprofloxacin

portion of the drug bound to serum protein (which determines how *much* drug can be filtered as serum bound proteins usually cannot be filtered due to size exclusion), and the urine pH (*the maximum concentration* that can be excreted into the urine).

- For drugs that are **weak acids,** alkalinize urine with bicarbonate to increase clearance.
- For drugs that are **weak bases,** acidify urine with ammonium chloride to increase clearance.

Because most drugs are cleared by the kidneys, renal function (ie, GFR), is an important consideration when administering drugs.

Biliary Excretion

- Hepatic or biliary excretion is an important route of elimination for lipophilic drugs.
- Lipophilic drugs are solubilized in the bile, introduced into the small intestine, and ultimately excreted as feces. However, as fecal matter travels through the gastrointestinal tract, these drugs can be reabsorbed by the gut into the enterohepatic circulation and reenter the systemic circulation.

Clearance

Clearance = Rate of elimination of drug/Plasma drug concentration

Rate of Elimination

- See Figure 8-5.
- **Zero-order elimination:**
  - The starting concentration is irrelevant, and does not change the elimination rate. The rate of elimination is constant regardless of concentration, and the concentration decreases linearly with time. That is, a **constant amount** of drug is eliminated per unit of time.
  - Examples: Ethanol, phenytoin, aspirin at high doses.
- **First-order elimination:**
  - The rate of elimination is exponentially proportional to drug concentration. That is, a constant *fraction* of drug is eliminated per unit of time.
  - Concentration decreases exponentially with time.
  - Examples: Most drugs.

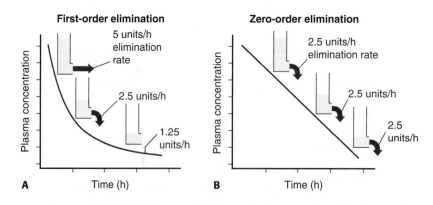

FIGURE 8-5. **Drug elimination rates.** (A) First-order elimination and (B) Zero-order elimination. (Modified with permission from Katzung BG, Trevor AJ. *Pharmacology: Examination & Board Review,* 5th ed. Stamford, CT: Appleton & Lange, 1985: 5.)

TABLE 8-4. Percentage of Steady State as a Function of Half-life

Number of Half-lives	1	2	3	3.3	4
Concentration (%)	50	75	87.5	90	93.75

HALF-LIFE

- Half-life ($t_{1/2}$) is the time required for the plasma drug concentration to decrease by 50% during elimination (reduction) or constant infusion (addition).
- A drug that is constantly infused reaches 94% of its steady-state plasma concentration after 4 half-lives (Table 8-4).
- Half-life is determined by the volume of distribution and clearance of the drug.

> **KEY FACT**
>
> $t_{1/2} = 0.7 \times V_d/CL$, where V_d is volume of distribution and CL is clearance.

DOSAGE CALCULATIONS

In the hospital, drugs are often administered in either loading or maintenance doses. The purpose of the **loading dose** is to achieve a desired drug plasma concentration rapidly when the clinical situation is urgent (eg, therapeutic levels of antiarrhythmic drug must quickly be reached during a potentially fatal arrhythmia event). **Maintenance doses,** on the other hand, are used once a drug has reached steady state, in order to offset the rate of clearance and maintain drug levels within the therapeutic window.

Loading Dose

- **Loading dose = $C_p \times V_d/F$,** where C_p = target plasma concentration, V_d = volume of distribution, and F = bioavailability.
- In urgent situations or when administering drugs with long half-lives, a large loading dose may be used to rapidly reach therapeutic plasma levels.

Maintenance Dose

- **Maintenance dose = $C_p \times CL/F$,** where C_p = target plasma concentration, CL = clearance, and F = bioavailability.
- To maintain a therapeutic concentration, the maintenance dose must be given to ensure that input = output.
- Patients with impaired hepatic or renal function often receive the same loading dose but a reduced maintenance dose.

> **KEY FACT**
>
> Loading dose = $C_p \times V_d/F$
> Maintenance dose = $C_p \times CL/F$

Toxicology

Table 8-5 lists in alphabetical order the most common toxic drugs, nondrug toxins, and their antidotes. For adverse reactions associated with drugs, see Table 8-7 in the next section.

CARBON MONOXIDE

MECHANISM

Binds to hemoglobin with much higher affinity than O_2, thereby inhibiting O_2 transport.

TABLE 8-5. Common Toxic Drugs, Nondrug Toxins, and Antidotes

DRUG OR TOXIN	ANTIDOTE
Acetaminophen	*N*-Acetylcysteine.
Anticholinergics	Physostigmine.
Anticholinesterases, organophosphates	Atropine, pralidoxime.
Arsenic, mercury, gold	Dimercaprol.
Aspirin	Sodium bicarbonate, alkalinization of urine, dialysis.
Benzodiazepines	Flumazenil.
β-Blockers	Glucagon, calcium gluconate, dextrose-insulin therapy.
Carbon monoxide	100% O_2, hyperbaric O_2.
Copper	D-Penicillamine.
Cyanide	Amyl nitrite, sodium thiosulfate, hydroxocobalamin.
Digitalis/digoxin	Antidigoxin Fab antibodies.
Ethylene glycol (antifreeze), methanol	Fomepizole, ethanol.
Heparin	Protamine.
Iron	Deferoxamine.
Isoniazid (INH)	Pyridoxine (vitamin B_6).
Lead	EDTA, dimercaprol.
Methemoglobinemia (drugs causing)	Methylene blue.
Opioids	Naloxone/naltrexone.
Quinidine	Hypertonic sodium bicarbonate, lidocaine, magnesium sulfate.
Strychnine	Benzodiazepines, neuromuscular blockade.
Theophylline	β-blockers, benzodiazepines.
Tissue plasminogen activator (tPA)	Aminocaproic acid.
Tricyclic antidepressants (TCAs)	Sodium bicarbonate, benzodiazepines.
Warfarin	Vitamin K, fresh frozen plasma.

EDTA = ethylenediaminetetraacetic acid.

EFFECTS

Headache, confusion, seizures, death.

ANTIDOTE

100% O_2, hyperbaric O_2.

CYANIDE

MECHANISM

Reacts with iron in cytochrome oxidase in mitochondria, thereby inhibiting electron transport and ATP formation.

EFFECTS

Tachycardia followed by brachycardia, hypotension, lactic acidosis, seizures, coma, and rapid death. O_2 utilization is diminished at the tissue level, and so venous O_2 concentration is elevated at higher than normal value and this is manifested as brighter red venous blood than normal.

ANTIDOTE

Amyl nitrite and sodium nitrite prevent and reverse binding of cyanide to cytochrome oxidase. Nitrites oxidize hemoglobin to methoxyhemoglobin, which binds cyanide. Sodium thiosulfate accelerates detoxification of cyanide to thiocyanate. Hydroxocobalamin chelates cyanide, forming cyanocobalamin.

ETHANOL

MECHANISM

Poorly understood. May exert effects at GABA receptors or by modifying ion channels in biologic membranes. Figure 8-6 illustrates the metabolism of ethanol.

EFFECTS

Euphoria, disinhibition, sedation, respiratory depression, pancreatitis, hepatitis, Wernicke-Korsakoff syndrome, gynecomastia, testicular atrophy, fetal alcohol syndrome.

ANTIDOTE

Benzodiazepines are used for acute withdrawal. Thiamine is used for prevention of Wernicke disease. Disulfiram is used to treat chronic alcoholism.

METHANOL

MECHANISM

Metabolized by alcohol dehydrogenase to formaldehyde, which is metabolized by aldehyde dehydrogenase to formic acid. Formic acid accumulation causes retinal and optic nerve toxicity.

EFFECTS

Blindness, metabolic acidosis, and death.

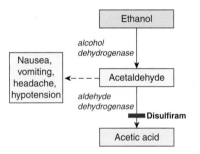

FIGURE 8-6. **Metabolism of ethanol.**

ANTIDOTE

Ethanol acts as a competitive substrate for alcohol dehydrogenase; fomepizole inhibits alcohol dehydrogenase.

HEAVY METALS

See Table 8-6.

STRYCHNINE

MECHANISM

Competitive antagonist of glycine in central nervous system (CNS), leading to loss of normal inhibitory tone and subsequent excitation.

EFFECTS

Seizure with contraction of all voluntary muscles, resulting in full extension of limbs and vertebrae (opisthotonos).

ANTIDOTE

Benzodiazepines and neuromuscular blockade.

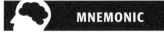

MNEMONIC

Clinical manifestations and treatment of LEAD poisoning:

Lead **L**ines on gingivae and epiphyses of long bones

Encephalopathy and **E**rythrocyte basophilic stippling

Abdominal pain and microcytic **A**nemia

Drops—wrist and foot drop from neuropathy; **D**imercaprol, **D**imercaptosuccinic acid and E**D**TA

TABLE 8-6. Heavy Metals (Arsenic, Cadmium, Iron, Lead, Mercury)

HEAVY METAL	MECHANISM OF TOXICITY	CLINICAL MANIFESTATIONS	ANTIDOTE
Arsenic	Interferes with oxidative phosphorylation.	*Early:* Garlic breath, bloody diarrhea. *Late:* Hair loss, neuropathy, hyperpigmentation, lung cancer.	Dimercaprol, dimercaptosuccinic acid, D-penicillamine.
Cadmium	Complexes with metallothionein.	Metallic taste, GI corrosive, renal and pulmonary disease.	Dimercaptosuccinic acid.
Iron	Direct GI corrosive; forms reactive oxygen species; disrupts oxidative phosphorylation.	Bloody diarrhea, coma, leukocytosis, hyperglycemia.	Deferoxamine.
Lead	Inhibits heme synthesis.	Anemia, abdominal pain, lead lines, motor neuropathy, encephalopathy.	Dimercaprol, EDTA, dimercaptosuccinic acid.
Mercury	Inhibits multiple enzyme processes.	Acute renal failure, pneumonitis, tremor, irrational behavior.	Dimercaptosuccinic acid, dimercaprol.

EDTA = ethylenediaminetetraacetic acid.

COMMON DRUG SIDE EFFECTS

Table 8-7 presents some commonly tested drug adverse effects and causative agents by organ system. This list is not comprehensive. Please refer to each organ system in the text for more details.

TABLE 8-7. Common Drug Reactions

SYSTEM	ADVERSE REACTION	DRUG	MNEMONIC
Neurologic	Cinchonism	Quinidine, quinine, aspirin.	
	Parkinsonism	Haloperidol, chlorpromazine, reserpine, MPTP.	
	Tardive dyskinesia	Antipsychotics, metoclopramide.	
	Extrapyramidal side effects	Chlorpromazine, thioridazine, haloperidol.	
	Seizures	Imipenem, antipsychotics, tricyclic antidepressants, lithium.	
Cardiovascular	Cardiac toxicity	Doxorubicin, daunorubicin.	
	Torsades de pointes	Class III (sotalol), class IA (quinidine) antiarrhythmics.	
	Coronary vasospasm	Cocaine.	
Pulmonary	Pulmonary fibrosis	**N**itrofurantoin. **B**leomycin. **B**usulfan. **A**miodarone.	**N**ot **B**eneficial for **B**reathing **A**ir
	Cough	ACE inhibitors.	
Gastrointestinal	Hepatitis	**H**alothane. **Is**oniazid.	**H**epatit**Is**
	Focal to massive hepatic necrosis	**V**alproic acid. **A**cetaminophen. **H**alothane. **A**manita mushroom.	**V**ariable **A**rea **H**epatic **A**ssassin
	Pseudomembranous colitis	Broad-spectrum antibiotics, (eg, clindamycin).	
	Gingival hyperplasia	Phenytoin.	
Renal	Lactic acidosis	Metformin, nucleoside reverse transcriptase inhibitors.	
	Tubulointerstitial nephritis	Sulfonamides, furosemide, methicillin, rifampin, NSAIDs (except aspirin).	
	Diabetes insipidus	Lithium, demeclocycline.	
	Fanconi syndrome	Expired tetracyclines, heavy metals.	

(continues)

TABLE 8-7. Common Drug Reactions *(continued)*

System	Adverse Reaction	Drug	Mnemonic
Heme	Hemolysis in G6PD-deficient individuals	**S**ulfonamides. **I**soniazid. **P**rimaquine, **P**yrimethamine, **I**buprofen, **N**itrofurantoin. **A**spirin. **D**apsone, **C**hloramphenicol.	**SIPPIN' A D**iet **C**oke
	Thrombosis	Oral contraceptives: Estrogens, progestins.	
	Agranulocytosis	**C**lozapine, **C**arbamazepine, **C**olchicine, propylthiouracil.	3 **C**'s
	Aplastic anemia	**C**hloramphenicol. **S**ulfonamides. **N**SAIDs gold salts. **B**enzene. **C**hlorpromazine.	**C**an't **S**ynthesize **N**ormal **B**lood **C**ells
Endocrine	Adrenocortical insufficiency	Glucocorticoid withdrawal.	
	Hot flashes	Tamoxifen.	
	Gynecomastia	**S**pironolactone. **D**igitalis. **C**imetidine. **E**strogen. Chronic **A**lcohol abuse. **K**etoconazole.	**S**ome **D**rugs **C**reate **E**xtremely **A**wesome **K**nockers
	Hyperprolactinemia	Tricyclic antidepressants, methyldopa, reserpine, phenothiazine.	
	SIADH	ACE inhibitors, SSRIs, vincristine, cyclophosphamide, carbamazepine, chlorpromazine.	
	Hypothyroidism	Lithium.	
Dermatologic	Photosensitivity	**S**ulfonamides. **A**miodarone. **T**etracyclines.	**SAT** for a photo
	Cutaneous flushing	**V**ancomycin (red man syndrome). **A**denosine. **N**iacin. **C**alcium channel blockers.	**VANC**
	Stevens-Johnson syndrome	**L**amotrigine. **E**thosuximide. **S**ulfonamides.	**LES**
	Gray baby syndrome	Chloramphenicol.	

TABLE 8-7.   Common Drug Reactions *(continued)*

System	Adverse Reaction	Drug	Mnemonic
Musculoskeletal	Tendonitis, tendon rupture, and cartilage damage	Fluoroquinolones.	
	Osteoporosis	Corticosteroids, heparin.	
Multiple	Ototoxicity and nephrotoxicity	Aminoglycosides, loop diuretics, cisplatin.	Toxic to **Poly**
	Neurotoxicity and nephrotoxicity	**Poly**myxi**Ns.**	**Ns:** Neuro/ nephrotoxic
Systemic	Anaphylaxis	Penicillin and many other drugs.	
	SLE-like syndrome	**H**ydralazine. **I**soniazid. **P**rocainamide, **P**henytoin. **P**enicillamine. Chlorpromazine, methyldopa, quinidine.	It's not **HIPPP** to have lupus
	Disulfiram-like reaction	Some **C**ephalosporins. **P**rocarbazine. **S**ulfonylureas. **Metro**nidazole.	**C**an't **P**ound **S**hots on the **Metro**
	Atropine-like side effects	Tricyclic antidepressants.	

ACE = angiotensin-converting enzyme; G6PD = glucose-6 phosphate dehydrogenase; MPTP = 1-methyl-4-phenyl-1,2,3,6-tetrahydropyridine; NSAID = nonsteroidal anti-inflammatory drug; SLE = systemic lupus erythematosus; SSRIs = selective serotonin reuptake inhibitors.

NOTES

INDEX

About the Senior Editors

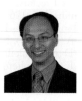

Tao Le, MD, MHS

Tao has been active in medical education for the past 19 years. As senior editor, he has led the expansion of *First Aid* into a global educational series. In addition, he is the founder of the *USMLERx* online test bank series as well as a cofounder of the *Underground Clinical Vignettes* series. As a medical student, he was editor-in-chief of the University of California, San Francisco, *Synapse*, a university newspaper with a weekly circulation of 9000. Tao earned his medical degree from the University of California, San Francisco, in 1996 and completed his residency training in internal medicine at Yale University and allergy and immunology fellowship training at Johns Hopkins University. At Yale, he was a regular guest lecturer on the USMLE review courses and an adviser to the Yale University School of Medicine curriculum committee. Tao subsequently went on to cofound Medsn and served as its chief medical officer. He is currently section cheif of adult allergy and immunology at the University of Louisville.

Kendall Krause, MD

Kendall is currently a resident in preventive medicine/public health at the University of Colorado. This is Kendall's third tour of duty with First Aid—she cut her teeth as a junior editor for *First Aid Cases for the USMLE Step 1* and senior editor on the first edition of the *First Aid for the Basic Sciences*. Kendall attended the Yale School of Medicine before completing her internship in emergency medicine at Massachusetts General and Brigham and Women's Hospitals. Kendall has acted as an articles editor for the *Yale Journal of Health Policy, Law, and Ethics*, and a contributor for the ABC News Medical Unit. Her current work is focused on health equity, evidence-based practice, and health care delivery and systems in resource limited settings.

About the Editor

Vinita Takiar, MD, PhD

Vinita has worked on a number of projects for First Aid, including three editions of *First Aid for USMLE Step 1* and *USMLERx Step 2 CK Qmax*. She also served as senior editor for the second edition of *First Aid Cases for the USMLE Step 1*. Vinita received both her MD and PhD from Yale, where she pursued basic science research evaluating a novel therapeutic target for polycystic kidney disease. She then completed her internship in the Yale Primary Care Internal Medicine Program. She is currently a resident in radiation oncology at the University of Texas, MD Anderson Cancer Center, where she hopes to further develop her interest in translational and applied basic science research along with her training in the clinic. When not pipetting or taking care of her patients, Vinita can be found "experimenting" in the kitchen, eating frozen yogurt, or relentlessly trying to solve the latest crossword puzzles.

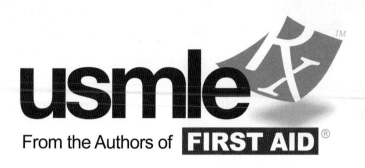
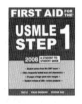